Bioinformatics and Human Genomics Research

Editor

Diego A. Forero, MD, PhD
Professor and Researcher
School of Health and Sport Sciences
Fundación Universitaria del Área Andina, Bogotá
Colombia

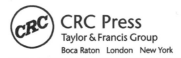

CRC Press
Taylor & Francis Group
Boca Raton London New York

CRC Press is an imprint of the
Taylor & Francis Group, an **informa** business

A SCIENCE PUBLISHERS BOOK

First edition published 2022
by CRC Press
6000 Broken Sound Parkway NW, Suite 300, Boca Raton, FL 33487-2742

and by CRC Press
4 Park Square, Milton Park, Abingdon, Oxon OX14 4RN

© 2022 Taylor & Francis Group, LLC
CRC Press is an imprint of Taylor & Francis Group, an Informa business

Library of Congress Cataloging-in-Publication Data
Names: Forero, Diego A., editor.
Title: Bioinformatics and human genomics research / editor, Diego A.
    Forero, Full Professor and Director of PhD Program in Health Sciences,
    School of Medicine, Universidad Antonio Nariño, Bogotá, Colombia.
Description: First edition. | Boca Raton : CRC Press, 2021. | Includes methods have led to
    a large number of published genome-wide studies in humans and animal models. In this
    context, recent tools from bioinformatics and computational biology have been fundamental
    for the analysis of these genomic studies. The book Bioinformatics and Human Genomics
    Research provides updated and comprehensive information about multiple approaches of
    the application of bioinformatic tools to research in human genomics. It covers strategies
    for analysis of genome-wide association studies, genome-wide expression studies, genome-
    wide DNA methylation, among other topics. It provides interesting strategies for data
    mining in human genomics, network analysis, prediction of binding sites for miRNAs
    and transcription factors, among other themes. Authors, from around the world, are
    recognized experts in bioinformatics and human genomics. Readers will find this book as
    quite useful for their in silico explorations, which would contribute to a better and deeper
    understanding of multiple biological processes and of pathophysiology of many human
    diseases"-- Provided by publisher.
Identifiers: LCCN 2021018860 | ISBN 9780367437602 (hardcover)
Subjects: LCSH: Bioinformatics. | Human genome--Research. | Genomics--Data processing.
Classification: LCC QH324.2 .B547315 2021 | DDC 570.285--dc23
LC record available at https://lccn.loc.gov/2021018860

ISBN: 978-0-367-43760-2 (hbk)
ISBN: 978-1-032-02893-4 (pbk)
ISBN: 978-1-003-00592-6 (ebk)

DOI: 10.1201/9781003005926

Typeset in Times New Roman
by Shubham Creation

Preface

A fundamental element in the development of this book was to provide an updated view of key concepts and methods of bioinformatics applied to human genomics research. As Editor, I invited researchers from around the globe (working in countries from America, Asia and Europe) with expertise in multiple methodologies and approaches of applied bioinformatics. I hope that the readers find this book useful and inspiring for future research in human genomics.

I appreciate the invitation of CRC Press and I thank my institution (Fundación Universitaria del Área Andina) for its support. In particular, I thank my Dean, Dr. Paola Ruiz Díaz, for her constant support and motivation.

Diego A. Forero
Editor

Contents

Chapter 1

Bioinformatics and Human Genomics Research: An Introduction

Diego A. Forero[1,2]* and
Yeimy González-Giraldo[3,4]

[1]Health and Sport Sciences Research Group, School of Health and Sport Sciences,
Fundación Universitaria del Área Andina, Bogotá, Colombia

[2]M.Sc. Program in Epidemiology, School of Health and Sport Sciences,
Fundación Universitaria del Área Andina, Bogotá, Colombia

[3]Center for Psychosocial Studies for Latin America and the Caribbean,
School of Psychosocial Therapies, Universidad Antonio Nariño. Bogotá, Colombia

[4]Departamento de Nutrición y Bioquímica, Facultad de Ciencias, Pontificia Universidad
Javeriana, Bogotá, Colombia

Human genomics has revolutionized research on the molecular basis of human diseases and phenotypes (Hindorff et al., 2018). High throughput sequencing and genotyping platforms (Ke et al., 2016; LaFramboise, 2009) have facilitated the analysis of the variability and expression of the whole genome in a large number of studies for common and rare disorders (Buniello et al., 2019), such as Alzheimer's disease (Tosto and Reitz, 2016), cancer (Hansen and Bedard, 2013), heart diseases (Reuter et al., 2020), autoimmune disorders (Maecker et al., 2012), hereditary syndromes (Kobayashi et al., 2013), etc. The current and future challenges for many researchers involve the analysis of a high volume o complex data (Finan et al., 2017). Although bioinformatics has been linked to the birth and consolidation of human genomics (Gauthier, 2019), the advances have been enormous and there is a constant need for the creation and refinement of more computational tools and resources.

In this book, a number of experts in bioinformatics (Gauthier et al., 2019) from around the world (Arcon et al., 2019; Baruah and Sharma, 2019; Carvajal-Rodriguez, 2018; Chandra, et al., 2010; Chen et al., 2019; de Anda-Jauregui and Hernandez-Lemus, 2020; Finan et al., 2017;

*Corresponding author: *dforero41@areandina.edu.co*

Iddamalgoda et al., 2016; Kumaran et al., 2019; Saxena and Sachin, 2018) have thrown light on the key aspects of bioinformatics applied to human genomics research. Over the decades, bioinformatics has allowed the knowledge and prediction of the structure and function of a large number of genes and proteins, as well as their regulation and interactions (Gauthier et al., 2019).

One of the starting points is the annotation of the genome—a process that allows the association of genomic sequence to biological function (Aken et al., 2016). There are automated and manual methods for performing the annotation of genomes, which are combined for completing and supplementing the tasks and results, as was realized in the ENCODE Project (Harrow et al., 2012). Considering the fundamental role of genome annotation for human research, in this book Gupta et al. have contributed a chapter on this important topic. Following the identification of the protein-coding genes there is the need to identify the function of such proteins. Bioinformatics methods have been implemented to predict these functions based on gene expression and proteomic data (Lee et al., 2007), amino acid sequences, protein structure information, and protein-protein interaction networks (Wang et al., 2018). An interesting overview about protein function prediction is given by Modak et al. in Chapter 3. In Chapter 4, Ramirez, has focused on bioinformatics and genomic data mining. Currently, there is a large amount of available data derived from high throughput studies, which might be useful for secondary analysis and for integration through several approaches, including data mining, which has been a powerful approach in human genomics. It allows generating new results and knowledge by extracting information from different datasets (Gudenas et al., 2019), and novel methods such as machine learning, have been implemented with this approach (Lin and Lane, 2017).

The study of RNA expression using high-throughput approaches brings a huge challenge for analyzing, interpreting, and sharing this data. Novel sequencing and microarray platforms have allowed the analysis of the expression of the entire genome (Hrdlickova et al., 2017) in different samples from patients and healthy subjects. These strategies have been useful to identify the molecular basis of a large number of diseases (Sweeney et al., 2016). A description of its analysis using in silico tools is presented by Tovar et al. in Chapter 5 on bioinformatics of genome-wide expression studies. This is a key topic, taking into account that depending on the techniques used, the analyses involve different tools and methods in order to obtain the results. For example, in the case of gene expression analysis using microarray platforms, after obtaining the raw intensities, it involves steps such as pre-processing, normalization, and differential expression analysis. On the other hand, RNA-seq requires a quality control analysis, alignment, generation of counts and analysis of differential gene expression (Wolff et al., 2018).

An analysis of variants in the entire genome or exome (Karczewski et al., 2020; Schwarze et al., 2018) has revolutionized human genomics. In this book, two chapters are dedicated to show the tools and programs used in that analysis. Salazar et al. provides a chapter about the analysis of whole-genome sequencing (WGS) data, which encompasses the analysis of exons, introns and intergenic regions. This is complemented by Kumaran's chapter about whole exome sequencing studies (WES); in these type of studies, only the exons (the coding regions) are analyzed. The WGS has been useful for identifying genetic variants involved in the pathogenesis of diseases and in the response to treatments (Bainbridge et al., 2011), such as anticoagulation treatment efficacy (Mizzi et al., 2014). In this context, the analysis of WES has been useful in identifying variants (in exons) that can be involved in the drug response, as it is shown in an analysis of patients with metastatic cancer (Beltran et al., 2015). Although WGS and WES approaches have several differences, both have advantages and disadvantages related to the cost, data analysis and results (Wang and Chen, 2020). Bereinstein et al. in their chapter discusses *in silico* prediction of the functional effects of variants, which is also useful for resequencing of candidate genes (Thusberg et al., 2011).

Regulation of gene expression encompasses several mechanisms at transcriptional and post-transcriptional levels, which include DNA methylation, transcription factors and microRNAs. In this book, four chapters describe the key computational tools and approaches for their analysis. Epigenomics is a hot topic in biomedical research and due to its complexity, its analysis has several challenges. Sharma et al.'s chapter deal with the analysis of genome-wide DNA methylation studies (Yong et al., 2016). In the last few years, there has been a growing number of studies about DNA methylation and its role in several diseases, which have found that this mechanism could play an important role in the etiology of them (Wockner et al., 2014). On the other hand, Navarro-Delgado et al. present a chapter on the prediction of transcription factor binding (Qin and Feng, 2017). Transcription factors are one of the most studied mechanisms of gene expression regulation at the transcriptional level. Non-coding RNAs represent a quite interesting category of genes, which are involved in the post-transcriptional regulation of gene expression (Beermann et al., 2016; Forero et al., 2019a). An important chapter of microRNA target prediction has been presented by Rawoof et al., this process is very useful to identify candidate target genes, which must subsequently be validated experimentally. Chandra et al. has contributed a chapter on the secondary structure of RNAs, which plays a key role in RNA translation, alternative splicing, processing and stability, and microRNA targeting (Vandivier et al., 2016).

Advanced analysis of omics data is very helpful for the identification of higher order dynamics (Lotfi Shahreza et al., 2018). Hernández-Lemus et al.'s chapter discusses the analysis of genomics data (Telenti et al., 2018). In order to identify the biological processes, molecular functions, pathways, and other categories associated with a gene set, functional enrichment analysis is performed when differentially expressed genes or SNPs associated with a disease are found using high-throughput techniques. Gomez-Romero et al.'s chapter is about bioinformatics and functional categories enrichment (Zhao et al., 2016). With the exponential growth of data from high-throughput techniques, integrative approaches for their analyses have been developed. Saxena et al.'s chapter discusses one of these approaches, meta-analysis, focusing on genomic data (Forero et al., 2019b). One of the key advantages of meta-analyses is the power to detect more reliable results, which can be generalizable (Ramasamy et al., 2008). Carvajal-Rodriguez et al.'s chapter is about correction for multiple testing, which is very important in bioinformatic analyses. Finally, in the last chapter, Barbosa et al. presents an important overview of bioinformatic analyses of genomics and cancers, which is a group of diseases which leads to a large burden of morbidity and mortality around the world.

In future, the role of open data and open software (Allen and Mehler, 2019; Forero, 2019; Gentleman et al., 2004) in human genomics research will be even more important. Publicly available genome-wide information with adequate annotation (Barrett et al., 2013; Brazma et al., 2001; Karczewski et al., 2020), will facilitate the identification and confirmation of genes and pathways for human diseases and related phenotypes (Forero et al., 2016). An adequate training of biological and biomedical researchers in basic advanced strategies of bioinformatics and computational biology will be key (Garmire et al., 2017). Teaching of programming languages, such as Python and R (Bassi, 2007; Eglen, 2009; Ekmekci et al., 2016), in undergraduate and postgraduate programs (Rubinstein and Chor, 2014) will also be helpful.

Acknowledgments

DAF has been supported by research grants from Colciencias. YG-G was previously supported by a PhD fellowship from Centro de Estudios Interdisciplinarios Básicos y Aplicados CEIBA (Rodolfo Llinás Program).

REFERENCES

Aken, B.L., S. Ayling, D. Barrell, L. Clarke, V., Curwen, S. Fairley, et al. (2016). The Ensemble gene annotation system. Database (Oxford), 2016. doi: 10.1093/database/baw093.

Allen, C. and D.M.A. Mehler. (2019). Open science challenges, benefits and tips in early career and beyond. PLoS Biol. 17(5): e3000246. doi: 10.1371/journal.pbio.3000246.

Arcon, J.P., C.P. Modenutti, D. Avendano, E.D. Lopez, L.A. Defelipe, F.A. Ambrosio, et al. (2019). AutoDock bias: Improving binding mode prediction and virtual screening using known protein-ligand interactions. Bioinformatics. 35(19): 3836–3838. doi: 10.1093/bioinformatics/btz152.

Bainbridge, M.N., W. Wiszniewski, D.R. Murdock, J. Friedman, C. Gonzaga-Jauregui, I. Newsham, et al. (2011). Whole-genome sequencing for optimized patient management. Sci. Transl. Med. 3(87): 87re83. doi: 10.1126/scitranslmed.3002243.

Barrett, T., S.E. Wilhite, P. Ledoux, C. Evangelista, I.F. Kim, M. Tomashevsky, et al. (2013). NCBI GEO: archive for functional genomics data sets--update. Nucleic Acids Res. 41(Database issue): D991–995. doi: 10.1093/nar/gks1193.

Baruah, M.M. and N. Sharma. (2019). *In silico* identification of key genes and signaling pathways targeted by a panel of signature microRNAs in prostate cancer. Med. Oncol. 36(5): 43. doi: 10.1007/s12032-019-1268-y.

Bassi, S. (2007). A primer on Python for life science researchers. PLoS Comput. Biol. 3(11): e199. doi: 10.1371/journal.pcbi.0030199.

Beermann, J., M.T. Piccoli, J. Viereck and T. Thum. (2016). Non-coding RNAs in development and disease: Background, mechanisms, and therapeutic approaches. Physiol. Rev. 96(4): 1297–1325. doi: 10.1152/physrev.00041.2015.

Beltran, H., K. Eng, J.M. Mosquera, A. Sigaras, A. Romanel, H. Rennert, et al. (2015). Whole-exome sequencing of metastatic cancer and biomarkers of treatment response. JAMA Oncol. 1(4): 466–474. doi: 10.1001/jamaoncol.2015.1313.

Brazma, A., P. Hingamp, J. Quackenbush, G. Sherlock, P. Spellman, C. Stoeckert, et al. (2001). Minimum information about a microarray experiment (MIAME)-toward standards for microarray data. Nat. Genet. 29(4): 365–371. doi: 10.1038/ng1201-365.

Buniello, A., J.A.L. MacArthur, M. Cerezo, L.W. Harris, J. Hayhurst, C. Malangone, et al. (2019). The NHGRI-EBI GWAS Catalog of published genome-wide association studies, targeted arrays and summary statistics 2019. Nucleic Acids Res. 47(D1): D1005–D1012. doi: 10.1093/nar/gky1120.

Carvajal-Rodriguez, A. (2018). Myriads: P-value-based multiple testing correction. Bioinformatics. 34(6): 1043–1045. doi: 10.1093/bioinformatics/btx746.

Chandra, V., R. Girijadevi, A.S. Nair, S.S. Pillai and R.M. Pillai. (2010). MTar: A computational microRNA target prediction architecture for human transcriptome. BMC Bioinformatics. 11: Suppl 1, S2. doi: 10.1186/1471-2105-11-S1-S2.

Chen, G., J.C. Ramirez, N. Deng, X. Qiu, C. Wu, W.J. Zheng, et al. (2019). Restructured GEO: Restructuring gene expression omnibus metadata for genome dynamics analysis. Database (Oxford), 2019. doi: 10.1093/database/bay145.

de Anda-Jauregui, G. and E. Hernandez-Lemus. (2020). Computational oncology in the multi-omics era: State of the art. Front. Oncol. 10: 423. doi: 10.3389/fonc.2020.00423.

Eglen, S.J. (2009). A quick guide to teaching R programming to computational biology students. PLoS Comput. Biol., 5(8): e1000482. doi: 10.1371/journal.pcbi.1000482.

Ekmekci, B., C.E. McAnany and C. Mura. (2016). An introduction to programming for bioscientists: A Python-based primer. PLoS Comput. Biol. 12(6): e1004867. doi: 10.1371/journal.pcbi.1004867.

Finan, C., A. Gaulton, F.A. Kruger, R.T. Lumbers, T. Shah, J. Engmann, et al. (2017). The druggable genome and support for target identification and validation in drug development. Sci. Transl. Med. 9(383): doi: 10.1126/scitranslmed.aag1166.

Forero, D.A., A. Wonkam, W. Wang, P. Laissue, C. Lopez-Correa, J.C. Fernandez-Lopez, et al. (2016). Current needs for human and medical genomics research infrastructure in low and middle income countries. J. Med. Genet. 53(7): 438–440. doi: 10.1136/jmedgenet-2015-103631.

Forero, D.A. (2019). Available software for meta-analyses of genome-wide expression studies. Curr. Genomics. 20(5): 325–331. doi: 10.2174/1389202920666190822113912.

Forero, D.A., Y. Gonzalez-Giraldo, L.J. Castro-Vega and G.E. Barreto. (2019a). qPCR-based methods for expression analysis of miRNAs. Biotechniques. 67(4): 192–199. doi: 10.2144/btn-2019-0065.

Forero, D.A., S. Lopez-Leon, Y. Gonzalez-Giraldo and P.G. Bagos. (2019b). Ten simple rules for carrying out and writing meta-analyses. PLoS Comput. Biol. 15(5): e1006922. doi: 10.1371/journal.pcbi.1006922.

Garmire, L.X., S. Gliske, Q.C. Nguyen, J.H. Chen, S. Nemati, J.D. Van Horn, et al. (2017). The training of next generation data scientists in biomedicine. Pac Symp Biocomput, 22, 640–645. doi: 10.1142/9789813207813_0059.

Gauthier, J., A.T. Vincent, S.J. Charette and N. Derome. (2019). A brief history of bioinformatics. Brief. Bioinform. 20(6): 1981–1996. doi: 10.1093/bib/bby063.

Gentleman, R.C., V.J. Carey, D.M. Bates, B. Bolstad, M. Dettling, S. Dudoit, et al. (2004). Bioconductor: Open software development for computational biology and bioinformatics. Genome Biol. 5(10): R80. doi: 10.1186/gb-2004-5-10-r80.

Gudenas, B.L., J. Wang, S.Z. Kuang, A.Q. Wei, S.B. Cogill and L.J. Wang. (2019). Genomic data mining for functional annotation of human long noncoding RNAs. J. Zhejiang Univ. Sci. B. 20(6): 476–487. doi: 10.1631/jzus.B1900162.

Hansen, A.R. and P.L. Bedard. (2013). Clinical application of high-throughput genomic technologies for treatment selection in breast cancer. Breast Cancer Res. 15(5): R97. doi: 10.1186/bcr3558.

Harrow, J., A. Frankish, J.M. Gonzalez, E. Tapanari, M. Diekhans, F. Kokocinski, et al. (2012). GENCODE: The reference human genome annotation for The ENCODE Project. Genome Res. 22(9): 1760–1774. doi: 10.1101/gr.135350.111.

Hindorff, L.A., V.L. Bonham, L.C. Brody, M.E.C. Ginoza, C.M. Hutter, T.A. Manolio, et al. (2018). Prioritizing diversity in human genomics research. Nat. Rev. Genet. 19(3): 175–185. doi: 10.1038/nrg.2017.89.

Hrdlickova, R., M. Toloue and B. Tian. (2017). RNA-Seq methods for transcriptome analysis. Wiley Interdiscip Rev RNA. 8(1): 10.1002/wrna.1364. doi:10.1002/wrna.1364.

Iddamalgoda, L., P.S. Das, A. Aponso, V.S. Sundararajan, P. Suravajhala and J.K. Valadi. (2016). Data mining and pattern recognition models for identifying inherited diseases: challenges and implications. Front. Genet. 7: 136. doi: 10.3389/fgene.2016.00136.

Karczewski, K.J., L.C. Francioli, G. Tiao, B.B. Cummings, J. Alfoldi, Q. Wang, et al. (2020). The mutational constraint spectrum quantified from variation in 141,456 humans. Nature. 581(7809): 434–443. doi: 10.1038/s41586-020-2308-7.

Ke, R., M. Mignardi, T. Hauling and M. Nilsson. (2016). Fourth generation of next-generation sequencing technologies: Promise and consequences. Hum. Mutat. 37(12): 1363–1367. doi: 10.1002/humu.23051.

Kobayashi, D., S. Sallaam and R.A. Humes. (2013). Tetralogy of fallot with complete DiGeorge syndrome: Report of a case and a review of the literature. Congenit. Heart Dis. 8(4): E119–126. doi: 10.1111/j.1747-0803.2012.00694.x.

Kumaran, M., U. Subramanian and B. Devarajan. (2019). Performance assessment of variant calling pipelines using human whole exome sequencing and simulated data. BMC Bioinformatics. 20(1): 342. doi: 10.1186/s12859-019-2928-9.

LaFramboise, T. (2009). Single nucleotide polymorphism arrays: a decade of biological, computational and technological advances. Nucleic Acids Res. 37(13): 4181–4193. doi: 10.1093/nar/gkp552.

Lee, D., O. Redfern and C. Orengo. (2007). Predicting protein function from sequence and structure. Nat. Rev. Mol. Cell. Biol. 8(12): 995–1005. doi: 10.1038/nrm2281.

Lin, E. and H.Y. Lane. (2017). Machine learning and systems genomics approaches for multi-omics data. Biomark. Res. 5: 2. doi: 10.1186/s40364-017-0082-y.

Lotfi Shahreza, M., N. Ghadiri, S.R. Mousavi, J. Varshosaz and J.R. Green. (2018). A review of network-based approaches to drug repositioning. Brief Bioinform. 19(5): 878–892. doi: 10.1093/bib/bbx017.

Maecker, H.T., T.M. Lindstrom, W.H. Robinson, P.J. Utz, M. Hale, S.D. Boyd, et al. (2012). New tools for classification and monitoring of autoimmune diseases. Nat. Rev. Rheumatol. 8(6): 317–328. doi: 10.1038/nrrheum.2012.66.

Mizzi, C., B. Peters, C. Mitropoulou, K. Mitropoulos, T. Katsila, M.R. Agarwal, et al. (2014). Personalized pharmacogenomics profiling using whole-genome sequencing. Pharmacogenomics. 15(9): 1223–1234. doi: 10.2217/pgs.14.102.

Qin, Q. and J. Feng. (2017). Imputation for transcription factor binding predictions based on deep learning. PLoS Comput. Biol. 13(2): e1005403. doi: 10.1371/journal.pcbi.1005403.

Ramasamy, A., A. Mondry, C.C. Holmes and D.G. Altman. (2008). Key issues in conducting a meta-analysis of gene expression microarray datasets. PLoS Med. 5(9): e184. doi: 10.1371/journal.pmed.0050184.

Reuter, M.S., R.R. Chaturvedi, E. Liston, R. Manshaei, R.B. Aul, S. Bowdin, et al. (2020). The cardiac genome clinic: Implementing genome sequencing in pediatric heart disease. Genet. Med. 22(6): 1015–1024. doi: 10.1038/s41436-020-0757-x.

Rubinstein, A. and B. Chor. (2014). Computational thinking in life science education. PLoS Comput. Biol. 10(11): e1003897. doi: 10.1371/journal.pcbi.1003897.

Saxena, A. and K. Sachin. (2018). A network biology approach for assessing the role of pathologic adipose tissues in insulin resistance using meta-analysis of microarray datasets. Curr. Genomics. 19(7): 630–666. doi: 10.2174/1389202919666180726125645.

Schwarze, K., J. Buchanan, J.C. Taylor and S. Wordsworth. (2018). Are whole-exome and whole-genome sequencing approaches cost-effective? A systematic review of the literature. Genet. Med. 20(10): 1122–1130. doi: 10.1038/gim.2017.247.

Sweeney, T.E., L. Braviak, C.M. Tato and P. Khatri. (2016). Genome-wide expression for diagnosis of pulmonary tuberculosis: A multicohort analysis. Lancet Respir. Med. 4(3): 213–224. doi: 10.1016/S2213-2600(16)00048-5.

Telenti, A., C. Lippert, P.C. Chang and M. DePristo. (2018). Deep learning of genomic variation and regulatory network data. Hum. Mol. Genet. 27(R1): R63–R71. doi: 10.1093/hmg/ddy115.

Thusberg, J., A. Olatubosun and M. Vihinen. (2011). Performance of mutation pathogenicity prediction methods on missense variants. Hum. Mutat. 32(4): 358–368. doi: 10.1002/humu.21445.

Tosto, G. and C. Reitz. (2016). Genomics of Alzheimer's disease: Value of high-throughput genomic technologies to dissect its etiology. Mol. Cell. Probes. 30(6): 397–403. doi: 10.1016/j.mcp.2016.09.001.

Vandivier, L.E., S.J. Anderson, S.W. Foley and B.D. Gregory. (2016). The conservation and function of RNA secondary structure in plants. Annu. Rev. Plant Biol. 67: 463–488. doi: 10.1146/annurev-arplant-043015-111754.

Wang, L., J. Law, S.D. Kale, T.M. Murali and G. Pandey. (2018). Large-scale protein function prediction using heterogeneous ensembles. F1000 Res. 7. doi: 10.12688/f1000research.16415.1.

Wang, H. and R. Chen. (2020). Whole-exome sequencing and whole-genome sequencing. pp. 27–39. *In*: X.R. Gao (ed.), Genetics and Genomics of Eye Disease. Academic Press.

Wockner, L.F., E.P. Noble, B.R. Lawford, R.M. Young, C.P. Morris, V.L. Whitehall, et al. (2014). Genome-wide DNA methylation analysis of human brain tissue from schizophrenia patients. Transl Psychiatry, 4, e339. doi: 10.1038/tp.2013.111.

Wolff, A., M. Bayerlova, J. Gaedcke, D. Kube and T. Beissbarth. (2018). A comparative study of RNA-Seq and microarray data analysis on the two examples of rectal-cancer patients and Burkitt Lymphoma cells. PLoS One. 13(5): e0197162. doi: 10.1371/journal.pone.0197162.

Yong, W.S., F.M. Hsu and P.Y. Chen (2016). Profiling genome-wide DNA methylation. Epigenet. Chromatin. 9: 26. doi: 10.1186/s13072-016-0075-3.

Zhao, H., D. Fan, D.R. Nyholt and Y. Yang. (2016). Enrichment of SNPs in functional categories reveals genes affecting complex traits. Hum. Mutat. 37(8): 820–826. doi: 10.1002/humu.23007.

CHAPTER 2

Bioinformatics of Genome Annotation

Dinesh Gupta* and Rahila Sardar

Translational Bioinformatics Group
International Centre for Genetic Engineering and Biotechnology (ICGEB)
New Delhi, India

1 WHAT IS GENOME ANNOTATION?

After performing the genome assembly with adaptor trimming and filtering for good quality sequences, the next step is assigning biological information to the raw sequence data called genome annotation such as function, pathway, location, size, molecular weight and other attributes. This includes providing annotation to protein-coding genes as well as non-coding genes. This allows us to identify ORFs, introns, exons, repetitive regions, regulatory elements, etc.

Development of genome annotation strategies started in the year 1990, with the launch of the Human Genome Project with an aim to sequence and decipher all 3 billion letters of a human genome. The first draft of the human genome was published in 2001 with computational annotation for 30,000 to 40,000 protein-coding genes from 22 pairs of autosomes and the X and Y sex chromosomes in a genome of 2.9 billion bases.

Since then, there has been significant progress in the efficiency of genome annotation pipelines, with the development of better bioinformatics algorithms, tools and availability of reference genomes. The growth of NCBI sequence data for eukaryotic organisms clearly shows that annotation and also re-annotation of organisms is exponentially increasing with time.

Despite the availability of more efficient and faster automated annotation pipelines, manual annotation is still performed to improve the quality of automatic annotations.

The annotation pipelines and its quality are also dependent on the sequencing technologies used. An overview of new sequencing technologies is presented in the following section (Fig. 1).

*Corresponding author: *dinesh@icgeb.res.in*

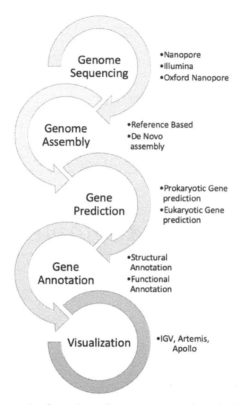

Figure 1 Overview of genome annotation pipeline.

2   EMERGENCE OF NEXT GENERATION SEQUENCING TECHNOLOGIES

Genome sequencing and genomics research are developing gradually after the report of the first human genome sequence in 2001 (International Human Genome Sequencing Consortium, 2001, 2004). Small genomes like bacteria and fungi can be easily assembled and annotated with fewer amounts of resources within a limited time whereas performing such tasks for higher genomes require more computation resources and longer periods. Assembly and annotation of eukaryotic genomes take few months up to years where no reference genomes can be used (Dominguez Del Angel et al., 2018). However, with the progress in bioinformatics tools and emerging new sequencing techniques, it is now more expedient and convenient to assemble and annotate large eukaryotic genomes (Jansen et al., 2017). Nonetheless, obtaining high-quality genome assembly and annotation is still a major challenge.

Since 2001, NGS technology has been developed which allows us to sequence genome, exomes, proteomes and gene panels much faster with less error rate in a cost-effective way (Goodwin, et al., 2016). Several sequencing platforms can be classified into three main types based on the coverage and genome sequencing technique. The first type, e.g., Illumina and Ion Torrent platforms, are based on finding the clonally amplified target and Pac Bio and Oxford Nanopore technology that uses single-molecule detection per reaction. The second type consists of sequencing by synthesis and direct measurement of DNA which is used by Illumina, Ion Torrent, and Pacific Biosciences platforms. The third type is based on either optical detection, for example, Illumina and Pacific Biosciences platforms, or non-optical detection for base read call. Currently, a hybrid genome sequencing platform is also available which relies on taking advantage of the different types of sequencing platforms (Koren et al., 2012).

Current sequencing methods to perform whole-genome sequencing are categorized mainly into two categories based on the length of the nucleotide sequence produced or sequence 'read with their advantages and disadvantages, shown in Table 1. Choosing the appropriate technology according to the query plays a crucial role in downstream analysis.

Table 1   Currently used sequencing strategies with their advantages and disadvantages

Parameters	Illumina-MiSeq	NextSeq 500	HiSeq 2500	PacBioRSII	GSFLX
Read length	2*300bp	2*150bp	2*150bp	3000bp	700bp
Run Time	5–65 hours	up to 30 hours	up to 6 days	30 min	23 hours
Gb/Run	0.3–15 GB	30–120 GB	50–1000 GB	3 GB	~1 GB
Million Reads	~25 million	~400 million	~2 billion	~0.5 million	
Advantage	High throughput/cost	High throughput/cost	High throughput/cost	Longest read length	Long read length
Disadvantage	Long run time	Long run time	Long run time	High error rate	The high error rate in homopolymer

3   GENOME ASSEMBLY AND ANNOTATION: AN OVERVIEW

Genome assembly refers to the process of arranging the raw reads into the correct order as they are naturally packed. Accurate assembly of the genome is the key step before beginning successful annotation. Genome assembly can be performed in two ways: reference-based assembly, or *de novo* assembly. For reference-based assembly, a known pre-sequenced and the assembled genome is used for mapping with a newly sequenced genome (Fig. 2). Bowtie and bwa are widely used tools for mapping and genome assembly (Langmead and Salzberg, 2012).

For example: Bowtie is an ultra-fast short-read aligner too, which helps in mapping and assembly. It aligns a large number of short sequencing reads to a reference sequence. For the longer read with the above, Bowtie 2 is used, which is generally faster, more sensitive, and uses less memory than Bowtie. There are various popular assemblers developed for the assembly of small and large genomes from the sequencing data from various platforms, as shown in Table 2.

Table 2   Widely used genome assemblers (El-Metwally et al., 2013a; Schlebusch and Illing, 2012)

Software	Algorithm	Operating systems	Sequencer	Genome specificity	Input
Edena	Greedy	L, W	Illumina	Small genomes	Paired-end and single-end
CABOG	Overlap/Layout/Consensus	Linux, Mac, Darwin	Mixed	Large genomes	Paired-end
SGA	Overlap/Layout/Consensus	Linux, Mac	Illumina	Large genomes	Paired-end
Euler	De bruijn	Linux	454+Sanger	Large genomes	Paired-end and unpaired
Velvet	De bruijn	Linux, Mac, Cygwin	Illumina	Small genomes	Paired-end and single-end
Soap denovo	De bruijn	Linux	Illumina	Large genomes	Paired
Abyss	De bruijn	All OS	Illumina	Large genomes	Paired-end and single-end
Newbler	Overlap/Layout/Consensus	Linux, Centos	454	Large genomes	Paired-end

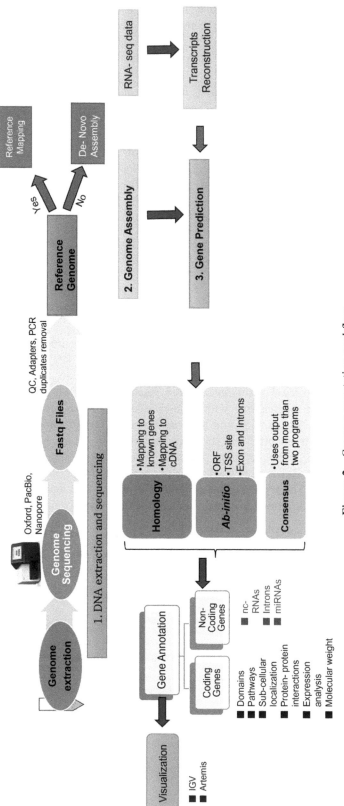

Figure 2   Genome annotation workflow.

Accurate assembly with good assembly statistics is the initial step that should be considered before annotation of genomes. N50 is a measurement parameter often used to evaluate the genome assembly characteristics (Dominguez Del Angel et al., 2018).

Various bioinformatics tools that are available to evaluate the quality of genome assemblies such as Quast (Gurevich et al., 2013), Reapr (Hunt et al., 2013), FRCBam (Vezzi et al., 2012) and BUSCO (Simão et al., 2015) are very useful.

4   REPEAT IDENTIFICATION

Repetitive DNA consists of hundreds to thousands of repeated sequence motifs and estimated to contribute around ~30% of the total genome. Repetitive regions are mainly classified into microsatellites, i.e., short tandem repeats (STRs) or simple sequence repeats (SSRs), minisatellites and satellite DNAs (Richard et al., 2008) according to their size. Most of them are found to be located in centromeres, telomeres, and dispersed throughout the genome (Pelley, 2012). Eukaryotic genomes such as human are highly repetitive, constituted of around 47% of repeats throughout the genome (International Human Genome Sequencing Consortium, 2001).

Complete fragments of repeats are found occasionally because the borders of repeats are not well defined and often inserted within other repeats, also found to be poorly conserved across genomes. This leads to complication in genome assembly and annotation. For accurate annotation, repeats need to be correctly identified and annotated. Several tools till now have been developed to do such analysis which is based on two methods, i.e., homology-based (Buisine et al., 2008; Han and Wessler, 2010) and *de novo*-based repeats identification approach (Flynn et al., 2020). Repeat identification, its masking and annotation thus plays a significant role in accurate genome annotation projects. Some of the recent tools are RepeatModeler2 (Flynn et al., 2020), RepeatAnalyzer (Catanese et al., 2016), Red (Girgis, 2015) and TAREAN (Novák et al., 2017).

5   GENE PREDICTION

Computational gene prediction is the essential stage for the functional annotation of genes and genomes. Through decades significant progress has been made to predict prokaryotic genes. But eukaryotic gene prediction is still more challenging due to the presence of coding as well as non-coding regions (Xiong, 2006).

Discovery of gene includes identification of ORFs, introns and exons in the case of eukaryotic genomes. In prokaryotes, DNA is transcribed into mRNA by the process of transcription as translated into proteins known as translation without being modified. Whereas, in eukaryotic organisms, the transcription process involves the removal of introns by the process of splicing followed by other necessary modifications. This complexity in the eukaryotic genomes cause gene prediction much more difficult as compared to prokaryotic genomes (Wang et al., 2004). Gene prediction can be broadly characterized into homology-based and *ab initio*-based gene prediction (Fig. 2).

5.1   Homology-based Gene Prediction

Sequence similarity or homology-based approach is where the given genome is used to discover similarity in gene sequences between ESTs (expressed sequence tags), proteins, and spliced variants. This approach is based on the fact that coding regions are more evolutionarily conserved than non-coding regions. After similarity-based EST and protein identification, the next step is to infer the function of the region. EST-based similarity search led to the identification of only small portions of gene sequence which often led to difficulties in complete gene prediction for the given region (Wang et al., 2004). NCBI, Ensembl and Celera have recently added EST sequences for exon and transcript predictions.

There are various similarity-based gene prediction tools that have been developed, BLAST is a widely-used tool for homology-based gene finders. It performs a similarity search by first cutting down the input sequence into a series of DNA or protein sequences and then searches against a local or NCBI database. Local and global alignment of BLAST are the two main algorithms used for gene prediction. genBlast program, which is based on local alignments, has two programs, viz. genBlastA and genBlastG (She et al., 2009; Medema and Breitling, 2013). genBlastA performs local alignments by BLAST and WU-BLAST and identifies groups of high-scoring segment pairs (HSPs). However, genBlastG is a fast homology-based gene finding tool that uses the output from geneBlastA as the input to define gene models. Homology-based prediction is a fast and accurate way of identifying gene models.

(i) *Ab initio* Methods

Ab initio gene predictions do not rely on external evidences such as EST and protein alignments. They extract gene information by generating mathematical models and identifying their intron-exon pattern. This method can help in the identification of gene regions that are located in boundaries which include promoters and start and stop codons. But only relying on the *ab initio* method for gene prediction generates more false positives and cannot predict splice variants and 5′ – 3′ UTRs. To improve the accuracy of *ab initio* method tools like TwinScan (Korf et al., 2001), FGENESH (Solovyev et al., 2006), Augustus (Nachtweide and Stanke, 2019), GAZE and SNAP use external evidences (Korf, 2004).

5.2   Evidence-based Predictions

To better predict the genes with stronger evidence RNA-seq data can be used. RNA-seq data plays a significant role in improvising the accuracy of gene annotations, as this generates evidence for the presence of exons, splice sites and alternative splicing events. This can be performed in two ways: first by assembling the reads by *de novo* assemblers such as ABySS, SOAPdenovo and Trinity and then align it to the reference genome using TopHat, GSNAP followed by generation of transcripts using Cufflinks (Yandell and Ence, 2012).

6   ANNOTATION AND TYPES OF ANNOTATIONS

Genome annotation is typically divided into two types: structural annotation and functional annotations. Structural annotation describes the sequence features of genes such as CDS, ORFs, TSS, exons and introns whereas functional annotation describes as attaching functional information to the genes such as domains, pathways and others which is described in the forthcoming sections.

Genes are the heritable material transferred from parents to offspring. Genes are further distinguished into coding and non-coding genes.

6.1   Non-coding Genes

There are only ~1.5% of the genes that code for proteins while the remaining 98.5% constitutes the non-coding genes for the human genome and was previously referred to as junk DNA with no biological role (Lander, 2011). The amount of coding and non-coding DNA varies significantly across species. As mentioned, non-coding genes were earlier referred to as junk DNA with no biological role but now they are reported to have a significant role in regulating gene expression (Rinn and Chang, 2012).

ncRNAs are broadly classified into two groups that include small RNAs (sRNAs) and lncRNAs. Further, sRNAs consist of microRNA (miRNAs), Pi-interacting RNAs (piRNAs), short interfering RNAs (siRNAs), small nucleolar RNAs (snoRNAs) and other short RNAs (sRNAs) (Gomes et al., 2013).

Annotation techniques for non-coding RNA (ncRNA) are less efficient as techniques for protein-coding genes. But with the advancement in technology and software, several programs have been developed for the identification and annotation of non-coding RNAs. Recently, various studies have shown the process of how miRNAs interact with their targets, i.e., mRNAs, long non-coding RNAs (lncRNAs), pseudogenes and circular RNAs (circRNAs) (Tay et al., 2014). Among the other classes of sRNAs, microRNAs (or miRNAs) have been well studied that are known to regulate essential biological processes such as gene expression regulation and gene silencing in animals as well as plants. The biogenesis of miRNA in animals and plants is different and involve different types of proteins (Chen et al., 2018). There are a variety of tools and databases that have been developed specifically for plant and animal miRNAs and are used for the identification of miRNAs, their targets and cleavage sites (Table 3).

Table 3 Bioinformatics tools for miRNA identification with their targets

Software/Databases	Animals	Plants
Annotation	miRbase Rfam miRIAD	miRBase
Identification	miRDeep MiRSan	miRPlant MicroPC
Cleavage site	PHDcleav LBsSizecleav	miRNA Digger
Disease/Stress	miR2Disease HMDD	PASmiRHMDD
Target Discovery	miRanda TargetScan TarBase	TarBase psRNATarget

ENCODE and FANTOM are projects which are focused on systematic annotation and functional characterization of non-coding RNA (ncRNA) genes. One method to identify ncRNA genes is based on the identification of conserved secondary structures and motifs. Tools like tRNAscan-SE (Lowe and Eddy, 1997) and Snoscan perform such analysis (Schattner et al., 2005).

6.2 Coding Genes

Genes that code for proteins are called coding genes, also known as CDS. With the accumulation of protein sequences from proteomics and genomics data, the functional annotation of protein sequences with high accuracy is a daunting task. Functional annotation includes identification of domains, pathways, gene ontology analysis, protein-protein interaction, structural analysis and domain identification. Till now there are many tools and bioinformatics databases that have been developed for the functional analysis of proteins as shown in Fig. 3. Some of them are discussed below in Table 4.

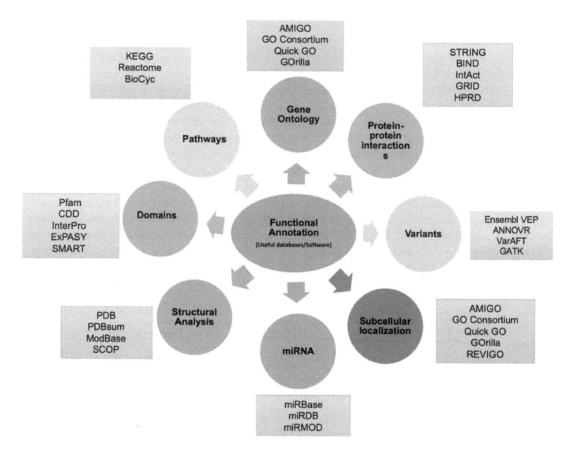

Figure 3   Bioinformatics tools/databases used in functional annotation of genes.

Table 4   Useful databases for functional annotation of proteins

Trembl	Description	Link
	RefSeq Protein	
SwissProt	Manually curated protein sequence database which strives to provide a high level of annotation with a minimal level of redundancy and high level of integration with other databases.	https://www.uniprot.org/
	Computationally annotated with records that await full manual annotation.	https://www.uniprot.org/
	The Reference Sequence (RefSeq) collection provides a comprehensive, integrated, non-redundant, well-annotated set of sequences, including genomic DNA, transcripts, and protein set of reference sequences including genomic, transcript, and protein.	https://www.ncbi.nlm.nih.gov/refseq/
UniProt	Comprehensive, high-quality and freely accessible resource of protein sequence and functional information.	https://www.uniprot.org/
	Structure database	
PDB	Provides information about the 3D shapes of proteins, nucleic acids, and complex assemblies.	https://www.rcsb.org/

Trembl	Description	Link
PDBsum	Overview of the contents of each 3D macromolecular structure deposited in the Protein Data Bank.	http://www.ebi.ac.uk/thornton-srv/databases/cgi-bin/pdbsum/GetPage.pl?pdbcode=index.html
ModBase	Database of annotated comparative protein structure models, containing models for more than 3.8 million unique protein sequences.	https://modbase.compbio.ucsf.edu/modbase-cgi/index.cgi
SCOP	Comprehensive structural and evolutionary relationships between all proteins whose structure is known.	http://scop.mrc-lmb.cam.ac.uk/
Domains information		
Pfam	Collection of protein families, represented by multiple sequence alignments and hidden Markov models (HMMs).	https://pfam.xfam.org/
CDD	Collection of well-annotated multiple sequence alignment models for ancient domains and full-length proteins. available as position-specific score matrices (PSSMs) for fast identification of conserved domains in protein sequences.	https://www.ncbi.nlm.nih.gov/cdd
InterPro	Functional analysis of proteins by classifying them into families and predicting domains and important sites.	https://www.ebi.ac.uk/interpro/
ExPASY	Access to scientific databases and software tools (i.e., resources) in different areas of life sciences including proteomics, genomics, phylogeny, systems biology, population genetics, transcriptomics, etc.	https://www.expasy.org/
SMART	Allows the identification and annotation of genetically mobile domains and the analysis of domain architectures.	http://smart.embl-heidelberg.de/
Subcellular localization		
CELLO	CELLO is a multi-class SVM classification system to predict subcellular localization.	http://cello.life.nctu.edu.tw/
PSORT	PSORT is a computer program for the prediction of protein localization sites in cells.	https://psort.hgc.jp/
iPSORT	iPSORT is a subcellular localization site predictor for N-terminal sorting signals. It will predict whether it contains a Signal Peptide (SP), Mitochondrial Targeting Peptide (mTP), or Chloroplast Transit Peptide (cTP).	http://ipsort.hgc.jp/
ngLOC	Software and web server for predicting protein subcellular localization in prokaryotes and eukaryotes.	http://ngloc.unmc.edu/
TargetP-2.0	TargetP-2.0 server predicts the presence of N-terminal presequences: signal peptide (SP), mitochondrial transit peptide (mTP), chloroplast transit peptide (cTP) or thylakoid luminal transit peptide (luTP).	http://www.cbs.dtu.dk/services/TargetP/
signalP	SignalP 5.0 server predicts the presence of signal peptides and the location of their cleavage sites in proteins from Archaea, gram-positive bacteria, gram-negative bacteria and Eukarya.	http://www.cbs.dtu.dk/services/SignalP/

Table 4. Contd....

Table 4   Useful databases for functional annotation of proteins (Contd. ...)

Trembl	Description	Link
Gene ontology		
AMIGO	Web-based set of tools for searching and browsing the Gene Ontology database.	http://amigo.geneontology.org/amigo
GO Consortium	The main aim of GO Consortium is to develop a comprehensive, computational model organism.	http://geneontology.org/
Quick GO	QuickGO is a fast web-based browser of the Gene Ontology and Gene Ontology annotation data.	https://www.ebi.ac.uk/QuickGO/
GOrilla	GOrilla is a tool for identifying and visualizing enriched GO terms in ranked lists of genes.	http://cbl-gorilla.cs.technion.ac.il/
REVIGO	REVIGO is a web server that summarizes lists of GO terms by finding a representative subset of the GO terms using a simple clustering algorithm that relies on semantic similarity measures.	http://revigo.irb.hr/
Variant annotation		
Ensembl VEP	VEP determines the effect of your variants (SNPs, insertions, deletions, CNVs or structural variants) on genes, transcripts, and protein sequence, as well as regulatory regions.	https://asia.ensembl.org/Tools/VEP
wANNOVAR	ANNOVAR is a rapid, efficient tool to annotate functional consequences of genetic variation from high-throughput sequencing data identify whether SNPs or CNVs cause protein-coding changes and the amino acids that are affected.	http://wannovar.wglab.org/
VarAFT	VarAFT provides experiments' quality, annotates, and allows the filtration of VCF files. Data from multiple samples may be combined to address different Mendelian Inherited Disorders, Population Genetics or Cancers.	https://varaft.eu/
GATK	It is developed by Broad Institute,and offers the toolkit which provides wide variety of tools with a primary focus on variant discovery and genotyping.	https://software.broadinstitute.org/gatk/
miRNA database		
miRBase	miRBase is a biological database of microRNA sequences with their detailed annotations.	http://www.mirbase.org/
miRDB	It is an online resource for microRNA target prediction and functional annotations.	http://mirdb.org/
miRMOD	It is a GUI-based tool to predict modifications in miRNAs.	http://bioinfo.icgeb.res.in/miRMOD/
Transcription factors		
CiSBP	It is a library of transcription factor (TF) and transcription factor binding motifs (TFBS) and specificities.	http://cisbp.ccbr.utoronto.ca/index.php
JASPAR	It is an open-access database of curated non-redundant transcription factor (TF) binding profiles stored as position frequency matrices (PFMs) and TF flexible models (TFFMs) for TFs across multiple species in six taxonomic groups.	http://jaspar.genereg.net/

Trembl	Description	Link
ApicoTFDB	It is a web repository of apicomplexan transcription factors and transcription-associated co-factors.	http://bioinfo.icgeb.res.in/PtDB/
AnimalTFDB	It is a comprehensive resource for annotation and prediction of animal transcription factors.	http://bioinfo.life.hust.edu.cn/AnimalTFDB/
Protein-protein interactions		
IntAct	It is an open-source EMBI-EBI database of 1059311 curated molecular interactions.	http://www.ebi.ac.uk/intact
STRING	It is a database consisting of known and predicted protein-protein interactions consisting of both direct (physical) and indirect (functional) associations.	https://string-db.org/
DIP	It constitutes experimentally determined interactions between proteins.	https://dip.doe-mbi.ucla.edu/

7 PROTEIN SEQUENCE ANNOTATION AND DATABASES

The basic function of a protein can only be extracted from its primary sequence. The correct protein sequence is the prior and foremost thing that is required for the functional annotation of proteins. Many protein sequences are incorrect due to errors in sequencing and/or false ORF prediction. Incorrect protein sequence leads to false annotation like domains, sites of interactions, pathways and other downstream analysis (Bridge et al., 2008). There are a large number of databases that are available for protein sequence retrieval. These databases mainly consist of two types of information: protein sequences repositories and protein sequence annotation databases. Protein sequence repositories contain protein sequence information and also provide sequences that are newly sequenced but with no annotations of sequences. These databases also have a large number of redundant sequences with different record id's. There are other freely available repositories of protein sequences and annotation (discussed below).

(i) UniProtKB
UniProt Knowledgebase (UniProtKB) is a manually curated protein database divided into two sections: Swiss-Prot, where each entry is reviewed and manually annotated, and TrEMBL, which consists of unreviewed and automatically annotated entries, as shown in Fig. 4. UniProt is the central open access repository of protein sequences with its annotation.

The UniProt Consortium was formed as a collaboration between the European Bioinformatics Institute (EBI), the Protein Information Resource (PIR) and the Swiss Institute of Bioinformatics (SIB). The main aim behind UniProt's development was to provide a high-quality functional annotation of proteins which are curated and reviewed manually. Every three weeks UniProt is updated with new annotations and entries (http://www.uniprot.org).

(ii) SwissProt
SwissProt was established by the Department of Medical Biochemistry at the University of Geneva in collaboration with the European Molecular Biology Laboratory (EMBL). Since 1987, it is maintained by the Swiss Institute of bioinformatics (SIB) and the European Bioinformatics Institute (EBI). SWISS-PROT is a repository of protein sequences with their complete annotations.

SWISS-PROT consists of protein sequence entries in its format.

With every sequence entry, three main data are available, i.e., the sequence information, bibliographical and the taxonomic data.

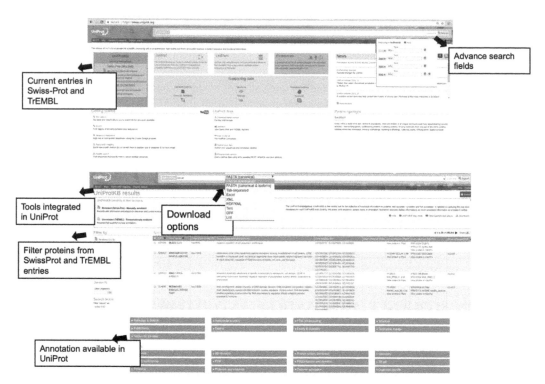

Figure 4   Protein annotation utilities in the UniProt database.

Also, annotation with every protein sequence is present, which includes post-translational modifications, variant information, protein domain, protein structure, functions of protein and associated disease with protein are available. This database has protein annotations with less redundancy and is also integrated with other useful sequence-related databases (nucleic acid sequences, protein sequences and protein tertiary structures) that make SWISS-PROT highly useful and unique as compared to other protein sequence database. Since 2002, this database is maintained by the UniProt consortium which can be accessed using the UniProt website. Currently, there are 562,253 protein sequence entries available at SWISS-PROT. Among them, there are 20,365 entries for humans, 17, 038 for mouse, 15, 952 for *A. thaliana,* 8,094 for rat and 6721 for *S. cerevisiae* available in the current version of the database (Release 2020_2).

(iii) TREMBL (EMBL)

TREMBL, (Translated EMBL) is a very large protein database which is a supplement of SwissProt that consists of computer translations of EMBL nucleotide sequence entries. Translation of sequences is not always correct, therefore the proteins predicted in the TrEMBL database are poorly annotated. In the year 1999 Release 11 of TrEMBL was developed to translate all 3,79,000 CDSs in the EMBL Nucleotide Sequence Database release 58. Amongst these, around 119 000 of CDS were reported in SWISS-PROT, and therefore, removed from TrEMBL. To remove redundancy the remaining sequences were merged automatically with the new method. There are 4, 180, 690, 447 of TrEMBL entries in the current release, i.e., 2020_2 of UniProtKB.

(iv) RefSeq

NCBI Reference Sequence (RefSeq) database is another popular and freely accessible protein sequence and annotation. This database consists of a large number of curated, non-redundant and annotated sequences of DNA, RNA, and protein.

Refseq includes species from taxonomically different groups which include viruses, archaea, bacteria, and eukaryotes. Every entry in Refseq was retrieved and dependent on the sequence submitted to the International Nucleotide Sequence Database Collaboration (INSDC). Refseq entries can be retrieved by searching other interlinked NCBI resources such as PubMed, Nucleotide, Protein, Gene, and Map Viewer. RefSeq was developed to provide high standard functional annotation consisting of locations of SNPs found in medical records with no redundancy.

8 PROTEIN DOMAIN ANNOTATION

A domain can be defined as a conserved portion in protein sequence which can form a semi-independent 3D structure in proteins. They play a role in specific protein functions genetically evolving and transfer them within different organisms. Several protein families are known to have arisen from a common ancestor by attaining a different combination of domains (George and Heringa, 2002). The identification of these conserved domains is crucial to understand the function of proteins. Popular methods like the Hidden Markov Model (HMM) and PSI-BLAST are widely used to detect domains in a protein sequence.

(i) Pfam

Pfam is a database comprising curated protein families, defined by conserved Hidden Markov Model (HMM) profiles. The database can be accessed via servers in the UK (http://pfam.sanger. ac.uk/) and the USA (http://pfam.janelia.org/).

HMM is defined as a class of probabilistic models that are used to predict homology. Profiles can be generated by aligning a predefined set of defined family-representative sequences. In the Pfam database the profile HMM is searched against a large number of sequences obtained from UniProt Knowledgebase (UniProtKB) to identify all instances of the protein family. These HMM profiles are searched using the HMMER software. There is a predefined threshold that is set for each family to remove false positives called a 'gathering threshold'. Sequences that are above these thresholds are aligned to the defined HMM profiles to generate the full alignment. The entries which are curated by Pfam called Pfam-A entries. The main aim of the Pfam database is to include the maximum number of protein sequences representing the fewest number of models.

Each Pfam entry is tagged with one of the types—family, domain, motif, repeat, coiled-coil, or disordered—representing the functional unit class. In the current release (release 32) there are 17,929 protein families. With comparison to the structural classification database, namely, the Evolutionary Classification of Protein Domains (ECOD) by Pfam community, there is an addition of 825 new families. Moreover, each Pfam entry is now connected to the Sequence Ontology (SO).

(ii) Conserved Domain Database (CDD)

Conserved Domains can be described as regions in the sequence that have a similar or exact pattern of amino acid in a variety of organisms. These conserved domain patterns in the sequence can be achieved by performing multiple sequence alignment. CDD is a part of the NCBI Entrez search and retrieval system and is cross-linked with NCBI databases such as Entrez/protein, Entrez/Gene, 3D-structure (MMDB), NCBI BioSystems, PubMed and PubChem. For improving bacterial genome annotations there exists NCBIfam in CDD which is a set of HMM models (PMC6943070). In CDD, high-confidence (specific) domain annotation is used to differentiate between superfamily and subfamily domain architectures. CDD collects data from five other major resources including Pfam, SMART, COGs, TIGRFAMs and PRKs. Data can be downloaded in ASN Text, XML, JSON, BLAST Text format.

(iii) InterPro

InterPro is a freely accessible software available at https://www.ebi.ac.uk/interpro/. This database is useful in the classification of proteins into families by predicting their domains and other important sites. For the classification of proteins, Interpro relies on different predictive models referred to as 'signature' collected from several different databases that are the part of Interpro consortium.

9 DATABASES OF PATHWAY ANNOTATION

KEGG: Kyoto Encyclopedia of Genes and Genomes was developed by Minoru Kanehisa in the year 1995 in Japan by the Ministry of Education, Science, Sports and Culture in Japan and is available at https://www.genome.jp/kegg/pathway.html. KEGG database consists of high-level annotation, i.e., genomic to the molecular level annotation of biological systems. It provides detailed diagrammatic representation in the form of a network for genes, proteins, drugs and chemicals involved in various biological processes and diseases depicted in Fig. 5.

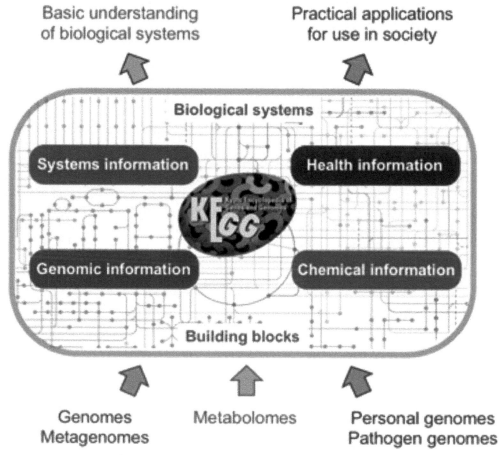

Figure 5   Annotation utilities in KEGG database.
Source: https://www.kegg.jp/kegg/kegg1a.html

The KEGG database resource comprises 18 databases that are broadly classified into four main categories that include system, chemical, genomic and health information and currently with 537, 18,701, 23,360, 1,011 entries (Table 5).

Table 5 Statistics of different modules in KEGG pathways with their number of entries till 1-05-2020

	Systems information	
KEGG PATHWAY	Pathway maps, reference (total)	537 (706,980)
KEGG BRITE	Functional hierarchies, reference (total)	200 (249,044)
KEGG MODULE	KEGG modules	394
	Reaction modules	41
	Genomic information	
KEGG ORTHOLOGY	KEGG Orthology (KO) groups	23,360
	KEGG organisms	6,542
KEGG GENOME	(541 eukaryotes, 5683 bacteria, 318 archaea)	
	KEGG selected viruses	341
KEGG GENES	(including 3,969 addendum, 372,625 viral)	3,15,92,703
KEGG SSDB	Best hit relations within GENES	3,80,05,47,33,157
	Bi-directional best hit relations within GENES	19,06,32,72,100
	Chemical information	
KEGG COMPOUND	Metabolites and other small molecules	18,701
KEGG GLYCAN	Glycans	11,040
KEGG REACTION	Biochemical reactions	11,416
	Reaction class	3,165
KEGG ENZYME	Enzyme nomenclature	7,736
	Health information	
KEGG NETWORK	Disease-related network elements	1,011
	Network variation maps	114
KEGG VARIANT	Human gene variants	416
KEGG DISEASE	Human diseases	2,421
KEGG DRUG	Drugs	11,264
	Drug groups	2,277
KEGG ENVIRON	Crude drugs and health-related substances	864

10 PROTEIN-PROTEIN INTERACTION DATABASES

It is important to identify the interaction between proteins because proteins do not work alone, instead, they interact with other proteins and form a network of interactions. There are various experimental techniques which have been developed to identify such interactions.

Yeast two-hybrid (Y2H) system and affinity purification followed by mass spectrometry (AP-MS) are two popular methods used to identify physical interactions. Various bioinformatics databases have been developed which consists of protein-protein interactions (PPI) information from various experimental as well as prediction methods. PPI information is visualized in the form of graphs with nodes as proteins and edges as an interaction between nodes.

(i) STRING

STRING database is a widely used database comprising known and predicted protein-protein interactions from experimental data, text mining, predictions and literature. The current version of the STRING database (11.0) has PPI of 24,584,628 proteins from 5090 organisms. Among them, 4445 are from bacteria, 477 from eukaryotes and 168 from Archae. The STRING resource is available online at https://string-db.org. STRING databases include physical (direct) as well as functional (indirect) interactions. STRING 11.0 has one important new feature where users can upload complete genome-wide datasets and perform gene-set enrichment analysis such as Gene Ontology and KEGG pathway analysis.

IntAct: This database was developed by EMBL-EBI. IntAct is freely available at http://www.ebi.ac.uk/intact and is an open-source database consisisting of molecular interactions extracted from either the literature or from direct data depositions.

(ii) DIP

The Database of Interacting Proteins consists of experimentally verified PPI and is available at http://dip.doe-mbi.ucla.edu. The DIP database provides three-level details: protein information protein-protein connections information and details of experiments detecting the protein-protein interactions. The protein information table contains protein identification codes from the SWISS-PROT, PIR and GenBank sequence databases, as well as each protein's gene name, description, enzyme code and cellular localization if known.

11   GENE ONTOLOGY ANALYSIS

Gene Ontology was developed in the year 1998 by a consortium of researchers working on the genomes of three model organisms: *Drosophila melanogaster* (fruit fly), *Mus musculus* (mouse), and *Saccharomyces cerevisiae* (brewer's or baker's yeast). Gene Ontology (GO) provides functional details associated with gene or gene products in detail. GO mainly consists of three types of information that include molecular function, biological process and cellular localization associated with every gene.

- *Molecular Function*:   Molecular function involves different activities that are present at the molecular level such as "catalysis" or "transport". Activities that can be accomplished by individual gene products such as proteins or RNA or activities that are performed by molecular complexes consist of multiple gene products fall under the molecular function category.
- *Biological Process*:   The larger processes or 'biological functions' performed by multiple molecular activities fall under this category, such as DNA repair or signal transduction.
- *Cellular Component*:   Unlike the other two classes this class does not provide information on processes but rather cellular anatomy. It provides information on the cellular location of gene products where it performed various functions (e.g., mitochondrion, ribosome, Golgi and others).

Till now a number of databases have been developed for GO identification.

One of the main important repositories is the Gene Ontology Consortium and is available at http://geneontology.org/ number of model organisms GOs. The Gene Ontology (GO) consortium is the world's largest knowledgeable database of information with regard to the functions of genes. As of June 2020, the GO consortium contains 44,441 GO terms, 7,975,639 annotations, and 1,558,956 gene products from 4,611 species.

The main aim behind GO Consortium is to develop an up-to-date, comprehensive, database of biological systems functional annotations from the molecular level, biological pathways and cellular level.

12   GENOME/ORGANISM-SPECIFIC ANNOTATION DATABASES

Genome-specific databases are biological databases developed to provide in-depth annotations for a specific model organism. These databases allow scientists to perform various integrated analysis in a single platform. These kinds of databases also provide a platform to scientists from the same fields for discussions and updates related to a specific organism's information such as latest publications, new achievements, related conferences and meetings, etc.

Some of the widely used organism-specific databases that have been developed until now, are discussed below in Table 6.

Table 6 Genome/Organism-specific annotation databases

Annotation database	*Description*	*No. of species*	*Link to database*
JGI-Genome	The Department of Energy (DOE) Joint Genome Institute (JGI) is a national user facility with massive-scale DNA sequencing and analysis capabilities dedicated to advancing genomics for bioenergy and environmental applications particular class of organisms.	3500	https://genome.jgi.doe.gov/portal/
TAIR	Complete genome sequence along with gene structure, gene product information, gene expression, DNA and seed stocks, genome maps, genetic and physical markers, publications, and information of Arabidopsis genomes.	1	https://www.arabidopsis.org/
Rice Genome Annotation project	Annotation data for the rice genome.	12	http://rice.plantbiology.msu.edu/
dictyBase	dictyBase includes the complete genome sequence, ESTs, and the literature relevant to Dictyostelium species.	4	http://dictybase.org/
UCSC genome	The UCSC Genome Browser is an on-line, and downloadable, genome browser developed by the University of California, Santa Cruz. This database consists of genome sequencing data from different species and model organisms, with their annotations.	105	https://genome-asia.ucsc.edu/cgi-bin/hgGateway?redirect=manualandsource=genome.ucsc.edu
Vertebrate and Genome Annotation Project (Vega)	(VEGA) the database is a biological database for annotating genes or regions of vertebrate genomes.	10	http://vega.archive.ensembl.org/index.html
GeneDB	The resource provides a portal to genome sequence and annotation data, which is primarily generated by the Pathogen Genomics group at the Wellcome Trust Sanger Institute. It combines data from completed and ongoing genome projects with curated annotation, which is readily accessible from a web-based resource.	41	https://www.genedb.org/
EupathDB	Database of *insilico* and experimental data of eukaryotic pathogens.	170+	https://eupathdb.org/eupathdb/
WormBase	Database providing biological information, of *Caenorhabditis elegans* with other nematodes.	196	https://www.wormbase.org
GENCODE	The goal is to identify and classify all gene features in the human and mouse genomes with high accuracy based on biological evidence.	2	https://www.gencodegenes.org/
FlyBase	This resource provides genetic, genomic and functional information on *D. melanogaster* and other fly species.	1	https://flybase.org/

13   GENOME PROPERTIES INFLUENCING ASSEMBLY AND ANNOTATION

We should check various genome properties which have an effect on quality of the downstream analysis. These include:

(i) Quality and purity check of extracted DNA
Contaminants such as phenol, salt and ethanol should be removed before proceeding with DNA sequencing. The introduction of such salts and alcohols may produce nicks in the DNA which makes it fragile. DNA becomes fragile due to other factors too such as using inappropriate storage such asstorage of DNA at above –20 degrees Celsius which causes DNA degradation. RNA contamination in the DNA samples also plays a major role in DNA structural integrity. This results in an overabundance of nucleic acid molecules concentration.

(ii) Choosing an appropriate sequencing technology
If you are working for new genome assembly and annotation, longer reads producing sequencing should be used such as Nanopore, PacBio, etc. For improving the assembly and annotation of specific genomes, sequencing platforms generating shorts reads need to be considered. This will help in filling the gaps which were not yet properly assembled.

(iii) DNA repeats
DNA repeats occur in multiple copies in different locations in the genome and influences significantly the genome assembly statistics. The main reasons behind it is similar reads are produced from different repeats which ultimately confuses the assembly tools which are not able to distinguish them properly (Phillippy et al., 2008). This can further result in a poor assembly where repeats from different regions assemble incorrectly. It can be avoided by choosing sequencing technology which produces longer reads.

(iv) GC-content
Bias in the GC content of various organisms have been observed. This bias in GC content has shown to cause low or no coverage in that region of the genome (Chen et al., 2013). Therefore, it is suggested that while working with these types of genome, sequencing technology which does not consider that bias (i.e., Pac-Bio or Nanopore) is recommended.

14   ANNOTATION FILE FORMATS

The file after complete genome annotation is called the GFF format. GFF file format is used for representing genes with their structural and functional features such as protein domains, pathways, interactions, structure and localization. It is in a tab-delimited format with 9 fields. Other file formats are gene transfer format (GTF), BED, GenBank, and EMBL. GFF file format does not include gene sequence information whereas BED and GenBank contain sequence information with annotations.

15   AUTOMATED ANNOTATION PIPELINES

Manual annotation of genomes cannot keep pace with the genome data explosion witnessed in recent years, hence, several automated and semi-automated pipelines for performing annotations have been developed to speed up the genome annotation process (Table 7).

Table 7 Automated annotation softwares for prokaryotes and eukaryotes

Software	Organisms	Link
MAKER2	Both	https://www.yandell-lab.org/software/maker.html
NCBI Eukaryotic Annotation Pipeline	eukaryotic genomes	https://www.ncbi.nlm.nih.gov/genome/annotation_euk/
NCBI prokaryotic Annotation Pipeline	Prokaryotic genomes	https://www.ncbi.nlm.nih.gov/genome/annotation_prok/
Kobas 3.0	covering 5,945 species	http://kobas.cbi.pku.edu.cn/kobas3
ENSEMBLE	annotate over 70 different vertebrate species	http://www.ensembl.org/index.html
RAST	Prokaryotic genomes	https://rast.nmpdr.org/
PROKKA	Prokaryotic genomes	http://www.bioinformatics.net.au/software.prokka.shtml

(i) RAST

In 2008, the RAST (Rapid Annotation using Subsystem Technology) annotation software was developed to annotate bacterial and archaeal genomes (Aziz et al., 2008). It uses manually curated gene annotations from the SEED database onto newly submitted genomes and then helps in identifying genomic features (i.e., protein-encoding genes and RNA) and annotating their functions. RAST has become popular for consistent and accurate annotation of microbial genomes. The RAST community currently consists of ~10,000 active users who contributed an average of 1,170 microbial genomes per week in the year 2014. To make RAST a more useful tool with advancements in bioinformatics that is both customizable and extensible to the RAST tool kit (RASTtk), a modular version of RAST was developed (Brettin et al. 2015). This pipeline enables researchers to customize their annotation pipelines. RASTtk offers many softwares for the identification and annotation of genomic features. RASTtk also allows batch submission of genomes with the ability to customize the annotation pipeline during batch submissions. This is the first major software restructuring of RAST since its inception. RASTtk is available at the RAST website (http://rast.nmpdr.org).

(ii) MAKER

MAKER is an open access easy-to-use genome annotation pipeline. The main purpose behind this pipeline is to independently annotate and create databases for smaller eukaryotic and prokaryotic genomes. MAKER performs gene annotation by identification of repeats, ESTs alignment and proteins to the query genome which generates *ab initio* gene predictions and automatically converts these data into gene annotation database. The input for MAKER is minimum and its output can be directly uploaded into a GMOD database. MAKER has proven to be extremely useful for scientists with minimal bioinformatics experience during handling sequencing projects from a model organism.

With the advent of second-generation sequencing technologies, more genomes have been sequenced and it is becoming difficult to handle such an enormous amount of data. Techniques like mRNA-seq generate large amounts of data but they have a great advantage in improving genome annotation quality. Therefore, it is necessary to convert the output of the annotation pipeline into a genome database. To address the challenges faced while annotating second-generation sequencing data, MAKER 2 was developed. This is an updated version of MAKER which is an improvement upon the *de novo* annotation capacities of MAKER and integrates multiple *ab initio* prediction tools. The main feature of MAKER2 is the integration of the Annotation Edit Distance (AED) metric to improve annotation quality and database management. To scale up and handle the data of any size this pipeline supports distributed parallelization on computer clusters via MPI.

MAKER2 pipeline can be run on computers with UNIX based operating systems such as Linux and Darwin in Mac OS X.

(iii) Galaxy

Galaxy is a widely used, web-based genomic workbench that enables users to perform computational analyses of genomic data. The Galaxy Genome Annotation (GGA) Project is focused on supporting genome annotation inside the Galaxy workspace. GGA project consists of various teams, tool and suites that are working together to bring extensive and easy to use Genome Annotation experience for galaxy users.

Galaxy developed a docker available at https://github.com/galaxy-genome-annotation/docker-galaxy-genome-annotation which provides end-to-end solutions for genome annotation. The docker has tools for Assembly (Spades, Mira), Structural Prediction (Glimmer, Augustus), Functional Prediction (BLAST+, InterProScan, BLAST, Diamond, Blast2GO), various Utilities (FASTA manipulation tools, EMBOSS), tools for Comparative Genomics (CD-Hit, ClustalW, AntiSmash, mummer), and Visualization tools (Apollo Tools, JBrowse-in-Galaxy, JBrowse-in-Galaxy Extras, Triple Admin tools, Circos).

(iv) G-OnRamp

G-OnRamp is a user-friendly system web-based platform for collaborative, end-to-end annotation of eukaryotic genomes using UCSC Assembly Hubs and JBrowse/Apollo genome browsers (Liu et al., 2019). It integrates the Galaxy platform, over 25 community and custom bioinformatics tools and the UCSC and JBrowse/Apollo genome browsers to create a single platform for annotation. The data used in this browser is from evidence collected from sequence alignments, *ab initio* gene predictors, RNA-Seq data and repeats identification. G-OnRamp is available from the GitHub repository at https://github.com/goeckslab.

(v) Ensembl

The Ensembl gene annotation system is a very popular annotation system that has been used to annotate over 70 different vertebrate species from a large number of genome projects. Moreover, it produces automatic annotation for the human and mouse GENCODE gene sets. The annotation in this pipeline is based on the alignment of protein sequences, ESTs, cDNAs, and RNA-seq reads, to the reference genome to generate transcript models (Aken et al., 2016). By filtering and assessing and of the selected transcripts ultimately forms the final gene set, which becomes available on the Ensembl website. Ensembl database can be accessed at http://www.ensembl.org/index.html.

16   COMMERCIAL SOFTWARE FOR GENOME ANNOTATION

Genious Prime is acommercial software developed by biomatters that provides easy to use solution for genome annotation for users with less bioinformatics expertise. Geneious Prime includes genome annotation features and reports that include the structure and function of various genomic regions, such as genes, CDS's (coding sequences), exons, introns, 5'- 3' UTR's, tRNA's, rRNA's, ORF's (open-reading frames), etc. Geneious can be easily installed on a local workstation. It does not require high RAM for example, for Illumina data roughly 1 GB of RAM will be required to assemble a data set of 1 million reads. Raw FastQ files and the reference genome can be directly imported into Geneious, used for sequence alignment of the sample against the reference genome and downstream annotation analysis. It provides a graphical visualization of genome analysis such as genome assembly statistics, domain and pathway information.

Other softwares are Blast2GO and CLC workbench which are also highly used for genome annotation (Smith, 2015) and provides graphical details (Table 8).

Table 8 Some popular commercial softwares for annotation

Software	Company	Free trial (days)	Operating systems	Plug-ins	Workflows
CLC Genomics Workbench	CLC bio, Qiagen	30	M, W, L	Yes	Yes
CodonCode Aligner	CodonCode	30	M, W	No	No
Geneious	Biomatters	14	M, W, L	Yes	Yes
Full Lasergene Suite	DNASTAR	30	M, W	Yes	Yes
Blast2GO	biobam	30	M, W, L	Yes	Yes
NextGENe	Softgenetics	35	W	No	No
Sequencher	Gene Codes	30	M, W	Yes	No

17 DATA VISUALIZATION

Data visualization is one of the important steps during genomic data analysis. High throughput sequencing and array-based profiling generate a large quantity of diverse genomic data. Such diversity in the data types created major challenges to the visualization tools. Several genomics data visualization tools have been developed such as Tablet, IGV and Artemis.

(i) Integrative Genomics Viewer (IGV)
Integrative Genomics Viewer (IGV) is a commonly used visualization tool developed by Broad Institute that enables visualization of diverse, large-scale genomic data sets (Thorvaldsdottir et al., 2013). It is a web-based application and can be easily installed on the desktop. IGV advancement began in 2007 in consequence of a need by the Cancer Genome Atlas (TCGA) undertaking to visualize copy number variations, gene expression and clinical information. It supports the integration of a wide range of genomic data types that includes aligned sequences, variant data, gene expression, methylation and genomic annotations. The current version of IGV supports several file formats such as GFF, BAM, BED, FASTA, GTF, MAF, VCF and others. It consumes minimal desktop requirements. Besides, IGV also allows collaborators to load and share data locally or remotely using the internet. IGV is available at www.broadinstitute.org/igv

(ii) Artemis
Artemis is a very popular DNA sequence visualization and annotation tool developed by Sangers Institute for analyzing the genomes of bacteria, archaea and lower eukaryote (Rutherford et al., 2000). It allows the visualization of results from any sequence analysis such as NGS data and its six-frame translation. It is implemented in Java and can be run on any suitable platform. It uses sequences and annotations in EMBL, GenBank and GFF format. Another version of Artemis is ACT (Artemis comparison tool), which is a Java-based application for displaying pairwise comparisons between two or more DNA sequences.

ACT can be utilized to identify and analyze regions of similarity and distinction among genomes and to investigate conservation of synteny with regard to the complete sequences and their annotation (Carver et al., 2005).

Artemis is available at https://www.sanger.ac.uk/tool/artemis/

ACT is available at https://www.sanger.ac.uk/tool/artemis-comparison-tool-act/

(iii) Apollo

Apollo is an application for annotating genome sequences and provides an interactive tool to allow biological experts to edit and create gene models (Lewis et al., 2002). The first version of Apollo was a standalone desktop application.

But with the advancement in software development, Apollo was also upgraded and took advantage of new technologies to provide a better experience to users. In the year 2010 Apollo changed to running inside a web browser. The latest version of Apollo provides new interface features that include support for real-time collaboration, allowing users to edit the same encoded features at the same time also show the updates made by other researchers in the same region (Dunn et al., 2019). This feature of Apollo allows users to integrate it into multiple genomic analysis pipelines and diverse laboratory workflow platforms.

18   MAKING DATA PUBLICLY AVAILABLE

Annotating and publishing research paper is not just the end of the solution. Submitting the annotation data to publicly available repositories is also necessary, which will probably be used to help annotate other genomes.

Some popular databases for submitting your annotations are GenBank, EMBL-EBI and Ensembl; or users can also submit to organism-specific genome databases.

REFERENCES

Aken, Bronwen L., et al. (2016). The ensembl gene annotation system. Database: The Journal of Biological Databases and Curation. 2016: baw093. https://doi.org/10.1093/database/baw093.

Aziz, Ramy K., et al. (2008). The RAST server: Rapid annotations using subsystems technology. BMC Genomics. 9(1): 75.

Brettin, T., et al. (2015). RASTtk: A modular and extensible implementation of the RAST algorithm for building custom annotation pipelines and annotating batches of genomes. Sci. Rep. 5(1): 8365.

Bridge, A.J., A.-L. Veuthey and N.J. Mulder (2008). Resources for functional annotation. pp. 139–164. *In*: D. Frishman and A. Valencia (ed.). Modern Genome Annotation. Vienna: Springer Vienna. http://link.springer.com/10.1007/978-3-211-75123-7_8 (June 11, 2020).

Buisine, N., H. Quesneville and V. Colot (2008). Improved detection and annotation of transposable elements in sequenced genomes using multiple reference sequence sets. Genomics. 91(5): 467–475.

Carver, T.J. et al. (2005). ACT: The artemis comparison tool. Bioinformatics. 21(16): 3422–3423.

Catanese, H.N., K.A. Brayton and A.H. Gebremedhin (2016). RepeatAnalyzer: A tool for analysing and managing short-sequence repeat data. BMC Genomics. 17(1): 422. https://doi.org/10.1186/s12864-016-2686-2.

Chen, Y.-C. et al. (2013). Effects of GC bias in next-generation-sequencing data on *de novo* genome assembly. PLoS ONE. 8(4): e62856.

Chen, L. et al. (2018). Trends in the development of MiRNA bioinformatics tools. Briefings in Bioinformatics. 20(5): 1836–1852. https://academic.oup.com/bib/advance-article/doi/10.1093/bib/bby054/5047127 (June 11, 2020).

Dominguez Del Angel, V. et al. (2018). Ten steps to get started in genome assembly and annotation. F1000Research 7: 148.

Dunn, N.A. et al. (2019). Apollo: Democratizing genome annotation. PLoS Comput. Biol. 15(2): e1006790.

El-Metwally, Sara, Taher Hamza, Magdi Zakaria, and Mohamed Helmy (2013a). Next-generation sequence assembly: Four stages of data processing and computational challenges. PLoS Comput. Biol. 9(12): e1003345.

Flynn, J.M. et al. (2020). RepeatModeler2 for automated genomic discovery of transposable element families. Proceedings of the National Academy of Sciences. 117(17): 9451–9457.

George, R.A. and J. Heringa (2002). Protein domain identification and improved sequence similarity searching using PSI-BLAST. Proteins: Structure, Function, and Genetics. 48(4): 672–681.

Girgis, H.Z. (2015). Red: An intelligent, rapid, accurate tool for detecting repeats de-novo on the genomic scale. BMC Bioinformatics. 16(1): 227.

Gomes, A., S. Nolasco, and H. Soares (2013). Non-Coding RNAs: Multi-tasking molecules in the cell. Int. J. Mol. Sci. 14(8): 16010–16039.

Goodwin, S., J.D. McPherson and W.R. McCombie (2016). Coming of age: Ten years of next-generation sequencing technologies. Nat. Rev. Genet. 17(6): 333–351.

Gurevich, A., V. Saveliev, N. Vyahhi and G. Tesler (2013). QUAST: Quality assessment tool for genome assemblies. Bioinformatics. 29(8): 1072–1075.

Han, Y. and S.R. Wessler (2010). MITE-Hunter: A program for discovering miniature inverted-repeat transposable elements from genomic sequences. Nucleic Acids Res. 38(22): e199.

Hunt, M., et al. (2013). REAPR: A universal tool for genome assembly evaluation. Genome Biol. 14(5): R47.

International Human Genome Sequencing Consortium (2001). Initial sequencing and analysis of the human genome. Nature. 409(6822): 860–921.

International Human Genome Sequencing Consortium (2004). Finishing the euchromatic sequence of the human genome. Nature. 431(7011): 931–945.

Jansen, H.J. et al. (2017). Rapid de novo assembly of the european eel genome from nanopore sequencing reads. Sci. Rep. 7(1): 7213.

Koren, S. et al. (2012). Hybrid error correction and de novo assembly of single-molecule sequencing reads. Nat. Biotechnol. 30(7): 693–700.

Korf, I., P. Flicek, D. Duan and M.R. Brent (2001). Integrating genomic homology into gene structure prediction. Bioinformatics. 17(Suppl 1): S140–S148.

Korf, I. (2004). Gene finding in novel genomes. BMC Bioinformatics. 5: 59.

Lander, E.S. (2011). Initial impact of the sequencing of the human genome. Nature. 470(7333): 187–197.

Langmead, B. and S.L. Salzberg (2012). Fast gapped-read alignment with bowtie 2. Nature Methods. 9(4): 357–359.

Lewis, S. et al. (2002). Apollo: A sequence annotation editor. Genome Bio. 3(12): research0082.1.

Liu, Y. et al. (2019). G-OnRamp: A galaxy-based platform for collaborative annotation of eukaryotic genomes. Bioinformatics. 35(21): 4422–4423.

Lowe, T.M. and S.R. Eddy (1997). tRNAscan-SE: A program for improved detection of transfer RNA genes in genomic sequence. Nucleic Acids Res. 25(5): 955–964.

Medema, M.H., E. Takano and R. Breitling (2013). Detecting sequence homology at the gene cluster level with MultiGeneBlast. Mol. Biol. Evol. 30(5): 1218–1223.

Nachtweide, S. and M. Stanke (2019). Multi-genome annotation with AUGUSTUS. pp. 139–160. *In*: M. Kollmar (ed.). Gene Prediction, Methods in Molecular Biology. Springer New York. http://link.springer.com/10.1007/978-1-4939-9173-0_8 (June 11, 2020).

Novák, P. et al. (2017). TAREAN: A computational tool for identification and characterization of satellite DNA from unassembled short reads. Nucleic Acids Res. 45(12): e111.

Pelley, J.W. (2012). Elsevier's Integrated Review Biochemistry, 2nd Ed. Elsevier, Philadelphia, PA.

Phillippy, A.M., M.C. Schatz and M. Pop (2008). Genome assembly forensics: Finding the elusive mis-assembly. Genome Biol. 9(3): R55.

Richard, G.-F., A. Kerrest and B. Dujon (2008). Comparative genomics and molecular dynamics of dna repeats in eukaryotes. MMBR. 72(4): 686–727.

Rinn, J.L. and H.Y. Chang (2012). Genome regulation by long noncoding RNAs. Annual Review of Biochemistry. 81(1): 145–166.

Rutherford, K., J. Parkhill, J. Crook, T. Horsnell, P. Rice, M.A. Rajandream, et al. (2000). Artemis: sequence visualization and annotation. Bioinformatics. 16(10): 944–945.

Schattner, P., A.N. Brooks and T.M. Lowe. (2005) The TRNAscan-SE, Snoscan and SnoGPS web servers for the detection of TRNAs and SnoRNAs. Nucleic Acids Res. 33(Web Server): W686–W689.

Schlebusch, S. and N. Illing (2012). Next generation shotgun sequencing and the challenges of *de novo* genome assembly. S. Afr. J. Sci. 108(11/12): 8.

She, R., J.S. Chu, K. Wang, J. Pei, and N. Chen. (2009). GenBlastA: Enabling BLAST to identify homologous gene sequences. Genome Res. 19(1): 143–149.

Simão, F.A. et al. (2015). BUSCO: Assessing genome assembly and annotation completeness with single-copy orthologs. Bioinformatics. 31(19): 3210–3212.

Smith, D.R. (2015). Buying in to bioinformatics: An introduction to commercial sequence analysis software. Briefings Bioinf. 16(4): 700–709.

Solovyev, V., P. Kosarev, I. Seledsov and D. Vorobyev. (2006). Automatic annotation of eukaryotic genes, pseudogenes and promoterstitle found. Genome Biol. 7(Suppl 1): S10.

Tay, Y., J. Rinn and P.P. Pandolfi (2014). The multilayered complexity of CeRNA crosstalk and competition. Nature. 505(7483): 344–352.

Thorvaldsdottir, H., J.T. Robinson and J.P. Mesirov (2013). Integrative genomics viewer (IGV): High-performance genomics data visualization and exploration. Briefings Bioinf. 14(2): 178–192.

Vezzi, F., G. Narzisi and B. Mishra (2012). Reevaluating assembly evaluations with feature response curves: GAGE and assemblathons. PLoS ONE 7(12): e52210.

Wang, Z., Y. Chen and Y. Li (2004). A brief review of computational gene prediction methods. Genomics, Proteomics & Bioinformatics. 2(4): 216–221.

Xiong, J. (2006). Essential Bioinformatics. Cambridge: Cambridge University Press. http://ebooks.cambridge.org/ref/id/CBO9780511806087 (June 11, 2020).

Yandell, M. and D. Ence (2012). A beginner's guide to eukaryotic genome annotation. Nat. Rev. Genet. 13(5): 329–342.

CHAPTER 3

Protein Function Prediction: Human Sequences and Structures

Sonal Modak[1] and Jayaraman Valadi[2]*

[1]Lead Domain Engineer, Life Sciences and Healthcare Unit,
Persistent Systems Inc., Santa Clara, CA 95054, USA
e-mail: samurai.modak@gmail.com

[2]Department of Center for Informatics, School of Natural Sciences (SoNS),
Shiv Nadar University, Greater Noida, Uttar Pradesh 201314, India
e-mail: jayaraman.valadi@snu.edu.in

and

Flame University, Pune-412115, India
e-mail: valadi@gmail.com

1 INTRODUCTION

With the sequencing of newer genomes there is an increasing gap between documented and annotated protein sequences. This gap is increasing at a much fast rate everyday. There is an urgent need for accurate functional annotation of proteins. This need is much more important for human-related proteins. In the beginning, a few decades ago, functional annotations were mainly done with multiple sequence alignment techniques. These methods, however, have certain pitfalls, including excessive computational requirements due to the heuristic nature of the algorithms and performance degradation for low similarity sequences. With the advent of machine learning methodologies, various tools and techniques have been developed by various researchers for alignment-free annotation of protein functions. These techniques include extraction of a plethora of domain-dependent features and descriptors differing in size and information content. A need arose for selecting a subset of features with the highest information content and discarding noisy features. Several feature selection techniques have been developed

---

Corresponding author: jayaraman.valadi@snu.edu.in

to achieve this purpose. Appropriate classification and regression techniques with different levels of complexity and rigors have been developed alongside for robust prediction tasks. Several data bases and webservers have also been developed for ready use by practitioners, researchers and academicians. In this review we have discussed about all the above aspects in detail with special reference to human-related proteins, wherever necessary we have given illustrations and tables for ready reference.

2 CLASSIFIERS FOR BUILDING PREDICTION MODELS

In this section we will discuss some important classifiers used in functional annotations.

2.1 Support Vector Machines (SVMs) for Classification

Support Vector Machines (SVMs) can be used for both supervised and unsupervised learning tasks. SVM classifiers are formulated from statistical learning theory by Vapnik (Mika et al., 1999). For binary classification problems, SVM builds a linear maximum margin hyperplane defined by the following equation:

$$\mathbf{w} \bullet \mathbf{x_i} + b = 0 \qquad (1)$$

where $\mathbf{x_i}$ represents the vector of input attributes, b the bias and $\mathbf{w}$ represents the weight vectors.

For linearly separable examples, SVM creates such a linear hyperplane which maximizes the margin and is defined as the distance between the hyperplane and the nearest examples belonging to both classes. This can be formulated as a weight vector norm minimization problem with suitable constraints. The convex quadratic optimization problem obtains the optimized vectors solely defined by the examples falling on the margins. These examples are known as support vectors and hence the name Support Vector Machines. This quadratic convex optimization problem is highly desirable because it provides a unique solution as opposed to several classifiers which get trapped into the local minima. This aspect has driven researchers in various fields to employ support vector machines.

For non-, linearly separable problems, SVM converts the data into a higher dimension. Thereafter it employs a linear hyperplane. Such a transformation can create intractability difficulties. SVM overcomes this by defining the kernel functions. These functions connect the dot products in higher dimensional space to functions of dot products in the input space. Kernel functions facilitate all computations to be carried out in the original space itself. Kernel functions must be positive, definite along with Hilbert Space axioms to be satisfactory. The usual kernel functions employed in typical classification tasks are: Polynomial, Gaussian Radial Basis Function (RBF), and Multi-layer Perceptron kernel functions. We have in bioinformatics domain several domain-dependent kernels. For increasing generalization capabilities, a soft margin formulation is used. In this formulation a modified convex quadratic optimization problem is formulated. This formulation incorporates a cost parameter to handle trade-off between margin maximization and misclassification error.

2.2 Decision Tree Algorithms

Decision trees are tree-structured algorithms which progressively divide the original data set into smaller and smaller subsets. They start with a head node in which the most informative feature and most optimal split point of that attribute are used to divide the data into smaller subsets. The split can be binary or multiway. This splitting is continued at the intermediate nodes in the same way. At every stage the most informative attribute is used for node splitting. This process continues until the leaf nodes are reached. The splitting is done from a node to the children nodes so that the children nodes are purer than the original parent. Several criteria like Gini Index, entropy and misclassification error are used by different authors to evaluate the quality of splits. Splitting is stopped when

(i) the attributes of examples in that node do not differ much in their values and

(ii) when the number of examples are less than a previously defined threshold. The fully grown trees are finally subjected to pruning which helps in avoiding overfitting and increasing generalization capabilities

Protein function prediction plays a vital role in the sensitive procedure of drug development. Though drug discovery process is labour intensive and expensive, efficient computational methods can be used to reduce the labour, time as well as cost associated with this process. In such a flow, decision trees can be used as classifiers, which can learn classification rules from the given training data which are used to predict functions of unknown proteins. Sandhu et al., worked on enhancing the use of decision trees as classifiers for Human Protein Function (HPF) prediction based on sequence derived features (Singh et al., 2007). In the work, decision tree is created by HPF predictor by using training data by processing sequence derived features and known functional classes of protein sequences. The test data is used to compute percentage accuracy of the decision tree created. The highlighted advantage of usingsequence derived features in this study is that new prediction technique creates decision trees with depth of thirteen nodes, as compared to decision trees with depths of two nodes using existing techniques. The large depth of the tree has led to the consideration of more number of tests before functional class assignment and has thus resulted in more accurate predictions. For the same test data, the percentage accuracy of the new HPF predictor is 72% and that of the existing prediction technique is 44%.

2.3 Random Forest Algorithm

Random Forest (RF) is an ensemble of decision tree classifiers (Breiman, 2001; Liaw and Weiner, 2002; Cutler et al., 2007). With an improved bagging version, RF employs two kinds of randomness while growing trees. In the first, bootstrap sampling with replacement is used in each decision tree. The other randomness is in selection of a subset of attributes in node splitting; it employs a predetermined random subset of trees in each tree. Every split and split point is optimized by various measures like Gini Index, Entropy and misclassification error. Each tree is grown to full size and pruning is not carried out . The overall prediction is made averaging the prediction of individual trees. As bootstrap sampling is employed, roughly one-third of the examples are left unused by each tree; these instances are known as Out of Bag (OOB) examples. RF performance can be estimated by CV measures as well as by estimating OOB error measures. Accuracy of prediction depends upon the performance of each tree and the correlation between the trees. An optimal value of subset of features used in each tree will provide the best trade-off. Such a trade-off will enhance generalization capabilities of RF. RF has several advantages: (a) two different feature rankings can be embedded in the algorithm, (b) the algorithm can be used to remove outliers, (c) the algorithm can be effectively used for missing values imputation. RF has been found to be a very robust classification algorithm and has found uses in different function prediction tasks.

2.3.1 Variable selection using random forests

Random Forests can also be used to find out the most informative attributes embedded in the algorithm itself. This is done by permuting each feature column and finding the mean decrease in performance of the OOB estimates. This raw importance score is an estimate of the contribution of this feature in the data set performance. The other measures the grand weighted average of the mean decrease in Gini measure, an attribute during split into different trees. This mean decrease in Gini importance score has also been found to be an effective way of scoring attributes.

2.4 Neural Network Algorithms

Artificial Neural Networks mimic this cooperative functioning of the neurons in the brain by connecting the inputs of a given data (input neurons) to the required outputs of a specific task through a series of layers of neurons (Zurada, 1992). A typical ANN architecture consists of an input layer, 1 or 2 hidden layers and an output layer. The inputs are weighted and then passed to each of the neurons in the first hidden layer. These are summed, squashed (non-linearly mapped), weighted and then passed to the next hidden layer of neurons. These are summed and further squashed by activation function, summed up and sent to the output layer. Every input example is fed through the layers, following the same procedure. The network output is compared with the actual output and overall error is computed. The weights are revised using back propagation algorithm. The procedure is repeated until the total error in minimized. The working of ANN is schematically shown in Fig. 1.

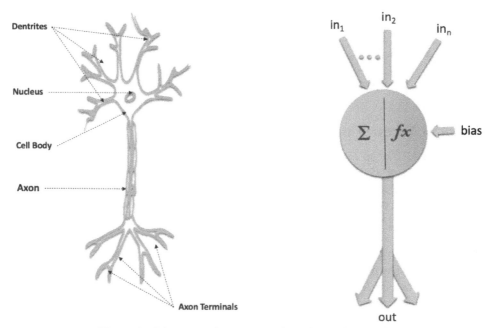

Figure 1   Diagrammatic representation of neural network.

2.5 Deep-neural Networks

The conventional neural networks are shallow and at most contain two hidden layers. Depth differentiate deepneural networks are different from conventional neural networks. They have many hidden layers in their configurations. Additionally, deep neural networks train on distinct levels of features in each layer. With increasing depth, the levels of features learned are higher. With increase in depth, the complexity of features learnt increases due to a built-in aggregation and recombination mechanism. Convolutional neural network (CNN) is a very popular class of deep neural networks and finds applications in analysis of visual imagery. CNNs, like shallow, consists of layers of receive input data, aggregates a weighted sum and propagates through an appropriately selected activation function. The output received from the last layer of hidden neurons is compared with the actual output and the weights are corrected using back propagation algorithm.

In deep neural networks, the input is a multi-channelled image. For an RGB image, say of size 32×32×3, is input to CNN. This input is subjected to a series of convolution operations in CNN with several filters each having random weights. These convolve over the image, as shown in Fig. 2. Assume that a 5×5×3 filter slides over the complete image covering all possible unique 5×5×3 subsets of the image; on every convolution operation the resulting output (WT.X + B) is a scalar (one number), where W.X represents the dot product between weights and inputs. Similarly, for every other dot product taken we obtain a scalar output. It is easy to compute that 28×28 unique image subsets are to be convolved. A single filter after a complete convolution operation provides an output of size 28×28×1, shown in Fig. 3. The convolution layer consisting of six filters will provide six feature maps. Hence, we will obtain a combined size of 28×28×6. Each filter is independently convolved with the image with the shape of the filter map obtained being 28×28×1. This is diagrammatically represented in Fig. 4. The architecture consisting of several convolution layers in sequence will look like as shown in Fig. 5.

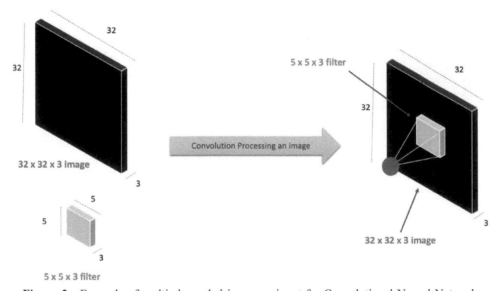

Figure 2 Example of multi-channeled image as input for Convolutional Neural Network.

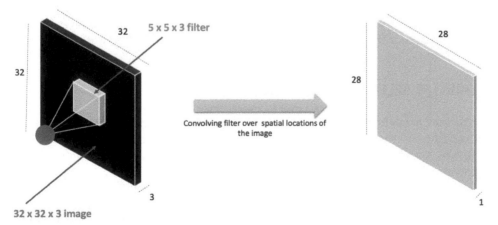

Figure 3 Convolution operation with a single filter.

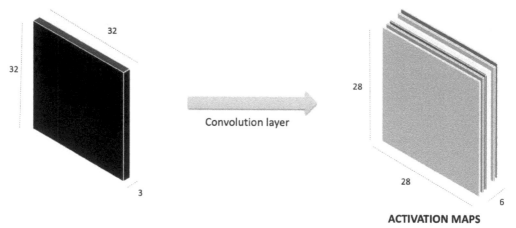

Figure 4   Output of multiple feature maps in a Convolutional Neural Network.

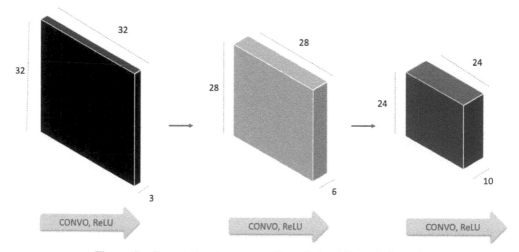

Figure 5   Convolution layers in a Convolutional Neural Network.

It may be noticed that with each layer there is a thickening and thinning of the breadth. The pooling layer is another important building block of CNN. This layer is provided mainly to down samples the image and progressively reduce the size and hence the parameters to learn. This pooling layer effectively works on each feature map. CNN also has different activation functions and ReLU is the most used in CNNs. Finally, the fully connected layer of neurons converts the image to a linear structure similar to conventional neural networks.

3   ATTRIBUTE SELECTION

Not all attributes are informative in data sets. Features which are non-informative will act as noise, do not have discriminative power, and interfere with the classification process. Hence the model will have very little predictive accuracy. In protein function identification in viral biology, several sequence and structural features can be extracted (Ma and Huang, 2008; Saey et al., 2007). For example the AA, dipeptide and tri-peptide compositional features put together amount to 8400 in number and not all of them will be important in a particular function annotation task. To select a subset of informative features by brute force, we need to evaluate a huge number of subsets of features which becomes computationally time consuming. Various feature/attribute selection methods are available to simplify the process of subset selection. Feature selection techniques help us to avoid overfitting and improve model performance to provide faster and more cost-effective models; they also provide invaluable domain information. However, feature selection techniques have to employ appropriate search techniques, and additional level of complexity and computational cost. Feature selection techniques differ from one another in the way they incorporate this search in the added space of feature subsets in the model selection. These methods can be broadly classified as filter, wrapper and embedded methods.

3.1 Filter Ranking Methods

Filter ranking methods employ appropriate heuristics to rank the features of a given data set. Once the features are ranked, top ranking feature subsets can be used for classification, discarding the rest of the redundant features. Mutual information, student t-test, correlation-based feature selection (CFS), Minimum Redundancy-Maximum Relevance (mRmR) and Uncorrelated Shrunken Centroid (USC) algorithm are some of the popular filter ranking methods.

3.2 Wrapper Methods

Filter methods are very fast and can provide an estimate of accuracies of informative features. As they are not accurate, different wrapper methods are used in literature. Conventional wrapper methods include forward selection and backward selection algorithms. In forward selection, in the first iteration, the most relevant attribute providing maximum classification performance is selected. In the next iteration, along with the selected feature in the first iteration, the next most relevant feature is identified by combining each of the remaining features with the already selected feature. In the rest of the iterations this procedure is repeated with an additional feature added progressively. In backward selection the reverse operation is conducted removing the least relevant feature at every iteration and employing a procedure similar to forward selection.

Genetic algorithms, Ant Colony Optimization or other swarm intelligent methods are also used profusely for attribute selection. These methods mimic natural processes for any given optimization problem. The idea is to use only a fraction of all possible combinations to arrive close to the optimal feature set. Biogeography-based optimization (BBO) is another method which mimics the natural processes of immigration and emigration of populations. Srivatsava et al. employed BBO based feature selection for MHC Class I Peptide Binding Prediction with Support Vector Machines and Random Forests as classifiers (Srivatsava et al., 2013).

3.3 Embedded Methods

In embedded class of feature selection techniques, feature ranking facility is embedded in the algorithm itself. SVM recursive feature elimination (SVMRFE) and the two random forest ranking methodologies are examples of embedded methods. In SVMRFE the hyperplane is built with all features initially and the attribute having lowest absolute weight is removed. This attribute has the lowest relevance with the classification. This process is repeated until only one attribute is left. Thus, for a data with 'n' features 'n' different experiments are needed to rank the features which is much less than that required for conventional recursive methods.

4 DOMAIN FEATURES FOR FUNCTION ANNOTATION

Domain information can be given to the machine learning algorithm in a variety of ways. These may includesequence derived and structure based. Several sequence-based features can be extracted. These include amino acid, dipeptide and k-mer features, evolutionary information in the form of position-specific scoring matrix (PSSM), predicted structural information, sequence conservation score, annotations of functional sites, network properties, etc.

4.1 Sequence Composition-based Features

Sequence features represent domain knowledge extracted from protein sequences. The simplest, most popular and most widely used features are composition-based features. These descriptors convert unequal length protein alphabet from various sequences in the data set into equal length attributes. Such equal length attribute extraction is very convenient because they can be readily employed as input to various classifiers. Figure 6 enlists broad categorization of feature based on composition of peptides and amino acid properties in protein sequences. Some of the commonly employed descriptors are described in detail below:

4.1.1 Amino acid composition

Amino acid composition (AAC) can be defined as a fraction of each amino acid present in a peptide sequence. AAC can be computed using the following equation:

$$AAC(i) = \frac{Frequency\ of\ amino\ acid(i)}{Length\ of\ the\ peptide} \tag{2}$$

where i can be any natural amino acid. The AAC is very attractive as it represents the domain information in the form of a very small number of constant length input vectors. In the same way dipeptide and higher k-mer compositions can be extracted from the primary sequences. Once these descriptors are extracted, they can be represented in a stacked form vector as input features. As all of them may not have predictive power, an attribute selection method is commonly employed to identify the most informative features.

4.1.2 Atomic composition

Atomic Composition (ATC) is the frequency count of each atom (C, H, N, O, and S) present in the given peptide sequence. Kumar et al. (Kumar et al., 2015) discusses details about the number and types of atoms in naturally occurring amino acids. In this study ATC features were employed for antihypertensive peptides design. The ATC has a fixed length of five features.

4.1.3 Pseudo amino acid composition

Pseudo amino acid composition (PseAAC) was first employed by Kuo-Chen Chou in 2001 (Chou, 2001). Similar to conventional amino acid composition method, this characterizes proteins using a matrix of frequencies to represent protein sequences. Additionally, the method provides additional information to include local features, such as correlation between residues of different distances. As a consequence, the amino acid frequencies contain a set containing more than 20 discrete descriptors. The additional components incorporate sequence-order information and various pseudo-components. Over the period of time, different variants of iPseAA composition were developed to address several kinds of problems in proteins and protein-related systems. Inspired by PseAAC, Lin et al. (2015) have incorporated g-gap dipeptide composition.

4.1.4 Examples of sequence composition-based features

Cancer is a pathological condition which is characterized by uncontrolled cell division, invading or spreading to other parts of the body. Due to the complex and heterogenous nature of this dreadful disease, development of effectual anticancer therapies havebecome one of the most prevalent area of research (Basith et al., 2017). Cancer treatment by conventional methods like radiotherapy and chemotherapy are expensive. Moreover, the side effects of these methods are deleterious to normal cells. Peptide-based cancer therapy has emerged as one of the most promising approaches dues to its several advantages. These peptides can have high specificity, increased capability for tumor penetration, and minimal toxicity under normal physiological conditions (Harris et al., 2013). Anticancer peptides (ACPs) are peptides capable of use as therapeutic agents to treat various cancers. Recent studies demonstrated the selectivity of ACPs toward cancer cells without affecting normal physiological functions, making them a potentially valuable therapeutic strategy (Thundimadathil, 2012; Vlieghe et al., 2010). ACPs have cationic amphipathic structures composed of 5–30 amino acid residues. These structures are capable of interacting with the anionic lipid membrane of cancer cells, thereby enabling selective targeting (Gaspar et al., 2013; Yan and Liu, 2016). Manavalan et al. demonstrated prediction of anticancer peptides based on machine learning algorithm (Manavalan et al., 2017). SVM and Random Forest-based machine learning methods were employed for the prediction of ACPs using the features calculated from the amino acid sequence. In this study, features were extracted based on amino acid composition, dipeptide composition, atomic composition, and physicochemical properties. These features have been thoroughly discussed in Section 4.1. The training dataset contained 450 ACPs and 450 non-ACPs sequences. SVM yielded an average accuracy of 88.2% with Matthews correlation coefficient of 0.750, while Random Forest outperformed with 94.6% of accuracy and Matthews correlation coefficient of 0.885.

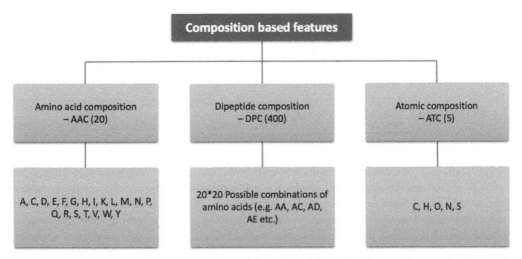

Figure 6 Overview features based on composition of peptides and amino acid properties in protein sequence.

Similar work was done by Hasan et al. in identifying an uncharacterized protein sequence as phosphorylated protein. It has been already established that protein phosphorylation potentially plays a vital role in regulating protein function and conformation (Hasan et al., 2017). For prediction of multi-label phosphorylated proteins, the authors developed a novel computational tool termed 'iMulti-HumPhos'. The first step was to extract three different sets of features from protein sequences. Individual kernel functions were defined for each set of features. Using multiple kernel learning, these kernels were later combined into a single kernel. Lastly, a combination of SVMs was employed where each SVM was trained with a combined kernel to achieve construction of a multi-label predictor. The features considered in this study includes Amino Acid Composition (AAC), Dipeptide Composition (DC), and Sequential evolution feature representation: data of the Position-Specific Scoring Matrix (PSSM). In this study, the authors observed that the iMulti-HumPhos predictor performed significantly better than the existing predictor, i.e., Multi-iPPseEvo (Qiu et al., 2017). iMulti-HumPhos achieves 0.5855 for multi-label accuracy, which is also higher than other predictors. The webserver for iMulti-HumPhos is hosted at http://research.ru.ac.bd/iMulti-HumPhos/.

The most abundant form of genetic variation is single nucleotide polymorphism (SNP). Eventually they can lead to change in amino acid due to missense mutation, and is thus often referred to as single amino acid polymorphism (SAP) (Yip et al., 2004). Not all the amino acid substitutions lead to deleterious diseases, most of them are neutral substitutions and they are believed to cause phenotypic differences between individuals. There are studies interrelating protein structure with its function and revealing evidences that single amino acid substitutions are responsible for certain disease types (Gong and Blundell, 2010; Sunyaev et al., 2000). Some studies also suggested that about 60% of Mendelian disease is caused by amino acid substitutions (Botstein and Risch, 2003; Gong and Blundell, 2010).

4.2   Structural Features

The structural properties of macromolecules provide a more accurate description of the actual environment or the neighborhood of a residue. These properties are extracted from the 3D structures of the molecules. Most common features in this category are:

(i)   Secondary structure types, viz. α-helix, β-strand and coil

(ii)   dihedral angle

(iii)   hydrogen bond

(iv)   3D distance of a mutation residue position to other functional sites.

One limitation of this approach is that the feasibility of feature extraction is dependent on the availability of a 3D structure of the protein. DSSP (Kabsch and Sander, 1983) is often used to determine structural annotation from PDB file (Berman et al., 2000).

4.2.1   Examples of use of structural features

Amino acids in the core of proteins are relatively conserved compared with those in the solvent accessible regions (Hubbard and Blundell, 1987; Worth and Blundell, 2009). Catalytic amino acids responsible for enzymatic reactions are also well conserved throughout evolution. Thus, mutations tend to occur in amino acid residues where evolutionary pressure is relatively relaxed and where they can remain in the population. Gong et al. catalogued structural and functional features of proteins that restrain genetic variations leading to single amino acid substitutions (Gong and Blundell, 2010). In this work, the authors used the features from the structural environments of amino acid variants, namely, side-chain solvent accessibility, main-chain secondary structure, and hydrogen bonds from a side chain to a main chain or other side chains. These features were extracted from three categories of datasets, viz. Mendelian disease-related variants, neutral polymorphisms and cancer somatic mutations. In this detailed study, the focus was on the amino acid substitutions located at functionally important sites involved in protein-protein interactions, protein-ligand interactions or catalytic activity of enzymes. With supporting evidences, the authors concluded that the occurrence of amino acid variants is affected by the structural and functional restraints.

Solvent accessibility property has been shown to be the one of the most powerful attributes in predicting function, which is evident from the work done by Dobson et al. (Dobson et al., 2006) and Saunders and Baker (Saunders and Baker, 2002). In one, study by Ye et al. investigated different definitions of solvent accessibilities (Ye et al., 2007). For determination of protein function, they considered solvent accessibilities by calculating the absolute and relative solvent accessibilities of all atoms, total side chain, main chain, non-polar side chain and all-polar side chain. A novel approach was developed by defining a new attribute, the structural neighbor profile, to comprise a 20-D vector of the counts of different types of residues found in the 3D vicinity of a site: a count was obtained for each of the 20 residue types; a residue was considered as a 'Neighbor' if one or more of its heavy atoms fell within a specific radius around the C atom of the residue at the center. We calculated the structural neighbor profiles for both the wild-type and variant residue positions. Further, authors built a support vector machines (SVMs) classifier employing a carefully selected set of new and previously published attributes. Through a strict protein-level 5-fold cross-validation, an overall accuracy of 82.61%, and an MCC of 0.60 was attained.

The first step in computational biology approach is to generate the data from a biological source, which can further be used to deduce meaningful evidences to support a study. Post-genomic era has an abundance of a large volume of sequencing data, but tasks like providing accurate function annotation, has always been a challenge. The most common approaches are based on looking for similarity in orthologous sequences. A major disadvantage of such methods is that it cannot address problems like annotating distant protein sequences or orphan protein sequences. Jones et al. used feature characteristics of protein sequence to address the problem of performing function prediction (Cozzetto et al., 2016). For this machine-learning based approach, the authors also developed a user-friendly web server using Gene Ontology Annotations (Ashburner et al., 2000). This server processes query amino acid sequences as input for generating gene ontology termed predictions. The most important part of the pipeline flow is to start with generating descriptors for query sequence. This feature set is based on predicted properties like transmembrane regions, post-translational modification patterns, cellular localization and secondary structures (Lobley et al., 2008). Though prediction algorithms can process single amino acids, but in this, for transmembrane and disorder features, secondary structures, algorithms processing PSI-BLAST profiles, can make more accurate predictions. Thus, in this case, data from uniref90 (Apweiler et al., 2004) was used to generate three separate PSI-BLAST profiles. The resulting output was translated in feature descriptors defining all the attributes in the query sequence. SVMs were employed to screen the normalized feature matrix, whose classifier output was a binary decision value. Finally, the probability and decision values were used to deduce gene ontology terms and reported annotations along with the confidence scores. In this exciting study, the authors demonstrated an alternative to homology inference-based methods by integrating data from many different sources.

4.3 Annotations from Database

The functional sites on the structure of proteins execute their biological functions. Most likely a protein loses its function if the neighboring residues of the functional sites alter the structure. Therefore, annotation of functional sites is an important feature. There are various studies demonstrating use of sequence and 3D distances between mutation position and functional sites as features to predict the functional impact on protein due to sequence mutation (Gong and Blundell, 2010; Bromberg et al., 2008; Adzhubei et al., 2010; Bromberg and Rost, 2007).

4.3.1 Examples of annotations as features

In many of the examples, we saw that predicting the unknown protein function protein interaction information is an emerging area of research in the field of bioinformatics. It is a well accepted fact that proteins execute critical functions in essentially all biological processes. Computational methods like gene neighborhood, sequence and structure, protein-protein interactions (PPI), etc. have naturally created a larger impact in the field of protein function prediction than the biological-based experimental methods. On the same lines Nasipuri et al. demonstrated an approach to determine the functions of unannotated proteins, by utilizing their neighborhood properties in PPI network on the basis of the fact that neighbors of a particular protein have similar functions (Saha et al., 2017). Here the authors used Gene Ontology (GO) dataset of humans obtained from UniProt database. GO system used involved three categories, namely: (i) Cellular-component, (ii) Molecular-function and (iii) Biological process. There is a possibility that each protein may be annotated by several GO terms in each category, thus every GO term of three categories were ranked based on the maximum number of occurrences in each of them. Then 10% of proteins belonging to the top 15 GO terms in each of three categories were selected as unannotated while the remaining 90% proteins were chosen as training samples using random sub-sampling technique. In this comparative study, performance of the proposed approach relatively performed much better than the other existing methods in unannotated protein function prediction.

Sequencing of phenotyped clinical subjects will soon become a method of choice in studies of the genetic causes of Mendelian and other complex diseases. Adzhubei et al. presented a new method and the corresponding software tool, PolyPhen-2 (http://genetics.bwh.harvard.edu/pph2/) for predicting the damaging effects of missense mutations (Adzhubei et al., 2010). PolyPhen-2 is different from the earlier tool PolyPhen-1 in the set of predictive features, the alignment pipeline and the method of classification. PolyPhen-2 uses eight sequence-based and three structure-based predictive features, which were selected automatically by an iterative greedy algorithm. The majority of these features involve comparison of a property of the wild-type (ancestral, normal) allele and the corresponding property of the mutant (derived, disease-causing) allele. The alignment pipeline selects a set of homologous sequences using a clustering algorithm and then constructs and refines its multiple alignment. The most informative predictive features characterize how likely the two human alleles are to occupy the site, given the pattern of amino-acid replacements in the multiple-sequence alignment; how distant the protein harboring the first deviation from the human wildtype allele is from the human protein; and whether the mutant allele originated at a hypermutable. The functional importance of an allele replacement is predicted from its individual features by a naive Bayes classifier. For a false positive rate of 20%, PolyPhen-2 achieved true positive prediction rates of 92% and 73% on two different datasets used.

Many non-synonymous single nucleotide polymorphisms (nsSNPs) in humans are suspected to impact protein function. Bromberg et al. proposed the method SNAP (screening for non-acceptable polymorphisms) that predicts the functional effects of single amino acid substitutions. SNAP was developed using annotations extracted from PMD, the Protein Mutant Database (Kawabata et al., 1999; Nishikawa et al., 1994). SNAP identifies over 80% of the non-neutral mutations at 77% accuracy and over 76% of the neutral mutations at 80% accuracy at its default threshold. Each prediction is associated with a reliability index that correlates with accuracy and thereby enables the observererto zoom into the most promising predictions.

4.4 Physicochemical Properties

Physicochemical properties include a number of features, such as introduction of an inflexible proline into a beta strand, replacement of a hydrophobic side-chain by hydrophilic substances or vice versa, a charged residue into a buried position, and over-packing of a pocket in the protein by changing the size of the residue, the hydrophobicity difference between original and mutated residues (Saha et al., 2017). Several approaches for predicting the functional impact of SAP were developed based on physicochemical properties (Apweiler et al., 2004; Bromberg and Rost, 2007; Care et al., 2007; Hubbard and Blundell, 1987). It represents the physicochemical class of residues present in a given peptide sequence. The percentage compositions for amino acids can be calculated based on different categories. Table 1 enlists the amino acid residues belonging to different groups:

Table 1 Categorical distribution of amino acid residues as per the physiochemical properties

Property	Amino acid symbol
Polar	D, E, R, K, Q, N
hydrophobic	C, V, L, I, M, F, W
charged	D, E, K, H, R
aliphatic	I, L, V
aromatic	F, H, W, Y
positively charged	H, K, R
negatively charged	D, E
tiny	A, C, D, G, S, T
small	E, H, I, L, K, M, N, P, Q, V
large	F, R, W, Y

Along with these categories, one more important property is *peptide mass* (Chen et al., 2016; Sanders et al., 2011; Tyagi et al., 2013).

Many of these properties have been encoded as descriptors individually and with various combinations for different function identification problems. Gromiha et al. have considered the AAIndex1 currently containing 544 amino acid indices (Rawat et al., 2020). Each entry consists of an accession number, a short description of the index, the reference information and the numerical values for the properties of 20 amino acids.

We have provided a link to the corresponding PubMed entries of each AAIndex entry, instead of a link to the LitDB literature database that we originally used. In addition, each entry contains cross-links to other entries with an absolute value for the correlation coefficient of 0.8 or larger. The links enable the users to identify a set of entries describing similar properties. In some instances, the values are not reported for all 20 amino acids.

The AAIndex2 currently contains 94 amino acid substitution matrices: 67 symmetric matrices and 27 non-symmetric matrices. The format of the entry is almost the same as that of AAIndex1 except that it contains 210 numerical values (20 diagonal and $20 \times 19/2$ off-diagonal elements) for a symmetric matrix and 400 or more numerical values for a non-symmetric matrix (some matrices include a gap or distinguish two states of cysteine). In the previous release, each symmetric matrix, which is triangular in shape, was folded into a 10×21 table for the purpose of saving space, and columns were separated by space characters. In the present release, symmetric matrices are not folded, and the delimiter of the columns has been changed into a tab character for making easier parsing of the entry.

The AAIndex3 section currently contains 47 amino acid contact potential matrices: 44 symmetric matrices and 3 non-symmetric matrices. The format of the entry is almost the same as that of AAIndex2.

4.4.1 Example of physicochemical properties as features

An important genetic process in molecular biology is 'translation', which is directly linked with synthesis of peptide sequences. In the process, the messenger RNA (mRNA) carries information which is decoded by the ribosome complex. Rules of genetic code are followed to produce a specific protein (or peptide) chain (Jackson et al., 2010). The initiation of peptide chain synthesis starts with identification of proper start position on mRNA. This site where the translation is initiated is called the Translation Initiation Site (TIS). In-depth genome analysis includes identification of the TIS. Computational methods proposed in this regard do not consider the global or long-range sequence-order effects of DNA, and hence their prediction quality is limited. To address this inadequacy, Chen et al. developed a new predictor called 'iTIS-PseTNC' incorporating the physicochemical properties into the pseudo trinucleotide composition (Chen et al., 2014). The physicochemical properties considered by the authors included: (i) numerical values of hydrophobicity, (ii) hydrophilicity, and (iii) sidechain mass of the peptide chains. The genome coordinates of the annotated translation initiation sites in the human genome were obtained from the TIS database (TISdb) at http://tisdb.human.cornell.edu (Wan and Qian, 2014). iTIS-PseTNC predictor correctly identified 195 TIS and 194 non-TIS and yielded accuracy of 97%. As a web server, iTIS-PseTNC is freely accessible at http://lin.uestc.edu.cn/server/ iTIS-PseTNC.

4.5 Network Features

Structure-function relationship of a protein can also be studied by representing the protein structures as networks. In this type of depiction, the vertices of the network are the amino acid residues, while the edges are their interactions. Network representation has proved to be a prevailing tool to study complex networks of interacting amino acid residues since it provides noteworthy insights into the organization of protein structure and the regulation of protein function (Li et al., 2011a).

4.5.1 Example of use of network feature

With the advent of cutting edge sequencing technologies, the sequence data is readily available to the research community. The most studied sequence variations are the Non-synonymous SNPs (nsSNPs), which are often referred to as Single Amino acid Polymorphisms (SAPs). This type of sequence variation accounts for the majority of human inherited diseases. Though SAPs are often associated with certain diseases, they are not always deleterious. Thus, distinguishing neutral SAPs with deleterious one, is extremely important. As discussed in the above sections, sequence-based or structure-based features are the most popular approaches. Huang et al. believe that: the likelihood of relating a SAP to a disease is based on the fact that the presence of SAP within a region of protein, alters the sequence and eventually its structure (Huang et al., 2010). They consider this as a better rationale for deleterious SAP prediction. So they developed a prediction method to find out the deleterious SAPs-based hybrid properties and protein interaction network. In this interesting study, the authors used 472 features such as network, sequential and structural features to characterize SAPs. Optimal feature set was obtained using Incremental Feature Selection (IFS) and mRmR methods, while the prediction model employed in this study was the Nearest Neighbor Algorithm (NNA). Prediction model using 263 optimized features yielded jackknife cross-validation of 83.27% accuracy. This prediction model with optimized features performed well even when tested with independent datasets with an accuracy of 80%. Moreover, this work demonstrated that accurate prediction can also be achieved using network features.

For analyzing association of nsSNPs with diseases, the most accepted approach is to explore sequence and evolutionary information. To evaluate the potential of structural information, Cheng et al. developed a structure-based approach called Bongo (Bonds ON Graph) for prediction of structural effects of nsSNPs (Cheng et al., 2008). In this work, authors used graph measures of residue–residue interaction networks to identify the residues that are critical for maintaining the structural stability of proteins. This approach showed considerably good performance with an outstandingly low false positive rate by identifying the mutations that cause both local and global structural effects. The highlight of this study was a positive predictive value of 78.5%, which was attained for prediction of 506 disease-associated nsSNPs. This study is an important example of association between structural changes resulting from nsSNPs and their pathological consequences.

There are several notable instances where complex networks were used effectively in proteomics. One of the most important reasons for the success of this approach is that the topology network representation of the protein structures provides innovative perception of protein folding mechanism. Yizhou et al. developed a new feature to reveal the correlations

Table 2 Illustrative examples of features employed in human protein function identification

S. no.	Reference	Brief description of work	Feature used
1.	iTIS-PseTNC: A sequence-based predictor for identifying translation initiation site in human genes using pseudo trinucleotide composition (Chen et al., 2014)	**Purpose:** Identifying translation initiation site in human genes **Method:** SVM was used with regularization parameter C and the kernel width parameter c was optimized via an optimization procedure using a grid search, and their actual values were obtained in the current study were C = 8 and c = 0.125, respectively. The probability score obtained from SVM was used to make predictions.	physicochemical properties of amino acids: a. their numerical values of hydrophobicity b. hydrophilicity c. sidechain mass
2.	iMulti-HumPhos: a multi-label classifier for identifying human phosphorylated proteins using multiple kernel learning based support vector machines (Hasan et al., 2017)	**Purpose:** Identifying an uncharacterized protein sequence as phosphorylated protein **Method:** iMulti-HumPhos was developed to predict multi-label phosphorylated proteins by: a. Extract 3 different set of features from protein sequences. b. Individual kernel functions were defined for each set of features. Using multiple kernel learning, these kernels were later combined into single kernel. c. Lastly, a combination of SVMs were employed where each SVM was trained with combined kernel to achieve construction of a multi-label predictor.	a. Amino Acid Composition (AAC) b. Dipeptide Composition (DC) c. Sequential evolution feature representation: data of the Position-Specific Scoring Matrix (PSSM)
3.	Alpha influenza virus infiltration prediction using virus-human protein–protein interaction network (Khorsand et al., 2020)	**Purpose:** Predict protein-protein interactions between human proteins and Alphainfluenzavirus proteins **Method:** Five different categories of features were used each in a separate model. Combination of these features were performed by choosing random features among all existing features for training 10 other models. All these 15 models were constructed by different classifiers to obtain divers base classifiers.	A. Amino acid sequence-based features: a. Amino acid composition (AAC) b. Dipeptide Composition (DC) B. Nucleotide sequence-based features a. GC content b. Codon usage c. Relative synonymous codon usage (RSCU) d. Codon adaption index (CAI) e. Stacking energy f. Interaction energy C. Physicochemical properties : a. Hydrophobicity b. Hydrophilicity c. Polarity d. Polarizability

Table 2 Contd....

Table 2 Illustrative examples of features employed in human protein function identification (Contd....)

S. no.	Reference	Brief description of work	Feature used
			e. Side chain volume
			f. Solvent-accessible surface area
			g. Net charge index of residue side chains
			D. Gene Ontology semantic similarity
			a. Cellular compartment (CC)
			b. Molecular function (MF)
			c. Biological process (BP)
			E. Network topology-based features
			a. Degree (connectivity)
			b. Neighborhood connectivity
			c. Shortest paths
			d. Shared neighbors
			e. Stress centrality
			f. Topological coefficients
			g. Closeness centrality
			h. Radiality
4.	Predicting rRNA-, RNA-, and DNA-binding proteins from primary structure with support vector machines (Yu et al., 2006)	**Purpose:** Prediction of protein function. **Method:** SVM was used to build three binary classifiers to predict rRNA-, RNA-, and DNA-binding proteins. Self-consistency test and jackknife test were used to measure the performance of SVM classifiers.	Feature vector was assembled from encoded representations of sequence amino acid composition and tabulated residue properties including hydrophobicity, predicted secondary structure, predicted solvent accessibility, normalized Van Der Waals volume, polarity, and polarizability.
5.	Prediction models of human plasma protein binding rate and oral bioavailability derived by using GA–CG–SVM method (Ma et al., 2008)	**Purpose:** Develop prediction models of human plasma protein binding rate (PPBR) and oral bioavailability (BIO). **Method:** Support vector machine (SVM) method combined with genetic algorithm (GA) for feature selection and conjugate gradient (CG) method for parameter optimization (GA–CG–SVM), has been employed to develop prediction models.	Following 29 descriptors were finalized for building the SVM model: a. constitutional descriptors (5) b. topological descriptors (3) c. Walk and path counts (1) d. connectivity indices (1) e. geometrical descriptors (1) f. RDF descriptors (3) g. atom-centred fragments (9) h. edge adjacency indices (2) i. molecular properties (2) j. functional group counts (2)

S. no.	Reference	Brief description of work	Feature used
6.	A Random Forest Sub-Golgi Protein Classifier Optimized via Dipeptide and Amino Acid Composition Features (Lv et al., 2019)	**Purpose:** Random forests sub-Golgi protein classifier, rfGPT, was developed gain insight into the malfunction of the Golgi apparatus and its relationship to various genetic and neurodegenerative diseases. **Method:** The rfGPT used 2-gap dipeptide and split amino acid composition for the feature vectors and was combined with the synthetic minority over-sampling technique (SMOTE) and an analysis of variance (ANOVA) feature selection method.	Amino acid and peptide composition and their derived features AAC features: k-Gapped Dipeptides Composition Split Amino Acid Composition
7.	Prediction of human protein function according to Gene Ontology categories. (Jensen et al., 2003)	**Purpose:** Prediction of protein function for a subset of classes from the Gene Ontology classification scheme. **Method:** Standard feed-forward neural networks with a single layer of hidden neurons was used for training the model.	Sequence derived protein features
8.	Inferring Function Using Patterns of Native Disorder in Proteins (Lobley et al., 2007)	**Purpose:** Evaluate potential contribution of protein disorder in predicting protein function using standard Gene Ontology (GO) categories. **Method:** Sequence-based pattern analysis was performed to demonstrate that functions of intrinsically disordered proteins are position and length dependent. Feature vectors were constructed using these dependencies to quantify the contribution of disorder in human protein function prediction using SVM classifiers.	Disorder Feature Encoding Scheme: Protein was considered disordered if it contained a contiguous stretch of predicted disordered residues of 30 amino acids. GO categories were identified that were over-represented with disordered proteins as a positive control set of categories likely to be associated with protein disorder features.
9.	Support Vector Machine-based Method for Subcellular Localization of Human Proteins Using Amino Acid Compositions, Their Order, and Similarity Search. (Garg et al., 2005)	**Purpose:** Prediction of subcellular localization (cytoplasm, mitochondrial, nuclear, and plasma membrane) of human proteins. **Method:** SVM-based modules for predicting subcellular localization using traditional amino acid and dipeptide $(i + 1)$ composition. To gain further insight, a hybrid module (hybridI) was developed based on amino acid composition, dipeptide composition, and similarity information.	a. Amino Acid Composition, b. Traditional Dipeptide Composition $(i + 1)$, c. Multivariate Adaptive Regression Splines, d. Compositions of Amino Acid Properties: (i) nonpolar aliphatic amino acids (ii) polar uncharged amino acids (iii) aromatic amino acids (iv) negatively charged amino acids (v) positively charged amino acids
10.	Prediction of protein-protein interactions between viruses and human by an SVM model (Cui et al., 2012)	**Purpose:** Prediction of protein-protein interactions from amino acid sequences. **Method:** SVM model was built to predict human proteins that interact with virus proteins.	Protein sequence of variable length in a frequency vector of fixed length, which encodes the relative frequency of three consecutive amino acids of a sequence.

Table 2 Contd....

Table 2   Illustrative examples of features employed in human protein function identification (Contd....)

S. no.	Reference	Brief description of work	Feature used
11.	Prediction of Function Changes Associated With Single-Point Protein Mutations Using Support Vector Machines (SVMs) (Gao et al., 2009)	**Purpose:** Prediction protein function changes associated with amino acid substitutions using only sequence information. **Method:** With three SVM classifiers, the authors investigated three local properties within a local window on a protein sequence, namely' residue composition (IP-SVMI), hydrophobic interaction (IP-SVM2), and evolutionary property (SM-SVM).	local sequence features ofproteins: a. residue composition b. hydrophobic interaction c. evolutionary property
12.	Support vector machines for predicting rRNA-, RNA-, and DNA-binding proteins from amino acid sequence (Cai and Lin, 2003)	**Purpose:** Protein function prediction using SVM and the pseudo-amino acid composition, a collection of non-linear features extractable from protein sequence. **Method:** SVM was employed to build classifiers for protein function. Authors have implemented three SVMs for binary classification of rRNA-, RNA- and DNA-binding proteins, respectively.	Pseudo-amino acid composition of a protein was used as a 40-dimensional input feature vector for SVM
13.	Predicting the insurgence of human genetic diseases associated to single point protein mutations with support vector machines and evolutionary information (Capriotti et al., 2006)	**Purpose:** Prediction method based on SVMs that starting from the protein sequence information can predict whether a new phenotype derived from a non-synonymous coding SNPs (nsSNP) can be related to a genetic disease in humans. **Method:** SVM-Sequence and SVM-Profile are cast in a unique workflow with a decision tree method (HybridMeth) that allows adopting either SVM-Sequence or SVM-Profile, depending on the presence or absence of a sequence profile of the sequence at hand, respectively.	The input vector consists of 40 values: the first 20 (the 20 residue types) explicitly define the mutation by setting to -1 the element corresponding to the wild-type residue and to 1 the newly introduced residue (all the remaining elements are kept equal to 0). The last 20 input values encode for the mutation sequence environment (again the 20 elements represent the 20 residue types).
14.	A novel method for protein secondary structure prediction using dual-layer SVM and profiles (Guo et al., 2004)	**Purpose:** Protein secondary structure prediction based on the dual-layer support vector machine (SVM) and position-specific scoring matrices (PSSMs). **Method:** A prediction model was developed using SVM's, whose performance was further improved by combining PSSM profiles with the SVM analysis. The PSSMs were generated from PSI-BLAST profiles, which contain important evolution information.	classical local coding scheme of the protein sequences with a sliding window. PSI-BLAST matrix with n rows and 20 columns can be defined for single sequence with n residues.

S. no.	Reference	Brief description of work	Feature used
15.	Feature Selection and the Class Imbalance Problem in Predicting Protein Function from Sequence (Al-Shahib et al., 2005)	**Purpose:** Use of machine learning to predict protein function directly from amino acid sequence features. **Method:** Predicting protein function from sequence can be significantly improved by a. performing full (100%) under sampling of the majority class, b. using feature-selected data and c. generating support vector machine (SVM) classifiers.	Diverse sequence-related features were extracted and calculated, including amino acid composition, amino acid pair ratios, protein length, molecular weight, isoelectric point, hydropathicity and aliphatic index. A total of 433 features were used.
16.	Loss of Protein Structure Stability as a Major Causative Factor in Monogenic Disease (Yue et al., 2005)	**Purpose:** Testing the hypothesis that destabilization of protein structure is a major factor in human monogenic disease. **Method:** A set of structural effects, such as reduction in hydrophobic area, overpacking, backbone strain, and loss of electrostatic interactions, is used to represent the impact of single residue mutations on protein stability. A support vector machine (SVM) was trained on a set of mutations causative of disease, and a control set of non-disease-causing mutations.	Combined sequence and structure strategies to varying degrees. Sunyaev predicted the effect of mis-sense mutations using empirically derived rules which make use of a variety of data, such as functional information, hydrophobic propensity, side-chain volume change and transmembrane location,8 together with sequence information.
17.	MLACP: machine-learning-based prediction of anticancer peptides (Manavalan et al., 2017)	**Purpose:** Machine learningbased prediction of anticancer peptides. **Method:** Support vector machine- and random forest-based machine-learning methods for the prediction of ACPs using the features calculated from the amino acid sequence.	amino acid composition, dipeptide composition, atomic composition, and physicochemical properties.
18.	DPP-PseAAC: A DNA-binding protein prediction model using Chou's general PseAAC (Rahman et al., 2018)	**Purpose:** Identification of DNA-binding proteins. **Method:** Extraction of meaningful information directly from the protein sequences, without any dependence on functional domain or structural information. After feature extraction, Random Forest (RF) model was employed to rank the features.	position independent and position specific: a. Amino Acid Composition (AAC) b. Dipeptides (Dip) c. Tripeptides d. n-gapped-dipeptides (nGDip) e. Position specific n-grams (PSN)

Table 2 Contd....

Table 2 Illustrative examples of features employed in human protein function identification (Contd....)

S. no.	Reference	Brief description of work	Feature used
19.	Mem-PHybrid: Hybrid features-based prediction system for classifying membrane protein types (Hayat and Khan, 2012)	**Purpose:** Two-layer novel membrane protein prediction system. **Method:** Mem-PHybrid is based on a hybrid feature extraction strategy and SVM. The physicochemical and SAAC features were combined to exploit the discrimination power of both feature extraction strategies.	Physico-chemical properties of proteins: a. hydrophobicity b. normalized van der Waals volume c. polarity d. polarization e. charge f. secondary structure g. solvent accessibility
20.	Mito-GSAAC: mitochondria prediction using genetic ensemble classifier and split amino acid composition (Afridi et al., 2012)	**Purpose:** Identification of new mitochondrial proteins. **Method:** Authors trained different individual classifiers on several feature extraction strategies. First, mitochondria protein sequences are converted into features using the feature extraction strategies. These features are finally provided to the different individual classifiers for training and prediction performance for each individual classifier is determined.	amino acid composition, dipeptide composition, pseudo amino acid composition, and split amino acid composition (SAAC)
21.	FFPred 3: feature-based function prediction for all Gene Ontology domains (Cozzetto et al., 2016)	**Purpose:** Assignment of Gene Ontology terms to human protein chains. **Method:** Authors used machine-learning approach to perform function prediction in protein feature space using feature characteristics predicted from amino acid sequence. The features are scanned against a library of support vector machines representing over 300 Gene Ontology (GO) classes and probabilistic confidence scores returned for each annotation term.	secondary structure, transmembrane helices, intrinsically disordered regions, signal peptides and other motifs

Table 3 Examples of web servers for human protein function identification

Server	Purpose	Features used	Reference Link
AGVGD (Tavtigian et al., 2006)	Predicting functional impact of SAPs	multiple sequence alignments	http://agvgd.iarc.fr/index.php
VirulentPred (Garg and Gupta, 2008)	Prediction method for virulent proteins in bacterial pathogens	amino acid composition, dipeptide composition, higher order dipeptide composition, and Position Specific Iterated BLAST (PSI-BLAST)	http://bioinfo.icgeb.res.in/virulent/
PRINTR (Wang et al., 2008)	Prediction of RNA binding sites in proteins	Sequence-derived, structure information	http://210.42.106.80/printr/.
CyclinPred (Kalita et al., 2008)	Predicting Cyclin Protein Sequences	amino acid composition, dipeptide composition, secondary structure composition and PSI-BLAST generated Position Specific Scoring Matrix (PSSM) profiles	http://bioinfo.icgeb.res.in/cyclinpred
RBPPred (Zhang and Liu, 2017)	Predicting RNA-binding proteins	physicochemical properties with the evolutionary information	http://rnabinding.com/RBPPred.html.
topoSNP (Zhang and Liu, 2017 (Stitziel et al., 2004)	Predicting Functional Impact of SAPs	sequence conservation and multiple sequence alignments	http://gila.bioengr.uic.edu/snp/toposnp/
FFPred 3 (Cozzetto et al., 2016)	Assignment of Gene Ontology terms to human protein chains	secondary structure, transmembrane helices, intrinsically disordered regions, signal peptides and other motifs	http://bioinf.cs.ucl.ac.uk/ffpred
MutPred Splice (Mort et al., 2014)	Prediction of exonic variants that disrupt splicing	evolutionary attributes, structural attributes, functional attributes	http://mutdb.org/mutpred
MutationTaster (Schwarz et al., 2010)	Evaluation of disease- causing potential of sequence alterations	evolutionary conservation, splice-site changes, loss of protein and changes of amount of mRNA.	http://www.mutationtaster.org/
KvSNP (Stead et al., 2011)	Predicting the effect of genetic variants in voltage-gated potassium channels	Conservation score, subfamily membership, hydrophobicity, predicted secondary structure, predicted solvent Accessibility, predicted change in stability, predicted solvent accessibility	http://www.bioinformatics.leeds.ac.uk/KvDB/KvSNP.html

between residues using a protein structure network (Li et al., 2011b). In this attempt to quantify the effects of several key residues on catalytic residues, a power function was used to model interactions between the residues. The results indicated that focusing on a few residues is a feasible approach to identifying the catalytic residues. The spatial environment surrounding a catalytic residue was analyzed in a layered manner. Feature analysis revealed satisfactory performance for the features used, which were combined with several conventional features in a prediction model for catalytic residues using a comprehensive data set from the Catalytic Site Atlas. Values of 88.6% for sensitivity and 88.4% for specificity were obtained by 10-fold cross-validation. These results suggest that these features reveal the mutual dependence of residues and are promising for further study of structure–function relationship.

5   WEB SERVER

Researchers have developed local tools or online servers to provide the service of predicting the function of proteins in various different applications. All these tools have been implemented on the basis of acceptable predictive capabilities of the method employed. Table 3 shows some of the web servers based on SVM models that are used in protein function prediction.

As in many other areas, decisions play an important role also in medicine, especially in medical diagnostic processes. Decision support systems helping physicians are becoming a very important part in medical decision making, particularly in those situations where decision must be made effectively and reliably. Since conceptual simple decision-making models with the possibility of automatic learning should be considered for performing such tasks, decision trees are a very suitable candidate. They have been already successfully used for many decision-making purposes. As in many other areas, decisions play an important role also in medicine, especially in medical diagnostic processes. Decision support systems helping physicians are becoming a very important part in medical decision making, particularly in those situations where decision must be made effectively and reliably. Since conceptual simple decision-making models with the possibility of automatic learning should be considered for performing such tasks, decision trees are a very suitable candidate. They have been already successfully used for many decision-making purposes.

6   CONCLUDING REMARKS

Protein being such a complex macromolecule, offers numerous aspects of feature definition, ranging from sequence to structure. In this review, we elucidated numerous sequences-based characteristic features of proteins which are explored in several studies for constructing protein function prediction models. We have enlisted several examples where some set features outperformed over others, indicating that use of feature set depends on the problem statement. We have also listed some of the important methods employed in feature selection. We have tried to cover different examples which are mostly focused critical research areas that directly or indirectly touch human life. Out of all the studies, the area which has been explored the most by the research community is predicting the effect of mutations in humans, which ultimately alters the function of protein. We have also listed large number of case studies and examples of protein function predictions.

REFERENCES

Adzhubei, I.A., S. Schmidt, L. Peshkin, V.E. Ramensky, A. Gerasimova, P. Bork, et al. (2010). A method and server for predicting damaging missense mutations. Nature Methods. 7(4): 248–249.

Afridi, T.H., A. Khan and Y.S. Lee (2012). Mito-GSAAC: Mitochondria prediction using genetic ensemble classifier and split amino acid composition. Amino Acids. 42(4): 1443–1454.

Al-Shahib, A., R. Breitling and D. Gilbert (2005). Feature selection and the class imbalance problem in predicting protein function from sequence. Applied Bioinformatics. 4(3): 195–203.

Apweiler, R., A. Bairoch, C.H. Wu, W.C. Barker, B. Boeckmann, S. Ferro, et al. (2004). UniProt: The universal protein knowledgebase. Nucleic Acids Research. 32(Suppl_1): nD115–119.

Ashburner, M., C.A. Ball, J.A. Blake, D. Botstein, H. Butler, J.M. Cherry, et al. (2000). Gene ontology: Tool for the unification of biology. Nature Genetics. 25(1): 25–29.

Basith, S., M. Cui, S.J. Macalino and S. Choi (2017). Expediting the design, discovery and development of anticancer drugs using computational approaches. Current Medicinal Chemistry. 24(42): 4753–4778.

Berman, H.M., J. Westbrook, Z. Feng, G. Gilliland, T.N. Bhat, H. Weissig, et al. (2000). The protein data bank. Nucleic Acids Research. 28(1): 235–242.

Botstein, D. and N. Risch (2003). Discovering genotypes underlying human phenotypes: Past successes for mendelian disease, future approaches for complex disease. Nature Genetics. 33(3): 228–237.

Breiman, L. (2001). Random forests. Machine Learning. 45(1): 5–32.

Bromberg, Y. and B. Rost (2007). SNAP: Predict effect of non-synonymous polymorphisms on function. Nucleic Acids Research. 35(11): 3823–3835.

Bromberg, Y., G. Yachdav and B. Rost (2008). SNAP predicts effect of mutations on protein function. Bioinformatics. 24(20): 2397–2398.

Cai, Y.D. and S.L. Lin (2003). Support vector machines for predicting rRNA-, RNA-, and DNA-binding proteins from amino acid sequence. Biochimica et Biophysica Acta (BBA)-Proteins and Proteomics. 1648(1-2): 127–133.

Capriotti, E., R. Calabrese and R. Casadio (2006). Predicting the insurgence of human genetic diseases associated to single point protein mutations with support vector machines and evolutionary information. Bioinformatics. 22(22): 2729–2734.

Care, M.A., C.J. Needham, A.J. Bulpitt and D.R. Westhead (2007). Deleterious SNP prediction: be mindful of your training data!. Bioinformatics. 23(6): 664–672.

Chen, W., P.M. Feng, E.Z. Deng, H. Lin and K.C. Chou (2014). iTIS-PseTNC: A sequence-based predictor for identifying translation initiation site in human genes using pseudo trinucleotide composition. Analytical Biochemistry. 462: 76–83.

Chen, W., H. Ding, P. Feng, H. Lin and K.C. Chou (2016). iACP: A sequence-based tool for identifying anticancer peptides. Oncotarget. 7(13): 16895.

Cheng, T.M., Y.E. Lu, M. Vendruscolo, P. Lio and T.L. Blundell (2008). Prediction by graph theoretic measures of structural effects in proteins arising from non-synonymous single nucleotide polymorphisms. PLoS Computational Biology. 4(7).

Chou, K.C. (2001). Prediction of protein cellular attributes using pseudo-amino acid composition. Proteins: Structure, Function, and Bioinformatics. 43(3): 246–255.

Cozzetto, D., F. Minneci, H. Currant and D.T. Jones (2016). FFPred 3: Feature-based function prediction for all gene ontology domains. Sci. Rep. 6: 31865.

Cui, G., C. Fang and K. Han (2012). Prediction of protein-protein interactions between viruses and human by an SVM model. BMC Bioinformatics. 13: S5. https://doi.org/10.1186/1471-2105-13-S7-S5.

Cutler, D.R., T.C. Edwards Jr, K.H. Beard, A. Cutler, K.T. Hess, J. Gibson, et al. (2007). Random forests for classification in ecology. Ecology. 88(11): 2783–2792.

Dobson, R.J., P.B. Munroe, M.J. Caulfield and M.A. Saqi (2006). Predicting deleterious nsSNPs: An analysis of sequence and structural attributes. BMC Bioinformatics. 7(1): 217.

Gao, S., N. Zhang, G.Y. Duan, Z. Yang, J.S. Ruan and T. Zhang (2009). Prediction of function changes associated with single-point protein mutations using support vector machines (SVMs). Human Mutation. 30(8): 1161–1166.

Garg, A., M. Bhasin and G.P. Raghava (2005). Support vector machine-based method for subcellular localization of human proteins using amino acid compositions, their order, and similarity search. Journal of Biological Chemistry. 280(15): 14427–14432.

Garg, A. and D. Gupta (2008). VirulentPred: A SVM based prediction method for virulent proteins in bacterial pathogens. BMC Bioinformatics. 9(1): 62.

Gaspar, D., A.S. Veiga and M.A. Castanho (2013). From antimicrobial to anticancer peptides. A review. Frontiers in Microbiology. 4: 294.

Gautam, A., K. Chaudhary, R. Kumar, A. Sharma, P. Kapoor, A. Tyagi, et al. (2013). *In silico* approaches for designing highly effective cell penetrating peptides. Journal of Translational Medicine. 11(1): 74.

Gong, S. and T.L. Blundell (2010). Structural and functional restraints on the occurrence of single amino acid variations in human proteins. PLoS ONE 5(2): e9186. https://doi.org/10.1371/journal.pone.0009186

Guo, J., H. Chen, Z. Sun and Y. Lin (2004). A novel method for protein secondary structure prediction using dual-layer SVM and profiles. PROTEINS: Structure, Function, and Bioinformatics. 54(4): 738–743.

Han, J., J. Pei and M. Kamber (2011). Data Mining: Concepts and Techniques. Elsevier.

Harris, F., S.R. Dennison, J. Singh and D.A. Phoenix (2013). On the selectivity and efficacy of defense peptides with respect to cancer cells. Medicinal Research Reviews. 33(1): 190–234.

Hasan, M.A., S. Ahmad and M.K. Molla (2017). iMulti-HumPhos: a multi-label classifier for identifying human phosphorylated proteins using multiple kernel learning based support vector machines. Molecular BioSystems. 13(8): 1608–1618.

Hayat, M. and A. Khan (2012). Mem-PHybrid: Hybrid features-based prediction system for classifying membrane protein types. Analytical Biochemistry. 424(1): 35–44.

Huang, T., P. Wang, Z.Q. Ye, H. Xu, Z. He, K.Y. Feng, et al. (2010). Prediction of deleterious non-synonymous SNPs based on protein interaction network and hybrid properties. PLoS ONE 5(7): e11900. https://doi.org/10.1371/journal.pone.0011900

Hubbard, T.J. and T.L. Blundell (1987). Comparison of solvent-inaccessible cores of homologous proteins: Definitions useful for protein modelling. Protein Engineering, Design and Selection. 1(3): 159–171.

Jackson, R.J., C.U. Hellen and T.V. Pestova (2010). The mechanism of eukaryotic translation initiation and principles of its regulation. Nature Reviews Molecular Cell Biology. 11(2): 113–127.

Jensen, L.J., R. Gupta, H.H. Staerfeldt and S. Brunak (2003). Prediction of human protein function according to Gene Ontology categories. Bioinformatics. 19(5): 635–642.

Kabsch, W. and C. Sander (1983). Dictionary of protein secondary structure: pattern recognition of hydrogen-bonded and geometrical features. Biopolymers: Original Research on Biomolecules. 22(12): 2577–2637.

Kalita, M.K., U.K. Nandal, A. Pattnaik, A. Sivalingam, G. Ramasamy, M. Kumar, et al. (2008). CyclinPred: a SVM-based method for predicting cyclin protein sequences. PLoS ONE 3(7): e2605. https://doi.org/10.1371/journal.pone.0002605

Kawabata, T., M. Ota and K. Nishikawa (1999). The protein mutant database. Nucleic Acids Research. 27(1): 355–357.

Khorsand, B., A. Savadi, J. Zahiri and M. Naghibzadeh (2020). Alpha influenza virus infiltration prediction using virus-human protein–protein interaction network. Mathematical Biosciences and Engineering. 17(4): 3109.

Kumar, R., K. Chaudhary, J.S. Chauhan, G. Nagpal, R. Kumar, M. Sharma, et al. (2015). An *in silico* platform for predicting, screening and designing of antihypertensive peptides. Sci. Rep. 5: 12512.

Li, Y., G. Li, Z. Wen, H. Yin, M. Hu, J. Xiao, et al. (2011a). Novel feature for catalytic protein residues reflecting interactions with other residues. PLoS ONE 6(3): e16932. https://doi.org/10.1371/journal.pone.0016932

Li, Y., Z. Wen, J. Xiao, H. Yin, L. Yu, L. Yang, et al. (2011b). Predicting disease-associated substitution of a single amino acid by analyzing residue interactions. BMC Bioinformatics. 12(1): 14.

Liaw, A., and M. Wiener (2002). Classification and regression by Random Forest. R. News. 2(3): 18–22.

Lin, H., W.X. Liu, J. He, X.H. Liu, H. Ding and W. Chen. (2015). Predicting cancerlectins by the optimal g-gap dipeptides. Sci. Rep. 5(1): 1–9.

Lobley, A., M.B. Swindells, C.A. Orengo and D.T. Jones (2007). Inferring function using patterns of native disorder in proteins. PLoS Comput Biol 3(8): e162. https://doi.org/10.1371/journal.pcbi.0030162

Lobley, A.E., T. Nugent, C.A. Orengo and D.T. Jones (2008). FFPred: An integrated feature-based function prediction server for vertebrate proteomes. Nucleic Acids Research. 36(Suppl. 2): W297–W302.

Lv, Z., S. Jin, H. Ding and Q. Zou (2019). A random forest sub-Golgi protein classifier optimized via dipeptide and amino acid composition features. Frontiers in Bioengineering and Biotechnology. 7: 215.

Ma, S. and J. Huang (2008). Penalized feature selection and classification in bioinformatics. Briefings In Bioinformatics. 9(5): 392–403

Ma, C.Y., S.Y. Yang, H. Zhang, M.L. Xiang, Q. Huang and Y.Q. Wei (2008). Prediction models of human plasma protein binding rate and oral bioavailability derived by using GA–CG–SVM method. Journal of Pharmaceutical and Biomedical Analysis. 47(4-5): 677–682.

Manavalan, B., S. Basith, T.H. Shin, S. Choi, M.O. Kim and G. Lee (2017). MLACP: Machine-learning-based prediction of anticancer peptides. Oncotarget. 8(44): 77121.

Mika, S., B. Schölkopf, A.J. Smola, K.R. Müller, M. Scholz and G. Rätsch (1999). Kernel PCA and de-noising in feature spaces. pp. 536–542. In: MS Kearns and SA Solla and DA Cohn (eds). Advances in Neural Information Processing Systems 11. MIT Press.

Mort, M., T. Sterne-Weiler, B. Li, E.V. Ball, D.N. Cooper, P. Radivojac, et al. (2014). MutPred Splice: machine learning-based prediction of exonic variants that disrupt splicing. Genome Biology. 15(1): R19.

Nishikawa, K., S. Ishino, H. Takenaka, N. Norioka, T. Hirai and T. Yao (1994). Constructing a protein mutant database. Protein Eng. 7(5): 733. doi: 10.1093/protein/7.5.733.

Qiu, W.R., Q.S. Zheng, B.Q. Sun and X. Xiao (2017). Multi-iPPseEvo: A Multi-label classifier for identifying human phosphorylated proteins by incorporating evolutionary information into Chou's general PseAAC via grey system theory. Molecular Informatics. 36(3): 1600085.

Rahman, M.S., S. Shatabda, S. Saha, M. Kaykobad and M.S. Rahman (2018). Dpp-pseaac: A DNA-binding protein prediction model using Chou's general PseAAC. Journal of Theoretical Biology. 452: 22–34.

Rawat, P., R. Prabakaran, S. Kumar and M.M. Gromiha (2020). AggreRATE-Pred: A mathematical model for the prediction of change in aggregation rate upon point mutation. Bioinformatics. 36(5): 1439–1444.

Saey, Y., I. Inza and P. Larrañaga (2007). A review of feature selection techniques in bioinformatics. Bioinformatics. 23(19): 2507–2517.

Saha, S., P. Chatterjee, S. Basu and M. Nasipuri (2017). Gene ontology based function prediction of human protein using protein sequence and neighborhood property of PPI network. pp. 109–118. *In*: Proceedings of the 5th International Conference on Frontiers in Intelligent Computing: Theory and Applications. Springer, Singapore.

Sanders, W.S., C.I. Johnston, S.M. Bridges, S.C. Burgess and K.O. Willeford (2011). Prediction of cell penetrating peptides by support vector machines. PLoS Comput. Biol. 7(7): e1002101. doi: 10.1371/journal.pcbi.1002101

Saunders, C.T. and D. Baker (2002). Evaluation of structural and evolutionary contributions to deleterious mutation prediction. Journal of Molecular Biology. 322(4): 891–901.

Schwarz, J.M., C. Rödelsperger, M. Schuelke and D. Seelow (2010). MutationTaster evaluates disease-causing potential of sequence alterations. Nature Methods. 7(8): 575–576.

Singh, M., P.K. Wadhwa and P.W. Sandhu (2007). Human protein function prediction using decision tree induction. International Journal of Computer Science and Network Security. 7(4): 92–98.

Srivastava, A., S. Ghosh, N. Anantharaman and V.K. Jayaraman (2013). Hybrid biogeography based on simultaneous feature selection and MHC class I peptide binding prediction using support vector machines and random forests. Journal of Immunological Methods. 387(1-2): 284–292

Stead, L.F, I.C. Wood and D.R. Westhead (2011). KvSNP: Accurately predicting the effect of genetic variants in voltage-gated potassium channels. Bioinformatics. 27(16): 2181–2186.

Stitziel, N.O., T.A. Binkowski, Y.Y. Tseng, S. Kasif and J. Liang (2004). TopoSNP: A topographic database of non-synonymous single nucleotide polymorphisms with and without known disease association. Nucleic Acids Research. 32(Suppl. 1): D520–D522.

Sunyaev, S., V. Ramensky and P. Bork (2000). Towards a structural basis of human non-synonymous single nucleotide polymorphisms. Trends in Genetics. 16(5): 198–200.

Tavtigian, S.V., A.M. Deffenbaugh, L. Yin, T. Judkins, T. Scholl, P.B. Samollow, et al. (2006). Comprehensive statistical study of 452 BRCA1 missense substitutions with classification of eight recurrent substitutions as neutral. Journal of Medical Genetics. 43(4): 295–305.

Thundimadathil, J. (2012). Cancer treatment using peptides: Current therapies and future prospects. Journal of Amino Acids.

Tyagi, A., P. Kapoor, R. Kumar, K. Chaudhary, A. Gautam and G.P. Raghava (2013). *In silico* models for designing and discovering novel anticancer peptides. Sci. Rep. 3: 298.

Vlieghe, P., V. Lisowski, J. Martinez and M. Khrestchatisky (2010). Synthetic therapeutic peptides: Science and market. Drug Discovery Today. 15(1-2): 40–56.

Wan, J. and S.B. Qian (2014). TISdb: A database for alternative translation initiation in mammalian cells. Nucleic acids research. 42(D1): D845–D850.

Wang, Z. and J. Moult (2001). SNPs, protein structure, and disease. Human Mutation. 17(4): 263–270.

Wang, Y., Z. Xue, G. Shen and J. Xu (2008). PRINTR: Prediction of RNA binding sites in proteins using SVM and profiles. Amino Acids. 35(2): 295–302.

Worth, C.L. and T.L. Blundell (2009). Satisfaction of hydrogen-bonding potential influences the conservation of polar sidechains. Proteins: Structure, Function, and Bioinformatics. 75(2): 413–429.

Yan, M. and Q. Liu (2016). Differentiation therapy: A promising strategy for cancer treatment. Chinese Journal of Cancer. 35(1): 3.

Ye, Z.Q., S.Q. Zhao, G. Gao, X.Q. Liu, R.E. Langlois, H. Lu, et al. (2007). Finding new structural and sequence attributes to predict possible disease association of single amino acid polymorphism (SAP). Bioinformatics. 23(12): 1444–1450.

Yip, Y.L., H. Scheib, A.V. Diemand, A. Gattiker, L.M. Famiglietti, E. Gasteiger E, et al. (2004). The Swiss-Prot variant page and the ModSNP database: a resource for sequence and structure information on human protein variants. Human Mutation. 23(5): 464–70.

Yu, X., J. Cao, Y. Cai, T. Shi and Y. Li (2006). Predicting rRNA-, RNA-, and DNA-binding proteins from primary structure with support vector machines. Journal of Theoretical Biology. 240(2): 175–184.

Yue, P., Z. Li and J. Moult (2005). Loss of protein structure stability as a major causative factor in monogenic disease. Journal of Molecular Biology. 353(2): 459–473.

Zhang, X. and S. Liu (2017). RBPPred: Predicting RNA-binding proteins from sequence using SVM. Bioinformatics. 33(6): 854–862.

Zurada, J.M. (1992). Introduction to Artificial Neural Systems. West Publishing Company, St. Paul.

CHAPTER 4

Bioinformatics and Genomic Data Mining

Juan Camilo Ramírez*

Universidad Antonio Nariño, Facultad de Ingeniería de Sistemas,
Bogotá, Colombia

1 GENOMICS, BIOINFORMATICS AND DATA MINING: AN OVERVIEW

Genomics is the branch of biology that studies genomes, i.e. any organism's full set of genes and how these interact with one another in order to produce observable phenomena at the phenotype level. This is in contrast to *genetics*, which generally studies genes and their effects individually. Considerable advances in sequencing technology in the recent years have resulted in an explosive growth of genomic and proteomic data. Given the massive amounts of information stored in a single genome, genomics generally relies on the use of computational tools in order to analyse these data and subsequently derive biological interpretations from them. *Bioinformatics* is the interdisciplinary field devoted to the design, use and application of mathematical and computational techniques for the analysis of biological data in order to identify patterns, derive generalizations, or make predictions from these, e.g., prediction of disease risk from gene expression (Huet et al., 2018; Shedden et al., 2008; Zhou et al., 2018) as well as prediction of genes or protein structures (Lomsadze et al., 2018; Senior et al., 2020), among others applications. Thus scientific interest in this field has seen an increase in recent years with the growing availability of genomic and proteomic data.

Bioinformatics makes extensive use of various subdisciplines of computer science, namely, *data mining, machine learning, deep learning, data science*, and *big data*, which are all closely related to each other with each exhibiting significant overlap with the rest. Data mining refers to the application of statistical methods and algorithms in order to discover interesting

---

*Corresponding author: *juan.ramirez@uan.edu.co*

patterns in large amounts of data, which would otherwise be a very difficult and impractical task to achieve through manual means. Machine learning, as the name implies, refers to the study and design of computer algorithms that are able to learn from data in order to make generalizations or predictions from them, with deep learning being a more advanced form of this discipline. On the other hand, data science and big data are loosely and frequently defined as the extraction of useful knowledge through the analysis of large, complex, raw and unstructured data, as well as the storage and manipulation of these in such large amounts that would not be manageable through traditional, computational means. There is no universal agreement on the difference between these disciplines, or where the boundary should be placed between any two of them, given that all refer to the study of data, generally in large volumes. Nevertheless, some distinctions can be unequivocally made. Data mining focuses more on the discovery of previously unknown patterns, relationships and anomalies that are present in large amounts of data. Classical textbook examples of data mining applications include the discovery of unknown patterns found in historical purchase data and the identification of new associations that could indicate customer purchasing behaviour in the future that could be exploited commercially. For this reason, data mining is frequently used in retail in order to identify buying patterns and trends. On the other hand, machine learning and deep learning focus on the design of algorithms that can learn from and make predictions about the data, without human intervention and in more general contexts than data mining, while keeping the emphasis on the optimization of the learning task. Data science and big data can be defined as umbrella terms encompassing methods for the elucidation of insights in data of such volumes that make them not manageable through traditional computational means. Furthermore, all these disciplines are related to, and widely considered to overlap significantly with, statistical inference. However, while the main purpose of statistical inference is to discover underlying properties from a data population, along with an estimate of the uncertainty of these, data mining, machine learning and deep learning are more concerned about learning how to make predictions from raw pieces of information, which necessarily implies some degree of inference as well, whereas data science and big data are more concerned with the descriptive and manoeuvrability aspects of the data.

Applications of data mining, machine learning, deep learning, data science and big data are varied and dependent on the area. In the particular case of bioinformatics, the purpose frequently is to build a mathematical model from biological data, e.g., from gene expression measurements, in order to make predictions about similar observations, previously unseen by the model. Common applications include the prediction of an organism's risk of developing a given disease based on gene expression levels (Bashiri et al., 2017; Park et al., 2020; Salem et al., 2017), differential gene expression analysis (Blanco et al., 2019; Spies et al., 2019), gene clustering (Gulisija and Plotkin, 2017; Zareizadeh et al., 2018) and identification of gene regulatory networks (Carey et al., 2018; Mochida et al., 2018; Ni et al., 2016). Other ambitious applications include, but are not limited to, the prediction of gene expression (Dong et al., 2012), gene locations (Mathé et al., 2002), regulatory regions (Fernandez and Miranda-Saavedra, 2012), an organism's genetic response to a medication (Wang et al., 2011) or health status (Kourou et al., 2015), the effect of single-nucleotide polymorphisms on gene regulation (Zhou and Troyanskaya, 2015), among many others. The application of machine learning and related areas, such as data mining and deep learning, on biological data accelerates the understanding of complex diseases, for instance, cancer or diabetes, and eventually lead to automated diagnostic tools in medicine, among other advancements (Baldi and Brunak, 2001; Chicco, 2017; Larranaga et al., 2006).

This chapter is targeted towards readers from the biological sciences with a basic understanding of programming and statistical inference methods, and aims to provide a friendly, yet effective introduction to common applications of data mining on genomic analysis using software tools and libraries freely available online. The chapter is structured as follows. Section 2 describes briefly the type of genomic data available nowadays and the current technology to acquire these as well as the public databases and repositories where these can be found. Section 3 provides an introduction into *classification analysis*, one of the most common problem types addressed through data mining, particularly on the analysis of genomic data. Section 4 provides a brief introduction to the programming language Python along with a summary of the procedures to be followed for the installation of a work environment in this language with freely available packages and libraries required for genomic data analysis. Section 5 presents an example of how to use machine learning with Python in order to conduct classification analysis on genomic data from a public repository for the prediction of cancer types from patient's gene expression. Section 6 describes other methods of applications of data mining and data analysis and genomics. Finally, Section 7 presents a summary of the chapters with the most important take aways.

2 GENOMIC DATA AND SEQUENCING TECHNOLOGY

One of the greatest scientific achievements of the late twentieth century is the *Human Genome Project* (HGP), an international and multidisciplinary endeavour aimed at mapping the full sequence of genes found in the human DNA, documenting the functional roles of each. Since strictly speaking there is no single human genome, with each person having their unique genome, HGP aimed to provide a single sequence from the integrated mappings obtained from a limited number of individuals. The results obtained from the HGP included, among many others, the revelation that the human genome comprises more than 20,000 genes, which is a significantly lower figure than thought earlier by the academic community at the time, with prior estimates ranging between 50,000 and 100,000. This collaborative effort had its origins in 1984, followed by several years of planning after which the project officially started in 1990 and ended on 14 April 2003. Various sources of funding from around the world contributed to the completion of the project, particularly the National Institutes of Health[1] in the United States. One of the main legacies of the HGP and related initiatives is the massive and growing amount of genomic data that can be used to expand the current understanding of the inner workings of an organism, e.g., an individual's response to a pathogen, such as a virus, or to a novel medication. This has numerous applications in a variety of fields, such as molecular medicine and biology. Specialized databases exist to store these data, many of which are freely accessible to the general public on the internet. Examples of these include the Gene Expression Omnibus[2] (GEO), the DNA Data Bank of Japan[3], the European Molecular Biology Laboratory's repository[4], and GenBank[5], Other publicly-available repositories exist, albeit less specialized on biological data that nonetheless store some genomics-related datasets, including Kaggle[6] and the UCI Machine Learning Repository[7].

Currently there are various technologies that allow the sequencing, either partial or in full, and posterior analysis of genomic data. This mass quantification of gene transcripts is frequently used, for instance, in intervention studies, e.g., experiments where one tissue sample has been exposed to a stimulus, such as a pathogen or medication, and its expression levels are assessed and contrasted against those of a similar sample, referred to as the control, where no stimulus has been applied. These experiments are conducted in order to quantify the effectiveness of novel medications or the host organism's response to an infection, for instance. Experiments

---

[1]National Institutes of Health (https://www.nih.gov/).

[2]Gene Expression Omnibus (https://www.ncbi.nlm.nih.gov/geo/).

[3]DNA Data Bank of Japan (https://www.ddbj.nig.ac.jp/).

[4]European Molecular Biology Laboratory's repository (https://www.embl.org/).

[5]GenBank (https://www.ncbi.nlm.nih.gov/genbank/).

[6]Kaggle (https://www.kaggle.com/).

[7]UCI Machine Learning Repository (https://archive.ics.uci.edu/ml/).

based on the sequencing of a single individual are referred to as *personal genomics*. The most common methods used nowadays for the collection of genomic data include *DNA microarrays* and *next-generation sequencing* (NGS). DNA microarrays are laboratory devices designed for the simultaneous quantification of up to thousands of gene transcripts from a single tissue sample and have for years been the standard tool in experiments designed for the characterization of gene expression variation across different biological conditions. Each consists of a grid where each probe allows the hybridization of a known DNA or oligonucleotide target with a matching RNA sample that has previously been reverse-transcribed and labeled. On the other hand, next generation sequencing (NGS), also known as *high–throughput sequencing*, is a set of related technologies that allow the examination of the entire genome without requiring a predefined set of targets. This is achieved through the process of synthesis, where DNA polymerase incorporates a set of nucleotides. All this, in contrast to microarrays, which are based on hybridization and return results only for those regions of the transcriptome for which their probes have been specifically designed. Even though NGS technologies offer a more modern and powerful option than microarrays, the choice between the two depends mainly on the experiment to be conducted, especially considering that the latter is generally more affordable than the former.

Given the large amount of data collected by microarray experiments, systematic errors frequently occur which may lead to variation in the reported values even for identically replicated experiments. These errors, which may originate from dye intensity effects among other, may make two different arrays or samples not directly comparable. These problems are corrected through a process known as *normalization*, which is a pre-processing step normally required in order to make microarray data comparable and thus plays an important role in the earlier stages of the analysis of these. The main purpose of this procedure is to remove the sources of noise in the gene expression levels measurements. However, no single, universally-accepted method or algorithm exists for achieving this, and the results of the subsequent analysis may depend remarkably on the method used (Park et al., 2003; Quackenbush, 2002; Yang et al., 2001). Normalization may consist of statistical methods (Kerr et al., 2000; Wolfinger et al., 2001), locally weighted scatterplot smoothing (LOWESS) (Cleveland, 1979), subset normalization (Chen et al., 2003), local regression (Kepler et al., 2002), iterative estimation of coefficients (Wang et al., 2002), non-linear methods (Workman et al., 2002), data scaling as well as averaging duplicated values. and can be visualized through an *MA plot*, which can be produced using software tools such as Excel, R, or MATLAB. Genomic data is typically stored in plain text using standardized formats and submitted to publicly-available repositories such as the Gene Expression Omnibus, GenBank or Kaggle for reference and posterior re-use by the academic community. Section 5 presents an example of data mining analysis for the prediction of cancer types from gene expression data stored in text format and available on Kaggle using the modelling technique introduced in Section 3 as well as the software tools presented in Section 4.

3   CLASSIFICATION ANALYSIS

In data mining, as well as in machine learning, *classification analysis* refers to the task of automatically identifying the appropriate *category*, alternatively called the *label* or *class*, for each one of a set of *items*, also called *observations* or *data points*, from a predefined set of known categories. One example of a classification problem is the task of learning how to automatically categorize emails either as *"spam"* or *"not spam"*. In this example, each email is an observation and the possible categories are *"spam"* or *"not spam"*. The purpose of classification analysis is to design a computer program, referred to as the *model* or the *classifier*, that can be trained in order to later be able to identify automatically the class of any new observation. During training, the model is presented with as many observations as possible whose correct categories are already known, with these known observations being called *training data* or *labelled data*, and then *learns* to identify the characteristics of each observation that are predictors of its class. In the case of the emails, for instance, the model would be fed many example emails, some known to be spam and some others known to not be spam, and would be expected to learn to identify the characteristics present in those messages that are known to be spam, e.g., their structure, writing style or their use of certain words, and to differentiate them from those messages whose characteristics indicate they are not spam. Another common application of classification analysis consists of facial recognition, i.e., learning to identify a specific person's face from a set of photos (the observations) who are already known to belong to one of two categories, namely, *"person is present in the photo"* and *"person is not present in the photo"*, where the process of training is analogous. Another example is the automated classification of cancer types based on gene expression read through DNA microarrays, such as in the study conducted by Golub et al. (1999), who train a model in order to automatically categorize patients' acute leukemias as either *acute lymphoblastic leukemia* (ALL) or *acute myeloid leukemia* (AML). During training, the model is given the gene expression data of various patients (the observations) with known diagnoses, either ALL or AML (the categories), and learns to identify the common characteristics present in these data that serve as predictors of either condition. Regardless of the problem being addressed through classification analysis, these characteristics refer to quantifiable properties observed in each item and are often referred to as *features, attributes, independent variables* or *explanatory variables*. The model learns to use these to predict automatically any item's correct category, which is normally referred to as *class*, as explained earlier, or, less frequently, as *dependent variable*. These features may be variables of different types and domains, including real-valued (e.g., a real number to refer to a patient's blood pressure), integer valued (e.g., an integer to represent a patient's age), ordinal (e.g., "low" or "normal" or "high", another way to refer to a patient's blood pressure), or categorical (e.g., "masculine" or "feminine" to refer to a patient's gender). Once the model has been sufficiently trained it is able to use these features in order to predict, with reasonable accuracy, the category of a message not seen before, as in the example of the email classification, or the patient's cancer typein the leukemia example. From the perspective of machine learning, classification analysis is called *supervised learning* because training of the model is conducted over data for which the labels or categories are already known, e.g., the emails which are known to be either spam or not. There are other types of machine learning techniques, also used frequently in data mining, where these labels are neither available nor needed during training, such as *clustering analysis* (described in Section 6), that are thus referred to as *unsupervised learning*.

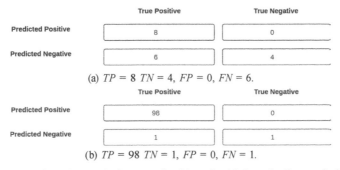

(a) *TP* = 8 *TN* = 4, *FP* = 0, *FN* = 6.

(b) *TP* = 98 *TN* = 1, *FP* = 0, *FN* = 1.

Figure 1 Two examples of a confusion matrix. Plotted with http://onlineconfusionmatrix.com/.

The supreme goal of any classification model, regardless of the specifics of the underlying problem, is to be able to make reliable predictions for future or previously unseen data, e.g., future emails or photos or patients not seen before. Frequently, more than one model is trained over the same labelled data using different learning algorithms and parameterizations of these and then the reliability of each candidate model is evaluated after training in order to assess its predictive performance and choose the best. Various training-evaluation strategies exist, with the choice for each particular problem being normally made prior to training the model and with the most basic of these consisting of randomly partitioning the labelled data into two independent subsets, namely, the *training dataset* and the *testing dataset*. As their names suggest, the former is used first to train the model while the latter is subsequently used to evaluate how accurate the predictions of the resulting model are. Various evaluation metrics are normally used during and after the training of the candidate models in order to determine which of these performs best at the task of generalizing from the training data and identifying the relationships between the items' features and their corresponding categories, which would ultimately lead to better predictions and insights on future previously unseen data. Each one of these evaluation metrics, all computed from the number of correct and mistaken predictions made by the model during testing, has its own meaning and interpretation and can be summarized briefly as follows, for the sake of simplicity, assuming that there are only two classes, which can be referred to as the *positive class* and the *negative class*. It should be noted first, however, that the use of the words "positive" and "negative" in this context is neutral and should not be interpreted as the value or desirability of the class being referred to. In the context of predicting the risk of developing a disease, for instance, the "positive" class could refer to those patients who are "diseased" or in high risk whereas the "negative" class might refer instead to those who are "healthy" or that exhibit a low risk. The number of *true positives* (TP) is the number of observations from the testing dataset where the model correctly predicts the positive class, i.e., the situation where the model predicts the positive class for an observation that is already known to truly belong to this category, whereas the number of *false positives* (FP), also known as *type I error* in statistics, is the number of observations from the testing dataset where the model incorrectly predicts the positive class, i.e., the situation where the model mistakenly predicts the positive class for an observation that is known to actually belong to the negative category. The number of *true negatives* (TN) and *false negatives* (FN), the latter being known also as *type II error* in statistics, are defined analogously. These four metrics are generally tabulated in a *confusion matrix* in order to visualize the performance of the model, as illustrated in Fig. 1. The confusion matrix is simply a table that outlines the predictions made by the model during testing and contrasts them with the corresponding actual values. Also known as the error matrix, it is used in data mining as well as in machine learning and statistics. Figure 1(a) illustrates a confusion matrix from a model evaluated over 18 observations, where 14 of these were known to belong to the positive class and the remaining 4 were known to belong to the negative class. The matrix shows that the model correctly predicted the class of all the negative observations (i.e., $TN = 4$ and $FP = 0$) as well as the correct class of 8 of the positive observations ($TP = 8$), having mistakenly identified the 6 remaining as negative ($FN = 6$). Figure 1(b), on the other hand, depicts a performance evaluation where the test data was composed of 100 examples, 99 of which truly belonged to the positive class whereas the remaining one example belonged to the negative class, and where the classifier under examination commits one false negative and zero false positives.

More descriptive metrics, computed from the false and negative predictions, can be briefly described as follows. A classifier's *accuracy* is defined as the ratio of correct predictions made by the model as shown in Eqn. (1). Accuracy can often be used as an easily interpretable heuristic or rule of thumb to assess immediately whether a model is being trained correctly and how it may perform generally on unseen data. Even though this metric may seem as an intuitive evaluation method it has some limitations, especially when the training data is imbalanced, e.g., when there are only two possible classes in the data with a significant discrepancy between the number of observations belonging to one class and the number of observations belonging to the other, such as in the example depicted in Fig. 1(b). The main drawback from this is that with a training strategy that emphasizes the maximization of this metric, the model may simply 'learn' to indiscriminately predict always the class with the most observations, without actually generalising from the features of these, since this blind approach would still result mostly in correct predictions and hence result in high accuracy scores. For instance, a classifier that ignores the features of all observations and predicts always the positive class would obtain an almost perfect accuracy score in the training data used in the example depicted in Fig. 1(b). Therefore, accuracy is reliable as a performance metric mainly when there are approximately equal number of samples belonging to each class.

$$\text{Accuracy} = \frac{TP + TN}{TP + TN + FP + FN} \tag{1}$$

Precision and *recall* are robust metrics of predictive performance to be used when the classes in the input data are imbalanced, in contrast to accuracy. Both are based on the concept of *relevance*, from the information retrieval theory (Maron and Kuhns, 1960; Schamber, 1994). Algebraically, precision is calculated by dividing the number of true positives by the total number of positive results predicted by the classifier, as shown in Eqn. (2), while recall is calculated by dividing the number of true positives by the number of all relevant samples, i.e., all samples that should have indeed been identified as positive, including those the model failed to retrieve, as shown in Eqn. (3). Precision can be interpreted as the ratio of observations classified by the model as positive that are actually positive whereas recall is indicative of the number of all truly positive observations that are correctly predicted as such by the classifier. A related metric is the *specificity*, shown in Eqn. (4), which is the ratio of true negatives, i.e., the proportion of true negatives that are correctly predicted as such by the classifier.

$$\text{Precision} = \frac{TP}{TP + FP} \tag{2}$$

$$\text{Recall} = \frac{TP}{TP + FN} \tag{3}$$

$$\text{Specificity} = \frac{TN}{TN + FP} \tag{4}$$

Two metrics that provide a balanced view of the classifier's predictive performance are *F*1 and the receiver operating characteristic curve, also known simply as *ROC curve* or *ROC AUC*. *F*1, whose algebraic definition is depicted in Eqn. (5), provides an integrated measure of the evaluated classifier's precision and recall, consisting of the harmonic average of these two metrics. In this manner a model with perfect precision and recall is identified with an *F*1 score of 1, the maximum possible value. This metric can be interpreted then as a balanced measure of how precise the classifier is, in terms of the number truly positive observations it classifies correctly, as well as how robust it is, in terms of not failing to identify a significant number of truly positive observations as such. The *ROC* curve, on the other hand, is a plot of the false positive rate, also known as *sensitivity*, against the true positive rate, also known as *fallout* and shown in Eqn. (6), for various candidate discrimination thresholds between 0 and 1 and the area under, referred to as *ROC AUC*, provides an assessment of model's the predictive power as these thresholds are varied. Therefore, *ROC AUC* can be interpreted as a measure of the trade-off between the true positive rate and false positive rate for a predictive model using different probability thresholds. There are other metrics that are used less frequently, such as *mean absolute error*, *mean squared error*, *logarithmic loss*, among others. The choice of the evaluation metrics to use normally depends on the problem being solved and is a critical step in the design of the prediction model, since these influence how the performance of machine learning algorithms is measured and compared as well as the importance given by the model to the different characteristics in the data and ultimately the best learning algorithm to apply.

$$F1 = \frac{2TP}{2TP + FP + FN} \tag{5}$$

$$\text{Fallout} = 1 - \text{Specificity} = \frac{FP}{FP + TN} \tag{6}$$

Numerous learning techniques and algorithms exist for the implementation of classifiers, including *support vector machines* (SVMs) (Anaissi et al., 2016; Huang et al., 2018; Theera-Ampornpunt et al., 2016), *artificial neural networks* (ANNs) (Mobadersany et al., 2018; Zou et al., 2019), *logistic regression* (Staley et al., 2017; Wienbrandt et al., 2018), *decision trees* (Kretowski, 2019; Ludwig et al., 2018) and *random forests* (Acharjee et al., 2016; Ram et al., 2017), among others. However, this chapter will focus on SVMs, which can be briefly described as follows. When addressing a classification problem using this learning technique, each observation is represented as a point in an *N*-dimensional space, *N* being the number of features, and the objective of the support vector machine algorithm is to find the best *hyperplane* that distinctly separates points belonging to one class from the points belonging to the other. Hyperplanes are boundaries in the *N*-dimensional space can be used to discriminate the data points, which inevitably fall on either side of the hyperplane depending on the class each belongs to. The dimension of the hyperplane is also dependent on the dimensionality of the space, and hence on the number of features found in the training data. The hyperplane has a dimension of 1, i.e., it is a line, when the number of features is 2, i.e., when the space has two dimensions. If, instead, the space is 3-dimensional then the resulting hyperplane has two dimensions. Given any two classes of data points, there may be many possible hyperplanes that separate the two groups and the training algorithm is designed to find the best, namely, the one that imposes the greatest margin or the greatest possible distance between points in different groups. This is illustrated in Fig. 2, which depicts a hypothetical scenario with two-dimensional

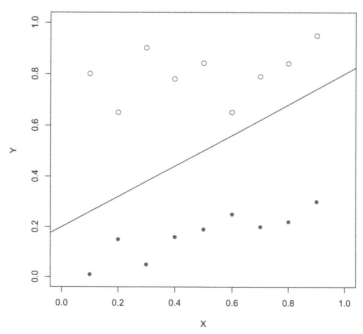

Figure 2   Graphical description of two classes (empty circles and solid circles) in a two-dimensional space being separated by a hyperplane (straight line).

data points, each with attributes x and y (i.e., the coordinate points in space), all distributed into two classes, namely *red* and *blue*. The solution support vector machine is the one that produces the hyperplane (i.e., a line, in this case) that best separates the members of the two categories and that thus serves as the decision boundary, i.e., anything on one side of the hyperplane is predicted to belong to one class while anything on the other side is predicted to belong to the other class. Analogous solutions are found through SVM training in problems with more than two dimensions or features.

Section 5 presents a simple programming example for the training and evaluation of a support vector machine designed to predict the type of cancer to be developed by a patient based on this person's gene expression. This is achieved using the programming tools introduced in Section 4.

4 THE PYTHON PROGRAMMING LANGUAGE AND LIBRARY SCIKIT-LEARN

Python[8] is a programming language used frequently for machine learning, data mining, data science, statistical computing, data analytics and scientific research, including in the biological sciences. It is arguably the most commonly used language in projects requiring data mining or machine learning and has become in recent years increasingly popular not only among computer and data scientists but also among biologists and statisticians, given its ease of use and smooth integration with other programming languages, such as C++, Java, SQL. For this reason, it is widely used by financial institutions and organizations for their internal research. In addition to these advantages, both Python and its most commonly used libraries and packages are free to download and use. What this means in practice is that both the language and most of its accompanying tools can be used for both academic and commercial purposes without having to pay for a usage licence. All these advantages make Python an attractive choice for any beginner wishing to get started with a powerful programming language regardless of the operating system used. Apart from its default features, Python allows the installation of *packages*. Each one of these is a structured collection of code, sometimes written in other programming languages, such as R and C, as well as documentation, and/or data for performing specific types of analyses.

Section 5 presents an example of the training and evaluation of a classifier for cancer type prediction from the patient's gene expression using Python and related libraries. In order to run the example, it is necessary to establish first a workstation in Python on a computer, which can be running any of the most common operating systems, such as Microsoft Windows, Mac OSX, or Ubuntu Linux. The easiest way to install both Python and the required libraries is by first installing Anaconda[9], which is a software package management system that facilitates the download and deployment of both Python and Python related packages and whose installer must be downloaded from its official website, which always contains the updated documentation and installation instructions for each operating system. The installer for Windows computers, for instance, is a .exe downloadable from the website and that must be executed on the destination machine using administrator rights. Generally, the default settings offered by the installer wizard should be used unless specific user requirements stipulate otherwise. For computers running other operating systems, similar instructions must be followed, and the up-to-date detail of these can be found in Anaconda's official website. Once the installation of Anaconda is complete, this package manager must then be used in order to install the required libraries,

---

[8]Python (https://www.python.org/).
[9]Anaconda (https://www.anaconda.com/).

namely scikit-learn[10], numPy[11] and pandas[12], using the instructions provided in each package's official website.

5   CLASSIFICATION OF CANCER TYPES FROM GENE EXPRESSION

This section presents an example of a classification problem showing how a classifier can be trained to predict the category of various cancer types from several patients' genomic data. The dataset was collected and published in the study conducted by Golub et al. (1999), which aimed at showing that cancer can be classified from a patient's gene expression measured through a DNA microarray, i.e., the experiment shows that tumors can be categorized into previously established classes using an appropriately trained classifier. The investigation conducted by these authors consisted of the implementation and training of various models for the automatic classification of cancer tumors as either *acute myeloid leukemia* (AML) or *acute lymphoblastic leukemia* (ALL) and their full dataset is freely available to the general public from Kaggle[13] and distributed in three files: data_set_ALL_AML_train.csv, containing the data for model training, data_set_ALL_AML_train.csv, containing the data for model testing, and actual.csv, containing the known labels of all patients in the study. Each line in the dataset consists of the expression of a single gene and each numbered column refers to a patient while the first two columns are the descriptors of the gene. The training data file contains the gene expression of patients 1 through 38 whereas the test data file contains the gene expression of patients 39 through 72, with each of all these having containing 7,129 values.

The classification example presented in this section is written in Python (version 2.7.16) using library scikit-learn (version 0.23) in order to implement a support vector machine (SVM) to make the cancer type prediction and the full code can be found in supplementary source file classification.py.[14] The purpose of this example is to classify patients as either diagnosed with AML or ALL from their genomic data using the SVM model. The code is divided into six steps that can be briefly described as follows.

The first line of the source file allow the import of the libraries required for the classification analysis to be performed. These are pandas and numPy, for data analysis and manipulation and sklearn (i.e., scikit-learn), which includes the machine learning algorithms to be used, namely, support vector machines. The lines of code that follow after this load the data from the input files, which, as described above, are divided into a training data file (data_set_ALL_AML_train.csv) and a test data file (data_set_ALL_AML_test.csv). As the names of these files clearly indicate, the former includes the data for the training of the classification model, a support vector machine in this case, whereas the latter contains the data to be used for evaluating the predictive performance of the models once the training of these has been completed. After this, the data found in these two files are merged into a single data structure, i.e., variable preprocessed_dataset, after which feature scaling is applied in order to reduce the large variability observable in the gene expression data so that these are in a comparable range. Furthermore, principal component analysis is applied in order to reduce the dimensionality of the data from their original 7,129 features to 38, with the latter figure having been identified as the one that explains around 90% of the variance in the dataset. Once the dataset has been fully pre-processed, the support vector machine model is trained. Prior to this, however, the best possible hyperparameters for

---

[10]scikit-learn (https://scikit-learn.org/).

[11]NumPy (https://numpy.org/).

[12]Pandas (https://pandas.pydata.org/).

[13]Gene expression dataset (Golub et al.) (https://www.kaggle.com/crawford/gene-expression/data).

[14]Online supplementary material (https://cutt.ly/Xc6lasz).

this model over these data are found first in order to optimize the learning process. This is what in machine learning and data mining is referred to as *hyperparameter optimization* or *hyperparameter tuning* and is fundamental for the training since these hyperparameters control the ability of the model to learn from the given data and there is no universal parameterisation that serves optimally in all situations. In classification.py this hyperparameter optimisation is achieved using function GridSearchCV from library scikit-learn. The optimal hyperparameters found are used to train the SVM model, which is subsequently evaluated in terms of various predictive performance metrics, namely, *ROC AUC*, *F*1, accuracy, precision, and recall. The confusion matrix is displayed, showing that the number of true positives is 8 and the number of true negatives is 4, whereas the number of false positives and negatives is 0 and 6, respectively. The performance metrics show that the model achieves a *ROC AUC* score of 0.7, which indicates that the SVM trained is effectively able to differentiate between cancer types, albeit within an error margin.

6 OTHER DATA MINING AND DATA ANALYSIS METHODS IN GENOMICS

While classification analysis is one of the most common applications of data mining and data analysis in genomics there are others that can be briefly described as follows. One of the most recurrent of these is *differential gene expression analysis* (DGEA), i.e., the identification of genes that are significantly down- or up-regulated in an intervention, experimental condition when contrasted to a control, since this is fundamental for the understanding of phenotypic variation (Costa-Silva et al., 2017; Finotello and Di Camillo, 2015; Salentijn et al., 2003; Sulkava et al., 2017; Zambonelli et al., 2016). More specifically, the purpose of a DGEA is the discovery of *differentially expressed genes* (DEG), i.e., those genes that exhibit statistically significant changes in their expression levels within a time period between two and more experimental conditions. Broadly speaking, DGEA consists of taking the normalized read count data and applying statistical tests in order to discover quantitative changes in expression levels between two or more experimental groups. Generally, DGEA consists of comparing the distribution of the gene expression data in one experimental condition, e.g., the samples taken from the control subject, against the distribution of corresponding data in the other condition, e.g., the intervention subject. No universal convention exists for determining when a gene is differentially expressed or not and this categorization may depend on the statistical methods used or the thresholds chosen, all of which there are many. In the same manner as in the methods used for the normalization of microarray data, different techniques for the detection of differentially expressed genes may lead to rather different results (Jaakkola et al., 2017; Rapaport et al., 2013). DGEA is commonly involved in investigations for the identification of a *gene regulatory network* (GRN), which refers to the set of regulatory interactions occurring between groups of genes and transcription factors (Davidson, 2010; Karlebach and Shamir, 2008). These interactions are fundamental for the activities played by the cell within the organism, including the morphogenesis. A GRN is frequently represented graphically as a directed graph indicating and quantifying how some groups of genes are up- or down-regulated by others. These networks can be inferred through the use of ordinary differential equations from the expression levels of individual genes or groups of genes (Carey et al., 2018). Investigations on this topic frequently attempt to identify GRNs in a variety of experimental settings, including those reflecting the organism's response to a pathogen, such as the human immunodeficiency virus (HIV) (Song et al., 2018), the influenza virus (Carey et al., 2018) or the *Bordetella pertussis* bacterium (Deng et al., 2019).

Gene clustering analysis is another method crucially employed when analyzing genomic data. Its purpose, broadly speaking, is to identify *clusters* (i.e., groups) of genes with similar expression patterns over time under the same experimental condition (Carey et al., 2018). In other words, the main purpose is to divide the genes in such a way that those with similar expression patterns fall into the same cluster whereas those with different patterns fall into different clusters. It can be considered an exploratory or descriptive method since it does not depend on previously established hypotheses nor on predefined categories or labels, in contrast to classification analysis (Section 3). Nevertheless, the general assumption is that genes exhibiting similar expression behaviour over time are likely to be either *co-functional*, i.e., share a biological function, or are *co-regulated*, i.e., promote the regulation of others in the same group. Therefore, clustering is useful to initialize data-driven hypotheses that can be examined more closely with complementary methods, such as functional gene annotation. These complementary methods are needed for a variety of reasons, one of which is the fact that there are many genes with unknown functions that may be discovered to be co-regulated with others with known functional roles. Clustering belongs to the type of techniques known as *unsupervised learning*, because it does not rely on previous knowledge about the data under examination, such as known categories or labels. Results obtained from clustering analysis may allow, for instance, to discover groups of genes that undergo similar a similar perturbation in response to a specific experimental condition. Some or many of the differentially expressed genes discovered during the DGEA may exhibit similar expression patterns over time and clustering analysis allows them to be grouped for further examination since they are likely to be playing related biological roles. Furthermore, this clustering reduces the dimensionality of the data for the subsequent identification of the gene regulatory network. The resulting clusters, however, may vary greatly in size. This is because while many co-expressed DEGs may effectively show the same temporal expressions patterns, others may be unique in their patterns (Carey et al., 2018). There are various types of clustering available in data mining, possibly the most commonly known of which is *k-means*, variants of which have been proposed for genomics analysis (Lam and Tsang, 2012). However, in genomics analysis it is common to use *hierarchical clustering analysis* (HCA) which, as the name clearly suggests, aims to identify gene clusters in an ordering or ranking, where the most similar of these are nested together from the bottom to the top (Qin et al., 2003). Examples of statistical analysis procedures in genomics that use hierarchical clustering include the one proposed by Carey et al. (2018) and others (Homayouni et al., 2005; Thalamuthu et al., 2006).

After identification of the DEGs and GRNs, a *gene set enrichment analysis* (GSEA) or *gene functional analysis* is normally conducted. GSEA is the process of determining the functional roles of a group of genes by looking up their known annotations. This is frequently done in order to derive biological interpretations from genomics data, e.g., in order to determine the biological processes involving a set of genes that were previously identified as differentially expressed (Subramanian et al., 2005). GSEA comprises the use of various statistical methods in order to identify classes or groups of genes that are significantly over-represented in the given set and that are likely to be participating together in the same biological processes. Various tools have been proposed for GSEA (Chen et al., 2013, 2009), the most common of which include the *Database for Annotation, Visualization and Integrated Discovery* (DAVID) (Huang et al., 2009; Sherman et al., 2009), which is freely available for public use online[15].

7 SUMMARY

- Bioinformatics is the discipline that aims to devise methods of storage and analysis of biological data, such as sequences and gene expression. Given the large amounts of data that can be collected in a single study as well as the individual volumes of these,

---

[15]Database for Annotation, Visualization and Integrated Discovery (DAVID) (https://david.ncifcrf.gov).

computational methods are required, mainly from branches of computer science, such as data mining as well as related areas, including machine learning, deep learning, data science and big data.

- One of the most common types of data mining is classification analysis, whose applications in genomics include, among others, disease type prediction from gene expression data. An example of this is provided in Section 5.

- Support vector machines are among the most powerful techniques for solving classification analysis problems and scikit-learn, for programming language Python, is one of the most widely used libraries for their implementation. Other classification techniques exist, including neural networks, random forests, decision trees, among many others.

REFERENCES

Acharjee, A., B. Kloosterman, R.G.F. Visser and C. Maliepaard (2016). Integration of multi-omics data for prediction of phenotypic traits using random forest. BMC Bioinformatics. 17(5): 180.

Anaissi, A., M. Goyal, D.R. Catchpoole, A. Braytee and P.J. Kennedy (2016). Ensemble feature learning of genomic data using support vector machine. PLoS One. 11(6): e0157330. doi: 10.1371/journal.pone.0157330.

Baldi, P. and S. Brunak (2001). Bioinformatics: The Machine Learning Approach. MIT Press.

Bashiri, A., M. Ghazisaeedi, R. Safdari, L. Shahmoradi and H. Ehtesham (2017). Improving the prediction of survival in cancer patients by using machine learning techniques: Experience of gene expression data: A narrative review. Iranian Journal of Public Health. 46(2): 165.

Blanco, J.L., M. Gestal, J. Dorado and C. Fernandez-Lozano (2019). Differential gene expression analysis of RNA-seq data using machine learning for cancer research. pp. 27–65. *In*: G. Tsihrintzis, M. Virvou, E. Sakkopoulos and L. Jain (eds). Machine Learning Paradigms. Learning and Analytics in Intelligent Systems, vol 1. Springer, Cham.

Carey, M., J.C. Ramírez, S. Wu and H. Wu (2018). A big data pipeline: Identifying dynamic gene regulatory networks from time-course gene expression omnibus data with applications to influenza infection. Statistical Methods in Medical Research. 27(7): 1930–1955.

Chen, Y.-J., R. Kodell, F. Sistare, K.L. Thompson, S. Morris and J.J. Chen (2003). Normalization methods for analysis of microarray gene-expression data. Journal of Biopharmaceutical Statistics. 13(1): 57–74.

Chen, J., E.E. Bardes, B.J. Aronow and A.G. Jegga (2009). ToppGene suite for gene list enrichment analysis and candidate gene prioritization. Nucleic Acids Research. 37: W305–W311.

Chen, E.Y., C.M. Tan, Y. Kou, Q. Duan, Z. Wang, G.V. Meirelles, et al. (2013). Enrichr: Interactive and collaborative HTML5 gene list enrichment analysis tool. BMC Bioinformatics. 14(1): 128.

Chicco, D. (2017). Ten quick tips for machine learning in computational biology. BioData Mining. 10(1): 35.

Cleveland, W.S. (1979). Robust locally weighted regression and smoothing scatterplots. Journal of the American Statistical Association. 74(368): 829–836.

Costa-Silva, J., D. Domingues and F.M. Lopes (2017). RNA-Seq differential expression analysis: An extended review and a software tool. PLoS One. 12(12): e0190152. doi: 10.1371/journal.pone.0190152

Davidson, E.H. (2010). The Regulatory Genome: Gene Regulatory Networks in Development and Evolution. Elsevier.

Deng, N., J.C. Ramirez, M. Carey, H. Miao, C.A. Arias, A.P. Rice, et al. (2019). Investigation of temporal and spatial heterogeneities of the immune responses to *Bordetella pertussis* infection in the lungs and spleen of mice via analysis and modeling of dynamic microarray gene expression data. Infectious Disease Modelling, 4: 215–226.

Dong, X., M.C. Greven, A. Kundaje, S. Djebali, J.B. Brown, C. Cheng, et al. (2012). Modeling gene expression using chromatin features in various cellular contexts. Genome Biology. 13(9): R53.

Fernandez, M. and D. Miranda-Saavedra (2012). Genome-wide enhancer prediction from epigenetic signatures using genetic algorithm-optimized support vector machines. Nucleic Acids Research. 40(10): e77.

Finotello, F. and B. Di Camillo (2015). Measuring differential gene expression with RNA-seq: challenges and strategies for data analysis. Briefings in Functional Genomics. 14(2): 130–142.

Golub, T.R., D.K. Slonim, P. Tamayo, C. Huard, M. Gaasenbeek, J.P. Mesirov, et al. (1999). Molecular classification of cancer: Class discovery and class prediction by gene expression monitoring. Science. 286(5439): 531–537.

Gulisija, D. and J.B. Plotkin (2017). Phenotypic plasticity promotes recombination and gene clustering in periodic environments. Nature Communications. 8(1): 1–11.

Homayouni, R., K. Heinrich, L. Wei and M.W. Berry (2005). Gene clustering by latent semantic indexing of MEDLINE abstracts. Bioinformatics. 21(1): 104–115.

Huang, D.W., B.T. Sherman and R.A. Lempicki (2009). Bioinformatics enrichment tools: Paths toward the comprehensive functional analysis of large gene lists. Nucleic Acids Res. 37(1): 1–13.

Huang, S., N. Cai, P.P. Pacheco, S. Narrandes, Y. Wang and W. Xu (2018). Applications of support vector machine (SVM) learning in cancer genomics. Cancer Genomics-Proteomics, 15(1): 41–51.

Huet, S., B. Tesson, J.-P. Jais, A.L. Feldman, L. Magnano, E. Thomas, et al. (2018). A gene-expression profiling score for outcome prediction disease in patients with follicular lymphoma: a retrospective analysis on three international cohorts. The Lancet. 19(4): 549.

Jaakkola, M.K., F. Seyednasrollah, A. Mehmood and L.L. Elo (2017). Comparison of methods to detect differentially expressed genes between single-cell populations. Briefings in Bioinformatics. 18(5): 735–743.

Karlebach, G. and R. Shamir (2008). Modelling and analysis of gene regulatory networks. Nature Reviews Molecular Cell Biology. 9(10): 770–780.

Kepler, T.B., L. Crosby and K.T. Morgan (2002). Normalization and analysis of DNA microarray data by self-consistency and local regression. Genome Biol. 3(7): RESEARCH0037. doi: 10.1186/gb-2002-3-7-research0037.

Kerr, M.K., M. Martin and G.A. Churchill (2000). Analysis of variance for gene expression microarray data. Journal of Computational Biology. 7(6): 819–837.

Kourou, K., T.P. Exarchos, K.P. Exarchos, M.V. Karamouzis and D.I. Fotiadis (2015). Machine learning applications in cancer prognosis and prediction. Computational and Structural Biotechnology Journal. 13: 8–17.

Kretowski, M. (2019). Multi-test decision trees for gene expression data. pp. 131–142. *In*: M. Kretowski (ed.). Evolutionary Decision Trees in Large-Scale Data Mining. Studies in Big Data, vol 59. Springer, Cham.

Lam, Y.K. and P.W.M. Tsang (2012). eXploratory K-Means: A new simple and efficient algorithm for gene clustering. Applied Soft Computing. 12(3): 1149–1157.

Larranaga, P., B. Calvo, R. Santana, C. Bielza, J. Galdiano, I. Inza, et al. (2006). Machine learning in bioinformatics. Briefings in Bioinformatics. 7(1): 86–112.

Lomsadze, A., K. Gemayel, S. Tang and M. Borodovsky (2018). Modeling leaderless transcription and atypical genes results in more accurate gene prediction in prokaryotes. Genome Research. 28(7): 1079–1089.

Ludwig, S.A., S. Picek and D. Jakobovic (2018). Classification of cancer data: Analyzing gene expression data using a fuzzy decision tree algorithm. pp. 327–347. *In*: C. Kahraman and Y. Topcu (eds). Operations Research Applications in Health Care Management. International Series in Operations Research & Management Science, vol 262. Springer, Cham.

Maron, M.E. and J.L. Kuhns (1960). On relevance, probabilistic indexing and information retrieval. Journal of the ACM. 7(3): 216–244.

Mathé, C., M.-F. Sagot, T. Schiex and P. Rouzé (2002). Current methods of gene prediction, their strengths and weaknesses. Nucleic Acids Research. 30(19): 4103–4117.

Mobadersany, P., S. Yousefi, M. Amgad, D.A. Gutman, J.S. Barnholtz-Sloan, J.E.V. Vega, et al. (2018). Predicting cancer outcomes from histology and genomics using convolutional networks. Proceedings of the National Academy of Sciences. 115(13): E2970–E2979.

Mochida, K., S. Koda, K. Inoue and R. Nishii (2018). Statistical and machine learning approaches to predict gene regulatory networks from transcriptome datasets. Frontiers in Plant Science. 9: 1770.

Ni, Y., D. Aghamirzaie, H. Elmarakeby, E. Collakova, S. Li, R. Grene, et al. (2016). A machine learning approach to predict gene regulatory networks in seed development in Arabidopsis. Frontiers in Plant Science. 7: 1936.

Park, T., S.-G. Yi, S.-H. Kang, S. Lee, Y.-S. Lee and R. Simon (2003). Evaluation of normalization methods for microarray data. BMC Bioinformatics. 4(1): 33.

Park, C., J. Ha and S. Park (2020). Prediction of Alzheimer's disease based on deep neural network by integrating gene expression and DNA methylation dataset. Expert Systems with Applications. 140: 112873.

Qin, J., D.P. Lewis and W.S. Noble (2003). Kernel hierarchical gene clustering from microarray expression data. Bioinformatics. 19(16): 2097–2104.

Quackenbush, J. (2002). Microarray data normalization and transformation. Nature Genetics. 32(4): 496–501.

Ram, M., A. Najafi and M.T. Shakeri (2017). Classification and biomarker genes selection for cancer gene expression data using random forest. Iranian Journal of Pathology. 12(4): 339.

Rapaport, F., R. Khanin, Y. Liang, M. Pirun, A. Krek, P. Zumbo, et al. (2013). Comprehensive evaluation of differential gene expression analysis methods for RNA-seq data. Genome Biology. 14(9): 3158.

Salem, H., G. Attiya and N. El-Fishawy (2017). Classification of human cancer diseases by gene expression profiles. Applied Soft Computing. 50: 124–134.

Salentijn, E.M.J., A. Aharoni, J.G. Schaart, M.J. Boone and F.A. Krens (2003). Differential gene expression analysis of strawberry cultivars that differ in fruit-firmness. Physiologia Plantarum. 118(4): 571–578.

Schamber, L. (1994). Relevance and information behavior. Annual Review of Information Science and Technology (ARIST). 29: 3–48.

Senior, A.W., R. Evans, J. Jumper, J. Kirkpatrick, L. Sifre, T. Green, et al. (2020). Improved protein structure prediction using potentials from deep learning. Nature. 577: 706–710.

Shedden, K., J.M.G. Taylor, S.A. Enkemann, M.-S. Tsao, T.J. Yeatman, W.L. Gerald, et al. (2008). Gene expression–based survival prediction in lung adenocarcinoma: A multi-site, blinded validation study. Nature Medicine. 14(8822).

Sherman, B.T., R.A. Lempicki, D.W. Huang, B.T. Sherman and R.A. Lempicki. (2009). Systematic and integrative analysis of large gene lists using DAVID bioinformatics resources. Nat. Protoc. 4(1): 44–57.

Song, J., M. Carey, H. Zhu, H. Miao, J.C. Ramírez and H. Wu (2018). Identifying the dynamic gene regulatory network during latent HIV-1 reactivation using high-dimensional ordinary differential equations. International Journal of Computational Biology and Drug Design. 11(1-2): 135–153.

Spies, D., P.F. Renz, T.A. Beyer and C. Ciaudo (2019). Comparative analysis of differential gene expression tools for RNA sequencing time course data. Briefings in Bioinformatics. 20(1): 288–298.

Staley, J.R., E. Jones, S. Kaptoge, A.S. Butterworth, M.J. Sweeting, A.M. Wood, et al. (2017). A comparison of Cox and logistic regression for use in genome-wide association studies of cohort and case-cohort design. European Journal of Human Genetics. 25(7): 854–862.

Subramanian, A., P. Tamayo, V.K. Mootha, S. Mukherjee, B.L. Ebert, M.A. Gillette, et al. (2005). Gene set enrichment analysis: A knowledge-based approach for interpreting genome-wide expression profiles. Proceedings of the National Academy of Sciences. 102(43): 15545–15550.

Sulkava, M., E. Raitoharju, M. Levula, I. Seppälä, L.-P. Lyytikäinen, A. Mennander, et al. (2017). Differentially expressed genes and canonical pathway expression in human atherosclerotic plaques– Tampere Vascular Study. Scientific Reports. 7(1): 1–10.

Thalamuthu, A., I. Mukhopadhyay, X. Zheng and G.C. Tseng (2006). Evaluation and comparison of gene clustering methods in microarray analysis. Bioinformatics. 22(19): 2405–2412.

Theera-Ampornpunt, N., S.G. Kim, A. Ghoshal, S. Bagchi, A. Grama and S. Chaterji (2016). Fast training on large genomics data using distributed support vector machines. pp. 1–8. *In*: 8th International Conference on Communication Systems and Networks (COMSNETS), 2016. IEEE.

Wang, Y., J. Lu, R. Lee, Z. Gu and R. Clarke (2002). Iterative normalization of cDNA microarray data. IEEE Transactions on Information Technology in Biomedicine. 6(1): 29–37.

Wang, L., H.L. McLeod and R.M. Weinshilboum (2011). Genomics and drug response. New England Journal of Medicine. 364(12): 1144–1153.

Wienbrandt, L., J.C. Kässens, M. Hübenthal and D. Ellinghaus (2018). 1,000 x Faster than PLINK: Genome-wide epistasis detection with logistic regression using combined FPGA and GPU accelerators. pp. 368–381. *In*: International Conference on Computational Science. Springer.

Wolfinger, R.D., G. Gibson, E.D. Wolfinger, L. Bennett, H. Hamadeh, P. Bushel, et al. (2001). Assessing gene significance from cDNA microarray expression data via mixed models. Journal of Computational Biology. 8(6): 625–637.

Workman, C., L.J. Jensen, H. Jarmer, R. Berka, L. Gautier, H.B. Nielser, et al. (2002). A new non-linear normalization method for reducing variability in DNA microarray experiments. Genome Biol. 3(9): research0048. doi: 10.1186/gb-2002-3-9-research0048.

Yang, Y.H., S. Dudoit, P. Luu and T.P. Speed (2001). Normalization for cDNA microarry data. pp. 141–152. *In*: M.L. Bittner, Y. Chen, A.N. Dorsel and E.R. Dougherty (eds). Microarrays: Optical Technologies and Informatics, vol. 4266. International Society for Optics and Photonics, Bellingham.

Zambonelli, P., M. Zappaterra, F. Soglia, M. Petracci, F. Sirri, C. Cavani, et al. (2016). Detection of differentially expressed genes in broiler pectoralis major muscle affected by White Striping–Wooden Breast myopathies. Poultry Science. 95(12): 2771–2785.

Zareizadeh, Z., M.S. Helfroush, A. Rahideh and K. Kazemi (2018). A robust gene clustering algorithm based on clonal selection in multiobjective optimization framework. Expert Systems with Applications, 113: 301–314.

Zhou, J. and O.G. Troyanskaya (2015). Predicting effects of noncoding variants with deep learning–based sequence model. Nature Methods. 12(10): 931–934.

Zhou, J., C.L. Theesfeld, K. Yao, K.M. Chen, A.K. Wong and O.G. Troyanskaya (2018). Deep learning sequence-based ab initio prediction of variant effects on expression and disease risk. Nature Genetics. 50(8): 1171–1179.

Zou, J., M. Huss, A. Abid, P. Mohammadi, A. Torkamani and A. Telenti (2019). A primer on deep learning in genomics. Nature Genetics. 51(1): 12–18.

CHAPTER 5

Bioinformatics of Genome-wide Expression Studies

Hugo Tovar[1]*, Diana E. Alvarez-Suarez[2],
Laura Gómez-Romero[1] and Enrique Hernández-Lemus[1,3]

[1]Computational Genomics Division, National Institute of Genomic Medicine, Mexico

[2]Medical Research Unit in Infectious Diseases, Hospital de Pediatría, CMN SXXI, Instituto Mexicano del Seguro Social, Mexico City, Mexico

[3]Center for Complexity Sciences, Universidad Nacional Autónoma de México, Mexico

1 INTRODUCTION

Genome-wide analysis of gene expression, also known as transcriptomics, is the study of all RNA transcripts in an individual or a population of cells. It has been used to refer to all RNAs or just protein-coding RNAs. Usually, based on data from high throughput sequencing or expression microarrays, it tries to find a specific combination of genes that are turned on (expressed) or turned off (repressed) and dictates cellular morphology (shape) of a particular cell or tissue type, condition, disease, or phenotype (Ralston and Shaw, 2008).

Gene expression is regulated by factors both internal and external. The interaction between these signals and the genome affects essentially all their molecular functions. External factors that regulate expression include environmental conditions, such as temperature, oxygen, small molecules, and secreted proteins. In the case of internal factors, cells communicate between them by sending and receiving secreted proteins, also known as growth factors, cytokines, morphogens, or signaling molecules (Adams, 2008). Gene expression is controlled by multiple molecular systems. This becomes more elaborate as one advance in evolutionary complexity.

*Corresponding author: *hatovar@inmegen.gob.mx*

Among the most important systems in eukaryotes are transcription factors. These are proteins that bind to specific DNA sequences and that can act independently or in concert (Harbison, 2004). In addition, another important system is that chromatin remodeling can allow or prevent transcriptional machinery from transiting to their DNA binding sites (Kornberg and Lorch, 1992; Mellor, 2005).

The first study to investigate the complete transcriptome of a cell type, published by Velculescu et al. (1997) describes 60,633 *Saccharomyces cerevisiae* transcripts using serial analysis of gene expression (SAGE) (Velculescu et al., 1997). With the increase in computational power and the successful advancement of bioinformatics, it became increasingly easy to analyze the vast amounts of data generated by high-throughput sequencing technologies (Jimenez-Chillaron et al., 2014). During the decade of 1980, the attempts to characterize the transcriptome increased (Pertea, 2012). From the decade of 1990 until the beginning of the 21st century, several techniques were developed to quantify the RNA of different cells or tissues, such as expressed tag sequences, serial gene expression analysis (SAGE), cap expression analysis genetics (CAGE) and massively parallel signature sequencing (MPSS) to identify portions of transcripts that were expressed (Brenner et al., 2000; Kodzius et al., 2006; Shiraki et al., 2003; Velculescu, 1995). However, the two techniques that dominated the field of transcriptomics were, expression microarrays and RNA-Seq. That is why this chapter will focus on the bioinformatics of these two types of experiments.

Microarrays and RNA-Seq experiments produce a large amount of data and need significant computing power to produce reliable results (Huber et al., 2015; Ritchie et al., 2015; Robinson et al., 2010; Smyth, 2005). The raw image output files from microarrays contain around 1 GB of information. These are generated through high-resolution images that require feature detection and spectral analysis (Govindarajan et al., 2012). The processed intensity files contain around 70 MB. To analyze this vast amount of data, statistical models are required to test assumptions involved in the design of microarrays, for example, several probes that target a single transcript can give information on the intron-exon structure of such transcript so a statistical model to aggregate this information would be required, or the normalization between samples by the background intensity per sample would be needed to compare different experiments (Gautier et al., 2004; Petrov and Shams, 2004; Ritchie et al., 2015).

RNA-Seq experiments, on the other hand, produce billions of short DNA sequences (reads) that need to be aligned against a reference genome made up of millions to billions of pairs of bases. *De novo* assembly of this number of reads requires the construction of highly complex sequence graphs (Haas et al., 2013). RNA-Seq operations are highly repetitive and benefit from parallel computing, indeed modern algorithms only require a medium desktop computer for simple transcriptomic experiments if no *de novo* assembly is required (Haas et al., 2013; Patro et al., 2017; Pertea et al., 2015). For example, using 30 million 100 bp length RNA-Seq readings for *Homo sapiens* samples[1] would be enough to capture its transcriptome accurately (Conesa et al., 2016; Hart et al., 2013). The fastq files in this example occupied, per sample, around 2 gigabytes of disk space. Count files are much smaller, as well as those intensity files generated for microarray.

Data analysis usually requires a combination of bioinformatics software tools that vary according to the experimental design and goals. The process can be broken down into four stages: quality control, alignment, quantification, and final analysis, to answer the research question (Verk et al., 2013). Most popular bioinformatics programs are run from a command-line interface, either

---

[1]The most studied organism. At the time of writing this, the GEO has 1,960,452 human transcriptome samples, while *Mus musculus*, the organism that follows it in the number of samples, has 900,070, less than half. Other organisms are *Rattus norvegicus* 98,920, *Arabidopsis thaliana* 61,563, *Drosophila melanogaster* 68,714, *Saccharomyces cere-visiae* 65,379 and *Danio rerio* 24,730.

in a Linux-like environment or within the R/Bioconductor (Huber et al., 2015; R Core Team, 2020) statistical environment[2].

2   TECHNOLOGIES

Although the questions that are often asked the most commonly used technologies to measure genome-wide expression coincide on many occasions, it is important to know details of each technology to know its scope and limitations as well as the characteristic biases of each one.

The first transcriptome annotations began with cDNA libraries in the 1980s. The advent of high-performance technologies led to faster and more efficient ways of obtaining data on the transcriptome. Two biological techniques are mainly used for genome-wide expression studies: 1) expression microarrays, a hybridization-based technique, and 2) RNA-seq, an approach based on high throughput sequencing (Cellerino and Sanguanini, 2018). RNA-seq is the method that the research community has chosen in the last decade (2010) based on its ability to discover novel transcripts, identify sequence variants, and its increased dynamic range on signal detection leading to increased fold change derived from expression levels (Raghavachari et al., 2012). However, expression microarrays are still used most of the time for their more accessible cost in large sample projects and their relative simplicity for preprocessing and analysis.

Single-Cell RNA-Seq (scRNA-seq) is a technology derived from RNA-Seq that is having a great adoption. scRNA-Seq is about to measure genome-wide expression within individual cells. For this reason, we have added a special section for this flourishing technique.

2.1   Microarrays Experiments

The first genome-wide expression studies were based on microarray techniques (also known as DNA chips). Techniques such as reverse transcriptase-polymerase chain reaction (RT-PCR) and Northern blot allow us to determine the expression of a few genes per experiment. But microarrays or "global expression profiling" allow us to measure genome-wide expression which helps to see the whole picture without having to focus only on some genes (Govindarajan et al., 2012). Microarrays consist of glass layers with spots in which they have grouped oligonucleotides, known as "probes"; each spot contains a known DNA sequence in a know position (Schena et al., 1995). Hybridization of complementary strands, the property of nucleic acids to specifically pair with another strand that is complementary, is the central principle of how microarrays work. Two chains highly complementary will have many tight non-covalent junctions between the two chains. Sequences with non-specific (non-complementary) junctions will be broken with a wash leaving only tightly paired chains attached (Govindarajan et al., 2012). Fluoroscent labeled target sequences that bind to a probe sequence generate a signal that is dependent on hybridization conditions (such as temperature) and washing after hybridization (Govindarajan et al., 2012). Transcript abundance is determined by estimating the fluorescence of these labeled

---

[2]*R* and *Bioconductor* have played a fundamental role in the history of Bioinformatics. *R* (Ross Ihaka and Robert Gentleman, New Zealand 1995) is a programming language and a statistical software environment. This gives it a great advantage for the world of Bioinformatics and is that non-literate users in informatics (Biologists, Biomedics, MDs, Biochemists, among others) begin by using their part of the environment and, by interacting with it, they learn to make use of the programming language. It is the point where biological knowledge meets computer knowledge. On the other hand, *Bioconductor* is an international initiative for the creative collaboration of exclusive Bioinformatics software based in *R* language. It is a free access database (with 2,041 packages on June 24, 2021) with the latest algorithms for bioinformatic analysis. Its great attraction for developers of bioinformatics methods is: being free software, ease of use and many information resources on the net.

target sequences (Barbulovic-Nad et al., 2006). The fluorescence intensity of each spot indicates the abundance of transcript for the specific sequence of that probe (Petrov et al., 2004). For microarray experiments, mRNA is collected from the samples. This mRNA is converted to cDNA to increase its stability and is labeled with colored fluorophores (generally red and green). The cDNA is spread over the microarray surface where it hybridizes with the oligonucleotides on the chip and a laser is used to scan it (Govindarajan et al., 2012).

A microarray generally contains enough oligonucleotides to represent all known genes; the new generations of expression microarrays now report not only mRNA but also miRNA, lncRNA, make an evaluation at the transcript level, not the gene level and report the presence of junctions between transcripts in order to determine splicing variants (for example the Affymetrix GeneChip[TM] Human Transcriptome Array 2.0 or HTA2.0). Also, some works have found that microarrays have a performance equal or even better in some respects than RNA-Seq (Romero et al., 2018; Zhang et al., 2015). However, the data obtained using microarrays do not provide information on unknown genes, mutations, or genetic alterations such as gene fusions. For these reasons, during the 2010s, the use of microarrays was reduced, at least in the field of research, in favor of RNA-Seq based on RNA sequencing.

2.1.1   Preprocessing Microarray Data

In any technology, low-level analysis or preprocessing is a crucial initial step before data analysis is performed. The purpose of preprocessing is to minimize the effects caused by technical variations and, as a result, allow the data to be comparable in order to find actual biological changes. In microarray technology, preprocessing removes systematic errors between arrays, introduced by labeling, hybridization, and scanning (Fujita et al., 2006; Shakya et al., 2010). Commonly, since the microarrays are printed by large companies such as Illumina or Thermo Fisher[3], these companies provide proprietary software for its customers for preprocessing and analysis of microarrays. Thermo Fisher offers Transcriptome Analysis Console (TAC) Software and Illumina offers a web-based service Basespace with a prepaid system. Both offer an analysis pipeline (Workbench) to analyze the results of their platforms. However, bioinformaticians prefer to use open-access tools such as those hosted in Bioconductor, a collaborative project for creating extensible software for computational biology and bioinformatics (Gentleman et al., 2004) based on R. Since the packages distributed by the manufacturers are easy to use, here we will focus on the packages and tools developed by the open-source software community that, although involving a higher learning curve, offer more transparency and flexibility than proprietary software; incidentally, a characteristic of fundamental importance for scientific research.

Figure 1 shows a typical expression microarray data preprocessing pipeline after being read and interpreted by the scanner. Some R packages know how to deal with the raw formats in which the intensity information of the probes is stored, most of the time this is a table in plain text with the name of the probe, the value of intensity, and maybe a p-value. In the case of Illumina[4] the raw files are txt files and in the case of the Termo Fisher/Affymetrix chips (hereafter referred to as Affymetrix arrays), the raw files are CEL files which can be either plain text or binary tables. For the raw files of Illumina's HumanHT-12 microarrays there is a package available in Bioconductor capable of dealing with the format of its intensity files called beadarray (Dunning et al., 2007). In the case of Affymetrix microarrays, more packages

---

[3]In 2016 Thermo Fisher Scientific Inc. acquired Affymetrix, Inc. and, with it, the most important line of microarrays on the market. Its Human Genome U133 microarray, which in its latest version can measure 47,000 transcripts which represent around 39,000 best-annotated genes, is the most common genome-wide expression microarray in the GEO database, in addition to the latest generation Affymetrix HTA2.0 microarray mentioned above.

[4]for example, the HumanHT-12 Expression BeadChip which has been discontinued to make way for its RNA-seq applications, but which, however, there are still around 90,000 samples available in the GEO.

are available but perhaps the most important are affy (Gautier et al., 2004) and oligo (Carvalho and Irizarry, 2010). Besides, there is another not so commonly used but newer package called affxparser (Bengtsson et al., 2020)[5]. After importing the raw files, a background correction is made, which includes a wide variety of methods. A background correction method should include any, if not all, of the following: correct background noise and processing effects, adjust binding of nonspecific DNA (cross-hybridization), and adjust expression estimates so that they fall on the proper scale (Bolstad, 2008). Background correction tools are affy and limma (Ritchie et al., 2015). Normalization is one of the most important steps in preprocessing. It involves eliminating unwanted non-biological variations that could exist between chips in a microarray experiment. There are two types of variation in a microarray, one that is related with the biological phenomena and the other that is not. The latter is known as obscuring variation or technical variation and is the one the standardization seeks to eliminate (Bolstad, 2008; Gautier et al., 2004; Ritchie et al., 2015). The source of the obscuring variation may include differences in the scanner configuration, the amounts of hybridized mRNA, the order in which the samples were processed, differences in operation between technicians, among many other factors. An important consideration to make when applying a normalization method is to account for how many genes are expected to change within a condition compared to how many genes are expected to change between conditions. Ideally, changes within one condition are expected to be minimal while they are expected to be larger between conditions. Moreover, in many cases treatments are not randomized or conditions are confused with the source of biological variance. For this reason, normalization is always executed on the total of the data as if it were a single group (Bolstad, 2008; Leek et al., 2010; Ritchie et al., 2015).

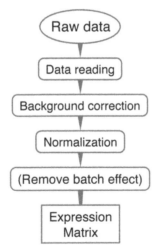

Figure 1 A preprocessing pipeline for Microarray data. Whether it is the result of a study or a meta-analysis, this process is followed for all samples involved in a project, both cases and controls. The flow starts with the intensity files of the microarray. The format of this file is specific to each manufacturer and, therefore, a suitable package must be found. The .CEL files characteristic of Affymetrix microarrays are well supported by packages affy (Gautier et al., 2004) and oligo (Carvalho and Irizarry, 2010). In the background correction step, the intensity detected around the probes is considered to try to adjust their intensity Silver: 2009. For Affymetrix microarrays, the package frma (McCall et al., 2010) performs normalization and background correction in one step. Depending on the experimental design, it will be necessary to eliminate the batch effect. See text for further explanation. The result is a matrix with the normalized expression for all samples.

---

[5]The authors of this work have not yet tested this software since we discovered it while writing this chapter.

However, there are cases where these elements of confusion are more important, as in the case of experiments where the samples are taken over a long time, or processed in different laboratories, or even where samples from different studies are being reused to re-analyze them in another context. In this cases, it is required to try to eliminate the batch effect. The term "batch" refers to the set of microarrays that are processed in one place for a short time. And the "batch effects" are the effects caused, not by the biological reason of the object of study, but by just the variations that imply being in different "batches" (Chen et al., 2011; Leek et al., 2010; Nygaard et al., 2015; Scherer, 2009). Suppose, for example, that all healthy patients are processed during the day and the sick patients at night. The effect of the disease will be confused with that of the processing hours. Figure 2 shows the expression density distribution of a study from multiple studies carried out with 880 microarrays of expression (819 corresponding to breast cancer tissue and 61 to adjacent normal tissue) (Tovar et al., 2015). Each one of the preprocessing stages affects the structure of the data. In this work, Combat (Johnson et al., 2007) (included in the sva (Leek et al., 2012) package) was used to remove the batch effect. This tool is one of the most used methods for it. Although Luo et al. (2010) found that the efficiency of the other methods available to remove the batch effect is very similar (Luo et al., 2010). It is worth mentioning that the expression microarray preprocessing analyzes (including the example of 880 samples) require a low computation capacity, so it can be run on a desktop computer.

2.2 RNA-seq Experiments

RNA sequencing is a next-generation sequencing technology. Unlike expression microarray, it does not require any prior knowledge and requires less RNA (Jimenez-Chillaron et al., 2014). RNA-seq, in addition to allowing a measurement of the relative amount of transcripts in an RNA sample (quantitative analysis), allows the discovery of new transcripts (qualitative analysis) (Cellerino and Sanguanini, 2018). The first work using the RNA-seq technique was published in 2006 (Bainbridge et al., 2006) however this work only generated 200,000 reads of 110 bp in length. Since a very high number of reads (the higher the better) is required for the high-throughput sequencing approach to be successful, the technology was not effective until Illumina (called Solexa at the time) developed a very short read technique (25 bp at the time) but with a number of total reads in the order of millions. Then, in 2008, three articles were published testing this technique (Mortazavi et al., 2008; Sultan et al., 2008; Wilhelm et al., 2008) that launched RNA-seq as the technique of choice for genome-wide transcriptomic research (McGettigan, 2013). Specifically, the technique implemented by Illumina, which was also adopted by laboratories such as the Broad Institute or the European Molecular Biology Laboratory-European Bioinformatics Institute (EMBL-EBI) that carry out large-scale projects such as The International Genome Sample Resource.

Cellerino and Sanguanini (2018) mention five advantages of RNA-Seq technology:

1. As already mentioned at the beginning of this section, in addition to quantitatively estimating the number of transcripts, you can describe them qualitatively.
2. The results have a resolution per base, which allows studying characteristics such as RNA editing or Single Nucleotide Polymorphisms (SNPs).
3. Since it does not require prior knowledge (as for the microarray expression tests), it is a potentially unbiased source of transcriptional information.
4. The results are generated in open formats and are not linked to a specific "hardware" allowing the quantification of transcripts regardless of the species and
5. Their simplicity has practically no limits, that is, with sufficient coverage, it would be possible to detect changes that happen in a single RNA molecule in a single cell.

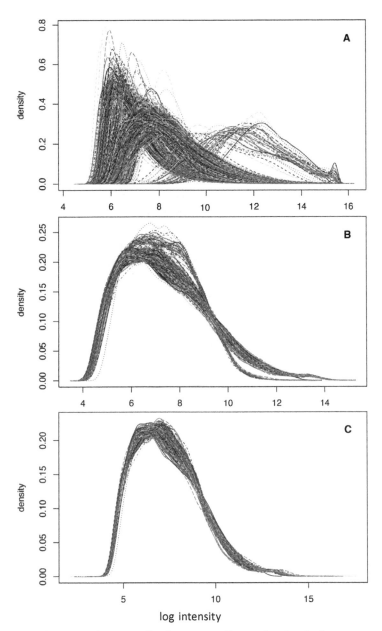

Figure 2 Expression microarray data normalization process. Expression data in three stages of advancement. In A you can see the density plot of the raw data corresponding to 880 samples from 10 different GEO datasets. In B, you can see the normalization made with the fRMA algorithm (McCall et al., 2010) implemented in the package frma in Bioconductor. Lastly, the ComBat algorithm (Johnson et al., 2007) implemented in the package sva also in Bioconductor to remove the batch effect (Tovar et al., 2015). Note the sudden change in density scale from A to B and the decrease of variability in C.

However, care must be taken not to find biological signals in transcriptional noise (Cellerino and Sanguanini, 2018).

The sequencing of the transcriptome of a biological sample consists of three steps: first, the RNA must be purified, then an RNA library must be synthesized and converted to cDNA, and finally, the library must be sequenced (Cellerino and Sanguanini, 2018). Regarding the purification step, the main problem is to extract the RNA of interest. There are three main categories of RNA: messenger RNA (mRNA) which encods proteins ($\gg$ 100 bp), long non-coding RNA ($>$ 100 bp, such as rRNA, snRNA, lncRNA) and short non-coding RNAs ($\ll$ 100 bp – tRNAs, miRNAs and related, snoRNAs, piRNAs, among others) (Cellerino and Sanguanini, 2018). It is necessary to take advantage of the specific characteristics of each of these types of RNA to be able to keep that specific portion; in this chapter we will focus on mRNA since it informs us about the genes that are being expressed in certain tissues. The implications that this step will have during bioinformatic analysis are primarily dealing with contamination, either from other organisms or from parts of unwanted RNA in the data. It will be common to find a significant proportion of rRNA (ribosomal RNA) in samples if this step is not carried out carefully.

The second step is the generation of the library. Some decisions taken at this step will greatly impact the way bioinformatics analysis is done. The generation of libraries is, essentially, the fragmentation of genetic material, generally by enzymatic methods. During this procedure, the size of the insert is decided, that is, the approximate size of the sequence fragments between adapter and adapter (between 50 and 300 bp commonly). An adapter is a short, asymmetric DNA fragment that is attached using a T4-RNA ligase to the ends of the sequencing fragments (Cellerino and Sanguanini, 2018). It is used both as a primer for elongation of sequencing fragments and to fix them to the plate. Since its sequence is known, it can be eliminated bioinformatically but in some circumstances (for example, libraries with very different fragment sizes) it could be prone to cause alignment problems. Likewise, in this step you choose whether the sequencing will be single-end or paired-end. Figure 3 illustrates the main differences between these strategies. Using the Paired-end technique, the boundaries of a fragment can be sequenced to facilitate the reconstruction of the original transcript. It is also very useful for detecting alternative splicing or even aberrant gene fusions trough bioinformatics methods (with tools such as FusionCatcher (Nicorici et al., 2014) or Star-Fusion (Haas et al., 2019). After fragmentation and binding of the primers, conversion to cDNA is carried out through a process commonly called reverse transcription-polymerase chain reaction (Rio, 2014; Salomon, 1995).

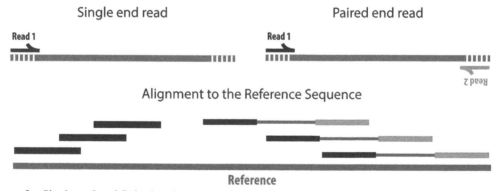

Figure 3 Single-end and Paired-end. In the paired-end strategy, it is sequenced in both chains without losing the information of the size of the reading. This helps in the reconstruction of the transcriptome through mapping.

The last part of the process, the sequencing by synthesis of the library, is carried out fully automated in the sequencer and is explained in great detail by Shendurre and Ji (2008). The sequencer generates files in fastq format (Cock et al., 2009) that, together with the fasta format, is the most popular format for distributing reference genomes are formats widely used in bioinformatics. The main characteristic of fastq format is that it reports the resulting sequence together with a quality score [Phred (Cock et al., 2009)] per base. This score is computed by the same sequencer. The Phred score will be used by the quality control tools to evaluate the sequencing process.

2.2.1 Preprocessing RNA-seq Data

As in microarrays data, the purpose of preprocessing RNA-seq data is to minimize the effects caused by technical variations and, as a result, allow the data to be comparable in order to find actual biological changes. Since RNA-seq technology is very different in many ways from microarrays technology, the preprocessing workflow is also different (Fig. 4).

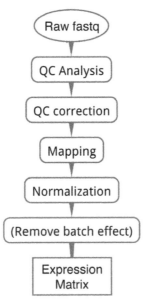

Figure 4 A preprocessing pipeline for RNA-seq data. The flow starts from the fastq files generated by the sequencer. Quality analysis is done on them. FastQC has become the standard of this step due to its speed and ease of use, in addition to generating a very complete and easy-to-view report. This report helps make decisions about what steps to take to improve the quality of the sequence. These corrections commonly include trimming the end of sequences or removing adapters or readings recognized as contamination. In addition to Trimmomatic, Trim Galore and Cutadapt mentioned in the text, we could also mention FASTX-toolkit and Seqtk (Shen et al., 2016) for being flexible tools that allow not only trimming fastq files but also help in many aspects of their manipulation. Mapping to a reference genome if one is available or to the de novo assembly in the opposite case. This alignment, as mentioned in the text, can be direct to the reference, or with splice-aware aligners or with pseudoaligners like the one used by Salmon (see later). Remove batch effect is an important step but its performance depends on the design of the experiment or the way of collecting the data. Although ComBat's algorithm can be used, it requires its specialized application for RNA-seq data in development in ComBat-seq (Zhang et al., 2020) or with new methods such as scBatch (Fei and Yu, 2020). The result is a matrix where the genes are in the lines and the samples are in the columns.

The first important change is the universal output format independent of the sequencer brand. This results in a ready-to-use sequencing format that can be interpreted by any of the available open-source software for all downstream processing steps. The quality control analysis evaluates the Phred score per base estimated by the sequencer. Generally, it is considered a good score if the Phred of a base exceeds the value of 28, an acceptable score if it is between 20 and 28 and bad if it is lower than 20. Other possible biases are evaluated such as: N content in the sequence (when the sequencer cannot determine which base is in a certain position reports an N), the uniform distribution of the four types of bases throughout the sequence (under the assumption that the probability of finding an A, T, G or C should be the same), and the distribution of kmers, that is, repeated sequences caused by external contamination during the sequencing process. The software widely used to evaluate these and other biases is FastQC (Andrews, et al., 2010) that generates a report per sample with graphs that are easy to read and interpret. As more massive experiments are done, other tools are required to concentrate the results for faster and more efficient inspection. To view many FastQC reports at the same time, tools such as MultiQC (Ewels et al., 2016) that also supports other data formats are very useful.

If the overall quality of the sequencing reads of a sample is not good, there is a way to increase the overall quality score. Due to the DNA polymerase dynamics, the latest synthetized bases from each read are those that carry the greatest number of errors. Cutting the final part of the reads with bioinformatics tools can help raise the overall quality score. It is also possible to search for and remove some adapters that have not been removed by the sequencer's internal data processing. Some popular tools to do these processes are Trimmomatic (Bolger et al., 2014) and Trim Galore which is a wrapper tool around Cutadapt (Martin, 2011). The most computationally demanding step is the alignment of the reads to a reference genome or transcriptome. Mapping an RNA-seq experiment would involve the matching of several tens of millions of short reads (30–100 bp) against a very large genome (on the order of billions of base pairs in the case of vertebrate species). There are three different alignment options:

Align only to the known transcriptome. It is faster but you can no longer find novel transcripts. Tools based on the Burrows-Wheeler Transform algorithm (Li and Durbin, 2009) such as BWA (Li and Durbin, 2009) or Bowtie (Langmead and Salzberg, 2012) can be used.

Splice-Aware Alignment Tools. We can not make a correct mapping of reads across splice junctions or detect alternative transcription if we do not consider splice-junction. We could align reads to the exons and splice junctions and then map them back to genomic coordinates if all exons and splice junctions were known. However, new transcripts of known genes are constantly being discovered as well as alternative splicing, therefore a splice-aware alignment is necessary (Williams et al., 2014). Splice-aware alignment allows identifying new genes or transcripts or even phenomena such as gene fusions (Conesa et al., 2016). Tools such as TopHat (Trapnell et al., 2009) or STAR (Dobin et al., 2012) or HISAT2 (Kim et al., 2019) are popular splice-aware aligners. And finally,

Assembled de novo, without reference. It is necessary when there is no reference genome. The transcriptome assembly is more complicated than the genome assembly since splicing variants of one gene can share exons with others and are difficult to resolve unambiguously. Tools like Trinity can be used in this case (Haas et al., 2013).

It is important to note that, up to this point, the fastq format has been used. However, the most frequently used format for reporting an alignment is SAM (Sequence Alignment Map) (Li and Durbin 2009) generated in the context of the 1000 genome project. SAM and its compressed version BAM (bgzf compression of a SAM) and CRAM (Fritz et al, 2011), is a text-based format that has a header starting with '@' before the alignment section. The alignment section has eleven mandatory fields, among which are: the sequence of the read itself, the position of the reference to which it aligns, the quality of its bases as well as the CIGAR (Concise Idiosyncratic Gapped Alignment Report) which encodes the changes required to transform the read into the reference sequence. SAM/BAM/CRAM files can be manipulated with the SamTools software (Li and Durbin 2009). For more details on the SAM format, see Li and Durbin 2009. A very useful piece of information when analyzing SAM files are their flags; the Broad institute offers a web tool to decode these flags.

Once the reads are aligned to the reference, the first analysis that can be done is to estimate how many reads are aligned to the region of a gene. This estimate is called a count. To estimate the counts per gene, a very useful tool is HTSeq (Anders et al., 2015). HTSeq reads the annotation files (format GFF o GTF) where the position of the genes in the genome is stored and, taking into account the alignment files, calculates how many reads fall on each gene. In addition to this, HTSeq estimates the quality of base-call files, calculating a coverage vector (how many reads per base does the experiment have) and exporting it for display in the Genome Browser.

Since genes have different sizes, normalization is required to make counts comparable. The usual normalization methods are:

- RPKM (Reads Per Kilobase per Million mapped reads) in which mapped reads are first normalized to RPM (Reads Per Million, divided by the total number of reads in the library scaled by the factor 10^6), to compare datasets at different sequencing depths, and then by gene length, assuming that a longer L gene is likely to produce a greater number of reads compared to a shorter S gene when the expression levels of S and L are equal.

- FPKM (Fragment Per Kilobase per Million mapped reads) have the same RPKM normalization ratio, however, it is used in paired-end RNA-seq, so that two paired reads (or a single unpaired one) are considered a single fragment and they are not counted twice.

- TPM (Transcript Per Million), in which the mapped reads are normalized first with the gene length and then with the total of the normalized reads scaled by the factor 10^6. TPM offers the advantage that the sum of the TPM for a given sample is always constant, regardless of the depth of the sequencing experiment (this is not true for RPKM values).

Once we have the counts, the type of normalization depends on the question we want to answer and the design of the experiment (Conesa et al., 2016). The tools most commonly used to normalize the count data are DESeq2 (Love et al., 2014), edge (Robinson et al., 2010) and glimma (Su et al., 2017). All of theme are based in R and available in the Bioconductor project. It is also worth mentioning that some of the most popular normalization methods for microarray data, such as limma (Law et al., 2018) or sva (Leek, 2014), were updated to deal with the RNA-seq data.

In recent years, different groups have developed workflows that integrate all the preprocessing. As an example, we will mention two tools. FastqPuri generates sequence quality reports by sample and by data set, integrating with graphs that facilitate decisions making for subsequent quality filtering. It also integrates tools to remove adapters and sequences from biological contamination. A very complete tool is Salmon (Patro et al., 2017). Salmon takes the fastq files, execute a quasi-mapping with a two-phase inference procedure, and returns the counts. It also integrates models that consider common attributes and biases in the RNA-seq data. So, it provides accurate expression estimates very quickly and while using little memory.

2.3 Single-Cell RNA-seq Experiments

The genome-wide expression technologies we have discussed so far use bulk RNA extracted from a tissue (bulk tissue). This technology is blind to cell type heterogeneity and to stochasticity of gene expression (Munsky et al., 2012; Raj and Oudenaarden, 2008; Stegle et al., 2015). When analyzing cells in bulk, we overlook subtle differences in molecular profiles and changes in individual cells that could be hidden in population variations (Kulkarni et al., 2019) (Fig. 5). The data produced from these bulk tissue assays have led to the identification of genes that are differentially expressed in different cell populations. But these genes could be doing different functions in the different cell types that make up the bulk tissue. In multicellular organisms, different cell types within the same population may have different roles and form subpopulations with different transcriptional profiles. Correlations in gene expression from different subpopulations can often be overlooked due to lack of subpopulation identification (Kanter and Kalisky, 2015). Single-cell RNA-seq (scRNA-seq) measures the expression levels of thousands of cells simultaneously. The technique is largely independent of prior knowledge of cell biology and allows for a fine-grained, detailed description of the cellular subtypes and cellular states of a tissue (Kashima et al., 2019). The scRNA-seq approaches have contributed to the discovery of new and rare cell types and subtypes; cellular heterogeneity within complex tissues; the presence and distribution of cellular states (e.g., phases of the cell cycle); and biological mechanisms in health and disease conditions (He et al., 2020).

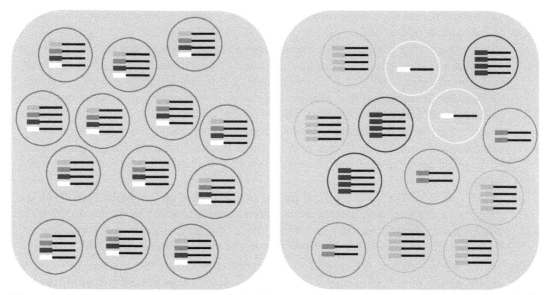

Figure 5 Bulk vs Single-Cell RNA-seq. Left side average gene expression profile of all cells in bulk tissue, on the right Single-Cell resolution gene expression profiles. This allows transcriptional differences between cell types to be analyzed separately, evidencing specific processes by cell type. (Modified from Chambers et al., 2018)

Examining the diversity of a cell population at this resolution was recently made possible, thanks to the development of high-throughput protocols for single-cell separation, for example the Fluidigm C1 platform (Xin et al., 2016), droplet microfluidics (Zilionis et al., 2016) and microwells (Han et al., 2018; Wadsworth et al., 2015) and complementary-DNA libraries with cell-specific barcodes (Pei et al., 2017; Perié et al., 2014). The methods for isolating individual cells for RNA sequencing vary depending on the number of cells they isolate (high-throughput or low-throughput) and how they select cells (biased or unbiased) (Cristinelli and Ciuffi, 2018; Gross et al., 2015). Dropletbased technologies are commonly used as an unbiased high-throughput solution (Prakadan et al., 2017). The three most used platforms are 10X Genomics Chromium, DropSeq and inDrop (Klein et al., 2015; Macosko et al., 2015; Zhang et al., 2018; Zheng et al., 2017). Each of these approaches uses microfluidics to label individual cells with individual beads that contain a unique barcode. Each mRNA transcript is also linked with a unique molecular identifier (UMI). This approach results in an array containing the absolute number of counts for each transcript in each cell (Kulkarni et al., 2019). Although the initial investment and operating costs are high, these platforms could expand the use of single-cell sequencing analysis for many laboratories and researchers (Kashima et al., 2019). The choice of platform depends on the objectives of the project: 10X Genomics Chromium is the most sensitive to detect the largest number of transcripts, but it is also the most expensive; DropSeq is generally less expensive, but less sensitive (fewer transcripts counted); inDrop may be ideal for detecting genes expressed at low levels due to its customizable parameters (Zhang et al., 2018).

2.3.1 Preprocessing scRNA-seq data

Single-cell data generated from many thousands of cells can reach greater orders of magnitude than that of typical genome-wide gene expression studies. Managing data of this magnitude presents computational and analytical challenges and requires High-performance computing (HPC) hardware, mass storage capacity, as well as specialized software. In general, single-cell data processing and many aspects of post-data analysis are not suitable for desktop computers. Parallel processing is critical due to the large size established by the number of cells sampled.

Furthermore, as scRNA-seq experiments get larger, the software must also scale up, and algorithms must be designed to handle exponential increases in data and complexity.

From the perspective of data analysis, the statistical properties of scRNA-seq data are different compared to the microarray or RNA-seq data, which means that many of the existing statistical and analytical methods are not always compatible. These differences have led researchers to build new approaches based on robust statistical methods commonly applied in fields such as population genetics, where analysis strategies designed to interrogate cohorts of tens of thousands of data are used. A problem associated with scRNA-seq is that the expression matrix is usually sparse (with many genes with a count of zero for gene expression). This phenomenon originates given the very low concentration of mRNA of the least expressed genes that, therefore, are not captured in the reverse transcription process. In general, of cell lysis, only 10–20% of total mRNA is detected (Grün et al., 2014; Stegle et al., 2015). Different strategies have been developed to alleviate this problem. We will mention only two of the most interesting ones: Markov Affinity-based Graph Imputation of Cells (MAGIC) (Dijk, et al., 2018) uses a diffusion operator to learn the underlying manifold and map cellular phenotypes to this manifold, restoring missing transcripts in the process. Archetypal-analysis for cell-tipe (ACTION) (Mohammadi et al., 2018) masks the universally expressed genes and then recalculates the transcriptional profile from the information of the genes that would be exclusive to the cell types studied.

There are currently as many preprocessing techniques as there are alternative technologies for obtaining single-cell data. Figure 6 offers a workflow that appears to be standard and is based on the analysis via three molecular identifiers: Sample Index (multiplex technology already present in RNA-seq), Unique Molecular Identification (UMI), and Cell Barcode. These three identifiers must be combined to get an accurate normalization.

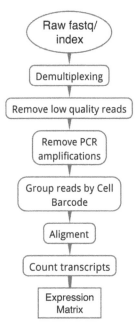

Figure 6 A preprocessing pipeline for Single-Cell RNA-seq data. Preprocessing begins with the fastq R1, R2, and Index files (optional depending on technology) returned by the sequencer. The first step is to sample the data (Demultiplexing) using the Sample Index. Next, the quality control is carried out, which first removes reeds with low quality. In order to remove overrepresented transcripts, the Unique Molecular Identification (UMI) is used to identify them from PCR amplifications. Reads are then grouped using the Cell Barcode and aligned using a splice-aware aligner like Kallisto (Bray et al., 2016) a splice-aware aligner designed for single-cell data. At the end collapse UMIs to count transcript by a cell. A matrix expression will be obtained with genes in the rows but with cells (not samples) in the columns.

While equipment manufacturers provide their own bioinformatics tools, such as Cell Ranger for Chromium, they focus on standard analysis leaving many particular applications out of the scope of these proprietary softwares. To overcome these problems, several bioinformaticians have developed new ways to interpret single-cell datasets (Kashima et al., 2019). Some examples of these efforts are scater (McCarthy et al., 2017) a Bioconductor package with a set of tools focused on quality control and visualization, Seurat (Butler et al., 2018) is another R package designed for QC, analysis, and exploration of single-cell RNA-seq data and ascend (Senabouth et al., 2019) a user-friendly standardization, cell expression, and differential expression software. They provide cutting-edge approaches to single-cell genomics data analysis and are complemented by comprehensive and easy-to-use tutorials and use case scenarios. Other software packages focus on normalization of expression data, visualization, single-cell genetics, and lineage tracing/ determination of cell fate. Many of these are cataloged at Awesome Single Cell, with new scRNA-seq software appearing frequently.

2.4 Genome-wide Expression Databases

Another way to obtain genome-wide expression data is through databases. It is increasingly clear to researchers that data sharing data is a very important part of research. Not only does it help make your results more reproducible, but it allows other researchers to look at the data produced with new eyes. Omics technologies in general and in particular transcriptomics generate large amounts of data and practically all journals request that authors place their data in some public database. Table 1 is a compendium of the best genome-wide expression databases. It is important to note that, although the data offered by most of these databases are already normalized, it is a good practice to explore and, when appropriate, renormalize the data, even more when it is intended to mix different datasets. It is also preferable to join datasets of the same technology.

3 INQUIRIES

So far we have obtained from all the technologies an expression matrix that contains the expression levels of the genes (in the lines) for each unit of analysis (samples or cells) in the columns. What kind of questions can we ask from this data? genome-wide expression data is used to study topics like cellular differentiation, transcription regulation, carcinogenesis, and biomarker discovery among others. Genome-wide expression studies are used by many other areas of biology such as biomedicine, proteomics, developmental biology, evolutionary biology, systems biology, among others. Each of them explores the genome-wide expression data with a different approach, but sometimes with the same goal. Here we will only recount those analyzes that have had the greatest impact during the development of the genome-wide expression study area.

3.1 Cluster and Principal Component Analysis

According to the expression of your genes, how do the elements of a study group differ? How many subgroups can be found according to their expressed genes? Cluster analysis and Principal Component Analysis (PCA) aim to answer these questions. These analyses are performed on a set of data that can come from one treatment or several, showing heterogeneity within a tissue, distinguishing cell types or expression patterns between different phenotypes. Cluster analysis is a series of algorithms that aim to make sets of elements whose characteristics are more similar between them than with others. In the case of the genome-wide expression experiments, the expression level of the genes of the samples (cell types in the case of scRNA-seq). The main

Table 1 Major genome-wide expression databases

Name	Site	Focus	Institution	Content	API*	Bioconductor package	Cite
ArrayExpress	ebi.ac.uk/arrayexpress	Functional genomics data	European Molecular Biology Laboratory-European Bioinformatics Institute	Microarray, RNA-seq	Yes	ArrayExpress	Athar et al., 2019
Expression Atlas	ebi.ac.uk/gxa/home	Gene and protein expression data across species and biological conditions	European Molecular Biology Laboratory-European Bioinformatics Institute	Microarray, RNA-seq	NA	ExpressionAtlas	Petryszak et al., 2015
Gene Expression Omnibus	ncbi.nlm.nih.gov/geo	Functional genomics data	National Center for Biotechnology Information, USA	Microarray, RNA-seq mainly	Yes	GEOmetadb GEOquery	Edgar et al., 2002
Genomic Data Commons	portal.gdc.cancer.gov	Cancer	National Cancer Institute, USA	Microarray, RNA-seq mainly	Yes	TCGAbiolinks	Grossman et al., 2016
Single Cell Expression Atlas	ebi.ac.uk/gxa/sc/home	Single cell gene expression across species	European Molecular Biology Laboratory-European Bioinformatics Institute	Single-Cell RNA-seq	NA	NA	Papatheodorou et al., 2019

*API is the acronym for Application Programming Interface, which is a software intermediary that allows two applications to talk to each other.

reason why there are many algorithms for cluster analysis is that there is not yet a consensus of what a "cluster" is and the different algorithms contain different philosophies of how the sets should be integrated (Estivill-Castro, 2002). One of the most representative works of the power of cluster analysis is the work of Perou et al. "Molecular portraits of human breast tumors" (Perou et al., 2000) defining the molecular signature used to identify the four subtypes of breast cancer and from which the PAM50 classification emerged (Perou et al., 2000; Sørlie et al., 2001). On the other hand, the Principal Component Analysis reduces the information on gene expression to the smallest and theoretically most coherent set. These "principal components" are the dominant patterns and represent the linear combination of the original variants (the expression of the genes). It is the analyst's responsibility to ask a question according to the data as well as being especially careful in interpreting the results, always considering the total variation captured by the first axes.

In Fig. 7, two graphs can be observed. First, a heatmap of the differential expression between patients with unilateral retinoblastoma vs those diagnosed with bilateral retinoblastoma. The objective of this analysis was to search for possible characteristic expression patterns that would help distinguish and diagnose the laterality of this cancer (Alvarez-Suarez et al., 2020). Both samples and genes (columns and lines, respectively) are ordered by similarity using a cluster analysis. This allows to compact those genes that are more characteristic of the most similar samples. In the second graph, a PCA is shown from the expression of all the differentially expressed genes and is only a visualization exercise, because, since it is made with the results of the differential expression analysis (see next section), it is obvious that the samples are separated according to their laterality.

3.2 Differential Expression

The most popular transcriptomic question are what genes are distinctive in the expression of one phenotype relative to another, e.g., diferentially expressed genes? In which biological processes are these differentially expressed genes enriched? How does expression differ between healthy versus sick tissue? How does expression differ between a treatment group of a drug versus its control? a genome-wide expression is the proper experiment required to answer this questions.

To obtain the differential expression between two groups it would seem simple to (1) estimate the density probability function that describes the distribution of the expression data, (2) estimate the variance, mean, median, and any other relevant parameter of each gene, and (3) calculate the *p*-value. However, there are strong obstacles to doing this: (a) the distribution of the expression of a gene throughout the samples is far from following a normal distribution, (b) the number of replicates is usually small, therefore the parameters that we consider relevant cannot be estimated with precision and (c) tens of thousands of genes are compared in an experiment, therefore it is essential to correct for multiple testing (Cellerino and Sanguanini, 2018).

Furthermore, each technology carries its difficulties. Thus, the most used approach for expression microarrays is to estimate differential expression with a Bayesian model like the one applied by the package limma (Ritchie et al., 2015). On the other hand, RNA-seq data is commonly modeled as a Negative Binomial assuming that most genes would not have differential expression. Besides, the mean and variance of the reparametrized distribution are usually calculated from the data as it is done by DESeq (Anders and Huber, 2010) and DESeq2 (Love et al., 2014). Moreover, the limma model transforms the RNA-seq data with voom (variance modeling at the observation-level) (Law, et al., 2014) a reparametrization of the data to make it appear as uniform as the microarray data. On the other hand, Single-Cell RNA-seq technology also uses models based on the negative binomial distribution [DESeq, edgaR (McCarthy et al., 2012) and SCDE (Kharchenko et al., 2014)] but it also considers new approaches such as the non-parametric earth mover's distance [SigEMD (Wang and Nabavi, 2017)] and zero-inflated negative binomial [DESingle (Miao et al., 2018)]. The resulting list of differentially expressed genes can then be analyzed in search of enriched biological processes using enrichment algorithms such as those discussed in chapter *Bioinformatics of functional categories enrichment*, in this same book. In Fig. 8 we can see again the retinoblastoma dataset shown in Fig. 7 (Alvarez-Suarez et al., 2020).

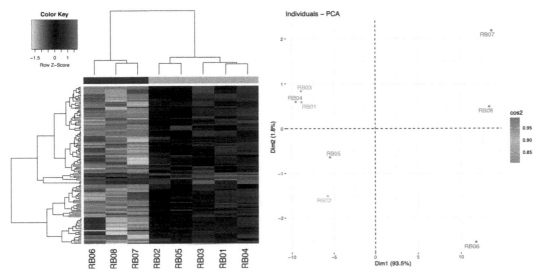

Figure 7 Cluster analyisis and PCA. A heatmap is the graphical representation of the intensity of a matrix. In this case, the left heatmap represents the intensity of expression of a matrix of genes differentially expressed between cancerous tissue of patients with unilateral retinoblastoma (left three sample's group) vs. patients diagnosed with bilateral retinoblastoma (rigth five sample's group) (Alvarez-Suarez et al., 2020). The best way to find patterns is to order the axes in such a way that groups are formed between which are more similar between them than with others. The dendrograms that this heatmap has above and to the left represents the similarity distance between the row and column elements. The PCA on the right was made with the data from the matrix represented in the heatmap and, therefore, show a clear separation between unilateral (RB06, RB07 and RB08) and bilateral (the rest) samples. This facilitates the visualization of how this analysis separates the elements summarizing the most important characteristics to reduce the greatest possible variance (Dim1 93.5 percent). You should not lose sight of how much variance each axis of the graph considers, to make decisions related to that amount. To make both figures, R was used with the following packages: for the heatmap ggplot2 heatmap2 (Wickham, 2016). To make the PCA, the function prcom included in R base (R Core Team, 2020) was used first and then, to graph, fviz_pca_ind a function from the package factoextra was used.

3.3 Gene Regulatory Networks

The coordinated behavior of a multitude of molecules, in particular, genes and their protein products, that determine the phenotypic conditions of a living cell can be represented as a gene regulatory network (GRN) (Barabási and Oltvai, 2004). GRN is a set of models derived from graph theory that describe this genetic expression in a population of cells in a unified way, under certain biological conditions at a given moment. In these representations, regulatory processes between molecules are represented by nodes and links. A GRN represents a systems biology approach to concerted gene expression, taking advantage of the growing number of genome-wide expression abundance data sets generated by high throughput methods discussed here. GRNs are usually displayed as either directed or undirected graphs in which nodes represent mRNA abundance and edges represent some form of regulatory relationship between the nodes. Since cells must continually adapt to changing conditions by altering their gene expression patterns, understanding the dynamic programs that a cell utilizes in response to internal or external stimuli is an important challenge in contemporary biology. These programs activate regulatory networks controlled by several transcription factors (Harbison et al., 2004) and may involve a large number of genes (Tovar et al., 2015).

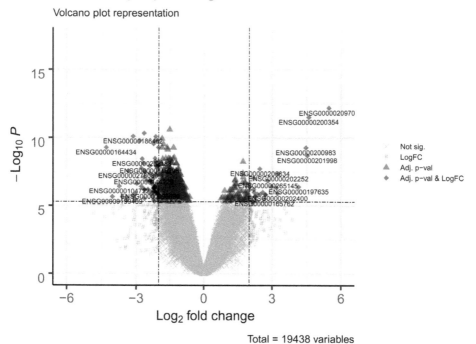

Total = 19438 variables

Figure 8 Representation of a differential expression analysis. A Volcanoplot is a representation of differential expression analysis. At a glance you can recognize if these genes are many or if they are mostly in over-expression or under-expression (as in this case), as well as the proportion of these. The figure was made with the EnhancedVolcano package (Blighe, 2020)

Network topology inference frequently involves deconvolution of interactions from the properties and dynamics of genome-wide expression of a specific cellular phenotype (Hernández-Lemus, 2013). In the last decade, many of these deconvolution methods have been applied to these systems. The method relies on the assumption that a strong statistical dependency between the expression of genes is an indication of a potential functional relationship (Wei et al., 2016). Among the most widely used are those known as co-expression networks, grouping algorithm networks, Bayesian methods, ordinary differential equations, and methods based on information theory (Bansal et al., 2007). All these methods face, to different degrees, different problems such as overfitting, high computational complexity, dependence on unrealistic network models, or much dependence on supplementary information not available for all biological models (Margolin et al., 2006). This last aspect is strongly related to the complexity of the models used to search for these networks. Biological models of greater complexity present especially two major problems: (1) a large number of variables with a lot of noise that results in the need for greater computational power and (2) the non-linearity of statistical dependencies, which results in many of the linear methods being unable to elucidate interactions between network elements (Hernández-Lemus and Rangel-Escareñõ, 2011).

For more details, please see the chapter *Bioinformatics and network analysis of biological data* in this book.

3.4 Master Regulation Analysis

A Transcriptional Master Regulator (TMR) is a Transcription Factor (TF) that is expressed at the beginning of the development of a phenotype or cell type, participates in the specifications of said phenotype regulating multiple downstream genes, by direct interaction or through gene cascades (Chan and Kyba, 2013). Transcriptional Master Regulators are responsible for the control of the entire genetic regulation program that defines a cell type (Affara et al., 2013; Basso et al., 2005; Han et al., 2004). TMRs can act on general cell processes (Hosking, 2012), but also on specific cellular phenotypes (Affara et al., 2013; Hinnebusch and Natarajan, 2002; Medvedovic et al., 2011). Understanding this organization and finding these regulatory genes is crucial in elucidating both normal cellular physiology and pathological phenotypes (Basso et al., 2005). The Master Regulation Analysis (MRA) is an example of integrating genomewide expression analyzes at different levels. MRA is based on two elements: (1) a transcriptional interaction network and (2) the expression profile of two related phenotypes. For example cancerous tissue and its corresponding adjacent tissue, or two states of transition/differentiation. The MRA seeks to identify those Transcription Factors responsible for the induction of one phenotype to another. For this, all the regulons (composed by all the targets of one TF) of each TF are extracted using the transcription network and it is evaluated if each regulon is enriched in the genes that are differentially expressed in both phenotypes through Gene Set Enrichment Analysis (GSEA, see chapter *Bioinformatics of functional categories enrichment*) (Subramanian et al., 2005). The TF with the highest score will be the one that controls the genes responsible for the phenotype. Although the interaction network can be generated without the need for expression data, the most commonly used strategy is to make an interaction network based on genome-wide expression (see chapter *Bioinformatics and network analysis of biological data*). Differentially expressed genes are obtained from comparing genome-wide expression data. This analysis has been used successfully to find Master Regulators mainly in cancer (Califano and Alvarez, 2016; Chu et al., 2016; Lefebvre et al., 2010; Smestad et al., 2019; Tovar et al., 2015) but it has also been used, for example, to find regulatory transcription factors of Psychiatric Disorders (Bristot et al., 2019) or, in the context of the COVID-19 pandemic, to find the master regulators of the SARS-CoV-2/ *Homo sapiens* interactome (Guzzi et al., 2020).

4 CONCLUDING REMARKS

Genome-wide expression studies are in an exciting moment of ascent. These will answer the molecular mechanisms of cell differentiation, the details of cell function, its response mechanisms to the environment, and also the mechanisms in which complex diseases such as cancer survives and are maintained. Like any other omics that is intimately linked with High Throughput Technologies, its relationship with bioinformatics is fundamental. Bioinformatics can be divided into two. On the one hand, some bioinformaticians design methods. They generate algorithms based on the peculiarities of data-generating technologies and their objective is to make tools that can function in most cases. On the other hand, some bioinformaticians use the methods. His challenge is to understand the study model and choose and implement the best algorithm for each particular case. Both require a thorough understanding of the particularities of both technologies and algorithms, and sometimes they jump from one function to another.

In this chapter, we made an overview of the most important transcriptomic technologies. The tools to process them and some of the most important topics in bioinformatic analysis. However, we must not forget that creativity is also required to find new forms, new topics, new research questions to expand our knowledge.

REFERENCES

Adams, J. (2008). The complexity of gene expression, protein interaction, and cell differentiation. Nature Education. 1(1): e110.

Affara, M., D. Sanders, H. Araki, Y. Tamada, B.J. Dunmore, S. Humphreys, et al. (2013). Vasohibin-1 is identified as a master-regulator of endothelial cell apoptosis using gene network analysis. BMC Genom. 14: 23.

Alvarez-Suarez, D.E., H. Tovar, E. Hernández-Lemus, M. Orjuela, S. Sadowinski-Pine, L. Cabrera-Munõz, et al. (2020). Discovery of a transcriptomic core of genes shared in 8 primary retinoblastoma with a novel detection score analysis. J. Cancer Res. Clin. Oncol. 146(8): 2029–2040. doi: 10.1007/s00432-020-03266-y.

Anders, S. and W. Huber (2010). Differential expression analysis for sequence count data. Genome Biol. 11(10): 1–12. doi:10.1186/gb-2010-11-10-r106. URL https://genomebiology.biomedcentral.com/articles/10.1186/gb-2010-11-10-r106.

Anders, S., P.T. Pyl and W. Huber (2015). Htseq-a python framework to work with high-throughput sequencing data. Bioinformatics. 31(2): 166–169. doi:10.1093/bioinformatics/ btu638.

Andrews, S., et al. (2010). Fastqc: a quality control tool for high throughput sequence data (2010).

Athar, A., A. Füllgrabe, N. George, H. Iqbal, L. Huerta, A. Ali, et al. (2019). Arrayexpress up-date-from bulk to single-cell expression data. Nucleic Acids Res. 47(D1): D711–D715. doi:10.1093/nar/gky964.

Bainbridge, M.N., R.L. Warren, M. Hirst, T. Romanuik, T. Zeng, A. Go, et al. (2006). Analysis of the prostate cancer cell line LNCaP transcriptome using a sequencing-by-synthesis approach. BMC Genom. 7(1): 246. doi: 10.1186/1471-2164-7-246.

Bansal, M., V. Belcastro, A. Ambesi-Impiombato and D. di Bernardo (2007). How to infer gene networks from expression profiles. Mol. Syst. Biol. 3.

Barabási, A.-L. and Z.N. Oltvai (2004). Network biology: understanding the cell's functional organization. Nat. Rev. Genet. 5(2): 101–113. doi:10.1038/nrg1272.

Barbulovic-Nad, I., M. Lucente, Y. Sun, M. Zhang, A.R. Wheeler and M. Bussmann, et al. (2006). Bio-microarray fabrication techniques—A review. Crit. Rev. Biotechnol. 26(4): 237–259. doi:10.1080/07388550600978358.

Basso, K., A.A. Margolin, G. Stolovitzky, U. Klein, R. Dalla-Favera and A. Califano (2005). Reverse engineering of regulatory networks in human B cells. Nat. Genet. 37(4): 382–390.

Bengtsson, H., J. Bullard and K.D. Hansen (2020). affxparser: Affymetrix file parsing SDK. R package version 1.62.0. https://github.com/HenrikBengtsson/affxparser.

Blighe, K., S. Rana and M. Lewis (2020). EnhancedVolcano: Publication-ready volcano plots with enhanced colouring and labeling. R package version 1.6.0. URL https://github.com/kevinblighe/EnhancedVolcano.

Bolger, A.M., M. Lohse and B. Usadel (2014). Trimmomatic: A flexible trimmer for Illumina sequence data. Bioinformatics. 30(15): 2114–2120. doi:10.1093/bioinformatics/btu170.

Bolstad, B. (2008). Preprocessing and normalization for affymetrix GeneChip expression microarrays. pp. 41–59. *In*: P. Stafford (ed.). Methods in Microarray Normalization, Drug Discovery Series/10. CRC Press.

Bray, N.L., H. Pimentel, P. Melsted and L. Pachter (2016). Near-optimal probabilistic RNA-Seq quantification. Nat. Biotechnol. 34(5): 525–527. doi:10.1038/nbt.3519.

Brenner, S., M. Johnson, J. Bridgham, G. Golda, D.H. Lloyd, D. Johnson, et al. (2000). Gene expression analysis by massively parallel signature sequencing (MPSS) on microbead arrays. Nat. Biotechnol. 18(6): 630–634. doi:10.1038/76469.

Bristot, G., M.A.D. Bastiani, B. Pfaffenseller, F. Kapczinski and M. Kauer-Sant'Anna (2019). Gene regulatory network of dorsolateral prefrontal cortex: A master regulator analysis of major psychiatric disorders. Mol. Neurobiol. 6(Suppl 1): 1–12. doi: 10.1007/s12035-019-01815-2. URL https://link.springer.com/article/10.1007/s12035-019-01815-2#citeas.

Butler, A., P. Hoffman, P. Smibert, E. Papalexi and R. Satija (2018). Integrating single-cell transcriptomic data across different conditions, technologies, and species. Nat. Biotechnol. 36(5): 411–420. doi: 10.1038/nbt.4096.

Califano, A. and M. J. Alvarez (2016). The recurrent architecture of tumour initiation, progression and drug sensitivity. Nat. Rev. Cancer. 17(2): 116–130. doi:10.1038/nrc.2016.124. URL http://www.nature.com.pbidi.unam.mx:8080/nrc/journal/vaop/ncurrent/full/nrc.2016.124.html

Carvalho, B.S. and R.A. Irizarry (2010). A framework for oligonucleotide microarray preprocessing. Bioinformatics. 26(19): 2363–2367. doi:10.1093/bioinformatics/btq431.

Cellerino, A. and M. Sanguanini (2018). Transcriptome Analysis, Introduction and Examples from the Neurosciences. Edizioni della Normale. ISBN: 978-88-7642-642-1.

Chambers, D.C., A.M. Carew, S.W. Lukowski and J.E. Powell (2018). Transcriptomics and single-cell RNA-sequencing. Respirology. 24(1): 29–36. doi:10.1111/resp.13412.

Chan, S.S. and M. Kyba (2013). What is a Master Regulator?. J. Stem Cell Res. Ther. 3: 114. doi:10.4172/2157-7633.1000e114.

Chen, C., K. Grennan, J. Badner, D. Zhang, E. Gershon, L. Jin, et al. (2011). Removing batch effects in analysis of expression microarray data: An evaluation of six batch adjustment methods. PloS one 6(2): e17238. doi:10.1371/journal.pone.0017238.

Chu, M., K. Yin, Y. Dong, P. Wang, Y. Xue, P. Zhou, et al. (2016). Tfdp3 confers chemoresistance in minimal residual disease within childhood t-cell acute lymphoblastic leukemia. Oncotarget. 8(1): 1405–1415. doi:10.18632/oncotarget.13630.

Cock, P.J.A., C.J. Fields, N. Goto, M.L. Heuer and P.M. Rice (2009). The sanger FASTQ file format for sequences with quality scores, and the Solexa/Illumina FASTQ variants. Nucleic Acids Res. 38(6): 1767–1771. doi:10.1093/nar/gkp1137.

Conesa, A., P. Madrigal, S. Tarazona, D. Gomez-Cabrero, A. Cervera, A. McPherson, et al. (2016). A survey of best practices for RNA-seq data analysis, Genome Biol. 17(1): 13. doi:10.1186/s13059-016-0881-8.

Cristinelli, S. and A. Ciuffi (2018). The use of single-cell RNA-seq to understand virus–host interactions. Curr. Opin. Virol. 29: 39–50. doi:10.1016/j.coviro.2018.03.001.

Dijk, D.v., R. Sharma, J. Nainys, K. Yim, P. Kathail, A.J. Carr, et al. (2018). Recovering gene interactions from single-cell data using data diffusion. Cell. 174(3): 716–729.e27. doi:10.1016/j.cell.2018.05.061.

Dobin, A., C.A. Davis, F. Schlesinger, J. Drenkow, C. Zaleski, S. Jha, et al. (2012). STAR: Ultrafast universal RNA-Seq aligner. Bioinformatics. 29(1): 15–21. doi:10.1093/ bioinformatics/bts635.

Dunning, M.J., M.L. Smith, M.E. Ritchie and S. Tavare (2007). Beadarray: R classes and methods for Illumina bead-based data. Bioinformatics. 23(16): 2183–2184. doi:10.1093/bioinformatics/btm311.

Edgar, R., M. Domrachev and A.E. Lash (2002). Gene Expression Omnibus: NCBI gene expression and hybridization array data repository. Nucleic Acids Res. 30(1): 207–210. doi:10.1093/nar/30.1.207.

Estivill-Castro, V. (2002). Why so many clustering algorithms: A position paper. ACM SIGKDD Explorations Newsletter. 4(1): 65–75. doi: 10.1145/568574.568575.

Ewels, P., M. Magnusson, S. Lundin and M. Käller (2016). MultiQC: Summarize analysis results for multiple tools and samples in a single report. Bioinformatics. 32(19): 3047–3048. doi:10.1093/bioinformatics/btw354.

Fei, T. and T. Yu (2020). Scbatch: Batch effect correction of RNA-Seq data through sample distance matrix adjustment. Bioinformatics. 36(10): 3115–3123. doi:10.1093/bioinformatics/btaa097.

Fritz, M.H.-Y., R. Leinonen, G. Cochrane and E. Birney (2011). Efficient storage of high throughput DNA sequencing data using reference-based compression. Genome Res. 21(5): 734–740. doi:10.1101/gr.114819.110.

Fujita, A., J. Sato, L. Rodrigues, C. Ferreira and M. Sogayar (2006). Evaluating different methods of microarray data normalization. BMC Bioinf. 7(1): 469. doi:10.1186/1471-2105-7-469.

Gautier, L., L. Cope, B.M. Bolstad and R.A. Irizarry (2004). affy—analysis of Affymetrix GeneChip data at the probe level. Bioinformatics. 20(3): 307–315. doi:10.1093/bioinformatics/btg405.

Gentleman, R.C., V.J. Carey, D.M. Bates, B. Bolstad, M. Dettling, S. Dudoit, et al. (2004). Bioconductor: Open software development for computational biology and bioinformatics. Genome Biol. 5(10): R80. doi:10.1186/gb-2004-5-10-r80.

Govindarajan, R., J. Duraiyan, K. Kaliyappan and M. Palanisamy (2012). Microarray and its applications. J. Pharm. BioAllied Sci. 4(Suppl 2): S310–S312. doi:10.4103/0975-7406.100283.

Gross, A., J. Schoendube, S. Zimmermann, M. Steeb, R. Zengerle and P. Koltay (2015). Technologies for single-cell isolation. Int. J. Mol. Sci. 16(8): 16897–16919. doi:10.3390/ ijms160816897.

Grossman, R.L., A.P. Heath, V. Ferretti, H.E. Varmus, D.R. Lowy, W.A. Kibbe, et al. (2016). Toward a shared vision for cancer genomic data. N. Engl. J. Med. 375(12): 1109–1112. doi:10.1056/nejmp1607591. URL https://www.nejm.org/doi/full/10.1056/NEJMp1607591

Grün, D., L. Kester and A.v. Oudenaarden (2014). Validation of noise models for single-cell transcriptomics. Nat. Methods. 11(6): 637–640. doi:10.1038/nmeth.2930.

Guzzi, P.H., D. Mercatelli, C. Ceraolo and F.M. Giorgi (2020). Master regulator analysis of the sars-cov-2/ human interactome. J. Clin. Med. 9(4): 982. doi:10.3390/jcm9040982.

Haas, B.J., A. Papanicolaou, M. Yassour, M. Grabherr, P.D. Blood, J. Bowden, et al. (2013). De novo transcript sequence reconstruction from RNA-seq using the Trinity platform for reference generation and analysis. Nat. Protoc. 8(8): 1494–1512. doi:10.1038/nprot.2013.084.

Haas, B.J., A. Dobin, B. Li, N. Stransky, N. Pochet, A. Regev (2019). Accuracy assessment of fusion transcript detection via read-mapping and de novo fusion transcript assembly-based methods. Genome Biol. 20(1): 213. doi:10.1186/s13059-019-1842-9.

Han, J.-D.J., N. Bertin, T. Hao, D.S. Goldberg, G.F. Berriz, L.V. Zhang, et al. (2004). Evidence for dynamically organized modularity in the yeast protein–protein interaction network. Nature. 430(6995): 88–93.

Han, X., R. Wang, Y. Zhou, L. Fei, H. Sun, S. Lai, et al. (2018). Mapping the mouse cell atlas by microwell-seq. Cell. 172(5): 1091–1107.e17. doi:10.1016/j.cell.2018. 02.001.

Harbison, C.T., D.B. Gordon, T.I. Lee, N.J. Rinaldi, K.D. Macisaac, T.W. Danford, et al. (2004). Transcriptional regulatory code of a eukaryotic genome. Nature. 431(7004): 99–104. doi:10.1038/ nature02800.

Hart, S.N., T.M. Therneau, Y. Zhang, G.A. Poland and J.-P. Kocher, (2013). Calculating sample size estimates for rna sequencing data. J. Comput. Biol. 20(12): 970–978. doi:10.1089/ cmb.2012.0283.

He, X., S. Memczak, J. Qu, J.C.I. Belmonte and G.-H. Liu (2020). Single-cell omics in ageing: A young and growing field. Nat. Metab. 2(4): 293–302. doi:10.1038/s42255-020-0196-7.

Hernández-Lemus, E. and C. Rangel-Escareñõ (2011). The role of information theory in gene regulatory network inference. pp. 109–144. In: P. Deloumeaux and J.D. Gorzalka (eds). Information Theory: New Research. Mathematics Research, Developments Series, Nova Publishing.

Hernández-Lemus, E. (2013). Further steps toward functional systems biology of cancer. Front. Physiol. 4: 256.

Hinnebusch, A.G. and K. Natarajan (2002). Gcn4p, a master regulator of gene expression, is controlled at multiple levels by diverse signals of starvation and stress. Eukaryotic Cell. 1(1): 22–32.

Hosking, R. (2012). mTOR: The Master Regulator. Cell. 149(5): 955–957.

Huber, W., V.J. Carey, R. Gentleman, S. Anders, M. Carlson, B.S. Carvalho, et al. (2015). Orchestrating high-throughput genomic analysis with bioconductor. Nat. Methods 12(2): 115–121. doi:10.1038/ nmeth.3252.

Jiménez-Chillarón, J.C., R. Díaz and M. Ramón-Krauel (2014). Omics tools for the genome-wide analysis of methylation and histone modifications. pp. 81–110. In: C. Simó, A. Cifuentes and V. García-Cañas (eds). Comprehensive Analytical Chemistry, vol 63. Elsevier. doi:10.1016/b978-0-444-62651-6.00004-0.

Johnson, W.E., C. Li and A. Rabinovic (2007). Adjusting batch effects in microarray expression data using empirical Bayes methods. Biostatistics. 8(1): 118–127. doi:10.1093/biostatistics/kxj037.

Kanter, I. and T. Kalisky (2015). Single cell transcriptomics: Methods and applications. Front. Oncol. 5: 53. doi:10.3389/fonc.2015.00053.

Kashima, Y., A. Suzuki and Y. Suzuki (2019). An Informative Approach to Single-Cell Sequencing Analysis. pp 81–96. *In*: Y. Suzuki (ed.). Single Molecule and Single Cell Sequencing. Advances in Experimental Medicine and Biology, vol 1129. Springer, Singapore. https://doi.org/10.1007/978-981-13-6037-4_6.

Kharchenko, P.V., L. Silberstein and D.T. Scadden (2014). Bayesian approach to single-cell differential expression analysis. Nat. Methods. 11(7): 740–742. doi:10.1038/nmeth.2967.

Kim, D., J.M. Paggi, C. Park, C. Bennett and S.L. Salzberg (2019). Graphbased genome alignment and genotyping with hisat2 and hisat-genotype. Nat. Biotechnol. 37(8): 907–915. doi:10.1038/s41587-019-0201-4.

Klein, A., L. Mazutis, I. Akartuna, N. Tallapragada, A. Veres, V. Li, et al. (2015). Droplet barcoding for single-cell transcriptomics applied to embryonic stem cells. Cell. 161(5): 1187–1201. doi:10.1016/j.cell.2015.04.044.

Kodzius, R., M. Kojima, H. Nishiyori, M. Nakamura, S. Fukuda, M. Tagami, et al. (2006). CAGE: Cap analysis of gene expression. Nat. Methods. 3(3): 211–222. doi:10.1038/nmeth0306-211.

Kornberg, R.D. and Y. Lorch (1992). Chromatin structure and transcription. Annu. Rev. Cell Biol. 8(1): 563–587. doi:10.1146/ annurev.cb.08.110192.003023.

Kulkarni, A., A.G. Anderson, D.P. Merullo and G. Konopka (2019). Beyond bulk: A review of single cell transcriptomics methodologies and applications. Curr. Opin. Biotechnol. 58: 129–136. doi:10. 1016/j.copbio.2019.03.001.

Langmead, B. and S.L. Salzberg (2012). Fast gapped-read alignment with Bowtie 2. Nat. Methods. 9(4): 357–359. doi:10.1038/nmeth.1923.

Law, C.W., Y. Chen, W. Shi and G.K. Smyth (2014). voom: precision weights unlock linear model analysis tools for RNA-Seq read counts. Genome Biol. 15(2): R29. doi:10.1186/gb-2014-15-2-r29.

Law, C.W., M. Alhamdoosh, S. Su, X. Dong, L. Tian, G.K. Smyth, et al. (2018). RNA-Seq analysis is easy as 1-2-3 with limma, glimma and edger. F1000Research. 5: 1408. doi:10.12688/f1000research.9005.3.

Leek, J.T., R.B. Scharpf, H.C. Bravo, D. Simcha, B. Langmead, W.E. Johnson, et al. (2010). Tackling the widespread and critical impact of batch effects in high-throughput data. Nat. Rev. Genet. 11(10): 733–739. doi:10.1038/nrg2825. URL http://www.nature.com/nrg/journal/v11/n10/full/nrg2825. html

Leek, J.T., W.E. Johnson, H.S. Parker, A.E. Jaffe and J.D. Storey (2012). The sva package for removing batch effects and other unwanted variation in high-throughput experiments. Bioinformatics. 28(6): 882–883. doi:10.1093/bioinformatics/bts034.

Leek, J. (2014). Svaseq: Removing batch effects and other unwanted noise from sequencing data. Nucleic Acids Res. 42(21): e161. doi: 10.1093/nar/gku864.

Lefebvre, C., P. Rajbhandari, M.J. Alvarez, P. Bandaru, W.K. Lim, M. Sato, et al. (2010). A human B-cell interactome identifies MYB and FOXM1 as master regulators of proliferation in germinal centers. Mol. Syst. Biol. 6(1): 1–10. doi:10.1038/msb.2010.31.

Li, H. and R. Durbin (2009). Fast and accurate short read alignment with Burrows-Wheeler transform. Bioinformatics. 25(14): 1754–1760. doi:10.1093/bioinformatics/btp324.

Love, M.I., W. Huber and S. Anders (2014). Moderated estimation of fold change and dispersion for RNA-Seq data with deseq2. Genome Biol. 15(12): 550. doi:10.1186/s13059-014-0550-8.

Luo, J., M. Schumacher, A. Scherer, D. Sanoudou, D. Megherbi, T. Davison, et al. (2010). A comparison of batch effect removal methods for enhancement of prediction performance using MAQC-II microarray gene expression data. Pharmacogenomics J. 10(4): 278–291. doi:10.1038/tpj.2010.57.

Macosko, E.Z., A. Basu, R. Satija, J. Nemesh, K. Shekhar, M. Goldman, et al. (2015). Highly parallel genome-wide expression profiling of individual cells using nanoliter droplets. Cell. 161(5): 1202–1214. doi:10.1016/j.cell. 2015.05.002.

Margolin, A.A., I. Nemenman, K. Basso, C. Wiggins, G. Stolovitzky, R. Favera, et al. (2006). ARACNE: An algorithm for the reconstruction of gene regulatory networks in a mammalian cellular context. BMC Bioinf. 7(Suppl 1): S7.

Martin, M. (2011). Cutadapt removes adapter sequences from high-throughput sequencing reads. EMBnet. Journal. 17(1): 10–12. doi:10.14806/ej.17.1.200.

McCall, M.N., B.M. Bolstad and R.A. Irizarry (2010). Frozen robust multiarray analysis (frma). Biostatistics. 11(2): 242–253. doi: 10.1093/biostatistics/kxp059.

McCarthy, D.J., Y. Chen and G.K. Smyth (2012). Differential expression analysis of multifactor RNA-seq experiments with respect to biological variation. Nucleic Acids Res. 40(10): 4288–4297. doi:10.1093/nar/gks042.

McCarthy, D.J., K.R. Campbell, A.T.L. Lun and Q.F. Wills (2017). Scater: pre-processing, quality control, normalization and visualization of single-cell RNA-seq data in R. Bioinformatics. 33(8): 1179–1186. doi: 10.1093/bioinformatics/btw777.

McGettigan, P.A. (2013). Transcriptomics in the RNA-seq era. Curr. Opin. Chem. Biol. 17(1): 4–11. doi:10.1016/j.cbpa.2012.12.008.

Medvedovic, J.J., A.A. Ebert, H.H. Tagoh and M.M. Busslinger (2011). Pax5: A master regulator of B cell development and leukemogenesis. Adv. Immunol. 111: 179–206.

Mellor, J. (2005). The dynamics of chromatin remodeling at promoters. Mol. Cell. 19(2): 147–157. doi:10.1016/j.molcel.2005.06.023.

Miao, Z., K. Deng, X. Wang and X. Zhang (2018). Desingle for detecting three types of differential expression in single-cell RNA-seq data. Bioinformatics. 34(18): 3223–3224. doi:10.1093/bioinformatics/bty332.

Mohammadi, S., V. Ravindra, D.F. Gleich and A. Grama (2018). A geometric approach to characterize the functional identity of single cells. Nat. Commun. 9(1): 1516. doi:10.1038/ s41467-018-03933-2.

Mortazavi, A., B.A. Williams, K. McCue, L. Schaeffer and B. Wold (2008). Mapping and quantifying mammalian transcriptomes by RNA-Seq. Nat. Methods. 5(7): 621–628. doi:10.1038/nmeth.1226.

Munsky, B., G. Neuert and A. v. Oudenaarden (2012). Using gene expression noise to understand gene regulation. Science. 336(6078): 183–187. doi:10.1126/science.1216379.

Nicorici, D., M. Satalan, H. Edgren, S. Kangaspeska, A. Murumagi, O. Kallioniemi, et al. (2014). FusionCatcher — a tool for finding somatic fusion genes in paired-end RNA-sequencing data. bioRxiv. 011650. doi:10.1101/011650.

Nygaard, V., E.A. Rødland and E. Hovig (2015). Methods that remove batch effects while retaining group differences may lead to exaggerated confidence in downstream analyses. Biostatistics. 17(1): 29–39. doi:10.1093/biostatistics/kxv027.

Papatheodorou, I., P. Moreno, J. Manning, A.M.-P. Fuentes, N. George, S. Fexova, et al. (2018). Expression atlas update: from tissues to single cells. Nucleic Acids Res. 48(D1): D77–D83. doi:10.1093/nar/gkz947.

Patro, R., G. Duggal, M.I. Love, R.A. Irizarry and C. Kingsford (2017). Salmon provides fast and bias-aware quantification of transcript expression. Nat. Methods. 14(4): 417–419. doi:10.1038/nmeth.4197.

Pei, W., T.B. Feyerabend, J. Rössler, X. Wang, D. Postrach, K. Busch, et al. (2017). Polylox barcoding reveals haematopoietic stem cell fates realized in vivo. Nature. 548(7668): 456–460. doi:10.1038/ nature23653.

Perié, L., P. Hodgkin, S. Naik, T. Schumacher, R. de Boer and K. Duffy (2014). Determining lineage pathways from cellular barcoding experiments. Cell Rep. 6(4): 617–624. doi:10.1016/j.celrep.2014.01.016.

Perou, C.M., T. Sørlie, M.B. Eisen, M.v.d. Rijn, S.S. Jeffrey, C.A. Rees, et al. (2000). Molecular portraits of human breast tumours. Nature. 406(6797): 747–752. doi:10.1038/35021093. URL http://www.nature. com/nature/journal/v406/n6797/full/ 406747a0.html

Pertea, M. (2012). The human transcriptome: An unfinished story. Genes. 3(3): 344–360. doi:10.3390/ genes3030344.

Pertea, M., G.M. Pertea, C.M. Antonescu, T.-C. Chang, J.T. Mendell and S.L. Salzberg (2015). StringTie enables improved reconstruction of a transcriptome from RNA-seq reads. Nat. Biotechnol. 33(3): 290–295. doi:10.1038/nbt.3122.

Petrov, A. and S. Shams (2004). Microarray image processing and quality control. J. VLSI Signal Process. Syst. Signal Image Video Technol. 38(3): 211–226. doi:10.1023/b:vlsi. 0000042488.08307.ad.

Petryszak, R., M. Keays, Y.A. Tang, N.A. Fonseca, E. Barrera, T. Burdett, et al. (2015). Expression atlas update–an integrated database of gene and protein expression in humans, animals and plants. Nucleic Acids Res. 44(D1): D746–D752. doi:10.1093/nar/gkv1045.

Prakadan, S.M., A.K. Shalek and D.A. Weitz (2017). Scaling by shrinking: Empowering single-cell "omics" with microfluidic devices. Nat. Rev. Genet. 18(6): 345–361. doi:10.1038/nrg.2017.15.

R Core Team (2020). R: A Language and Environment for Statistical Computing, R Foundation for Statistical Computing, Vienna, Austria (2020). URL https://www.R-project.org/

Raghavachari, N., J. Barb, Y. Yang, P. Liu, K. Woodhouse, D. Levy, et al. (2012). A systematic comparison and evaluation of high density exon arrays and RNA-seq technology used to unravel the peripheral blood transcriptome of sickle cell disease. BMC Med. Genomics. 5(1): 28. doi:10.1186/1755-8794-5-28.

Raj A. and A. v. Oudenaarden (2008). Nature, nurture, or chance: Stochastic gene expression and its consequences. Cell. 135(2): 216–226. doi: 10.1016/j.cell.2008.09.050.

Ralston, A. and K. Shaw (2008). Gene expression regulates cell differentiation. Nature Education. 1(1): e127.

Rio, D.C. (2014). Reverse transcription-polymerase chain reaction. Cold Spring Harb. Protoc. (11): 1207–1216. doi:10.1101/pdb. prot080887.

Ritchie, M.E., B. Phipson, D. Wu, Y. Hu, C.W. Law, W. Shiet al. (2015). limma powers differential expression analyses for RNA-sequencing and microarray studies. Nucleic Acids Res. 43(7): e47. doi:10.1093/nar/gkv007.

Robinson, M.D., D.J. McCarthy and G.K. Smyth (2010). edgeR: A Bioconductor package for differential expression analysis of digital gene expression data. Bioinformatics. 26(1): 139–140. doi: 10.1093/bioinformatics/btp616.

Romero, J.P., M. Ortiz-Estévez, A. Muniategui, S. Carrancio, F.J.D. Miguel, F. Carazo, et al. (2018). Comparison of RNA-seq and microarray platforms for splice event detection using a cross-platform algorithm. BMC Genom. 19(1): 703. doi:10.1186/s12864-018-5082-2.

Salomon, R.N. (1995). Introduction to reverse transcription polymerase chain reaction. Diagn. Mol. Pathol. 4(1): 2–3. doi: 10.1097/00019606-199503000-00002.

Schena, M., D. Shalon, R.W. Davis and P.O. Brown (1995). Quantitative monitoring of gene expression patterns with a complementary DNA microarray. Science. 270(5235): 467–470. doi:10.1126/science.270.5235.467.

Scherer, A. (2009). Batch Effects and Noise in Microarray Experiments. John Wiley & Sons, John Wiley & Sons.

Senabouth, A., S.W. Lukowski, J.A. Hernandez, S.B. Andersen, X. Mei, Q.H. Nguyen, et al. (2019).ascend: R package for analysis of single-cell RNA-Seq data. GigaScience. 8(8). doi:10.1093/gigascience/giz087.

Shakya, K., H.J. Ruskin, G. Kerr, M. Crane and J. Becker (2010). Advances in experimental medicine and biology. Adv. Exp. Med. Biol. 680: 139–147. doi:10.1007/978-1-4419 -5913-3_16.

Shen, W., S. Le, Y. Li and F. Hu (2016). Seqkit: A cross-platform and ultrafast toolkit for fasta/q file manipulation, PLoS ONE 11(10): e0163962. https://doi.org/10.1371/journal.pone.0163962.

Shendure, J. and H. Ji (2008). Next-generation DNA sequencing. Nat. Biotechnol. 26(10): 1135–1145. doi:10.1038/nbt1486.

Shiraki, T., S. Kondo, S. Katayama, K. Waki, T. Kasukawa, H. Kawaji, et al. (2003). Cap analysis gene expression for high-throughput analysis of transcriptional starting point and identification of promoter usage. Proc. Natl. Acad. Sci. U.S.A. 100(26): 15776–15781. doi:10.1073/pnas.2136655100.

Silver, J.D. M.E. Ritchie and G.K. Smyth (2008). Microarray background correction: Maximum likelihood estimation for the normal-exponential convolution. Biostatistics. 10(2): 352–363. doi: 10.1093/biostatistics/kxn042.

Smestad, J.A. and L.J. Maher (2019). Master regulator analysis of paragangliomas carrying SDHx, VHL, or MAML3 genetic alterations. BMC Cancer. 19(1): 1–19. doi:10.1186/s12885-019-5813-z. URL https://bmccancer.biomedcentral.com/articles/10.1186/s12885-019-5813-z

Smyth, G.K. (2005) limma: Linear models for microarray data. pp. 397–420. *In:* R. Gentleman, V.J. Carey, W. Huber, R.A. Irizarry and S. Dudoit (eds). Bioinformatics and Computational Biology Solutions Using R and Bioconductor. Statistics for Biology and Health. Springer, New York, NY. https://doi.org/10.1007/0-387-29362-0_23.

Sørlie, T., C.M. Perou, R. Tibshirani, T. Aas, S. Geisler, H. Johnsen, et al. (2001). Gene expression patterns of breast carcinomas distinguish tumor subclasses with clinical implications. Proc. Natl. Acad. Sci. U.S.A. 98(19): 10869–10874. doi:10.1073/pnas.191367098.

Stegle, O., S.A. Teichmann and J.C. Marioni (2015). Computational and analytical challenges in single-cell transcriptomics. Nat. Rev. Genet. 16(3): 133–145. doi:10.1038/nrg3833.

Su, S., C.W. Law, C. Ah-Cann, M.-L. Asselin-Labat, M.E. Blewitt and M.E. Ritchie (2017). Glimma: Interactive graphics for gene expression analysis. Bioinformatics. 33(13): 2050–2052. doi:10.1093/bioinformatics/btx094.

Subramanian, A., P. Tamayo, V.K. Mootha, S. Mukherjee, B.L. Ebert, M.A. Gillette, et al. (2005). Gene set enrichment analysis: A knowledge-based approach for interpreting genome-wide expression profiles. Proc. Natl. Acad. Sci. U.S.A. 102(43): 15545–15550. doi:10.1073/ pnas.0506580102.

Sultan, M., M.H. Schulz, H. Richard, A. Magen, A. Klingenhoff, M. Scherf, et al. (2008). A global view of gene activity and alternative splicing by deep sequencing of the human transcriptome. Science. 321(5891): 956–960. doi:10.1126/science.1160342.

Tovar, H., R. García-Herrera, J. Espinal-Enríquez and E. Hernández-Lemus (2015). Transcriptional master regulator analysis in breast cancer genetic networks. Comput. Biol. Chem. 59 Pt B: 67–77. doi:10.1016/j.compbiolchem.2015.08.007.

Trapnell, C., L. Pachter and S.L. Salzberg (2009). TopHat: Discovering splice junctions with RNA-Seq. Bioinformatics. 25(9): 1105–1111. doi:10.1093/bioinformatics/btp120.

Velculescu, V.E., L. Zhang, B. Vogelstein and K.W. Kinzler (1995). Serial analysis of gene expression. Science. 270(5235): 484–487. doi:10. 1126/science.270.5235.484.

Velculescu, V.E., L. Zhang, W. Zhou, J. Vogelstein, M.A. Basrai, D.E. Bassett, et al. (1997). Characterization of the yeast transcriptome. Cell. 88(2): 243–251. doi:10.1016/ s0092-8674(00)81845-0.

Verk, M.C.V., R. Hickman, C.M.J. Pieterse and S.C.M.V. Wees (2013). RNA-Seq: Revelation of the messengers. Trends Plant Sci. 18(4): 175–179. doi:10.1016/j.tplants.2013.02.001.

Wadsworth, M.H., T.K. Hughes and A.K. Shalek (2015). Marrying microfluidics and microwells for parallel, high-throughput single-cell genomics. Genome Biol. 16(1): 129. doi:10.1186/s13059-015-0695-0.

Wang, T. and S. Nabavi (2017). Differential gene expression analysis in single-cell RNA sequencing data, 2017. IEEE Int. Conf. Bioinf. Biomed. (BIBM). pp. 202–207. doi:10.1109/bibm.2017.8217650.

Wei, J., X. Hu, X. Zou and T. Tian (2016). Inference of genetic regulatory network for stem cell using single cells expression data, 2016. IEEE Int. Conf. Bioinf. Biomed. (BIBM). pp. 217–222. doi:10.1109/bibm.2016.7822521.

Wickham, H. (2016). ggplot2: Elegant Graphics for Data Analysis, Springer-Verlag New York. URL https://ggplot2.tidyverse.org

Wilhelm, B.T., S. Marguerat, S. Watt, F. Schubert, V. Wood, I. Goodhead, et al. (2008). Dynamic repertoire of a eukaryotic transcriptome surveyed at single-nucleotide resolution., Nature. 453(7199): 1239–1243. doi:10.1038/nature07002.

Williams, A.G., S. Thomas, S.K. Wyman and A.K. Holloway (2014). RNA-seq data: Challenges in and recommendations for experimental design and analysis. Curr. Protoc. Hum. Genet. 83(1): 11.13.1–11.13.20. doi:10.1002/0471142905.hg1113s83.

Xin, Y., J. Kim, M. Ni, Y. Wei, H. Okamoto, J. Lee, et al. (2016). Use of the fluidigm c1 platform for RNA-sequencing of single mouse pancreatic islet cells. Proc. Natl. Acad. Sci. U.S.A. 113(12): 3293–3298. doi: 10.1073/pnas.1602306113.

Zhang, W., Y. Yu, F. Hertwig, J. Thierry-Mieg, W. Zhang, D. Thierry-Mieg, et al. (2015). Comparison of RNA-seq and microarray-based models for clinical endpoint prediction. Genome Biol. 16(1): 133. doi:10.1186/s13059-015-0694-1.

Zhang, X., T. Li, F. Liu, Y. Chen, J. Yao, Z. Li, et al. (2018). Comparative analysis of droplet-based ultra-high-throughput single-cell RNA-seq systems. Mol. Cell. 73(1): 130–142.e5. doi: 10.1016/j.molcel.2018.10.020.

Zhang, Y., G. Parmigiani and W.E. Johnson (2020). Combat-seq: batch effect adjustment for RNA-Seq count data. bioRxiv. 2020.01.13.904730. doi:10.1101/2020.01.13.904730.

Zheng, G.X.Y., J.M. Terry, P. Belgrader, P. Ryvkin, Z.W. Bent, R. Wilson, et al. (2017). Massively parallel digital transcriptional profiling of single cells. Nat. Commun. 8(1): 14049. doi:10.1038/ncomms14049.

Zilionis, R., J. Nainys, A. Veres, V. Savova, D. Zemmour, A.M. Klein, et al. (2016). Single-cell barcoding and sequencing using droplet microfluidics. Nat. Protoc. 12(1): 44–73. doi:10.1038/nprot. 2016.154.

CHAPTER 6

Whole-genome Sequencing: From Samples to Variants and Beyond

Jose M. Lorenzo-Salazar[1], Adrián Muñoz-Barrera[1], Rafaela González-Montelongo[1] and Carlos Flores[1,2,3,4*]

[1]Genomics Division, Instituto Tecnológico y de Energías Renovables (ITER), Santa Cruz de Tenerife, Spain

[2]Research Unit, Hospital Universitario Nuestra Señora de Candelaria, Santa Cruz de Tenerife, Spain

[3]CIBER de Enfermedades Respiratorias, Instituto de Salud Carlos III, Madrid, Spain

[4]Instituto de Tecnologías Biomédicas (ITB), Universidad de La Laguna, Santa Cruz de Tenerife, Spain

1 INTRODUCTION

The use of whole-genome sequencing (WGS) theoretically allows the unbiased study of all types of genetic variation in the genome (Lappalainen et al., 2019), including rare and structural genetic variants (Ng and Kirkness, 2010). WGS and whole-exome sequencing (WES) have been shown as valuable and complementary methods for the discovery of the genetic causes of complex and rare diseases in the last decade (Pabinger et al., 2014; Worthey, 2017). However, compared to WES, WGS is aimed to assess genetic variation in the entire human genome, offering a more uniform depth of coverage and theoretically allowing to detect variants of any type irrespective of their genomic location. With time, Next Generation Sequencing technologies (NGS) have become affordable and efficient (Kuchenbaecker and Appel, 2018). Currently, the most widely used NGS technology is based on the short-read sequencing-by-synthesis popularized by Illumina, Inc., which can produce thousands of millions of short reads on a single experiment. NGS is

*Corresponding author: cflores@ull.edu.es

being challenged by the rapid development of promising Third-Generation Sequencing (TGS) technologies based on different sequencing mechanisms to obtain longer reads (Giani et al., 2020), such as Pacific Biosciences (PacBio) and Oxford Nanopore Technologies (ONT). This technological trend runs in parallel with the development of new bioinformatic tools, workflow and scripting languages, and management systems (Ekblom and Wolf, 2014) to foster the efficiency of computational NGS analysis.

In this chapter, we present a brief outline of the whole-genome library preparation, addressing the basic wet lab procedures to prepare the sample's DNA for the sequencing process. Then, we present an overview of NGS and TGS technologies, and their benefits for genetic discoveries. The next section presents a basic WGS workflow, pipeline scripting standards and languages, and state-of-the-art workflow editors. The central part of the chapter describes the numerous and complex steps involved in a WGS workflow for short variant discovery. In this part, we succinctly describe the algorithms, tools, file formats, and databases necessary to sustain the WGS workflows in the primary, secondary and tertiary analysis stages, with a main focus on germinal variation. The next section presents large-scale WGS projects and applications in population genomics, disease-oriented studies, use of low-coverage WGS, and clinical uses. The chapter finalizes with a summary of the challenges faced by WGS bioinformatics.

2 WHOLE-GENOME LIBRARY PREPARATION

2.1 Wet Lab Procedures

The advances in genomic research are linked to the development of new laboratory tools, typically integrating bench procedures from the "wet lab", with computational methods on the "dry lab" side to efficiently handle the massive sequencing data generated. Sequencing technologies have rapidly evolved over the last two decades accompanied by improvements in the methods for preparing nucleic acids for sequencing (Kozarewa et al., 2009; Quail et al., 2008). Developments have made it possible to deepen the knowledge of the genome in all areas of the biological and medical sciences.

The "wet lab" steps are critical for achieving reliable and robust sequencing results. Sequencing of the whole-genome requires the preparation of the DNA molecules following protocols that are technology-dependent to generate the so-called library. NGS approaches rely on native or amplified DNA for library preparation (Giani et al., 2020). Different approaches for the library preparation exist depending on the sequencing technology. Typically, a library preparation protocol for short-read sequencing requires the use of physical (mechanical shearing) or biochemical (enzymatic tagmentation) methods to break the DNA molecules into small fragments of a desired size, most commonly in the range of 125 to 700 base pairs (bp). Adapters are then ligated to the ends of each fragment. This step is usually followed by a DNA amplification step. The resulting library is multiplexed on a pool of samples and loaded in the sequencer flow cell.

During library preparation, several physical and biochemical effects may occur (shearing, oxidation, fragment-size shifts, adapter dimer and concatemer chain formation, etc.) causing library issues that will turn into suboptimal sequencing results. In addition, library preparation protocols that require amplification steps may generate sequence errors due to the polymerase activity, producing artifacts in downstream analyses (e.g., falsely called variants) and compromising the results. Besides, there are parts of the human genome not amenable for the sequencing process in the analysis stage, such as the centromere and telomeres of chromosomes, to name a few, as they contain long stretches of highly repetitive sequences, and genomic regions with variable-number of tandem repeats (VNTRs) and segmental duplications. In addition, sequence analysis of the fragments from regions of low sequence complexity frequently translates into unreliable results. Unfortunately, the human genome reference still lacks completeness and has a poor representation of the human genetic diversity in those regions. Long-read sequencing will be optimal for the analyses of these particularly complex regions.

2.2   Preservation of Samples

The preparation of high-quality sequencing libraries depends essentially on two main factors: the quantity and the quality of the starting DNA material. Moreover, the library preparation process should warrant the highest breath-of-coverage and the recovery of the original fragments obtained with the lowest bias. The chemistry and the sequencing technology determine the method of sequencing in each instrument. In such a way, NGS of the so-called second-generation focuses on obtaining short reads of the original or amplified DNA, whereas TGS usually aims for sequencing of long reads from unamplified molecules. Because of that, the second-generation sequencing implies a fragmentation step of the genomic DNA (gDNA) in homogeneous short fragments, whereas the TGS aims to preserve gDNA integrity to yield long reads.

Many research projects using biological samples typically use stored (biobanked) samples for research purposes. Therefore, it is essential that centers and researchers take into account the conservation conditions to maintain integrity of the material that allow applying downstream applications in research projects. The samples used in human WGS are provided mainly from biobanked extracted DNA, fresh tissue (blood, saliva, tissue biopsy, cells from primary cultures or transformed cells), tissues fixed in paraffin (FFPE) or preserved in ethanol (Robbe et al., 2018; Zar et al., 2019). As soon as the samples are collected, the gradual degradation begins. Therefore, it is crucial to maintain the adequate storage conditions to preserve integrity. The parameters that have the most significant impact on DNA conservation are the time and temperature at which the material is conserved. However, this depends not only on their long-term preservation but also on the collection, processing, and transportation to the laboratory for long-term storage. Some studies show that tissue maintenance at $-80°C$ preserves DNA stability over time (Chu et al., 2002). Others have described that DNA integrity is maintained for a decade if the tissue is saved in liquid nitrogen vapor (Qualman et al., 2004). The temperature recommendations for DNA depend on the expected storage period. The temperature varies between $+4°C$ for storage of fewer than two months and $-80°C$ for periods over one year (Camacho-Sanchez et al., 2013). If refrigeration of biological samples is not possible, nucleic acid preservation solutions at ambient temperature can be used that protect integrity and allow recovery of high molecular weight DNA for extended periods (Lee et al., 2012).

2.3   DNA Sources and Isolation

For a reliable analysis of the complete human genome, gDNA must be extracted in sufficiently pure amounts and preserving sufficient integrity. This essentially depends on the source of the sample (and the storage) and the methods used in the DNA extraction. Peripheral blood and FFPE samples are the most common gDNA sources for WGS (Trost et al., 2019). Blood samples minimize the risk of DNA degradation, whereas FFPE samples, which are more accessible in particular clinical settings, are much easier to prepare and to store, albeit formalin fixation results in DNA damage and considerable fragmentation. Formaldehyde, the component of formalin solutions, creates covalent bonds between DNA-DNA, DNA-RNA, or DNA-proteins and induces oxidation, deamination, and cyclic bases derivatives (Feldman, 1973; Karlsen et al., 1994). Formalin produces erroneous adenosine incorporations in the cytosine, in place of guanosine, causing an artificial C>T or G>A mutation (Srinivasan et al., 2002; Williams et al., 1999). In addition, crosslinks result in DNA fragmentation, which complicates the library preparation and the sequencing and analysis processes (Srinivasan et al., 2002). Some studies support that the type of formalin used and the time elapsed since the sample was fixed affects DNA quality and, thus, the resulting NGS data (Einaga et al., 2017; Nagahashi et al., 2017). Despite that, DNA from FFPE samples is valid material for WGS studies (Schweiger et al., 2009; Yost et al., 2012).

2.4 Library Preparation

Fragmentation of gDNA is usually the first step in standard WGS library preparation. For short-read sequencing technologies, the range of fragments is of several hundred bp at maximum, whereas the size range is wider and reaches several thousand bp or even Megabases (Mb) in TGS. The subsequent workflow will depend on the type of fragmentation. In general, later steps include end-repair and adapter ligation when a mechanical fragmentation procedure is used. The end-repair process is based on a set of enzymatic reactions that produce blunt ends with a complementary overhang for adapter ligation. The adapters contain solution-specific sequences that allow increasing the number of copies of the libraries by amplification, the attachment of fragments to the surface where the sequencing takes place using a free 3′ hydroxyl, and harboring the sequence indexes for multiple libraries to be pooled in a single experiment. On the other hand, in case of an enzyme-mediated fragmentation, the steps after fragmentation includes the indexing and the attachment of the adapters by amplification. After the adapters are attached, the library is subjected to size selection, most commonly using magnetic beads that are amenable for automation. It is a good practice to assess the library both for the concentration, using spectrofluorimetric methods (e.g., Qubit fluorometer, Thermo Fisher Scientific) or amplification-based methods (e.g., real-time quantitative polymerase chain reaction), and its size profile (e.g., TapeSation Systems, Agilent). Finally, indexed libraries need to be diluted to the recommended loading concentrations and pooled for sequencing. At this stage, the libraries must be combined to equimolar amounts in the pool to avoid large variations in the results because of their competition during the sequencing experiment. The number of libraries to be combined per pool depends on the design, the scale of the project, and the desired depth-of-coverage per sample.

Mechanical fragmentation methods include sonication or hydrodynamic shearing. The gold standard for random mechanical fragmentation is the acoustic shear by ultrasounds (Covaris). The acoustic energy induces cavitation (creation and continuous collapse of micro-bubbles) of the aqueous sample contained into a small glass vial. These localized forces break the DNA quickly, reproducibly, and under isothermal conditions. The device allows for controlling the shearing forces to fragment the gDNA to the desired size, yielding ranges between 150 and 5,000 bp. Acoustic shearing requires a small amount of initial gDNA of at least 100–200 ng, whereas the hydrodynamic shearing requires a range of 1–5 µg. Moreover, compared to hydrodynamic shear, acoustic shearing gives a uniform narrower size range of fragments and there is no sample loss. However, in addition to requiring a large investment for high-throughput, acoustic shearing can be a source of oxidative damage to the DNA that is known to produce sequencing artifacts (Costello et al., 2018).

Enzymatic fragmentation methods are currently based on the use of endonucleases or transposases. Many kits that ease the preparation of libraries are available, and among the most popular commercial enzymatic fragmentation kits are Fragmentase (New England Biolabs) and Nextera tagmentation (Illumina, Inc.). Fragmentase is a mix of two enzymes: one that randomly nicks double-stranded DNA, and a second one that cuts the strand opposite to the nicks to provide fragments between 100 and 800 bp, depending on the incubation times (Knierim et al., 2011). The Nextera kits (Illumina, Inc.) use enzymes called transposases that cut the gDNA into smaller fragments. During the fragmentation process, the transposases also ligate the adapter sequences to the DNA fragments in a single "cut and paste" step called tagmentation (Marine et al., 2011). Commercial transposases act in suspension as other enzymatic reactions or on solid surfaces where the enzymes are attached, such as bead-conjugated transposomes (Bruinsma et al., 2018). Illumina, Inc. commercializes kits based on on-bead tagmentation that works well with a wide gDNA input range (100–500 ng). As a consequence, its use saves time and the costs of the initial gDNA quantitation, as well as of the library quantitation and normalization before pooling and sequencing. The short sequences inserted by transposase are complementary to the tails of the primers used afterwards to add the adapter sequences with indexes using amplification. The final library includes all necessary components to later conduct bridge amplification on the flow cell surface and the subsequent sequencing on their platforms. Amplification generates sufficient quantities of DNA to allow accurate library quantification. Taken together, enzyme fragmentation is an efficient method that allows processing many samples simultaneously permitting automation, reducing sample loss, and requiring low sample input. As a drawback, it is known that transposases have sequence bias that may produce a non-random fragmentation, particularly in GC-rich regions, that could affect variant calling (Lan et al., 2015).

Multiplexing samples is the most common strategy for maximizing efficiency of a sequencing experiment. Briefly, libraries from each sample have a unique sequence index, and multiple libraries are pooled together for sequencing in the same run. Once sequenced, each read is assigned to the corresponding sample according to the unique index sequence in the pool. In this process, demultiplexing of results may lead to a misassignment of the index, which affects the quality of the data and may lead to artifacts. Library preparation is one of the steps in which the index swapping could occur due to errors in the manufacture or contamination of the oligonucleotides or the reagents during experimental handling. Sequencing errors on indexes are expected as well. On Illumina, Inc. platforms, especially those with patterned flow cells that use the clustering chemistry called exclusion amplification (ExAmp), a misassignment of the index occurs from low-level free index primers present in the pool. This index hopping can occur through free adapters that hybridize to the complementary sequence of 3' end of the adapter and is extended creating a new molecule with a unique index. This new index hopping strand is liberated from one nanowell and can seed another nanowells to generate a cluster for sequencing. The resulting read from this other cluster is then assigned to a different sample, and the evidence suggests that this occurs with a rate of 0.25–6% when using combinatorial dual index adapters (Costello et al., 2018). These events during clustering can have a severe impact if the aim is to detect somatic variation at low frequency, such as in liquid biopsy, tumor sequencing, or single cell sequencing (Costello et al., 2018; Vodák et al., 2018). The recommendations to minimize the level and effect of index hopping are to use an enzymatic treatment that blocks the extension of the free index primers together with some recommendations such as the storage of libraries individually at –20°C, pooling of libraries right before sequencing, and the use of unique dual indexing (UDI) pooling combinations. In general, library preparation methods that only involve ligation steps generate libraries with higher levels of index hopping than the methods that incorporate a subsequent amplification step. Also, libraries clustered on patterned flow cells using ExAmp cluster generation have higher rates of index hopping ($\leq 2\%$) compared to non-patterned flow cells with random bridge amplification ($\leq 1\%$) (white paper Illumina, Inc.). Therefore, the use of UDI mitigates misassignment of the index, allowing identification and filtering of swapped index reads in downstream analysis.

Either pipetting workstations or microfluidic systems can be used for automation of NGS library preparation. The use of liquid handling robots for library preparation allows high-throughput processing at the cost of limited flexibility regarding reagent savings. Microfluidic systems are more convenient in this sense because of miniaturization and lower investment costs, although there are not many options being commercialized. Illumina, Inc. and NuGEN (Tecan) commercialized electrowetting systems (Bowers et al., 2015; Coelho et al., 2017), although they are not currently marketed. Voltrax (ONT) is the most popular microfluidic system that currently allows automatic library preparation (Lu et al., 2016).

3   AN OVERVIEW OF THE NEXT GENERATION SEQUENCING PLATFORMS

3.1   Technologies by Read Length

There are three popular WGS strategies at the moment (Lappalainen et al., 2019): (1) short-read WGS using the Illumina, Inc. or MGI technologies (typically based on paired-end 150 bp reads with per-base errors in the range 0.1–0.5%); (2) single-end long-read WGS using single-molecule technologies from PacBio or ONT (typically 10–100 kb reads and per-base error rates of 1–15%, mostly consisting of insertions and deletions); and (3) linked-read WGS using the 10X Genomics technology (barcoded Illumina, Inc. short-reads from high-molecular weight DNA molecules) (Table 1).

Table 1   Overview of the main current sequencing technologies with WGS capabilities

Platform	Instrument	Maximum read length (bases)	Throughout per flow cell (Gbases)	Run time (h)	Observations
Illumina, Inc.	NextSeq550	2×150	120	12–30	
	NextSeq2000	2×150	300	24–48	Dual port run of SP flow cells
	HiSeq3000/4000	2×150	650–750	84	
	NovaSeq6000	2×250	6,000	13–44	Dual port run of SP flow cells
MGI	DNBSEQ-G50	2×100	10–150	66	
	DNBSEQ-G400	2×150	55–1,440	37	
	DNBSEQ-T7	2×150	6,000	24	
PacBio	Sequel I	> 80 kb	15	Up to 20	SMRT Cell 1M
	Sequel II	> 300 kb	100	Up to 30	SMRT Cell 8M
ONT	MinION Mk1B	Up to 2 Mb	50	max. 48	1 flow cell
	GridION Mk1	Up to 2 Mb	50	max. 48	5 flow cells
	PromethION 24/48	Up to 2 Mb	150	Up to 72	24/48 flow cells

Short-read WGS Illumina, Inc. technologies dominate the NGS market as it is used by most of the research and clinical groups because of the costs, accuracy, and throughput, with experiments frequently based on the HiSeq and NovaSeq sequencing platforms, producing reads of up to 150 bases. MGI technologies are becoming more popular in the last years because of the considerably reductions in cost and increase of throughput. In parallel, long-read technologies are especially relevant for *de novo* assembly of genomes (Gordon et al., 2016), long-distance haplotyping, and structural variant calling (Sedlazeck et al., 2018).

Some NGS methods use amplification during the library preparation step and the clustering of DNA fragments within flow cells. As the amplification is inefficient at extreme GC contents, regions with high or low GC content will be poorly covered. PacBio and ONT long-read sequencing technologies eliminate this bias by avoiding the amplification step (van Dijk et al., 2018), and can sequence DNA and RNA molecules while preserving base modifications (Depledge et al., 2019). PacBio and ONT have been leading the long-read sequencing market in the last decade, occupying a niche that short-read technologies can not satisfy alone. *De novo* assembly, detection of structural changes in the chromosomes, identification and mapping of transcript isoforms and post-transcriptional base modifications are among the most interesting applications of these TGS technologies (Amarasinghe et al., 2020).

3.2   Spectrum of Genetic Variation Covered

The genetic variation emerges from the comparison of one's DNA sequence with another sequence taken as a framework of reference. With such comparisons, one can typically identify the three categories of genetic variation defined by the size and the pattern of the changing sequence: short sequence variants (< 50 bp long), copy-number variants and a very diverse class of structural variants (> 50 bp) (Ho et al., 2020). Short sequence variants refer to the small changes in the sequence compared to a reference genome and includes single nucleotide variants (SNVs, also known as SNPs) and small insertions and deletions (indels). Copy-number variants (CNV) refer to the relative changes in the amount of a particular stretch of DNA sequence. Structural variants (SV) refer to the changes in the location and/or orientation of a particular DNA sequence. SVs range from ~50 bp to Mb, including inversions, inter- and intra-chromosomal translocations, mobile element insertions, multi-allelic CNVs, and segmental duplications (Ho et al., 2020). Indels and SVs are more likely to disrupt the biological function because they entail a larger portion of the sequence. When they affect the coding region of a gene, they can produce a codon reading frame shift and/or a loss/gain of a stop codon that predicts a large affectation of protein function (Lek et al., 2016). SNVs and indels comprise the vast majority of variants in the human population (Lappalainen et al., 2019). Estimates support that there are 4–5 million SNVs and 0.7–0.8 million indels in a typical comparison of a sample's WGS data versus the reference (Eichler, 2019; Taliun et al., 2021). Nonsynonymous or missense SNVs or in-frame indels lead to amino acid changes, which can be entirely benign, a modifier, or cause a severe disease (Lappalainen et al., 2019). Variants can also affect the gene regulation by affecting transcriptional and post-transcriptional regulatory elements.

The distinction between germline and somatic variants is also relevant to the design of the sequencing experiment for the variant discovery. Germline variants are present in every cell of an individual. In this case, the reference genome can be an external sequence source. Somatic variants refer to mutation events occurring in individual cells during the course of life. These can be caused by environmental exposure to mutagens such as radiation, cigarette smoke, harmful chemicals, among other causes. Therefore, somatic variation is present only in a subset of cells of our body. For that case, the analysis workflow typically includes sequences from a healthy tissue of the same subject as internal sequence reference for the variant calling.

3.3   The Human Reference Genome

A challenge for the variant discovery is the quality and completeness of the human reference genome (HRG). The completion of the first draft of the HRG in 2003 was a remarkable achievement in the history, establishing a standardized coordinate system for annotating genomic elements and comparing individual human genomes (Rakocevic et al., 2019). The HRG plays a relevant role in the WGS analysis workflow since it provides a scaffold for the mapping and assembly of sequencing reads. However, since it represents a mosaic of sequences from a few donors, it falls short in representing sequence variation of human populations (Eggertsson et al., 2017). The limits in the understanding of the complete spectrum of genetic variation stem not only from this and from the restrictions of the sequencing technology, but also from the difficulties in the variant discovery in our diploid genome (Huddleston and Eichler, 2016).

The reference version GRCh38, the latest build of the HRG that replaced the 3 Mb centromeric gaps on all chromosomes from the previous version with modeled centromeres, has expanded the repertoire of alternate contigs (ALT) representing the alternate haplotype, albeit most analysis tools make a limited use of them for now. In addition, the GRCh38 still has gaps and errors at repetitive and structurally diverse regions (Lappalainen et al., 2019). On top of it, all current HRGs are represented only by a single consensus linear DNA haplotype (i.e., are haploid) (Audano et al., 2019). As a consequence, the variant calling in WGS will be biased on individuals with local ancestry closely related to the reference genome at a particular locus. Another relevant drawback to consider is that novel sequences not present in the HRG will be missed after the mapping and alignment step. Therefore, many variant alleles will not be identified in particularly diverse loci (e.g., MHC, *MAPT*, *CYP2D6*, and KIR genes). Efforts have been made to build a gold standard for human genetic variations by focusing on haploid human genomes obtained from complete hydatidiform moles and applying alternative sequencing technologies to improve sensitivity over repetitive regions of the human genome (Huddleston et al., 2017; Li, et al., 2018a; Steinberg et al., 2014). This is the case of the *de novo* PacBio assemblies of two human cell lines that are homozygous across the whole genome, the so-called Sindyp genome. In 2019, the Telomere-to-Telomere Consortium (T2T) announced the gapless telomere-to-telomere *de novo* assembly of a human X chromosome for the first time (https://sites.google.com/ucsc.edu/t2tworkinggroup) using high-coverage, ultra-long-read ONT sequencing of the complete hydatidiform mole CHM13 genome (Eizenga et al., 2020; Miga et al., 2019).

The preponderance of data from European populations in human genetic studies has constrained the diversity of genomic variation identified so far. Recently, several *de novo* assemblies of human genomes have confirmed the hidden diversity of genomic variation in non-Europeans representing large ethnic groups, such as Koreans (Seo et al., 2016), Chinese Han (Du et al., 2019), Japanese (Nagasaki et al., 2019), and Ashkenazi (Shumate et al., 2020). However, the idea of a pangenome representing all relatively common DNA sequences and alleles in the human population has been considered in the last few years (Lappalainen et al., 2019). Genome graphs or variant graphs will be used to represent genome-wide allelic diversity (Garrison et al., 2018; Paten et al., 2017; Rakocevic et al., 2019). However, there is a current scarcity of analysis tools that can handle graph-based representations and they frequently require large computational resources.

4 WORKFLOWS FOR WHOLE-GENOME SEQUENCING DATA PROCESSING

A full NGS data analysis workflow is complex in nature because it comprises multiple serial and parallel analysis steps pipelining different software, tools and data files with user-defined parameters, and typically using several programming languages, file formats and databases. Typically, the user will find differences between the tools integrated in the workflows depending on the type of variants aimed to discover (Wu et al., 2016). Modern workflow frameworks provide advanced features, such as graphical user interfaces (GUI) to visualize quality controls and progress in real time, the use of containerized infrastructure-independent tools, support for running the pipelines in distributed clusters or in the cloud, etc. (Leipzig, 2017). A simplified WGS workflow has different stages, including the alignment-mapping of the reads and the variant calling. With data from TGS, the alignment stage can be substituted by a *de novo* assembly. An additional differentiation in a standard workflow is based on the nature of the studied variation: germline (Fig. 1) or somatic (Fig. 2).

In this section we will focus on a typical pipeline for WGS germline variant calling (Fig. 1). Following library preparation and sequencing, several preprocessing steps are conducted, sequences are aligned and mapped to a reference genome or are assembled *de novo* (i.e., without a reference). The workflow continues through the variant calling. Once the variants are called, they can be further analyzed in order to add relevant annotations and to infer biological functions. As a final step, variants are prioritized and classified based on different filtering or statistical techniques to investigate the relationship between the prioritized variation and the phenotype of interest. Depending on settings, it is possible to incorporate an additional validation step by means of orthogonal methods (e.g., Sanger sequencing) (Lincoln et al. 2019). High quality DNA library preparation is essential for accurate whole genome sequencing, but the sequencing and analysis steps are not error-free. Therefore, quality controls should be applied in the entire workflow. Further details of this general workflow are provided in the following sections.

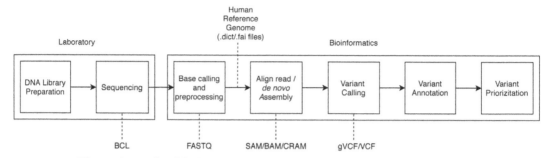

Figure 1   A simplified version of a WGS germline variant calling workflow.

A simplified version of a typical WGS workflow to study somatic alterations is shown in Fig. 2. A pair of normal or control and tumor samples from the same individual are sequenced, and can be compared to a *Panel-of-Normals* to identify and filter germline variants from the somatic alterations observed in the DNA from the same individual. It is also possible to use specialized somatic callers allowing an unpaired sample use. These variant callers are useful when matched normal samples are not available. Additional steps of contamination and tumor segmentation quality controls are also typically performed.

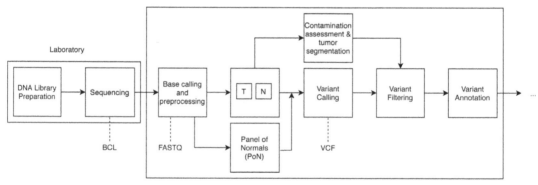

Figure 2   A simplified version of a WGS somatic variant calling workflow (T = tumor; N = Normal).

4.1   Workflow Languages and Editors

Advances in NGS in the last decade have resulted in a data deluge reaching the petabyte scale production every year (Baichoo et al., 2018), moving the bottlenecks from the sequencing side to the data analysis, transfer, storage, and backup. Automating the WGS workflow is a necessity to focus on interpreting the results or developing new methods, instead of in the complex technical details of the bioinformatic pipelines. Modern workflow management systems are able to communicate and adapt to High Performance Computing (HPC) and cloud-based systems (i.e., Google Life Sciences, Microsoft Azure), dealing with all type of job schedulers and execution engines (i.e., SLURM, PBS/Torque, LSF, Moab).

NGS workflows developed in the past has suffered from the lack of reproducibility and interoperability, challenging the portability across multiple infrastructures. A direct consequence of this is the proliferation of heterogeneous NGS analysis pipelines (Ewels et al., 2020). Among the most interesting properties of a state-of-the-art workflow is its flexibility to adapt to modifications and new data types, extensibility to integrate new tools and configurations, simplified setup and use, reproducibility of results, data types, user interfaces (command line or GUI), and availability (Federico et al., 2019).

4.1.1   Common workflow language

The Common Workflow Language (CWL) (https://www.commonwl.org) is one of the broadly adopted standards for describing workflows. CWL can be used to describe pipelines and computational tools, but can be also run on diverse bioinformatic infrastructures. It has been adopted by popular bioinformatics projects, such as Galaxy, Rabix, the genome analysis toolkit (GATK), and others. There are several executors supporting the use of CWL (Arvados, Toil). GATK adopted the CWL standards recently and their developers have rewritten the pipelines in WDL (https://github.com/gatk-workflows), a user-friendly scripting language maintained by the OpenWDL community (Box 1).

4.1.2   Nextflow

Nextflow is a domain-specific language (DSL) built on Groovy, developed at the Center for Genomic Regulation (https://www.nextflow.io). It enables scalable and reproducible scientific workflows (Box 1) using software containers with specific built-in features for bioinformatics (Baichoo et al., 2018). Nextflow offers a variety of exceptional features such as execution of workflows, Docker and Singularity containerization, and multiple executing engines including local execution, execution on clusters and in private and public clouds (Amazon EC2, Kubernetes, OpenStack).

WDL	*Nextflow*
```call MarkDuplicates { input: gatk="gatk", bam="/path/to/bam" ... } task MarkDuplicates { String gatk File bam ... command { ${gatk} --java-options ... \ MarkDuplicates \ -I ${bam} ... } output { ... } }```	```#!/usr/bin/env nextflow ... params.gatk="gatk" ... process MarkDuplicates { input: file(bam) ... output: ... script: """" $params.gatk --java-options ... \ MarkDuplicates \ -I $bam \ ... """" }```

Box 1   Examples of the coding structure in WDL (left) and Nextflow (right) for the MarkDuplicates step of the WGS workflow.

4.1.3 Workflow editors and pipeline builders

Workflows are usually programmed using two complementary approaches. On the one hand, one can use the command line, making a much more flexible workflow design, but requiring high-level bioinformatic skills and expertise that is not amenable for most researchers. This is the case with Nextflow (Di Tommaso et al., 2017) and Snakemake (Köster and Rahmann 2012). On the other hand, one can program the workflow by means of a GUI, offering limited flexibility to the user, as the exemplar case of Galaxy (Afgan et al., 2016).

Recently, several workflow editors have become popular to allow the user to combine both coding and graphical approaches (Sklarz et al., 2018). These state-of-the-art workflow editors include a GUI where the user can drag-and-drop modules (tools) and data inputs-outputs, which connect them to indicate the execution order and data flow (Fig. 3). The workflow editor allows the user to run the desired pipelines in local mode or to export it to a script that can be further edited or executed in a compatible framework. Examples of these modern workflow editors are BioDepot-workflow-builder out of Docker containers (https://github.com/BioDepot/BioDepot-workflow-builder; Hung et al., 2019), Seven Bridges' Rabix (https://rabix.io; Kaushik et al., 2017), Galaxy and Arvados with CWL, Toil with CWL/WDL (https://toil.readthedocs.io; Vivian et al., 2017), Sequanix with NGS Sequana Snakemake pipelines (http://sequana.readthedocs.io; Desvillechabrol et al., 2018), and DolphiNext under Nextflow (https://github.com/dolphinnext; Yukselen et al., 2020). Two interesting tools to build Nextflow pipelines from modular pre-configured blocks or templates are Flowcraft (https://github.com/assemblerflow/flowcraft) and

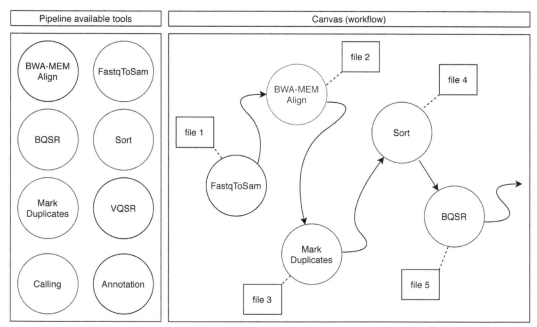

Figure 3   Scheme of a WGS workflow editor to build bioinformatic pipelines using a drag-and-drop graphical user interface.

Pipeliner (https://github.com/montilab/pipeliner; Federico et al., 2019). Other interesting tools are Omics Pipe (http://sulab.org/tools/omics-pipe; Fisch et al., 2015), Butler (https://github.com/llevar/butler; Yakneen et al., 2020), and GenPipes (https://github.com/c3g/GenPipes; Bourgey et al., 2019). Omics Pipe is an open-source modular web-based platform allowing the automation of several best practice multi-omics data analysis pipelines, such as the GATK-based variant-calling of WGS. Butler is a suite of tools to aid researchers to deploy and run workflows on multiple cloud computing platforms. Butler is being used in large projects such as the Pan Cancer

Analysis of Whole Genomes (PCAWG; ICGC/TCGA Pan-Cancer Analysis of Whole Genomes Consortium, 2020) and the Pan Prostate Cancer Group (https://panprostate.org). GenPipes is a Python-based workflow management system for pipeline development including a set of standardized analysis pipelines designed for HPC and cloud settings.

4.2 NGS Data Formats

Reference genomes are usually encoded in a text based FASTA format (Table 2). Chromosomes and contigs are identified and stored in single lines where the nucleotide sequences are represented using single-letter codes (A, C, G, T, or N). The data generated by the sequencer is stored in a vendor-dependent format. In the case of Illumina, Inc., raw data is stored on the sequencer workstation in Basecall format or BCL (Figs. 1 and 2), which is not human-readable. It is possible for the sequencer to output the data into a text file format or FASTQ (typically a compressed version or FASTQ.gz is used to reduce its size), a large file that stores the name of each read, the sequence and the base quality scores expressed in Phred-scale. For ONT technology, a more complex version of this format is FAST5 (based in the HDF5 format). Once the reads are aligned and mapped to the reference genome, the Sequence Alignment Map or SAM file is obtained. This format aggregates to the FASTQ information the alignment and mapping data, and additional metadata that some tools might require in the downstream analyses. SAM files are also very large in size. Therefore, a binary version of SAM, the BAM (Binary Alignment Map) is a common standard at this stage. It is also possible to use CRAM, a lossy compression format that require availability of the reference genome since CRAM only stores differences between the sample sequences and the reference genome. The WGS workflow produces a call set of variants in a VCF format, a tab-separated text format in which each variant is represented by one line (also in a more complex gVCF format). The first eight columns describe variant-level information such as genomic coordinate, the variant identifier, reference and alternatives alleles, etc. Further information can be retrieved from this link: https://www.ncbi.nlm.nih.gov/sra/docs/submitformats.

Table 2 Bioinformatic file formats used in WGS variant calling workflows

Format	URL
FASTA	https://zhanglab.ccmb.med.umich.edu/FASTA
FASTQ	https://www.ncbi.nlm.nih.gov/sra/docs/submitformats/#fastq-files
FAST5	http://simpsonlab.github.io/2017/02/27/packing_fast5
SAM/BAM	https://samtools.github.io/hts-specs/SAMv1.pdf
CRAM	https://samtools.github.io/hts-specs/CRAMv3.pdf https://genome.ucsc.edu/FAQ/FAQformat.html#format5.2
VCF 4.3	https://samtools.github.io/hts-specs/VCFv4.3.pdf https://academic.oup.com/bioinformatics/article/27/15/2156/402296
BED	https://genome.ucsc.edu/FAQ/FAQformat.html#format1
GFF	https://genome.ucsc.edu/FAQ/FAQformat.html#format3

5 WGS WORKFLOW FOR GERMINAL SHORT VARIANT DISCOVERY

In this central part of the chapter we will provide insights into the main steps of a state-of-the-art WGS workflow designed for the discovery of germline short variants following the GATK Best Practices recommendations. The WGS workflow to identify this type of variants in one individual or a cohort of individuals is presented in Fig. 4. The workflow is performed across three different stages defined as primary, secondary and tertiary analyses. Unless stated

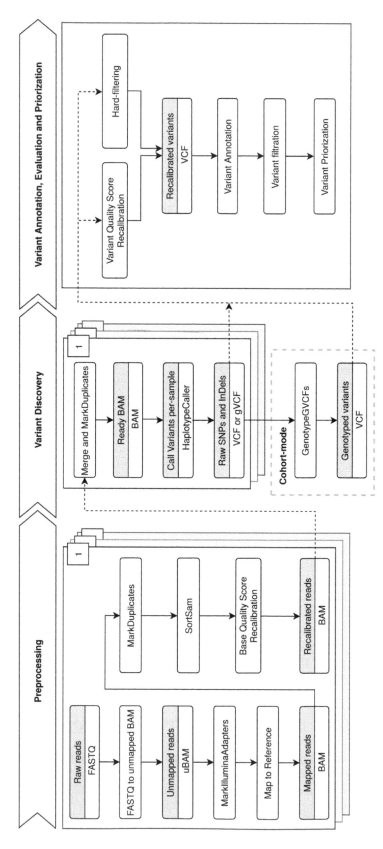

Figure 4 Detailed WGS workflow for germline short sequence variant discovery.

otherwise, the workflow analyzed in depth in this chapter focuses on Illumina, Inc. short-read technology to assess germline short sequence variation.

5.1 Primary Analysis

The nucleotide distribution across cycles is a useful quality control (QC) parameter for WGS and WES (Fig. 5), but not for amplicons or RNA-seq samples (Guo et al., 2014a). The distribution of the four nucleotides across all reads in a run should remain stable, except for some minor fluctuations that may be expected at the beginning of each read (depending on the DNA fragmentation method) and at the read end, since it is closely associated with base quality. The GC-content can also be used as a QC parameter. It varies across species and across the regions of the genome. The resulting depth-of-coverage and, thus, the proficiency of Illumina, Inc. sequencing technology is associated with the GC-content (Dohm et al. 2008), mainly in targeted sequencing experiments, which is linked to the coding sequence length (Oliver and Marín, 1996). Abnormal GC-content might be an indicator of sample contamination.

Other relevant QC account for the existence of index hopping or switching, mainly affecting Illumina, Inc. platforms using ExAmp chemistry and patterned flow cells (e.g., HiSeq 4000, HiSeq X and NovaSeq 6000). Index hopping represents an important issue in studies where adapter ligation is required, such as RNA-seq, or in the study of ancient degraded gDNA in which the resulting low coverage (Shapiro and Hofreiter, 2014) can be interfered by misassigned reads (Llamas et al., 2017). Multiplexing samples in sequencing experiments is a common practice. Samples are individually labelled with unique indexes (known molecular or oligonucleotides barcodes) that are embedded within one or both sequencing platform-specific adapters (van der Valk et al., 2020). Then, samples are pooled into a single DNA library and sequenced on the same lane or across lanes of a flow cell. Once the sequencing is carried out, demultiplexing allows the assignment of sequenced reads to the respective original sample. However, since multiplexing was introduced as part of the sequencing procedures, low rates of read misassignment across samples sequenced on the same lane have been reported (Costello et al., 2018; Larsson et al., 2018). The reported rate of read misassignment ranges from 0.25 to 7% (Li et al., 2019a). The use of a dual index system alleviates the index hopping issue and allows the filtering of reads that are likely misassigned. The extension of the index hopping can be computationally quantified by identifying reads with wrong index combinations provided those are present in a sample sheet used for demultiplexing (Fig. 5). In our own WGS experience based on DNA libraries prepared with the Nextera DNA Flex kit (Illumina, Inc.) and using dual indexes sequenced in a HiSeq 4000, the index hopping was estimated to be lower than 0.41%.

5.1.1 From sequence images to reads

The raw data produced by the sequencer is stored in a vendor-dependent binary format. The bioinformatic WGS workflow should start with the conversion of the raw data captured by the sequencer into strings of nucleotide calls (the reads) and the per base quality scores (Stein, 2011). Most laboratories use the base calling software provided by their NGS sequencer vendor. A major downside here is that base quality scores (stored in the so-called lookup tables) are not comparable across vendors. The base calling step can produce data in FASTQ format (one or two files in single- and paired-end experiments, respectively) per library in each lane of the flow cell or aggregated per sample across the flow cell through a process known as demultiplexing. This data is human readable, but it is not ready to be processed by the variant caller. Therefore, a series of preprocessing steps should be performed in order to prepare data for the downstream analyses. One of such preprocessing steps is the adapter removal and trimming of low-quality bases (Fig. 6). A number of classical bioinformatic tools for the BCL-to-FASTQ conversion and QC applied to this primary analysis are shown in Table 3.

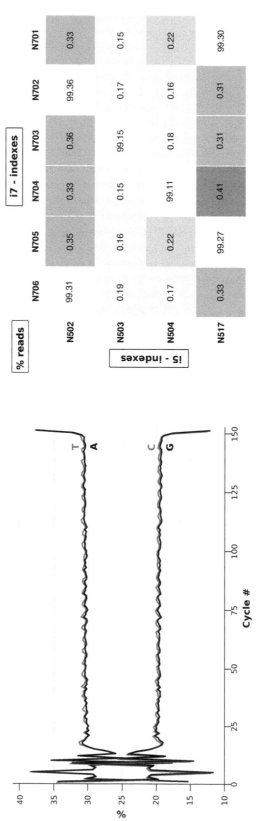

Figure 5 Representative plots of quality control steps in a WGS workflow. Nucleotide distribution typically observed when tagmentation is used in the library preparation (left). Index-hopping heatmap (right) computed after demultiplexing 6 WGS using combinations of 10 indexes (boxes with values above 99.0% represent the expected true index-combinations; numbers represent the percentage of reads showing a combination resulting from the intersection of rows and columns in the index-matrix).

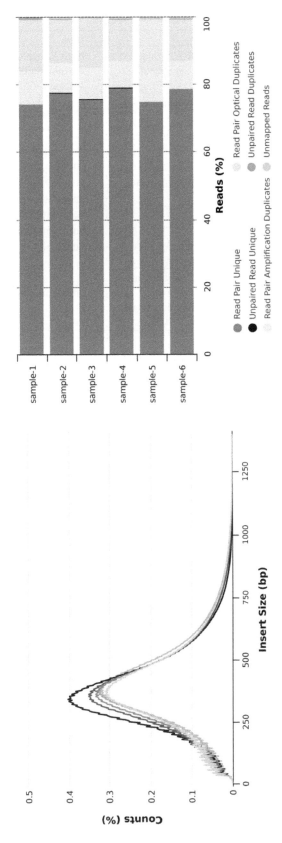

Figure 6 Representative plots of quality control steps in a WGS workflow. Insert-size distribution (left) of six WGS in an Illumina HiSeq 4000. MarkDuplicates statistics from a real WGS experiment (right).

Table 3   Bioinformatic tools used in the pre-processing steps of the WGS workflow

Tool	Task	Link
bcl2fastq	Conversion of base calls in BCL format to FASTQ files for Illumina, Inc. sequencing platforms.	https://emea.support.illumina.com/ downloads/bcl2fastq-conversion-software-v2-20.html
Cutadapt	Removal of adapter sequences, primers, poly-A tails and other types of unwanted sequence.	https://cutadapt.readthedocs.io/en/ stable
Trimmomatic	Read trimming.	http://www.usadellab.org/ cms/?page=trimmomatic
Qualimap	Facilitates QC of aligned sequencing data.	http://qualimap.bioinfo.cipf.es
FastQC	Pre-processing QC.	https://www.bioinformatics.babraham. ac.uk/projects/fastqc
MultiQC	Aggregation of multiple QC.	https://multiqc.info
MegaQC	Aggregation of multiple MultiQC.	https://github.com/ewels/MegaQC
PICARD	Conversion of base calls in BCL format to FASTQ files for Illumina, Inc. sequencing platforms. Manipulation of sequencing data and formats such as SAM/BAM/CRAM and VCF.	https://broadinstitute.github.io/picard

5.1.2   Read alignment against the human reference genome

WGS workflows dealing with short reads proceed with an alignment step against the reference genome, and mapping the reads against the reference using the so-called CIGAR structures (Concise Idiosyncratic Gapped Alignment Report). The alignment takes place using a fast indexing algorithm to identify potential matches in the reference sequence (Stein, 2011) such as the Burrows-Wheeler Transform (BWT). The widely known BWA, BOWTIE, and SOAP aligners use the BWT indexing for the task. This step, together with the variant calling step, exhibit strong levels of heterogeneity on the tools used and, therefore, on the results obtained by different users. This heterogeneity is particularly high for SVs. To minimize this variability, WGS data processing standards have been adopted that allow different groups to produce functionally equivalent results by harmonizing some of the main steps of the workflow (Regier et al., 2018). A number of aligners/mappers is shown in Table 4. It is worth mentioning that when selecting one of these tools, it is critical not only to understand the algorithmic capabilities and the accuracy, but also the level of technical support and the existing evidence indicating that it has been validated (Worthey, 2017). Besides, read alignment/mapping may lead to several complications. For example, the existence of gaps and low-complexity sequences or repeats in the reference sequence, and the existence of sample sequences that are absent from the reference, will produce unmapped or mismapped reads.

Among the tools (Table 4), most modern pipelines rely on BWA-MEM (Li and Durbin, 2009) for the alignment-mapping step, and a combination of tools for subsequent data processing. BWA will align the reads from the FASTQ files and will map them to generate a SAM or a binary BAM file. BWA-MEM has an ALT-aware version that can deal with the GRCh38 reference genome, rather than just the primary chromosomes (Li, 2013). Another aligner for nucleotide sequences, minimap2 (Li, 2018), has come recently into scene. It works with short reads, contig assembly and long noisy reads. Therefore, it can be used as a read aligner, a long-read overlapper, or a full-genome aligner.

Table 4 Widely adopted bioinformatic tools used for the alignment and mapping of reads

Tool	Task	Link
BWA	Short-read mapper	http://bio-bwa.sourceforge.net/ https://github.com/lh3/bwa
SOAP2	Short-read mapper	http://soap.genomics.org.cn/
BOWTIE2	Short-read mapper	https://github.com/BenLangmead/bowtie2
Novoalign	Short-read mapper (commercial)	https://anaconda.org/bioconda/novoalign http://www.novocraft.com/products/novoalign/
minimap2	Short- and long-read mapper	https://github.com/lh3/minimap2

Two QC parameters are worth considering in this step: the average (or median) depth and the percentage of the genome covered at a certain depth (Guo et al., 2014a). The theoretical coverage, estimated by the Lander-Waterman equation (Lander and Waterman, 1988) during the design of the sequencing experiment, can be easily skewed by high depth sequencing regions, especially in targeted sequencing experiments. Thus, a median depth or a measure of depth uniformity would be more robust statistics. A basic report of the alignment summary statistics can be easily obtained with Samtools (*idxstats* option) (Li et al., 2009), a suite of programs designed to interact with NGS derived data (http://www.htslib.org). PICARD also provide a complete set of metrics for QC such as *CollectRawWgsMetrics* and *CollectWgsMetricsWithNonZeroCoverage* (gathers metrics of coverage and performance of experiments).

5.1.3 Base quality score recalibration

The per-base quality score in each position of a read may be inaccurately estimated due to technology limitations (type of flow cell, chemistry used in the clustering, phasing, fading, fluorophore crosstalk, etc.). In addition, it covaries with features like the sequencing cycle and sequence context (DePristo et al., 2011), the flow cell lane, as well as with the tile, swath, and surface (top/bottom) of each lane. As many variant callers take into account the base quality score to improve the process, the quality score of each base must be recalibrated to account for those sequencing-technology dependent inaccuracies and covariation patterns. GATK runs the Base Quality Score Recalibration (BQSR) process in two steps. It first gathers covariate information from base calls in the dataset and builds an empirical error model from those data. Secondly, it applies the base quality adjustments to the original dataset based on that model and records the new base qualities into a recalibrated BAM file.

5.1.4 *De novo* assembly

Single Molecule Real Time (SMRT) sequencing platforms, such as ONT and PacBio, offer advantages for *de novo* assembly of genomes over other widely used short-read technologies. For example, ONT developments have led to an acceleration of the turnaround times and, more importantly, increases in the read length up to several thousand bp despite the high per base error rate. As a consequence, and with a combination with DNA extraction protocols to obtain high-molecular weight materials, the generation of long and ultra-long reads is facilitated nowadays. With this, ONT and other TGS platforms make possible to start assessing human genome variation from *de novo* assemblies (Shumate et al., 2020) that would be extremely discontinuous otherwise if using only short-read data (Magi et al., 2018).

5.1.4.1 *Strategies for de novo assembly*

Without having prior knowledge of the origin and structure of the genome to be reconstructed, *de novo* assembly algorithms manage to build contiguous, accurate and consensual sequences that represent as much as possible the genome of the analyzed individual. There are multiple strategies that can be followed when aiming for a *de novo* assembly. Each strategy, as well as the bioinformatic tools used, has diverse advantages and disadvantages. Therefore, the final approach will depend on the type and quality of the input reads, together with the size and complexity of the target genome. There are two main algorithmic strategies: one based on building a de Bruijn Graph (DBG), and the other one based on the Overlap Layout Consensus (OLC) algorithm. DBG is the graph algorithm based on k-mers approach. The first step of the assembly chooses a k-mer size and split the sequences into its k-mer components (Khan et al., 2018). Then, k-mers are paired overlapping by k-1 nucleotides constructing a directed graph (Miller et al., 2010). Because of the noise that is present in long reads, this approach has better results when it is used to assembly short reads. OLC is also a graph-based algorithm that is structured in three steps (Batzoglou, 2005), and is commonly used to assembly long reads:

1. First, the algorithm looks for the similarity between all sequences to discover possible overlaps and store the results in a pairwise-alignment file (PAF).
2. In the layout step, it builds the graph using the overlaps from the previous step, to yield an assembly file that contains all contigs.
3. Finally, in the consensus step, the most probable nucleotide sequence from each contig is selected using the assembly and the original raw data.

For now, both approaches still fail to build end-to-end chromosome sequences in human genomes. To solve that, a final step called *scaffolding* is needed to orient, order and concatenate contigs generated by the assembly step forming the scaffolds and using N's to fill the gaps between them (Wee et al., 2019). The use of the OLC algorithm or hybrid assemblies (combining data from different sequencing technologies or approaches) offers better quality over DBG alternatives to build *de novo* assemblies in terms of accuracy, performance and computing time (Sović et al., 2016). Some of the most frequently used tools for *de novo* assembly (including the hybrid mode) are shown in Table 5.

Table 5 Exemplar bioinformatic tools that can be combined for *de novo* genome assembly

Step	Tool	Description	Link
BaseCalling	Guppy	Data processing toolkit that contains basecalling algorithms.	https://github.com/nanoporetech
Filter reads	FiltLong	Quality filtering tool for long reads.	https://github.com/rrwick/Filtlong
Assembly Overlap (OLC)	Minimap2	Pairwise aligner used to find overlaps between long reads.	https://lh3.github.io/minimap2
Layout	Miniasm	Ultrafast *de novo* assembly for long noisy reads.	https://github.com/lh3/miniasm
Consensus	Racon	Consensus module for genome assembly of long uncorrected reads.	https://github.com/lbcb-sci/racon
Polishing	Medaka	Consensus tool to polish ONT data performed using neural networks.	https://github.com/nanoporetech/medaka
Hybrid assembly	HASLR	A fast tool for hybrid genome assembly of long and short reads.	https://github.com/vpc-ccg/haslr
Scaffolding	RaGOO	A tool to order and orient genome contigs alignments to a reference.	https://github.com/malonge/RaGOO
Quality Control	NanoPlot	Plotting tool for long read sequencing data and alignments.	https://github.com/wdecoster/NanoPlot
	QUAST	Quality Assessment Tool for Genome Assemblies.	http://quast.sourceforge.net/

New bioinformatic tools are permanently developed to adapt the WGS workflow and other applications to long-read technologies. A comprehensive list of available open-source tools for the different tasks can be found at https://long-read-tools.org.

5.1.4.2 *An example of a hybrid de novo assembly*

A popular approach to build a *de novo* assembly is based on the so-called hybrid approach, leveraging the power of short- and long-read technologies together. In this section, we present a simple workflow to complete a hybrid assembly using HASLR (Fig. 7), a fast hybrid assembler for long reads (Haghshenas et al., 2020). First, one establishes basic QC steps to evaluate the raw sequencing reads, those from ONT using NanoPlot (De Coster et al., 2018), and those from Illumina, Inc. using FastQC. Then, long reads can be filtered by quality and length using FiltLong.

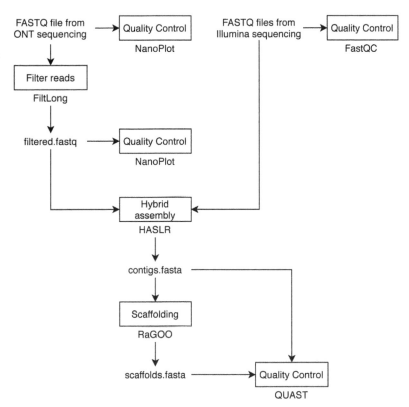

Figure 7 Schematic workflow to obtain a hybrid genome assembly using HASLR.

HASLR integrates different bioinformatic tools to perform the following steps:
1. Assembly of short reads using Minia (https://github.com/GATB/minia) to build Short Read Contigs (SRCs).
2. Find Unique Contigs (UCs).
3. Build a backbone graph using only the longest 25X depth-of-coverage of long reads.
4. Align UCs to long reads using minimap2.
5. Clean the graph discarding edges with less than 3 long reads.
6. Obtain consensus sequences using SPOA (https://github.com/rvaser/spoa).

The result of this is a FASTA file. The next step is to build the scaffolds, and that can be done using RaGOO. Then, its result can be compared against the HRG using QUAST in order to evaluate the quality of the assembly.

Table 6 shows a benchmark comparison between the hg19 HRG and WGS data belonging to an individual from the Canary Islands (Spain) assembled with HASLR and scaffolded with RaGOO. The number of DNA stretches (contigs and scaffolds) and the total assembled lengths are provided. The metrics were computed with QUAST.

Table 6 *De novo* assembly of a human Canary Islander genome

	Reference		Sample (contigs)		Sample (scaffolds)	
Length of the assembled stretch **(bp)**	*#contigs*	*assembled contig length* **(bp)**	*#contigs*	*contig assembly length* **(bp)**	*#scaffolds*	*scaffold assembly length* **(bp)**
≥ 1,000	93	3,137,161,264	2,934	2,737,712,212	39	2,738,146,596
≥ 10,000	92	3,137,157,002	2,282	2,734,865,263	37	2,738,133,599
≥ 25,000	89	3,137,105,510	1,958	2,729,575,446	33	2,738,060,346
≥ 50,000	62	3,136,052,357	1,638	2,717,994,864	30	2,737,943,784

The N50 statistic is a commonly used metric to assess the quality of the *de novo* assembly. It is defined as the largest length, L, for which the collection of all contigs of length ≥ L covers at least half of the assembly. To compute N50, the contig/scaffolds are first ordered by length from longest to shortest. Then, their lengths are sequentially summed starting from the longest, one contig/scaffold at a time, until the total sum equals half of the assembly length. N50 will be the length of the contig or scaffold where we stop the sum. Another useful metric is L50, defined as the number of contigs or scaffolds representing at least half of the assembly length. A summary of the assembly results based on contigs of size ≥ 3,000 bp is shown in Table 7.

Table 7 Summary of the hybrid *de novo* assembly of a human Canary Islander genome

Assembly parameter	*Reference*	*Sample, contig-based assembly*	*Sample, scaffold-based assembly*
Largest contig (bp)	249,250,621	34,750,177	229,689,446
Total length (bp)	3,137,161,264	2,737,196,331	2,738,146,596
GC-content (%)	40.94	40.80	40.80
N50 (bp)	146,364,022	7,816,942	140,437,715
N75 (bp)	115,169,878	3,071,497	107,000,639
L50 (#contigs)	9	104	8
L75 (#contigs)	14	250	13
Number of N's per 100 kbp	7,645.47	0.00	11.30

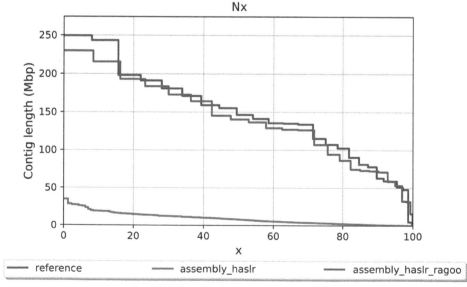

Figure 8 Plot of quality metrics for a hybrid *de novo* assembly of a human Canary Islander genome using the HASLR-RaGOO pipeline.

The quality of the assembly can be also represented graphically by plotting the length of the contig/scaffold against the Nx metric (where x ranges from 0 to 100%; Fig. 8). The Nx metric is defined as the largest contig length, L, such that using contigs of length L accounts for at least x% of assembly bases (Gurevich et al., 2013). The assembly of a Canary Islander whole-genome resulting from the pipeline using only HASLR and HASLR plus RaGOO shows a good concordance with the HRG hg19, with equivalent N50 and L50 values.

5.1.5 Duplicates

Most NGS protocols include amplification steps in the library preparation. The likelihood of increasing the amount of DNA and of duplicates raises with the number of amplification cycles. As a consequence, multiple reads originating from the same original DNA fragment might be sequenced. Unless the user has interest in amplicon sequencing where duplicates are desired (van der Auwera et al., 2013), these duplicated reads should be marked in WGS experiments to avoid biases in the results, for example to support the existence of a putative variant (Pabinger et al., 2014). Duplicates of DNA fragments may also develop during the clustering of libraries across the flow cell used in the ExAmp chemistry (Illumina, Inc.) and during the optical detection of sequences (optical duplicates). The user should consider those duplicates as non-independent observations and mark them as so as well. PICARD can be used to mark duplicates (a process known as 'dedupping') so that they are ignored later in the variant calling step. The dedupping is carried out per-sample on the full set of read groups (a read group, @RG, is a collection of tags that identify sequences). If a sequence from the same library is distributed into multiple read groups (i.e., tagged with different @RG because the library was multiplexed and sequenced across different lanes of a flow cell), the user can also use this step to aggregate the read group data into a single per-sample file. PICARD will produce a single sorted BAM file with the data from all the read groups belonging to the same sample (Fig. 4).

5.2 Secondary Analysis

5.2.1 Variant calling

Variant calling is central to any WGS data analysis workflow. The quality of the variant calling results from the obtained read alignments to the HRG impacts directly in downstream analyses. The bioinformatic tools for genome-wide variant identification can be grouped mainly into four categories (Pabinger et al., 2014): germline, somatic, CNV, and SV callers (Table 8). Tools for the identification of SVs can be further divided into those focused in CNVs and those specialized in the detection of large SVs, such as large indels, inversions, and translocations. The identification of germline variants is essential to discover the causes of both Mendelian and complex diseases. Genetic studies in cancer typically rely on the identification of somatic alterations by comparing tumor and normal sequences from the same individual.

Variant callers are frequently designed to be very sensitive, therefore being more tolerant to false positives than false negatives (Friedman et al., 2020). This is the case of the widely used GATK HaplotypeCaller, which has been designed to identify SNVs and indels with high sensitivity and accuracy. Samtools and the GATK-UnifiedGenotyper are among the so-called position-based or 'pileup' callers (Poplin et al. 2018), conceptually designed to identify mismatches between the aligned reads and the reference, and then sort them probabilistically taking into account the reported base quality and context prior for calling variants. These callers follow a Bayesian approach (Li et al., 2018b). A more refined approach is performed by the GATK-HaplotypeCaller (van der Auwera et al., 2013) and Platypus (Rimmer et al., 2014), designed to perform local realignments and *de novo* assembly to build theoretical haplotypes via DBG-like graphs from a consensus of the reads covering the genomic region of interest. The haplotype with the highest likelihood is considered to be the true sequence within that region, and variants contained in that haplotype will be called. Other variant callers offer:

- A combination of these two approaches: FreeBayes (Garrison and Marth, 2012), Fermikit (Li, 2015), and Octopus (Cooke et al., 2021).
- A completely different filtering strategy for variant candidates: xAtlas (Farek et al., 2018).
- A real-time mapping of reads obtained by the sequencer: HiLive2 (Loka and Renard, 2019).
- Use of Field Programmable Gate Arrays (FPGA), as the hardware-accelerated DRAGEN pipeline (Miller et al., 2015).
- A third-party Sentieon DNASeq variant calling workflow (Kendig et al., 2019).

Variant calling is challenging due to the numerous technical issues linked to the library preparation, sequencing platforms, preprocessing tools, incompleteness of the reference genome, misalignments, etc. State-of-the-art variant callers use a number of statistical techniques based on machine learning (Platypus, GATK-HaplotypeCaller, 16GT (Luo et al., 2017), FreeBayes, Strelka (Kim et al., 2018a), and VarsCan2 (Koboldt et al., 2012)), or deep learning such as convolutional neural networks in DeepVariant (Poplin et al., 2018) or in Clairvoyante (Luo et al., 2019) to model and solve these errors to accurately identify mismatches between reads and the reference genome caused by true genomic variants or by any error (Poplin et al., 2018).

Table 8   Some of the most widely used bioinformatic tools for variant calling

Tool	Type of variants	Link
GATK-HC	SNVs, indels	https://gatk.broadinstitute.org/hc
Platypus	SNVs, indels	https://github.com/andyrimmer/Platypus
Octopus	SNVs, indels	https://github.com/luntergroup/octopus
FreeBayes	SNVs, indels	https://github.com/ekg/freebayes
Fermikit	SNVs, indels, SVs	https://github.com/lh3/fermikit
DeepVariant	SNVs, indels, SVs	https://github.com/google/deepvariant
Clairvoyante	SNVs, indels, SVs	https://github.com/aquaskyline/Clairvoyante
Manta	Indels, SVs	https://github.com/Illumina/manta
Pisces	SNVs, Multi Nucleotide Variants (MNVs), indels (somatic)	https://github.com/Illumina/Pisces
Strelka2	SNVs, indels (germline/somatic)	https://github.com/Illumina/strelka
xAtlas	SNVs, indels	https://github.com/jfarek/xatlas
VarsCan2	SNVs, indels (germline/somatic)	http://dkoboldt.github.io/varscan
Medaka	SNVs, indels (ONT data)	https://github.com/nanoporetech/medaka
Longshot	SNVs, indels (ONT and PacBio data)	https://github.com/pjedge/longshot
NanoVar	SVs (ONT data)	https://github.com/benoukraflab/NanoVar
NanoCaller	SNVs, indels (ONT and PacBio data)	https://github.com/WGLab/NanoCaller

The output of the variant calling step is encoded in a VCF file (Fig. 9). Some of the widely used tools to read and operate on VCF files are VCFtools (https://vcftools.github.io; Danecek et al., 2011); BCFtools, which was designed to directly work with a binary representation of the variant call format (BCF) (http://samtools.github.io/bcftools); bedtools (https://bedtools. readthedocs.io; Quinlan and Hall, 2010; Quinlan, 2014), which include a suite of utilities to perform a wide range of tasks (merge, intersect, complement, etc.) with files in multiple formats (BAM, BED, GFF/GTF, VCF); and SnpSift (http://snpeff.sourceforge.net) to filter large genomic datasets. GATK also offers specialized tools for variant filtering and annotation. Routines such as *VariantFiltration* allows the filtering of variants based on INFO and FORMAT annotations already present in the VCF file by using Java EXpression Language, JEXL, filtering expressions (i.e., —*filterExpression* "*QUAL > 30 || MQ0 > 50*"). Other routines such as *VariantEval* and the PICARD *CollectVariantCallingMetrics* provide complementary diagnostic and quality metrics of the variant callset.

Comprehensive comparisons of pipelines for germline (Chen et al., 2019; Supernat et al., 2018) and somatic variant calling are available elsewhere (Chen et al., 2020; Xu, 2018).

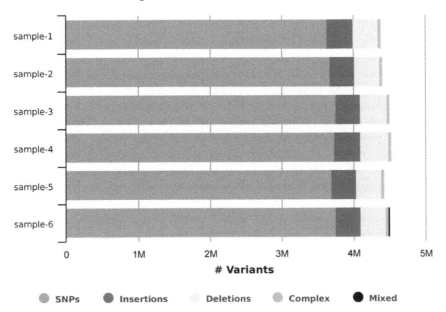

Figure 9   Distribution of the types of variants in a set of six human genomes after the variant calling.

5.2.2   Joint call of variants using a cohort of samples

The WGS workflow discussed in the previous sections were focused on the discovery of variants on a per-sample basis. In studies involving a number of individuals, such as those performed on family-pedigrees, large cohorts, biobank-scale or federated projects, a more refined variant calling may be used. A joint-call step, named Joint-Genotyping, of raw WGS data across the entire set of individual variant sites to increase sensitivity and accuracy is possible. This step is particularly useful in improving the sensitivity of the variant calling at low coverage positions. In the Join-Genotyping in cohort mode of the WGS workflow (see Fig. 4), the GATK-HaplotypeCaller is run in GVCF mode, a method that indicates that the variants must be emitted in a genomic VCF or gVCF format per-sample. The result of this process is a GVCF file per-sample containing the likelihoods for each possible genotype of the variant alleles. This special GATK variant calling methods adds a '<NON-REF>' allele symbol to each record of the gVCF file, holding the information for variant and non-variant sites. Once all the per-sample gVCF files are emitted and consolidated into a database by specialized GATK commands, the JointGenotyping is applied, resulting in individual VCF files (or a multisample VCF file) with improved sensitivity and accuracy. Further information on how modern WGS workflows perform the Joint-Genotyping are described elsewhere (Lappalainen et al., 2019; Poplin et al., 2018; Regier et al., 2018).

5.2.3   Quality control in the variant calling step

Assessing the quality of variant call results can be performed attending to distinct parameters computed from the variant callset itself, the most common being the transition-to-transversion ratio (Ti/Tv), the heterozygosity to non-reference homozygosity ratio (Het/HomAlt), and the total number of variable sites (estimated in about 4–5 M in a single WGS). The Ti/Tv ratio changes across the genome, but it is quite stable when comparing whole-genomes from individuals of different ancestry. On the contrary, the Het/HomAlt ratio varies notably by ancestry (Wang et al., 2015). Typically, Ti/Tv values are 3.0–3.3 for variants residing in exons (differs between synonymous and non-synonymous variants, Yang and Nielsen 1998; and about 2.0–2.2 in the non-coding regions of the genome, Bainbridge et al., 2011). Thus, Ti/Tv ratios are expected to be near 3.0 for WES and close to 2.0 for WGS (Guo et al., 2014b). Values differing from these figures may be cause for concern. The Het/HomAlt ratio is another good QC parameter and is expected to be ≤ 2.0 based on the Hardy-Weinberg equilibrium (Guo et al., 2014b). However, there is an indiscriminate use of Ti/Tv based on the assumption that novel variants should show the same ratio as the common variation. A relatively large number of variable sites, especially those with heterozygous genotypes, and a low Ti/Tv ratios among novel calls indicate the presence of likely false positives resulting from sequencing and alignment errors (DePristo et al., 2011). Other important QC parameters relevant for the assessment of the variant callset quality are the strand bias and allele balance. Theoretically, alleles at heterozygous sites should be supported by a balance of 50% of the reads aligning to the sites, meaning that approximately half of the reads are expected to support the reference allele while the other half are expected to support the alternative allele (Guo et al., 2014a), and found evenly distributed among both strands.

To identify somatic alterations in the WGS workflow, one typically aims to compare sequences between paired normal and tumor samples. The assessment of the variability is not so straightforward such as for detecting germline variants since the tumor sample might be contaminated by the normal tissue. If one identifies alternative alleles in the tumor but not in the matched normal at the same locus, the variant is identified as a somatic mutation in the tumor. Therefore, it is necessary to characterize the germline variation of each normal pair to clearly distinguish the somatic alterations.

If a WGS workflow is applied on a cohort of samples, once the VCF files are emitted from the variant calling step, more sophisticated QCs can be carried out to identify false calls and their possible sources:

- Ancestry QC based on the admixture using PLINK (https://www.cog-genomics.org/plink2; Purcell et al., 2007), ADMIXTURE (http://dalexander.github.io/admixture; Alexander, et al., 2009), or peddy (https://github.com/brentp/peddy; Pedersen and Quinlan, 2017).
- Kinship analysis to identify relatedness using KING (http://people.virginia.edu/~wc9c/ KING; Manichaikul et al., 2010) or PLINK. With these tools the user may assess sample cross-contamination and mislabeling. In this case, the Identity-By-Descent and genotype-concordance statistics can be used (in case SNP array data or other orthogonal data are available). Other tools such as verifyBamID (https://genome.sph.umich.edu/ wiki/VerifyBamID; Jun et al., 2012) and Somalier (https://github.com/brentp/somalier; Pedersen et al., 2020) are also useful for these tasks.
- Sex-check to identify discrepancies between the self-declared sex (if recorded) and the genetically estimated sex (based on PLINK or Somalier, for example). As a consequence, further investigation of samples with discordances (ambiguous sex assignment) might be recommended.

5.2.4 Refinement of variant calling results

Once the variant calling has finished, either from a single individual or from a cohort, it is necessary to further refine the callset to limit the false calls. QCs of the callset can improve the genotyping accuracy at common variants and minimize the false discovery rate at rare variants. Two different classes of methods exist to address this: filtering and classification methods. The filtering methods (hard filtering) define fixed thresholds depending on the type of variant (e.g., SNVs or indels) to several parameters to discard variants that are more likely to be false calls. Examples of these are: a high genotype missing call rate (> 5%), low mapping quality (MQ < 40), high allelic imbalance (usually > 60:40 or > 70:30 for reads supporting the REF:ALT alleles), low quality-by-depth (QD < 2), Fisher Strand bias statistic (> 60), StrandOddsRatio (> 3), among others (i.e., excess heterozygosity, RMSMappingQuality, MappingQualityRankSumTest, ReadPosRankSumTest). However, these thresholds are study-specific and manual fine-tuning is recommended. The classification methods rely on classical machine learning or deep learning techniques to identify most likely false calls. An example is the GATK Variant Quality Score Recalibration (VQSR) as part of its Best Practices recommendations. The approach applies Gaussian Mixture Models to embed the multidimensional space of annotations of the candidate variants. VQSR trains its models from curated variant databases such as The 1000 Genomes Project, HapMap, Omni, dbSNP, etc. One has to keep in mind that this procedure is slightly biased towards known variants and may discard novel variation due to generalization issues of the machine learning method (Li, et al., 2019a). However, the GATK VQSR allows the fine-tuning to a desired level of truth sensitivity and is less bias-prone than the hard filtering method (Van der Auwera et al., 2013).

Other machine learning-based methods exist for the refinement of the callset. The Genome Aggregation Database (GnomAD) uses a Random Forest algorithm for variant quality control in their recent releases, reformulating the GATK-style QD metric (qual/depth). FUWA (Li, et al., 2018b) is a decision-tree based machine learning Classification and Regression Tree (CART) relying in the dbSNP database. It has been applied to WGS, WES, and WGS at low coverage, showing improvements in sensitivity and specificity for SNVs and indels. An example of a combination of filtering and machine learning methods is the Random Forest algorithm approach built in ForestQC (Li, et al., 2019b). Convolutional Neural Network (CNNs) has also been used for filtering small genomic variants in short-read DNA sequence data (Friedman et al., 2020).

The refurbished version 4 of GATK also provides a modern algorithm to call variants in single samples using CNN filtering. Instead of using the WGS germline variant calling workflow based on the GATK-HaplotypeCaller plus VQSR, one may use the GATK CNN filtering. This new algorithm (GATK CNN 1-D or 2-D) encodes reference sequence, read data and variant annotations into tensors (a generalization of algebraic objects related to a vector space). This new version of GATK provides a set of precomputed models trained on highly validated callsets such as those from GIAB (https://github.com/genome-in-a-bottle), the Platinum Genomes (https://github.com/Illumina/PlatinumGenomes), and Syndip (https://github.com/lh3/CHM-eval).

5.2.5 Benchmarkings

Identifying variants with high quality and accuracy is a cornerstone in many applications, but particularly relevant in the clinical diagnosis. In consequence, bioinformatics benchmarking should be considered as an essential step for the assessment of the entire WGS workflow, by evaluating not only the pipeline performance but also the quality and accuracy of the data obtained. The benchmarking process should rely on standards and performance metrics directly computed from the NGS data (Box 2; Zook et al. 2019). The GIAB consortium provides genome reference materials such as the pilot genomes HG001 and HG002, and have developed benchmark datasets, cloud-based pipelines, and evaluation tools to optimize and validate results from NGS workflows (Zook et al., 2019). In 2016 and again in 2020, the US Food and Drug Administration (FDA) has organized several challenges to assess, compare, and improve techniques used in DNA sequencing by worldwide participants based on GIAB reference materials and datasets (https://precision.fda.gov/challenges). Other widely used dataset is the Platinum Genome reference (https://emea.illumina.com/platinumgenomes.html), corresponding to the NA12878 individual.

To assess the performance of a WGS workflow, we recommend following the Best Practices for benchmarking germline small variants in human calls (Krusche et al., 2019; Zook et al., 2019). One typically computes metrics such as the recall or sensitivity (the number of true-positive results over all samples that should be given a positive prediction), the precision (the number of true-positive results divided by the number of positive results predicted by the classifier), and the F1-score (the harmonic average of recall and precision) (Li et al., 2019). Frequently, a benchmarking study compares the performance of diverse pipelines and tools on simulated and/ or real specific data sets. Examples of SVs benchmarkings has become available in the last few years exposing the heterogeneity of variant calling methods derived for short- and long-read technologies (Cameron et al., 2019; Ho et al., 2020; Kosugi et al., 2019; Zook et al., 2020). Several concerns are associated to the available benchmark datasets (i.e. HG001). Such reference datasets are the consensus resulting from the calling of small variants and, in consequence, they are biased towards easy mappable regions (Li et al., 2018a), avoiding repetitive regions and segmental duplications. In addition, they are being used to train bioinformatic pipelines. Therefore, for the purpose of pipeline testing, another reference material is recommended. This is the case of the synthetic diploid call, which resulted in a new phased benchmark dataset, Syndip (synthetic diploid; Li et al., 2018a), resulting from *de novo* PacBio assemblies of two complete CHM-cells-derived from a hydatidiform mole.

Easy to use, but powerful, bioinformatic tools for assessing the benchmarking results are vcfeval, an advanced tool for comparison of VCF files from RT Genomics (https://github.com/ RealTimeGenomics/rtg-tools), and happy (https://github.com/illumina/hap.py), a tool to compare a VCF file against a gold standard dataset.

The Global Alliance for Genomics and Health and Genome in a Bottle: The Global Alliance for Genomics and Health (GA4GH; https://www.ga4gh.org) is a policy-framing and technical standards-setting organization, seeking to enable responsible genomic data sharing within a human rights framework. The GA4GH offers different toolkits to ease the access and adoption of open standards for genomic data security and sharing, and ready-to-use regulatory and ethics guidance for genomic and health-related data sharing. The Genome in a Bottle Consortium (GIAB; https://jimb.stanford.edu/giab) offers reference materials and data for human genome sequencing, as well as methods for genome comparison and benchmarking (Zook et al., 2016). Examples of these reference materials are the so-called human pilot genome sequences and results, NA12878 or HG001, and from Ashkenazi and Chinese trios. These data are unique among the National Institute of Standards and Technology materials and are the result of integrating results from twelve different sequencing technologies: BioNano Genomics, Complete Genomics paired-end and LFR, Ion Proton exome, ONT, PacBio, SOLiD, 10X Genomics GemCode WGS, and Illumina, Inc. exome and WGS paired-end, mate-pair, and synthetic long reads (Zook et al., 2016). They are widely used as validation tools in the context of WGS and WES analyses.

Box 2   The GA4GH and GIAB initiatives.

5.3   Tertiary Analysis

5.3.1   Annotation

Moving downstream in the WGS analysis workflow, the next step involves the annotation of the refined variant callset. This step is essential to provide functional information and disease-linked evidence (Wu et al., 2016). Thanks to the large-scale genome sequencing projects and the wide adoption of NGS in the clinical setting, diverse genetic information is being continuously generated and aggregated in public and private databases worldwide both for germline and somatic variants (Li et al., 2017). Depending on the type of annotations, one may want to use a variant-centric or a gene-centric annotation approach, querying information stored in specific databases.

Annotations to be considered may include basic variant information (Table 9) such as genomic location, gene symbol, variant type and frequency in selected populations, conservation scores, predicted functional and biological properties of the variant, the genomic region where it is located, transcript information, protein changes, nearby genes, and pre-computed *in silico* algorithm-based predictions, among others (Li et al., 2017). In addition to information from coding regions of the genome, the annotation step allows including specific information from noncoding transcripts, chromatin configuration, regulatory regions, DNase hypersensitivity sites, CpG islands, and population variation, among others (Armstrong et al., 2019).

Table 9 Repositories and data warehouses used to annotate basic variant information

Tool	Description	Link
NCBI Genome	Portal with information on genomes including sequences, maps, chromosomes, assemblies, and annotations.	https://www.ncbi.nlm.nih.gov/genome
UCSC table browser	Web-based tool to retrieve DNA sequence and associated data in a track.	http://www.genome.ucsc.edu/cgi-bin/hgTables
Ensembl Genomes	Ensembl genome database project.	http://ensemblgenomes.org/info
Ensembl Biomart	Web-based tool to extract of data from many Ensembl databases.	https://www.ensembl.org/biomart/martview
Locus Reference Genomic	Database of manually curated of stable genomic, transcript and protein reference sequences for reporting clinically relevant sequence variants.	https://www.lrg-sequence.org
RefSeqGene	Database with genomic sequences to be used as reference standards for well-characterized genes.	https://www.ncbi.nlm.nih.gov/refseq/rsg

The annotation step usually combines stand-alone and web-based tools and databases. Some of the most widely used annotation tools are ANNOVAR (https://annovar.openbioinformatics.org, Wang, Li, and Hakonarson, 2010), SnpEff (http://snpeff.sourceforge.net, Cingolani et al., 2012), the Ensembl Variant Effect Predictor VEP (https://ensembl.org/info/docs/tools/vep; McLaren et al., 2016), and stand-alone tools such as VarAFT (https://varaft.eu; Desvignes et al., 2018), VCF-Miner (http://bioinformaticstools.mayo.edu/research/vcf-miner; Hart et al., 2016), and VCFFilter (https://biomedical-sequencing.at/VCFFilter; Müller et al., 2017). A nice example of a collection of scripts dedicated to the annotation, filtering, and the prioritization of variants based on binary classification algorithms is VarSight (https://github.com/HudsonAlpha/VarSight; Holt et al., 2019).

These tools provide different annotations allowing the classification of variants according to distinct criteria: by variant type, by downstream impact (modifier, low, moderate, high; none/gain/loss of function), by functional class (silent, missense, nonsense), by type and region (exonic, intronic, intergenic, 5′ and 3′ UTR, regulatory, up/downstream; frameshift, splice site donor/acceptor, start gained/loss, stop gained/loss), etc., and also allow the use of pedigree-based information such as inheritance models. Frequently used databases are: ClinVar, a public archive of relationships reports based on evidences among human variations and phenotypes; the Online Mendelian Inheritance in Man database, a manually curated online catalog of human genes and genetic disorders; the Human Gene Mutation Database, a catalog of published germline mutations in nuclear genes that underlie, or are closely associated, with human inherited diseases; and COSMIC, the Catalogue of Somatic Mutations In Cancer, a database for exploring the impact of somatic mutations in human cancer. An overview of databases frequently used

Table 10 Databases for detailed annotation of variants

Tool	Description	Link
dbSNP	NCBI Short Genetic Variations database.	https://www.ncbi.nlm.nih.gov/snp
GnomAD	Genome Aggregation Database, a catalog of aggregated exome and genome variation from large-scale sequencing projects.	https://gnomad.broadinstitute.org
The 1000 Genomes Project	IGSR: The International Genome Sample Resource.	https://www.internationalgenome.org
dbVar	NCBI's database of human genomic Structural Variation.	https://www.ncbi.nlm.nih.gov/dbvar
HGMD	Catalog of known (published) gene lesions responsible for human inherited disease.	http://www.hgmd.cf.ac.uk/ac/index.php
ClinVar	Reports of the relationships among human germline rare variants and phenotypes, with supporting evidence.	https://www.ncbi.nlm.nih.gov/clinvar
ClinGen	Clinical relevance of genes and variants for use in precision medicine and research.	https://www.clinicalgenome.org
TOPMed	NHLBI Trans-Omics for Precision Medicine.	https://nhlbiwgs.org
OMIM	Online Mendelian Inheritance in Man.	https://www.omim.org
dbNSFP	Functional prediction and annotation of all potential non-synonymous single-nucleotide variants.	https://sites.google.com/site/jpopgen/dbNSFP
MCap	Mendelian Clinically Applicable Pathogenicity (M-CAP) Score.	http://bejerano.stanford.edu/mcap
CADD	Combined Annotation Dependent Depletion.	https://cadd.gs.washington.edu
Leiden Open Variation Database	Open source database designed to collect and display variants in the DNA sequence.	http://www.lovd.nl
COSMIC	Catalogue Of Somatic Mutations In Cancer.	https://cancer.sanger.ac.uk/cosmic
Ensembl Variant Effect Predictor (VEP)	Toolset for the analysis, annotation, and prioritization of genomic variants in coding and non-coding regions.	http://www.ensembl.org/info/docs/tools/vep
TCGA	The Cancer Genome Atlas Program.	https://www.cancer.gov/about-nci/organization/ccg/research/structural-genomics/tcga
ICGC	International Cancer Genome Consortium, Pan-Cancer Analysis of Whole Genomes (PCAWG).	https://dcc.icgc.org/pcawg
Open Target Genetics	Variant-gene-trait associations from UK Biobank and the GWAS Catalog.	https://genetics.opentargets.org
DECIPHER	Web-based database designed to share and compare phenotypic and genotypic, and in the interpretation of genomic variants.	https://decipher.sanger.ac.uk
Varsome	Variant knowledge community, data aggregator and variant data discovery tool.	https://varsome.com
Open Targets Platform	Resource for the integration of genetics, omics and chemical data to aid systematic drug target identification and prioritization.	https://www.targetvalidation.org

in the annotation step is shown in Table 10. A comprehensive list of databases and predictive algorithms have been described elsewhere (Gao et al., 2019; Li et al., 2017; Richards et al., 2015). Altogether, tools and databases allow a comprehensive analysis and prioritization of almost all classes of variants.

Once the WGS variant callset has been annotated, there is plenty of information to be used for filtering those variants that are more likely to be linked to the disease status from those with no effect on the phenotype under study. Annotation information can be also used to determine the clinical and functional impact of a variant and genomic feature in which the variant is located, as well as to estimate the allele frequency of the variant in a non-disease or disease population (Worthey, 2017).

5.3.2 Evaluation and prioritization of genomic variation

Variant interpretation has a paramount relevance in a clinical setting and represents a complex process out of the scope of this chapter (Fig. 10). A clinical-oriented WGS workflow should envisage an end-to-end automatic and validated pipeline to avoid human errors (Amendola et al., 2016).

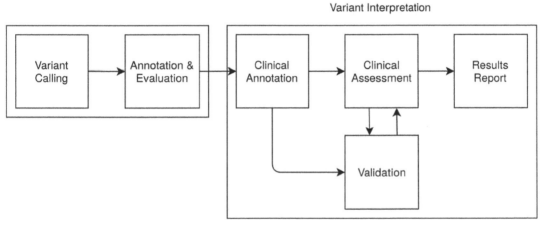

Figure 10 Pipeline steps related with the interpretation of the genomic variation. The variants in the VCF file are further analyzed to keep only those findings of clinical relevance (i.e., putative pathogenic or causal variants for example). Some of those findings may necessitate orthogonal validation.

Following the variant annotation step, each of the variants identified must be sufficiently annotated to perform a clinical interpretation. Each variant can be classified into a predefined category for clinical reporting (Worthey, 2017). In 2015, the American College of Medical Genetics and Genomics (ACMG) and the Association for Molecular Pathology (AMP) published guidelines for the assessment of variants in genes associated with Mendelian diseases (Richards et al., 2015). The current guidelines recommend the use of specific standard terminology to classify variants into five tiers and to define the evidence necessary for clinical interpretation: pathogenic, likely-pathogenic, uncertain significance (VUS), likely-benign, and benign. The ACMG-AMP variant interpretation criteria are diverse and relatively complex, ranging from computational and predictive to functional ones. Regarding the somatic alterations, in 2017 a joint consensus recommendation of the AMP, ACMG, and the College of American Pathologists (CAP) defined classified clinical evidence into four levels or tiers to evaluate the mutation clinical significance and actionability (Gao et al., 2019). From a clinical perspective, variants identified and annotated through a WGS workflow should also focus on the ACMG secondary findings list (Kalia et al., 2017) and genes of pharmacogenomic relevance as stated by the Clinical Pharmacogenetics Implementation Consortium (CPIC) standards (Crawford et al., 2019; Relling et al., 2017). More complete reviews of the standardization of NGS data and guidelines for the interpretation practices in the clinical setting are available (Dewey et al., 2014; Li et al., 2017; Lincoln et al., 2019; Lubin et al., 2017; O'Daniel et al., 2017; Strande et al., 2018; Watkins et al., 2019; Kim et al., 2020).

6   APPLICATIONS

6.1   Large-scale Whole-genome Sequencing Projects

A milestone in the era of the human genome sequencing was the 1000 Genomes Project (1000 Genomes Project Consortium et al., 2010). This project provided a comprehensive perspective of the genome variation across 2,504 individuals from 26 populations worldwide using a combination of low-coverage WGS, deep WES, and SNP array genotyping. According to the Phase III results, a typical individual genome differs from the reference human genome in 4–5 M sites and most of the variation consists of SNVs and indels, and an estimated number of 2,100–2,500 SVs.

Table 11   Some of the largest WGS initiatives

Project	Country	Link
100,000 Genomes Project	United Kingdom	https://www.genomicsengland.co.uk/about-genomics-england/the-100000-genomes-project
Australian Genomics Health Alliance (Australian Genomics)	Australia	https://www.australiangenomics.org.au
Initiative on Rare and Undiagnosed Diseases	Japan	https://www.amed.go.jp/en/program/IRUD
Genome Asia 100K	64 countries across Asia	https://genomeasia100k.org
European '1+ Million Genomes' Initiative	22 European countries	https://ec.europa.eu/digital-single-market/en/european-1-million-genomes-initiative
All of Us Research Program	USA	https://allofus.nih.gov
French Plan for Genomic Medicine 2025	France	http://pfmg2025.aviesan.fr
Dubai Genomics	United Arab Emirates	https://www.dha.gov.ae/en/Pages/DubaiGneomicsAbout.aspx
Saudi Human Genome Program	Saudi Arabia	https://www.saudigenomeprogram.org
Genome of the Netherlands Consortium	The Netherlands	http://www.nlgenome.nl
SweGen project	Sweden	https://swefreq.nbis.se
African Variation Genome Project	Sub-Saharan Africa	https://www.sanger.ac.uk/collaboration/african-genome-variation-project
Korean Personal Genome Project	Korea	http://kpgp.kr

In the last few years, technological advances have provided a momentum for large-scale WGS projects, frequently using low-to-intermediate depth-of-coverages (4 to 20X) (Telenti et al.,

2016) with some exceptions (1000 Genomes Project Consortium et al., 2010; Abel et al., 2020; Bergström et al., 2020; Gudbjartsson et al., 2015; Mallick et al., 2016; Lan et al., 2017; Nagasaki et al., 2015; Sherman et al., 2019; Shringarpure et al., 2017). To avoid the proven limitation of WGS in detecting rare variants, current WGS-based studies use a standard depth of >20X. Many international country- and federated-centric WGS initiatives are underway (Table 11). The NGS data produced by all these efforts will facilitate the assembly of new human reference genomes and will foster genome-wide studies in underrepresented populations.

The Exome Aggregation Consortium (ExAC) and GnomAD are among the largest initiatives to aggregate and harmonize NGS data obtained from WGS and WES projects. Using a web browser, it is possible to retrieve valuable data for SNVs, indels, and SVs from these two initiatives (Collins et al., 2020; Lek et al., 2016; Wang et al., 2020a).

6.2 WGS in Population Genomics

NGS data provided by WGS has extended the possibilities of the SNPs-based population genetic studies to the broad perspective of population genomics by increasing the number of genetic markers and allowing the development of new tools to deal with NGS data (Kelleher et al., 2019; Korneliussen et al., 2014). Segregating sites identified with WGS allows to infer finer population substructure, effective population sizes (Ne), demographic events and ancestry (e.g. bottlenecks and expansions, time of divergence, coalescence rates), levels of inbreeding, gene flow between populations (Bergström et al., 2020; Ekblom and Wolf, 2014;). In addition, WGS data has been used to reconstruct the human population history (Fan et al., 2019; Mallick et al., 2016), revealing how rare variants may impact in common diseases (Wu et al., 2016). Genome wide scans for selection can also be addressed using WGS data, as well as quantitative trait loci (QTL) fine mapping to detect loci responsible for local adaptation (Guillen-Guio et al., 2018; Steiner et al., 2013) and positive selection (Akbari et al., 2018).

6.3 WGS in Disease-oriented Studies

The use of WGS in a clinical setting is still complex and requires the interpretation of the expected average of 4–5 M variants per individual (Worthey, 2017), many of them classified as VUS or showing a non-functional or neutral effect (Lappalainen et al., 2019). Therefore, only a few variants with deleterious effects are expected in a human genome as a consequence of purifying selection (Karczewski et al., 2020). However, it is worth mentioning that variant frequency annotations have been involved in the diagnosis of many pathogenic or damaging alterations in gene function (Lacaze et al., 2019). Large-scale databases providing ancestry-based variant frequency information such as GnomAD and the TOPMed at the Bravo server (https://bravo.sph.umich.edu/freeze5/hg38) should be considered. Large regions of the human genome still remain inaccessible or '*dark*' to the traditional NGS technologies (Ebbert et al., 2019) because they are either unmappable or the tools fail in the aligning process. Therefore, identifying variants in these regions remains a challenge despite their likely implications on disease risk (i.e. neurological diseases such as amyotrophic lateral sclerosis, Alzheimer's disease, autism spectrum disorder).

6.4 Low Coverage WGS

Resequencing of human genomes at low coverage hinders the variant discovery because the reduced number of reads supporting a variant allele limits the performance of the caller (DePristo et al., 2011). In consequence, many variants will be missed from the callset. The 1000 Genomes Project (1000 Genomes Project Consortium et al., 2010) took advantage from this approach to reduce the costs, yet it is not currently a recommended approach if low frequency and rare variants are of interest (Panoutsopoulou et al., 2013). The continuously decreasing costs of WGS make NGS technologies affordable to projects with larger sample sizes and deep coverage. However, the use of low coverage WGS (lcWGS) has been shown to be as effective as variant imputation from SNP arrays (Homburger et al., 2019). lcWGS (0.1–0.5X) has also been useful to capture much of the common (>5%) and low-frequency (1–5%) variation across a human genome with comparable results as those obtained with SNP arrays in genome-wide association studies (GWAS) (Pasaniuc et al., 2012). lcWGS can discover > 95% of variants found by imputed SNP array data with an average minor allele concordance of 97% for common and low frequency variants (Gilly et al., 2019).

In the context of prenatal diagnosis, lcWGS has been used to detect mosaicism with higher resolution and sensitivity compared with those obtained with chromosome arrays (Wang et al., 2020b). SNP arrays routinely used in pharmacogenetic studies have also been challenged by the use of lcWGS. In a recent study, it has been shown that lcWGS provides high power for trait mapping when it is compared to most recent SNP arrays (Wasik et al., 2021). lcWGS followed by imputation supported an increase in GWAS statistical power and in accuracy for polygenic risk prediction at coverages >0.5X (Li et al., 2020). Genotype concordances between WGS data at > 13.7X depth and SNP array data were estimated at >99% (Kishikawa et al., 2019).

6.5 Clinical use of WGS

About 80% of rare diseases have a genetic basis. Therefore, they are suitable for the application of NGS technologies (Liu et al., 2019). Currently, clinical settings mostly end up combining chromosome microarrays (CMA) for CNV analysis, gene panels, and WES analysis (Meienberg et al., 2016; Stavropoulos et al., 2016), despite of the known limitations of the capture technology within GC-rich regions of the exome. WGS provides insights into the entire spectrum of human genomic variation, from the short variants to structural chromosomal anomalies, and therefore, can be useful in clinical settings (Scocchia et al., 2019). An improved distribution of sequencing quality parameters (Belkadi et al., 2015) and an improved diagnostic yield have been pointed out as the main benefits when compared with gene panels and WES, suggesting the use of clinical WGS (cWGS) as a first-tier diagnostic test (Lionel et al., 2018; Stavropoulos et al., 2016; Trujillano et al., 2017). From a technical point of view, it seems that WGS is better than WES for the most comprehensive genomic testing of Mendelian disorders (Meienberg et al., 2016). However, few studies comparing the diagnostic yield differences between WES and WGS in clinical settings have been published so far. From a cost perspective, the WES reanalysis seems to be recommended for now (Alfares et al., 2018). In genomic testing in cancer, the UK 100,000 Genomes Project is promoting a wider adoption of WGS, as well as other genomic strategies (e.g., pan-genomic markers, multi-omics and liquid biopsy) (Berner et al., 2019). Moreover, only a few health systems are adopting cWGS and it is not routinely used in the clinical practice for now (Bohannan and Mitrofanova, 2019; Evans et al., 2017). With the progressively decreasing costs of the sequencing technology, the bottleneck will continue moving away from the costs per-sequenced base and the analysis towards the variant interpretation (Worthey, 2017).

7   AVAILABLE SOLUTIONS

A large number of bioinformatic tools and pipelines have been developed and upgraded in the last few years to deal with WGS data. Some of them are cloud-based tools, while others were designed to be stand-alone. Their use can be hindered due to several limitations: many of them are operating system and version-dependent, require specific libraries, and compilations; some of them are not able to handle parallelization or require a lot of system resources (RAM memory, shared clusters, HPC and RAID systems, file systems specially designed to manage very big data files or a huge number of medium size data files, etc.); some were designed for academic use and lack of long-term support after the tool is published. As a consequence, it is common to find that the bioinformatic skills requirements for projects based on WGS are high, and it is not always possible to apply the default settings to the NGS data analysis to reproduce the results (Kwon et al., 2018).

One of the available solutions to solve these issues requires the wrapping of bioinformatic tools and environments (operating system, libraries, configuration files, auxiliary data files, etc.) in a package or '*image*' (Di Tommaso et al., 2015). Therefore, the user does not need either to install or compile code neither define a complex set of parameters, just retrieve the ready-to-run image from an appropriate web-hub, feed the corresponding NGS data files and run it into an isolated container (Kim et al., 2018b; Schulz et al., 2016). An example of this approach is Docker (Fig. 11), a solution to pack software and fix all its dependencies into the corresponding image. Docker images are registered and available at Docker Hub (https://hub. docker.com). Other solutions use Singularity (https://sylabs.io/docs) and Kubernetes (https:// kubernetes.io). The ORCA (the Genomics Research Container Architecture; https://github. com/bcgsc/orca) bioinformatic environment is presented as a Docker image containing over 625 bioinformatics tools and their dependencies as of June 2020 (Jackman et al., 2019). This containerization paradigm presents some downsides: the lack of standards for the distribution and sharing of images, multiple versioning, difficulties to integrate docker images into complex workflows when big data files are in place, etc.

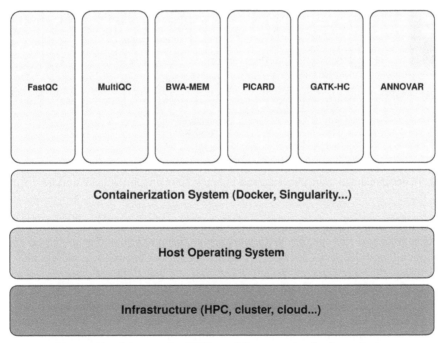

Figure 11 Scheme of a WGS workflow containerization solution.

Other solutions such as the virtualization technology are becoming deprecated in this context, because virtual machine images are typically very large, require a full copy of the operating system files, and recoding is not straightforward (Hinsen, 2014). A remarkable solution is the Biocontainers project (https://biocontainers.pro). It is a community-driven initiative providing infrastructure and guidelines to create, manage and distribute bioinformatics packages (e.g., Conda, https://anaconda.org/anaconda/conda) and containers (e.g., Docker, Singularity).

Some stand-alone solutions integrate many tools into a single server workbench, allowing the bioinformatic user to assemble pre-configured modular tools into pipelines, using a drag-and-drop GUI (Leipzig, 2017). Among the available solutions, Galaxy (https://usegalaxy.org), Apache-Taverna (https://taverna.incubator.apache.org), and ADAM (https://adam.readthedocs.io) are worth highlighting. They offer web-based interfaces and stand-alone clients to graphically create, edit and run workflows in local or cloud-environments.

Cloud-computing is another solution to host NGS workflows (Fig. 12), although it requires minimal bioinformatics expertise to setup and deploy the pipelines into computing infrastructures hosted in remote data centers. This solution is inexpensive in terms of subscriptions and per sample computation costs when a lot of samples must be processed. However, the bandwidths and transfer costs represent an issue to be considered. Examples of these solutions are the so-called *Infrastructures-as-a-Service* (IaaS) such as Amazon Web Services (AWS), Google Cloud Platform (GCP), and Microsoft Azure cloud platforms.

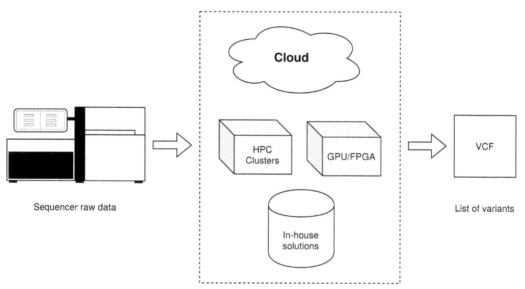

Figure 12 Conceptualization of the cloud and in-house solutions for a WGS workflow, from the sequencer raw data to the variant callset.

Apart from the desktop and web environments, commercial cloud-workbench solutions are also available to host and run specific WGS workflows taking advantage of the cloud computing power (Langmead and Nellore, 2018). This hybrid solution between a workbench and the cloud works under the paradigm of '*bringing the tools to the data*' of *Software-as-a-Service* (SaaS). Examples of these solutions are DNAnexus, Seven Bridges, and the Illumina BaseSpace Sequence Hub (Table 12). These solutions also provide Application Program Interfaces (API) to allow users to upload NGS data, launch pipelines, and download bulk results from the command line. Arvados offers a community and enterprise solutions based on the same concept of cloud-workbenching supporting AWS, GCP and Azure cloud platforms as well as on-premises installs.

An outstanding example of a cloud computing service combining all the advantages of the aforementioned solutions is Terra (formerly FireCloud; https://app.terra.bio), an open platform for secure and scalable workflow analysis on the cloud. Terra is a web-portal to make easier the access and sharing of code, pipelines, and data, offering the user workspaces where some workflows are already pre-configured for common use cases, without the need of writing code, along with example data suitable for testing and benchmarking. Another remarkable example of an open-source python-framework is Hail (https://hail.is), which leverages Apache Spark to process genomics data at the terabyte scale.

A last word in this section is devoted to data privacy and security. Most of data derived from human sequencing projects establish some security and regulation for accessing and sharing genomic data (i.e., the database of Genotypes and Phenotypes, dbGaP, and the EGA European Genome–Phenome Archive). Data access should be granted to users by robust password policies. Data storage and transfer should be protected by some level of encryption. Therefore, the selected bioinformatic solution should be aware of these issues. Of capital importance is data sovereignty, a major concern for international data transfers is most European countries according to the new General Data Protection Regulation (GDPR). The European ELIXIR initiative (https://elixir-europe.org) and the GA4GH have developed and adopted the Beacon API (https://beacon-project.io) as a discovery service for genetic variants that can be used worldwide while respecting the national data security jurisdiction of countries in the beacon-network.

Table 12 Advanced bioinformatic solutions for WGS workflows

Tool	Description	Link
Galaxy	Galaxy is an open, web-based platform for accessible, reproducible, and transparent computational research.	https://galaxyproject.org/use
Apache-Taverna	Suite of tools used to design and execute scientific workflows and aid in silico experimentation.	https://taverna.incubator.apache.org
Biocontainers	Provides the infrastructure and basic guidelines to create, manage and distribute bioinformatics packages (Conda) and containers (Docker and Singularity).	https://biocontainers.pro
Terra	Broad Institute secure, freely accessible cloud-based analysis portal.	https://app.terra.bio
Alibaba Cloud	Cloud platform (IaaS).	https://alibabacloud.com
AWS	Cloud platform (IaaS).	https://aws.amazon.com/ecs https://aws.amazon.com
Google Cloud Platform	Cloud platform (IaaS).	https://cloud.google.com
Microsoft Azure	Cloud platform (IaaS).	https://azure.microsoft.com
DNAnexus	Cloud-workbench (SaaS).	http://dnanexus.com
Illumina Sequence Hub BaseSpace	Cloud-workbench (SaaS).	https://basespace.illumina.com
Seven Bridges Genomics	Cloud-workbench (SaaS).	https://www.sevenbridges.com

8 WGS CHALLENGES

The WGS workflows present several challenges for the coming years (Table 13). From a cost-agnostic perspective, data governance and clinical translation are among the WGS workflow rate-limiting steps (Lightbody et al., 2019). From a technical point of view, there are still numerous aspects of the workflow that need a permanent revision and improvement, particularly the capabilities to efficiently store, access, share, and backup the data. Summed to the costs of sample preparation, sequencing, analyses and interpretation, and human resources, these elements contribute towards a more realistic assessment of the true cost of the per base NGS data (Liu et al., 2014; Sboner et al., 2011). With all this in mind, the user must carefully decide between building and adapting an ad hoc in-house bioinformatic solution or opt for commercialized third-party computational services (see Section 7).

Table 13   Main identified WGS challenges

Workflow step	Challenges
Workflow design	Availability and ease of use of open-source workflow editors with graphical user interfaces; Functional equivalency adopted in all steps of the workflow.
Computing solutions	Standardization of pipelines; Integration of containerized solutions within all-purpose shared clusters and HPC infrastructures.
Processing speed	Availability and costs of specialized hardware solutions for pipelining the workflow (FPGA, GPU, TPU solutions).
Integration of WGS data with other omics	Disconnection between NGS data from WGS workflows and other omics technologies that hinder disease biomarkers.
Sequencing	Sequencing traversing long-range SV; Reduction of the error rate in TGS; Size of NGS files; Costs of data storage and transfer; Reduction of total costs interpreted variant.
Reference genome	Improvements in the continuity; New reference materials not prone to caller-bias; Development of Pangenomes; Graph-representations to integrate diversity.
Read alignment	Improvements in the difficult to map regions and regions with low complexity.
Assembly	Graph-based assembly.
Variant calling	Improving the calling of SVs; Improving in speed, sensitivity and specificity; Scalability (Joint-Genotyping of hundreds of thousands of whole-genomes).
Variant refinement	Specificity improvements.
Variant annotation	Standardization of variant nomenclature; Prediction of effects in non-coding regions; Population biases.
Variant interpretation	Rules that can be easily followed (not all ACMG rules are of straightforward application); Predicted effects vs. biological causal effects.
Data transfer	Data transfer between local and cloud environments (vendor dependent).
Data size	Formats for lossy compression.
Data security & privacy (ethical concerns)	Privacy and security concerns (data access, data sharing, data querying); Data sovereignty.

Derived from the action of the WGS large-projects and the increasing number of sequenced genomes in cohort and disease-oriented studies, a number of computational issues need to be considered. One of these aspects are turnaround times, from the raw data at the sequencer side to a refined VCF file with high quality and accurate variants (Wu et al., 2016). The lack of standards for sample preparation, NGS sequencing and downstream analyses also represent challenging issues to the interpretation of NGS data (Hardwick et al., 2017). To this complex scenario of limiting conditions, one should add the technical issues derived from the current human genome reference (Eichler, 2019) described previously (see Section 3.3).

Another challenge, closely related to the data management bottlenecks, is the scale of the solution (see Section 7). A rational scalable strategy must be designed to host the requirements of the WGS workflow. Several solutions range from a shared-memory multicore architecture (typically for labs of small dimensions), the use of specialized hardware on HPC clusters (FPGA, GPU, tensor processing units — TPU) to accelerate machine learning workloads, the use of cloud scalable solutions, and containerization (Shi and Wang, 2019).

The variant calling process is one of the more demanding steps of the WGS workflow in terms of computational capabilities, mainly when dealing with a large number of genomes. As we have shown in the variant calling section (see Section 5.2), there exist a vast and diverse number of variant callers in terms of their mathematical algorithms and programming, ranging from the well know variant callers designed for germline variant identification to newer variant callers focused on the identification of somatic alterations (Bohannan and Mitrofanova, 2019). Frequently, the variant callers suffer from an imbalance in sensitivity and specificity, and low performance when variants with low allele frequencies are being studied. In line with these issues, the bioinformatic community has developed benchmarking reference materials, data and evaluation tools using simulated and real DNA sequences to develop standards at all levels of the WGS workflow.

Acknowledgements

The authors deeply acknowledge Manuel Cendagorta Galarza-López for unconditionally promoting and supporting our research projects and the support from Teide High-Performance Computing facilities from Instituto Tecnológico y de Energías Renovables (ITER). This work was supported by Ministerio de Ciencia e Innovación (RTC-2017-6471-1, AEI/FEDER, UE); Cabildo Insular de Tenerife (CGIEU0000219140); the agreement with ITER to strengthen scientific and technological education, training, research, development and innovation in Genomics, Personalized Medicine and Biotechnology (OA17/008); Consejería de Educación, Universidades, Cultura y Deportes, Gobierno de Canarias; and by Fundación CajaCanarias/Fundación Bancaria "La Caixa" (2018PATRI20).

REFERENCES

1000 Genomes Project Consortium, G.R. Abecasis, D. Altshuler, A. Auton, L.D. Brooks, R.M. Durbin, Richard, et al. (2010). A Map of Human Genome Variation from Population-Scale Sequencing. Nature. 467(7319): 1061–1073.

Abel, H.J., D.E. Larson, C. Chiang, I. Das, K.L. Kanchi, R.M. Layer, et al. (2020). Mapping and characterization of structural variation in 17,795 human genomes. Nature. 583: 83–89.

Afgan, E., D. Baker, M. van den Beek, D. Blankenberg, D. Bouvier, M. Čech, et al. (2016). The galaxy platform for accessible, reproducible and collaborative biomedical analyses: 2016 Update. Nucleic Acids Research. 44(W1): W3–W10.

Akbari, A., J.J. Vitti, A. Iranmehr, M. Bakhtiari, P.C. Sabeti, S. Mirarab, et al. (2018). Identifying the favored mutation in a positive selective sweep. Nature Methods. 15(4): 279–282.

Alexander, D.H., J. Novembre and K. Lange (2009). Fast model-based estimation of ancestry in unrelated individuals. Genome Research. 19(9): 1655–1664.

Alfares, A., T. Aloraini, L.-Al Subaie, A. Alissa, A.-Al Qudsi, A. Alahmad, et al. (2018). Whole-genome sequencing offers additional but limited clinical utility compared with reanalysis of whole-exome sequencing. Genetics in Medicine: Official Journal of the American College of Medical Genetics. 20(11): 1328–1333.

Amarasinghe, S.L., S. Su, X. Dong, L. Zappia, M.E. Ritchie and Q. Gouil (2020). Opportunities and challenges in long-read sequencing data analysis. Genome Biology. 21(1): 30.

Amendola, L.M., G.P. Jarvik, M.C. Leo, H.M. McLaughlin, Y. Akkari, M.D. Amaral, et al. (2016). Performance of ACMG-AMP variant-interpretation guidelines among nine laboratories in the clinical sequencing exploratory research consortium. American Journal of Human Genetics. 99(1): 247.

Armstrong, J., I.T. Fiddes, M. Diekhans and B. Paten (2019). Whole-genome alignment and comparative annotation. Annual Review of Animal Biosciences. 7: 41–64.

Audano, P.A., A. Sulovari, T.A. Graves-Lindsay, S. Cantsilieris, M. Sorensen, A.E. Welch, et al. (2019). Characterizing the major structural variant alleles of the human genome. Cell. 176(3): 663–675.e19.

Baichoo, S., Y. Souilmi, S. Panji, G. Botha, A. Meintjes, S. Hazelhurst, et al. (2018). Developing reproducible bioinformatics analysis workflows for heterogeneous computing environments to support african genomics. BMC Bioinformatics. 19(1): 457.

Bainbridge, M.N., M. Wang, Y. Wu, I. Newsham, D.M. Muzny, J.L. Jefferies, et al. (2011). Targeted enrichment beyond the consensus coding DNA sequence exome reveals exons with higher variant densities. Genome Biology. 12(7): R68.

Batzoglou, S. (2005). Algorithmic challenges in mammalian genome sequence assembly. *In*: M. Dunn, J. Jorde, P. Little, S. Subramaniam (eds). Encyclopedia of Genomics, Proteomics and Bioinformatics. Wiley, Hoboken, New Jersey.

Belkadi, A., Alexandre B., Y. Itan, A. Cobat, Q.B. Vincent, A. Antipenko, et al. (2015). Whole-genome sequencing is more powerful than whole-exome sequencing for detecting exome variants. Proceedings of the National Academy of Sciences of the United States of America. 112(17): 5473–5478.

Bergström, A., S.A. McCarthy, R. Hui, Md.A. Almarri, Q. Ayub, P. Danecek, et al. (2020). Insights into human genetic variation and population history from 929 diverse genomes. Science. 367(6484): eaay5012. https://doi.org/10.1126/science.aay5012.

Berner, A.M., G.J. Morrissey and N. Murugaesu (2019). Clinical analysis of whole genome sequencing in cancer patients. Current Genetic Medicine Reports. 7(2): 136–143.

Bohannan, Z.S. and A. Mitrofanova (2019). Calling variants in the clinic: Informed variant calling decisions based on biological, clinical, and laboratory variables. Computational and Structural Biotechnology Journal. 17: 561–569.

Bourgey, M., R. Dali, R. Eveleigh, K.C. Chen, L. Letourneau, J. Fillon, et al. (2019). GenPipes: An open-source framework for distributed and scalable genomic analyses. GigaScience. 8(6). https://doi.org/10.1093/gigascience/giz037.

Bowers, R.M., A. Clum, H. Tice, J. Lim, K. Singh, D. Ciobanu, et al. (2015). Impact of library preparation protocols and template quantity on the metagenomic reconstruction of a mock microbial community. BMC Genomics. 16: 856.

Bruinsma, S., J. Burgess, D. Schlingman, A. Czyz, N. Morrell, C. Ballenger, et al. (2018). Bead-linked transposomes enable a normalization-free workflow for NGS library preparation. BMC Genomics. 19(1): 722.

Camacho-Sanchez, M., P. Burraco, I. Gomez-Mestre and J.A. Leonard (2013). Preservation of RNA and DNA from mammal samples under field conditions. Molecular Ecology Resources. 13(4): 663–673.

Cameron, D.L., L.Di Stefano and A.T. Papenfuss (2019). Comprehensive evaluation and characterisation of short read general-purpose structural variant calling software. Nature Communications. 10(1): 3240.

Chen, J., X. Li, H. Zhong, Y. Meng and H. Du (2019). Systematic comparison of germline variant calling pipelines cross multiple next-generation sequencers. Sci. Rep. 9(1): 9345.

Chen, Z., Y. Yuan, X. Chen, J. Chen, S. Lin, X. Li, et al. (2020). Systematic comparison of somatic variant calling performance among different sequencing depth and mutation frequency. Sci. Rep. 10(1): 3501.

Chu, T.-Y., K.-S. Hwang, M.-H. Yu, H.-S. Lee, H.-C. Lai and J.-Y. Liu (2002). A research-based tumor tissue bank of gynecologic oncology: Characteristics of nucleic acids extracted from normal and tumor tissues from different sites. International Journal of Gynecological Cancer: Official Journal of the International Gynecological Cancer Society. 12(2): 171–176.

Cingolani, P., A. Platts, L.L. Wang, M. Coon, T. Nguyen, L. Wang, et al. (2012). A program for annotating and predicting the effects of single nucleotide polymorphisms, SnpEff: SNPs in the Genome of *Drosophila* Melanogaster Strain w1118; Iso-2; Iso-3. Fly. 6(2): 80–92.

Coelho, B., B. Veigas, E. Fortunato, R. Martins, H. Águas, R. Igreja, et al. (2017). Digital microfluidics for nucleic acid amplification. Sensors. 17(7). https://doi.org/10.3390/s17071495.

Collins, R.L., H. Brand, K.J. Karczewski, X. Zhao, J. Alföldi, L.C. Francioli, et al. (2020). A structural variation reference for medical and population genetics. Nature. 581: 444–451.

Cooke, D.P., D.C. Wedge and G. Lunter. (2021). A unified haplotype-based method for accurate and comprehensive variant calling. Nat Biotechnol. https://doi.org/10.1038/s41587-021-00861-3.

Costello, M., M. Fleharty, J. Abreu, Y. Farjoun, S. Ferriera, L. Holmes, et al. (2018). Characterization and remediation of sample index swaps by non-redundant dual indexing on massively parallel sequencing platforms. BMC Genomics. 19(1): 332.

Crawford, D.C., J.N.C. Bailey and F.B.S. Briggs (2019). Mind the gap: Resources required to receive, process and interpret research-returned whole genome data. Human Genetics. 138(7): 691–701.

Danecek, P., A. Auton, G. Abecasis, C.A. Albers, E. Banks, M.A. DePristo, et al. (2011). The variant call format and VCFtools. Bioinformatics. 27(15): 2156–2158.

De Coster, W., S. D'Hert, D.T. Schultz, M. Cruts and C. van Broeckhoven (2018). NanoPack: Visualizing and processing long-read sequencing data. Bioinformatics. 34(15): 2666–2669.

Depledge, D.P., K.P. Srinivas, T. Sadaoka, D. Bready, Y. Mori, D.G. Placantonakis, et al. (2019). Direct RNA sequencing on nanopore arrays redefines the transcriptional complexity of a viral pathogen. Nature Communications. 10(1): 754.

DePristo, M.A., E. Banks, R. Poplin, K.V. Garimella, J.R. Maguire, C. Hartl, et al. (2011). A framework for variation discovery and genotyping using next-generation DNA sequencing data. Nature Genetics. 43(5): 491–498.

Desvignes, J.-P., M. Bartoli, V. Delague, M. Krahn, M. Miltgen, C. Béroud, et al. (2018). VarAFT: A variant annotation and filtration system for human next generation sequencing data. Nucleic Acids Research. 46(W1): W545–W553.

Desvillechabrol, D., R. Legendre, C. Rioualen, C. Bouchier, J. van Helden, S. Kennedy, et al. (2018). Sequanix: A dynamic graphical interface for snakemake workflows. Bioinformatics. 34(11): 1934–1936.

Dewey, F.E., M.E. Grove, C. Pan, B.A. Goldstein, J.A. Bernstein, H. Chaib, et al. (2014). Clinical interpretation and implications of whole-genome sequencing. JAMA. 311(10): 1035–1045.

Di Tommaso, P., E. Palumbo, M. Chatzou, P. Prieto, M.L. Heuer and C. Notredame (2015). The impact of docker containers on the performance of genomic pipelines. PeerJ. 3: e1273.

Di Tommaso, P., M. Chatzou, E.W. Floden, P.P. Barja, E. Palumbo and C. Notredame (2017). Nextflow enables reproducible computational workflows. Nature Biotechnology. 35(4): 316–319.

Dohm, J.C., C. Lottaz, T. Borodina and H. Himmelbauer (2008). Substantial biases in ultra-short read data sets from high-throughput DNA sequencing. Nucleic Acids Research. 36(16): e105.

Du, Z., L. Ma, H. Qu, W. Chen, B. Zhang, X. Lu, et al. (2019). Whole genome analyses of chinese population and *de novo* assembly of a northern han genome. Genomics, Proteomics and Bioinformatics. 17(3): 229–247.

Ebbert, M.T.W., T.D. Jensen, K. Jansen-West, J.P. Sens, J.S. Reddy, P.G. Ridge, et al. (2019). Systematic analysis of dark and camouflaged genes reveals disease-relevant genes hiding in plain sight. Genome Biology. 20(1): 97.

Eggertsson, H.P., H. Jonsson, S. Kristmundsdottir, E. Hjartarson, B. Kehr, G. Masson, et al. (2017). Graphtyper enables population-scale genotyping using pangenome graphs. Nature Genetics. 49(11): 1654–1660.

Eichler, E.E. (2019). Genetic variation, comparative genomics, and the diagnosis of disease. The New England Journal of Medicine. 381(1): 64–74.

Einaga, N., A. Yoshida, H. Noda, M. Suemitsu, Y. Nakayama, A. Sakurada, et al. (2017). Assessment of the quality of DNA from various formalin-fixed paraffin-embedded (FFPE) tissues and the use of this DNA for next-generation sequencing (NGS) with no artifactual mutation. PloS One. 12(5): e0176280.

Eizenga, J.M., A.M. Novak, J.A. Sibbesen, S. Heumos, A. Ghaffaari, G. Hickey, et al. (2020). Pangenome graphs. Annual Review of Genomics and Human Genetics. 21: 139–162. https://doi.org/10.1146/annurev-genom-120219-080406.

Ekblom, R. and J.B.W. Wolf (2014). A field guide to whole-genome sequencing, assembly and annotation. Evolutionary Applications. 7(9): 1026–1042.

Evans, J.P., B.C. Powell and J.S. Berg. (2017). Finding the rare pathogenic variants in a human genome. JAMA. 317(18): 1904–1905.

Ewels, P.A., A. Peltzer, S. Fillinger, H. Patel, J. Alneberg, A. Wilm, et al. (2020). The Nf-Core framework for community-curated bioinformatics pipelines. Nature Biotechnology. 38(3): 276–278.

Fan, S., D.E. Kelly, M.H. Beltrame, M.E.B. Hansen, S. Mallick, A. Ranciaro, et al. (2019). African evolutionary history inferred from whole genome sequence data of 44 indigenous african populations. Genome Biology. 20(1): 82.

Farek, J., D. Hughes, A. Mansfield, O. Krasheninina, W. Nasser, F.J. Sedlazeck, et al. (2018). xAtlas: Scalable small variant calling across heterogeneous next-generation sequencing experiments. bioRxiv 295071. doi: https://doi.org/10.1101/295071.

Federico, A., T. Karagiannis, K. Karri, D. Kishore, Y. Koga, J.D. Campbell, et al. (2019). Pipeliner: A nextflow-based framework for the definition of sequencing data processing pipelines. Frontiers in Genetics. 10: 614.

Feldman, M.Ya. (1973). Reactions of nucleic acids and nucleodroteins with formaldehyde. Translated by A.L. Pumpiansky, Moscow. pp. 1–49. *In*: J.N. Davidson and W.E. Cohn (eds). Progress in Nucleic Acid Research and Molecular Biology, vol. 13. Academic Press.

Fisch, K.M., T. Meißner, L. Gioia, J.-C. Ducom, T.M. Carland, S. Loguercio, et al. (2015). Omics pipe: A community-based framework for reproducible multi-omics data analysis. Bioinformatics. 31(11): 1724–1728.

Friedman, S., L. Gauthier, Y. Farjoun and E. Banks (2020). Lean and deep models for more accurate filtering of SNP and INDEL variant calls. Bioinformatics. 36(7): 2060–2067.

Gao, P., R. Zhang and J. Li (2019). Comprehensive elaboration of database resources utilized in next-generation sequencing-based tumor somatic mutation detection. Biochimica et Biophysica Acta, Reviews on Cancer. 1872(1): 122–137.

Garrison, E. and G. Marth (2012). Haplotype-Based Variant Detection from Short-Read Sequencing. arXiv [q-bio.GN]. arXiv. http://arxiv.org/abs/1207.3907.

Garrison, E., J. Sirén, A.M. Novak, G. Hickey, J.M. Eizenga, E.T. Dawson, et al. (2018). Variation graph toolkit improves read mapping by representing genetic variation in the reference. Nature Biotechnology. 36(9): 875–879.

Giani, A.M., G.R. Gallo, L. Gianfranceschi and G. Formenti (2020). Long walk to genomics: History and current approaches to genome sequencing and assembly. Computational and Structural Biotechnology Journal. 18: 9–19.

Gilly, A., L. Southam, D. Suveges, K. Kuchenbaecker, R. Moore, G.E.M. Melloni, et al. (2019). Very low-depth whole-genome sequencing in complex trait association studies. Bioinformatics. 35(15): 2555–2561.

Gordon, D., J. Huddleston, M.J.P. Chaisson, C.M. Hill, Z.N. Kronenberg, K.M. Munson, et al. (2016). Long-read sequence assembly of the gorilla genome. Science. 352(6281): aae0344.

Gudbjartsson, D.F., H. Helgason, S.A. Gudjonsson, F. Zink, A. Oddson, A. Gylfason, et al. (2015). Large-scale whole-genome sequencing of the icelandic population. Nature Genetics. 47(5): 435–444.

Guillen-Guio, B., J.M. Lorenzo-Salazar, R. González-Montelongo, A. Díaz-de Usera, I. Marcelino-Rodríguez, A. Corrales, et al. (2018). Genomic analyses of human european diversity at the southwestern edge: Isolation, african influence and disease associations in the canary islands. Molecular Biology and Evolution. 35(12): 3010–3026.

Guo, Y., F. Ye, Q. Sheng, T. Clark and D.C. Samuels (2014a). Three-stage quality control strategies for DNA re-sequencing data. Briefings in Bioinformatics. 15(6): 879–889.

Guo, Y., S. Zhao, Q. Sheng, F. Ye, J. Li, B. Lehmann, et al. (2014b). Multi-perspective quality control of illumina exome sequencing data using QC3. Genomics. 103(5–6): 323–328.

Gurevich, A., V. Saveliev, N. Vyahhi and G. Tesler (2013). QUAST: Quality assessment tool for genome assemblies. Bioinformatics. 29(8): 1072–1075.

Haghshenas, E., H. Asghari, J. Stoye, C. Chauve and F. Hach (2020). HASLR: Fast hybrid assembly of long reads. iScience. 23(8): 101389.

Hardwick, S.A., I.W. Deveson and T.R. Mercer (2017). Reference standards for next-generation sequencing. Nat. Rev. Genet. 18(8): 473–484.

Hart, S.N., P. Duffy, D.J. Quest, A. Hossain, M.A. Meiners and J.-P. Kocher (2016). VCF-miner: GUI-based application for mining variants and annotations stored in VCF files. Briefings Bioinf. 17(2): 346–351.

Hinsen, K. (2014). ActivePapers: A platform for publishing and archiving computer-aided research. F1000Research. 3: 289.

Holt, J.M., B. Wilk, C.L. Birch, D.M. Brown, M. Gajapathy, A.C. Moss, et al. (2019). VarSight: Prioritizing clinically reported variants with binary classification algorithms. BMC Bioinformatics. 20(1): 496.

Homburger, J.R., C.L. Neben, G. Mishne, A.Y. Zhou, S. Kathiresan and A.V. Khera (2019). Low coverage whole genome sequencing enables accurate assessment of common variants and calculation of genome-wide polygenic scores. Genome Medicine. 11(1): 74.

Ho, S.S., A.E. Urban and R.E. Mills (2020). Structural variation in the sequencing era. Nat. Rev. Genet. 21(3): 171–189.

Huddleston, J. and E.E. Eichler (2016). An incomplete understanding of human genetic variation. Genetics. 202(4): 1251–1254.

Huddleston, J., M.J.P. Chaisson, K.M. Steinberg, W. Warren, K. Hoekzema, D. Gordon, et al. (2017). Discovery and genotyping of structural variation from long-read haploid genome sequence data. Genome Research. 27(5): 677–685.

Hung, L.-H., J. Hu, T. Meiss, A. Ingersoll, W. Lloyd, D. Kristiyanto, et al. (2019). Building containerized workflows using the BioDepot-workflow-builder. Cell Systems. 9(5): 508–514.e3.

ICGC/TCGA Pan-Cancer Analysis of Whole Genomes Consortium (2020). Pan-cancer analysis of whole genomes. Nature. 578(7793): 82–93.

Jackman, S.D., T. Mozgacheva, S. Chen, B. O'Huiginn, L. Bailey, I. Birol, et al. (2019). ORCA: A comprehensive bioinformatics container environment for education and research. Bioinformatics. 35(21): 4448–4450.

Jun, G., M. Flickinger, K.N. Hetrick, J.M. Romm, K.F. Doheny, G.R. Abecasis, et al. (2012). Detecting and estimating contamination of human DNA samples in sequencing and array-based genotype data. American Journal of Human Genetics. 91(5): 839–848.

Kalia, S.S., K. Adelman, S.J. Bale, W.K. Chung, C. Eng, J.P. Evans, et al. (2017). Recommendations for reporting of secondary findings in clinical exome and genome sequencing, 2016 update (ACMG SF v2.0): a policy statement of the american college of medical genetics and genomics. Genetics in Medicine: Official Journal of the American College of Medical Genetics. 19(2): 249–255.

Karczewski, K.J., L.C. Francioli, G. Tiao, B.B. Cummings, J. Alföldi, Q. Wang, et al. (2020). The mutational constraint spectrum quantified from variation in 141,456 humans. Nature. 581(7809): 434–443.

Karlsen, F., M. Kalantari, M. Chitemerere, B. Johansson, and B. Hagmar (1994). Modifications of human and viral deoxyribonucleic acid by formaldehyde fixation. Laboratory Investigation; a Journal of Technical Methods and Pathology. 71(4): 604–611.

Kaushik, G., S. Ivkovic, J. Simonovic, N. Tijanic, B. Davis-Dusenbery and Deniz Kural (2017). Rabix: An open-source workflow executor supporting recomputability and interoperability of workflow descriptions. Pacific Symposium on Biocomputing. Pacific Symposium on Biocomputing. 22: 154–165.

Kelleher, J., Y. Wong, A.W. Wohns, C. Fadil, P.K. Albers and G. McVean (2019). Inferring whole-genome histories in large population datasets. Nature Genetics. 51(9): 1330–1338.

Kendig, K.I., S. Baheti, M.A. Bockol, T.M. Drucker, S.N. Hart, J.R. Heldenbrand, et al. (2019). Sentieon DNASeq variant calling workflow demonstrates strong computational performance and accuracy. Frontiers in Genetics. 10: 736.

Khan, A.R., Md.T. Pervez, M.E. Babar, N. Naveed and Md. Shoaib (2018). A comprehensive study of *de novo* genome assemblers: Current challenges and future prospective. Evolutionary Bioinformatics. Online. 14: 1176934318758650.

Kim, S., K. Scheffler, A.L. Halpern, M.A. Bekritsky, E. Noh, M. Källberg, et al. (2018a). Strelka2: Fast and accurate calling of germline and somatic variants. Nature Methods. 15(8): 591–594.

Kim, Y.-M., J.-B. Poline and G. Dumas (2018b). Experimenting with reproducibility: A case study of robustness in bioinformatics. GigaScience. 7(7): giy077. https://doi.org/10.1093/gigascience/giy077.

Kim, H.J., H.J. Kim, Y. Park, W.S. Lee, Y. Lim and J.H. Kim (2020). Clinical genome data model (cGDM) provides interactive clinical decision support for precision medicine. Sci. Rep. 10(1): 1414.

Kishikawa, T., Y. Momozawa, T. Ozeki, T. Mushiroda, H. Inohara, Y. Kamatani, et al. (2019). Empirical evaluation of variant calling accuracy using ultra-deep whole-genome sequencing data. Sci. Rep. 9(1): 1784.

Knierim, E., B. Lucke, J.M. Schwarz, M. Schuelke and D. Seelow (2011). Systematic comparison of three methods for fragmentation of long-range PCR products for next generation sequencing. PloS One 6(11): e28240.

Koboldt, D.C., Q. Zhang, D.E. Larson, D. Shen, M.D. McLellan, L. Lin, et al. (2012). VarScan 2: Somatic mutation and copy number alteration discovery in cancer by exome sequencing. Genome Research. 22(3): 568–576.

Korneliussen, T.S., A. Albrechtsen and R. Nielsen (2014). ANGSD: Analysis of next generation sequencing data. BMC Bioinformatics. 15: 356.

Köster, J. and S. Rahmann (2012). Snakemake—a scalable bioinformatics workflow engine. Bioinformatics. 28(19): 2520–2522.

Kosugi, S., Y. Momozawa, X. Liu, C. Terao, M. Kubo and Y. Kamatani (2019). Comprehensive evaluation of structural variation detection algorithms for whole genome sequencing. Genome Biology. 20(1): 117.

Kozarewa, I., Z. Ning, M.A. Quail, M.J. Sanders, M. Berriman and D.J. Turner (2009). Amplification-free illumina sequencing-library preparation facilitates improved mapping and assembly of (G+C)-biased genomes. Nature Methods. 6(4): 291–295.

Krusche, P., L. Trigg, P.C. Boutros, C.E. Mason, F.M. De La Vega, B.L. Moore, et al. (2019). Best practices for benchmarking germline small-variant calls in human genomes. Nature Biotechnology. 37(5): 555–560.

Kuchenbaecker, K. and E.V.R. Appel (2018). Assessing rare variation in complex traits. Methods in Molecular Biology. 1793: 51–71.

Kwon, C., J. Kim and J. Ahn (2018). DockerBIO: Web application for efficient use of bioinformatics docker images. PeerJ. 6: e5954.

Lacaze, P., M. Pinese, W. Kaplan, A. Stone, M.-J. Brion, R.L. Woods, et al. (2019). The medical genome reference bank: A whole-genome data resource of 4000 healthy elderly individuals. Rationale and Cohort Design. EJHG. 27(2): 308–316.

Lander, E.S. and M.S. Waterman (1988). Genomic mapping by fingerprinting random clones: A mathematical analysis. Genomics 2(3): 231–239.

Langmead, B. and A. Nellore (2018). Cloud computing for genomic data analysis and collaboration. Nat. Rev. Genet. 19(4): 208–219.

Lan, J.H., Y. Yin, E.F. Reed, K. Moua, K. Thomas and Q. Zhang (2015). Impact of three illumina library construction methods on GC bias and HLA genotype calling. Human Immunology. 76(2): 166–175.

Lan, T., H. Lin, W. Zhu, T.C.A.M. Laurent, M. Yang, X. Liu, et al. (2017). Deep whole-genome sequencing of 90 han chinese genomes. GigaScience 6(9): 1–7.

Lappalainen, T., A.J. Scott, M. Brandt and I.M. Hall (2019). Genomic analysis in the age of human genome sequencing. Cell. 177(1): 70–84.

Larsson, A.J.M., G. Stanley, R. Sinha, I.L. Weissman and R. Sandberg (2018). Computational correction of index switching in multiplexed sequencing libraries. Nature Methods. 15(5): 305–307.

Lee, S.B., K.C. Clabaugh, B. Silva, K.O. Odigie, M.D. Coble, O. Loreille, et al. (2012). Assessing a novel room temperature DNA storage medium for forensic biological samples. Forensic Sci Int Genet. 6(1): 31–40.

Leipzig, J. 2017. A review of bioinformatic pipeline frameworks. Briefings Bioinf. 18(3): 530–536.

Lek, M., K.J. Karczewski, E.V. Minikel, K.E. Samocha, E. Banks, T. Fennell, et al. (2016). Analysis of protein-coding genetic variation in 60,706 humans. Nature. 536(7616): 285–291.

Lightbody, G., V. Haberland, F. Browne, L. Taggart, H. Zheng, E. Parkes, et al. (2019). Review of applications of high-throughput sequencing in personalized medicine: Barriers and facilitators of future progress in research and clinical application. Briefings Bioinf. 20(5): 1795–1811.

Li, H. and R. Durbin (2009). Fast and accurate short read alignment with burrows-wheeler transform. Bioinformatics. 25(14): 1754–1760.

Li, H., B. Handsaker, A. Wysoker, T. Fennell, J. Ruan, N. Homer, et al. (2009). The sequence alignment/map format and SAMtools. Bioinformatics. 25(16): 2078–2079.

Li, H. (2013). Aligning sequence reads, clone sequences and assembly contigs with BWA-MEM. [q-bio.GN]. arXiv. https://arxiv.org/abs/1303.3997..

Li, H. (2015). FermiKit: Assembly-based variant calling for illumina resequencing data. Bioinformatics. 31(22): 3694–3696.

Li, M.M., M. Datto, E.J. Duncavage, S. Kulkarni, N.I. Lindeman, S. Roy, et al. (2017). Standards and guidelines for the interpretation and reporting of sequence variants in cancer: A joint consensus recommendation of the association for molecular pathology, american society of clinical oncology, and college of american pathologists. JMD. 19(1): 4–23.

Li, H. (2018). Minimap2: Pairwise alignment for nucleotide sequences. Bioinformatics. 34(18): 3094–3100.

Li, H., J.M. Bloom, Y. Farjoun, M. Fleharty, L. Gauthier, B. Neale, et al. (2018a). A synthetic-diploid benchmark for accurate variant-calling evaluation. Nature Methods. 15(8): 595–597.

Li, Z., Y. Wang and F. Wang (2018b). A study on fast calling variants from next-generation sequencing data using decision tree. BMC Bioinformatics. 19(1): 145.

Li, Q., X. Zhao, W. Zhang, L. Wang, J. Wang, D. Xu, et al. (2019a). Reliable multiplex sequencing with rare index mis-assignment on DNB-based NGS platform. BMC Genomics. 20(1): 215.

Li, J., B. Jew, L. Zhan, S. Hwang, G. Coppola, N.B. Freimer, et al. (2019b). ForestQC: Quality control on genetic variants from next-generation sequencing data using random forest. PLoS Computational Biology. 15(12): e1007556.

Li, J.H., C.A. Mazur, T. Berisa and J.K. Pickrell (2020). Low-pass sequencing increases the power of GWAS and decreases measurement error of polygenic risk scores compared to genotyping arrays. Genome Res. 31(4): 529–537.

Lincoln, S.E., R. Truty, C.-F. Lin, J.M. Zook, J. Paul, V.H. Ramey, et al. (2019). A rigorous interlaboratory examination of the need to confirm next-generation sequencing-detected variants with an orthogonal method in clinical genetic testing. JMD. 21(2): 318–329.

Lionel, A.C., G. Costain, N. Monfared, S. Walker, M.S. Reuter, S.M. Hosseini, et al. (2018). Improved diagnostic yield compared with targeted gene sequencing panels suggests a role for whole-genome sequencing as a first-tier genetic test. Genetics in Medicine: Official Journal of the American College of Medical Genetics. 20(4): 435–443.

Liu, B., R.K. Madduri, B. Sotomayor, K. Chard, L. Lacinski, U.J. Dave, et al. (2014). Cloud-based bioinformatics workflow platform for large-scale next-generation sequencing analyses. Journal of Biomedical Informatics. 49: 119–133.

Liu, H.-Y., L. Zhou, M.-Y. Zheng, J. Huang, S. Wan, A. Zhu, et al. (2019). Diagnostic and clinical utility of whole genome sequencing in a cohort of undiagnosed chinese families with rare diseases. Sci. Rep. 9(1): 19365.

Llamas, B., G. Valverde, L. Fehren-Schmitz, L.S. Weyrich, A. Cooper and W. Haak (2017). From the field to the laboratory: Controlling DNA contamination in human ancient DNA research in the high-throughput sequencing era. STAR. 3(1): 1–14.

Loka, T.P., S.H. Tausch and B.Y. Renard (2019). Reliable variant calling during runtime of illumina sequencing. Sci. Rep. 9(1): 16502.

Lu, H., F. Giordano and Z. Ning (2016). Oxford nanopore MinION sequencing and genome assembly. Genomics, Proteomics and Bioinformatics. 14(5): 265–279.

Lubin, I.M., N. Aziz, L.J. Babb, D. Ballinger, H. Bisht, D.M. Church, et al. (2017). Principles and recommendations for standardizing the use of the next-generation sequencing variant file in clinical settings. JMD. 19(3): 417–426.

Luo, R., M.C. Schatz and S.L. Salzberg (2017). 16GT: A fast and sensitive variant caller using a 16-genotype probabilistic model. GigaScience. 6(7): 1–4.

Luo, R., F.J. Sedlazeck, T.-W. Lam and M.C. Schatz (2019). A multi-task convolutional deep neural network for variant calling in single molecule sequencing. Nature Communications. 10(1): 998.

Magi, A., R. Semeraro, A. Mingrino, B. Giusti and R. D'Aurizio (2018). Nanopore sequencing data analysis: State of the art, applications and challenges. Briefings in Bioinformatics. 19(6): 1256–1272.

Mallick, S., H. Li, M. Lipson, I. Mathieson, M. Gymrek, F. Racimo, et al. (2016). The simons genome diversity project: 300 genomes from 142 diverse populations. Nature. 538(7624): 201–206.

Manichaikul, A., J.C. Mychaleckyj, S.S. Rich, K. Daly, M. Sale and W.-M. Chen (2010). Robust relationship inference in genome-wide association studies. Bioinformatics. 26(22): 2867–2873.

Marine, R., S.W. Polson, J. Ravel, G. Hatfull, D. Russell, M. Sullivan, et al. (2011). Evaluation of a transposase protocol for rapid generation of shotgun high-throughput sequencing libraries from nanogram quantities of DNA. Applied and Environmental Microbiology. 77(22): 8071–8079.

McLaren, W., L. Gil, S.E. Hunt, H.S. Riat, G.R.S. Ritchie, A. Thormann, et al. (2016). The ensembl variant effect predictor. Genome Biology. 17(1): 122.

Meienberg, J., R. Bruggmann, K. Oexle and G. Matyas (2016). Clinical sequencing: Is WGS the better WES? Human Genetics. 135(3): 359–362.

Miga, K.H., S. Koren, A. Rhie, M.R. Vollger, A. Gershman, A. Bzikadze, et al. (2020). Telomere-to-telomere assembly of a complete human X chromosome. Nature. 585: 79–84.

Miller, J.R., S. Koren and G. Sutton (2010). Assembly algorithms for next-generation sequencing data. Genomics. 95(6): 315–327.

Miller, N.A., E.G. Farrow, M. Gibson, L.K. Willig, G. Twist, B. Yoo, et al. (2015). A 26-hour system of highly sensitive whole genome sequencing for emergency management of genetic diseases. Genome Medicine. 7: 100.

Müller, H., R. Jimenez-Heredia, A. Krolo, T. Hirschmugl, J. Dmytrus, K. Boztug, et al. (2017). VCF. Filter: Interactive prioritization of disease-linked genetic variants from sequencing data. Nucleic Acids Research. 45(W1): W567–W72.

Nagasaki, M., J. Yasuda, F. Katsuoka, N. Nariai, K. Kojima, Y. Kawai, et al. (2015). Rare variant discovery by deep whole-genome sequencing of 1,070 Japanese individuals. Nature Communications. 6: 8018.

Nagasaki, M., Y. Kuroki, T.F. Shibata, F. Katsuoka, T. Mimori, Y. Kawai, et al. (2019). Construction of JRG (Japanese Reference Genome) with single-molecule real-time sequencing. Human Genome Variation. 6: 27.

Nagahashi, M., Y. Shimada, H. Ichikawa, S. Nakagawa, N. Sato, K. Kaneko, et al. (2017). Formalin-fixed paraffin-embedded sample conditions for deep next generation sequencing. The Journal of Surgical Research. 220: 125–132.

Ng, P.C. and E.F. Kirkness (2010). Whole genome sequencing. Methods in Molecular Biology. 628: 215–226.

O'Daniel, J.M., H.M. McLaughlin, L.M. Amendola, S.J. Bale, J.S. Berg, D. Bick, et al. (2017). A survey of current practices for genomic sequencing test interpretation and reporting processes in us laboratories. Genetics in Medicine: Official Journal of the American College of Medical Genetics. 19(5): 575–582.

Oliver, J.L. and A. Marín (1996). A relationship between GC content and coding-sequence length. Journal of Molecular Evolution. 43(3): 216–223.

Pabinger, S., A. Dander, M. Fischer, R. Snajder, M. Sperk, M. Efremova, et al. (2014). A survey of tools for variant analysis of next-generation genome sequencing data. Briefings Bioinf. 15(2): 256–278.

Panoutsopoulou, K., I. Tachmazidou and E. Zeggini (2013). In search of low-frequency and rare variants affecting complex traits. Human Molecular Genetics. 22(R1): R16–R21.

Pasaniuc, B., N. Rohland, P.J. McLaren, K. Garimella, N. Zaitlen, H. Li, et al. (2012). Extremely low-coverage sequencing and imputation increases power for genome-wide association studies. Nature Genetics. 44(6): 631–635.

Paten, B., A.M. Novak, J.M. Eizenga and E. Garrison (2017). Genome graphs and the evolution of genome inference. Genome Research. 27(5): 665–676.

Pedersen, B.S. and A.R. Quinlan (2017). Who's who? detecting and resolving sample anomalies in human DNA sequencing studies with peddy. American Journal of Human Genetics. 100(3): 406–413.

Pedersen, B.S., P.J. Bhetariya, J. Brown, G. Marth, R.L. Jensen, M.P. Bronner, et al. (2020). Somalier: rapid relatedness estimation for cancer and germline studies using efficient genome sketches. Genome Med 12: 62.

Poplin, R., P.-C. Chang, D. Alexander, S. Schwartz, T. Colthurst, A. Ku, et al. (2018). A universal SNP and small-indel variant caller using deep neural networks. Nature Biotechnology. 36(10): 983–987.

Purcell, S., B. Neale, K. Todd-Brown, L. Thomas, M.A.R. Ferreira, D. Bender, et al. (2007). PLINK: A tool set for whole-genome association and population-based linkage analyses. American Journal of Human Genetics. 81(3): 559–575.

Quail, M.A., I. Kozarewa, F. Smith, A. Scally, P.J. Stephens, R. Durbin, et al. (2008). A large genome center's improvements to the illumina sequencing system. Nature Methods. 5(12): 1005–1010.

Qualman, S.J., M. France, W.E. Grizzle, V.A. LiVolsi, C.A. Moskaluk, N.C. Ramirez, et al. (2004). Establishing a tumour bank: Banking, informatics and ethics. British Journal of Cancer. 90(6): 1115–1119.

Quinlan, A.R. and I.M. Hall (2010). BEDTools: A flexible suite of utilities for comparing genomic features. Bioinformatics. 26(6): 841–842.

Quinlan, A.R. (2014). BEDTools: The swiss-army tool for genome feature analysis. Current Protocols in Bioinformatics. 47: 11.12.1–11.12.34.

Rakocevic, G., V. Semenyuk, W.-P. Lee, J. Spencer, J. Browning, I.J. Johnson, et al. (2019). Fast and accurate genomic analyses using genome graphs. Nature Genetics. 51(2): 354–362.

Regier, A.A., Y. Farjoun, D.E. Larson, O. Krasheninina, H.M. Kang, D.P. Howrigan, et al. (2018). Functional equivalence of genome sequencing analysis pipelines enables harmonized variant calling across human genetics projects. Nature Communications. 9(1): 4038.

Relling, M.V., R.M. Krauss, D.M. Roden, T.E. Klein, D.M. Fowler, N. Terada, et al. (2017). New pharmacogenomics research network: An open community catalyzing research and translation in precision medicine. Clinical Pharmacology and Therapeutics. 102(6): 897–902.

Richards, S., N. Aziz, S. Bale, D. Bick, S. Das, J. Gastier-Foster, et al. (2015). Standards and guidelines for the interpretation of sequence variants: A joint consensus recommendation of the american college of medical genetics and genomics and the association for molecular pathology. Genetics in Medicine: Official Journal of the American College of Medical Genetics. 17(5): 405–423.

Rimmer, A., H. Phan, I. Mathieson, Z. Iqbal, S.R.F. Twigg, WGS500 Consortium, et al. (2014). Integrating mapping-, assembly- and haplotype-based approaches for calling variants in clinical sequencing applications. Nature Genetics. 46(8): 912–918.

Robbe, P., N. Popitsch, S.J.L. Knight, P. Antoniou, J. Becq, M. He, et al. (2018). Clinical whole-genome sequencing from routine formalin-fixed, paraffin-embedded specimens: Pilot study for the 100,000 genomes project. Genetics in Medicine: Official Journal of the American College of Medical Genetics. 20(10): 1196–1205.

Sboner, A., X.J. Mu, D. Greenbaum, R.K. Auerbach and M.B. Gerstein (2011). The real cost of sequencing: Higher than you think! Genome Biology. 12(8): 125.

Schulz, W.L., T. Durant, A.J. Siddon and R. Torres (2016). Use of application containers and workflows for genomic data analysis. Journal of Pathology Informatics. 7(1): 53.

Schweiger, M.R., M. Kerick, B. Timmermann, M.W. Albrecht, T. Borodina, D. Parkhomchuk, et al. (2009). Genome-wide massively parallel sequencing of formaldehyde fixed-paraffin embedded (FFPE) tumor tissues for copy-number- and mutation-analysis. PLoS One. 4(5): e5548.

Scocchia, A., K.M. Wigby, D. Masser-Frye, M.D. Campo, C.I. Galarreta, E. Thorpe, et al. (2019). Clinical whole genome sequencing as a first-tier test at a resource-limited dysmorphology clinic in Mexico. NPJ Genomic Medicine. 4: 5.

Sedlazeck, F.J., H. Lee, C.A. Darby and M.C. Schatz (2018). Piercing the dark matter: Bioinformatics of long-range sequencing and mapping. Nat. Rev. Genet. 19(6): 329–346.

Seo, J.-S., A. Rhie, J. Kim, S. Lee, M.-H. Sohn, C.-U. Kim, et al. (2016). *De novo* assembly and phasing of a korean human genome. Nature. 538(7624): 243–247.

Shapiro, B. and M. Hofreiter (2014). A paleogenomic perspective on evolution and gene function: New insights from ancient DNA. Science 343(6169): 1236573.

Sherman, R.M., J. Forman, V. Antonescu, D. Puiu, M. Daya, N. Rafaels, et al. (2019). Assembly of a pan-genome from deep sequencing of 910 humans of african descent. Nature Genetics. 51(1): 30–35.

Shi, L. and Z. Wang (2019). Computational strategies for scalable genomics analysis. Genes. 10(12). https://doi.org/10.3390/genes10121017.

Shringarpure, S.S., R.A. Mathias, R.D. Hernandez, T.D. O'Connor, Z.A. Szpiech, R. Torres, et al. (2017). Using genotype array data to compare multi- and single-sample variant calls and improve variant call sets from deep coverage whole-genome sequencing data. Bioinformatics. 33(8): 1147–1153.

Shumate, A., A.V. Zimin, R.M. Sherman, D. Puiu, J.M. Wagner, N.D. Olson, et al. (2020). Assembly and annotation of an ashkenazi human reference genome. Genome Biology. 21(1): 129.

Sklarz, M., L. Levin, M. Gordon and V. Chalifa-Caspi (2018). NeatSeq-Flow: A lightweight high-throughput sequencing workflow platform for non-programmers and programmers alike. bioRxiv. https://doi.org/10.1101/173005.

Sović, I., K. Križanović, K. Skala and M. Šikić (2016). Evaluation of hybrid and non-hybrid methods for *de novo* assembly of nanopore reads. Bioinformatics. 32(17): 2582–2589.

Srinivasan, M., D. Sedmak and S. Jewell (2002). Effect of fixatives and tissue processing on the content and integrity of nucleic acids. The American Journal of Pathology. 161(6): 1961–1971.

Stavropoulos, D.J., D. Merico, R. Jobling, S. Bowdin, N. Monfared, B. Thiruvahindrapuram, et al. (2016). Whole genome sequencing expands diagnostic utility and improves clinical management in pediatric medicine. NPJ Genomic Med. 1: 15012.

Steinberg, K.M., V.A. Schneider, T.A. Graves-Lindsay, R.S. Fulton, R. Agarwala, J. Huddleston, et al. (2014). Single haplotype assembly of the human genome from a hydatidiform mole. Genome Research. 24(12): 2066–2076.

Steiner, C.C., A.S. Putnam, P.E.A. Hoeck and O.A. Ryder (2013). Conservation genomics of threatened animal species. Annual Review of Animal Biosciences. 1: 261–281.

Stein, L.D. (2011). An introduction to the informatics of 'next-generation' sequencing. Current Protocols in Bioinformatics. 36(1): 11.1.1–11.1.9.

Strande, N.T., S.E. Brnich, T.S. Roman and J.S. Berg (2018). Navigating the nuances of clinical sequence variant interpretation in mendelian disease. Genetics in Medicine: Official Journal of the American College of Medical Genetics. 20(9): 918–926.

Supernat, A., O.V. Vidarsson, V.M. Steen and T. Stokowy (2018). Comparison of three variant callers for human whole genome sequencing. Sci. Rep. 8(1): 17851.

Taliun, D., D.N. Harris, M.D. Kessler, J. Carlson, Z.A. Szpiech, R. Torres, et al. (2021). Sequencing of 53,831 diverse genomes from the NHLBI TOPMed Program. Nature. 590: 290–299.

Telenti, A., L.C.T. Pierce, W.H. Biggs, J. di Iulio, E.H.M. Wong, M.M. Fabani, et al. (2016). Deep sequencing of 10,000 human genomes. Proceedings of the National Academy of Sciences of the United States of America. 113(42): 11901–11906.

Trost, B., S. Walker, S.A. Haider, W.W.L. Sung, S. Pereira, C.L. Phillips, et al. (2019). Impact of DNA source on genetic variant detection from human whole-genome sequencing data. Journal of Medical Genetics. 56(12): 809–817.

Trujillano, D., A.M. Bertoli-Avella, K.K. Kandaswamy, M. Er Weiss, J. Köster, A. Marais, et al. (2017). Clinical exome sequencing: Results from 2819 samples reflecting 1000 families. EJHG. 25(2): 176–182.

van Dijk, E.L., Y. Jaszczyszyn, D. Naquin and C. Thermes (2018). The third revolution in sequencing technology. TIG. 34(9): 666–681.

van der Auwera, G.A., M.O. Carneiro, C. Hartl, R. Poplin, G.D. Angel, A. Levy-Moonshine, et al. (2013). From FastQ data to high confidence variant calls: The genome analysis toolkit best practices pipeline. Current Protocols in Bioinformatics 43: 11.10.1–11.10.33.

van der Valk, T., F. Vezzi, M. Ormestad, L. Dalén and K. Guschanski (2020). Index hopping on the illumina HiseqX platform and its consequences for ancient DNA studies. Mol. Ecol. Resour. 20(5): 1171–1181.

Vivian, J., A.A. Rao, F.A. Nothaft, C. Ketchum, J. Armstrong, A. Novak, et al. (2017). Toil enables reproducible, open source, big biomedical data analyses. Nature Biotechnology. 35(4): 314–316.

Vodák, D., S. Lorenz, S. Nakken, L.B. Aasheim, H. Holte, B. Bai, et al. (2018). Sample-index misassignment impacts tumour exome sequencing. Sci. Rep. 8(1): 5307.

Wang, K., M. Li and H. Hakonarson (2010). ANNOVAR: Functional annotation of genetic variants from high-throughput sequencing data. Nucleic Acids Research. 38(16): e164.

Wang, J., L. Raskin, D.C. Samuels, Y. Shyr and Y. Guo (2015). Genome measures used for quality control are dependent on gene function and ancestry. Bioinformatics. 31(3): 318–323.

Wang, Q., E. Pierce-Hoffman, B.B. Cummings, K.J. Karczewski, J. Alföldi, L.C. Francioli, et al. (2020a). Landscape of multi-nucleotide variants in 125,748 human exomes and 15,708 genomes. Nat. Commun. 11: 2539.

Wang, H., Z. Dong, R. Zhang, M.H.K. Chau, Z. Yang, K.Y.C. Tsang, et al. (2020b). Low-pass genome sequencing versus chromosomal microarray analysis: Implementation in prenatal diagnosis. Genetics in Medicine: Official Journal of the American College of Medical Genetics. 22(3): 500–510.

Wasik, K., T. Berisa, J.K. Pickrell, J.H. Li, D.J. Fraser, K. King, et al. (2021). Comparing low-pass sequencing and genotyping for trait mapping in pharmacogenetics. BMC Genomics. 22: 197.

Watkins, M., S. Rynearson, A. Henrie and K. Eilbeck (2019). Implementing the VMC specification to reduce ambiguity in genomic variant representation. AMIA Annu Symp Proc. 2020. 1226–1235.

Wee, Y., S.B. Bhyan, Y. Liu, J. Lu, X. Li and M. Zhao (2019). The bioinformatics tools for the genome assembly and analysis based on third-generation sequencing. Briefings in Functional Genomics. 18(1): 1–12.

Williams, C., F. Pontén, C. Moberg, P. Söderkvist, M. Uhlén, J. Pontén, et al. (1999). A high frequency of sequence alterations is due to formalin fixation of archival specimens. The American Journal of Pathology. 155(5): 1467–1471.

Worthey, E.A. (2017). Analysis and annotation of whole-genome or whole-exome sequencing derived variants for clinical diagnosis. Current Protocols in Human Genetics. 95: 9.24.1–9.24.28.

Wu, J., M. Wu, T. Chen and R. Jiang (2016). Whole genome sequencing and its applications in medical genetics. Quantitative Biology. 4(2): 115–128.

Xu, C. (2018). A review of somatic single nucleotide variant calling algorithms for next-generation sequencing data. Computational and Structural Biotechnology Journal. 16: 15–24.

Yakneen, S., S.M. Waszak, PCAWG Technical Working Group, M. Gertz, J.O. Korbel and PCAWG Consortium (2020). Butler enables rapid cloud-based analysis of thousands of human genomes. Nature Biotechnology. 38(3): 288–292.

Yang, Z. and R. Nielsen (1998). Synonymous and nonsynonymous rate variation in nuclear genes of mammals. Journal of Molecular Evolution. 46(4): 409–418.

Yost, S.E., E.N. Smith, R.B. Schwab, L. Bao, H. Jung, X. Wang, et al. (2012). Identification of high-confidence somatic mutations in whole genome sequence of formalin-fixed breast cancer specimens. Nucleic Acids Research. 40(14): e107.

Yukselen, O., O. Turkyilmaz, A.R. Ozturk, M. Garber and A. Kucukural (2020). DolphinNext: A distributed data processing platform for high throughput genomics. BMC Genomics. 21(1): 310.

Zar, G., J.G. Smith, M.L. Smith, B. Andersson and J. Nilsson (2019). Whole-genome sequencing based on formalin-fixed paraffin-embedded endomyocardial biopsies for genetic studies on outcomes after heart transplantation. PloS One. 14(6): e0217747.

Zook, J.M., D. Catoe, J. McDaniel, L. Vang, N. Spies, A. Sidow, et al. (2016). Extensive sequencing of seven human genomes to characterize benchmark reference materials. Scientific Data. 3(1): 160025.

Zook, J.M., J. McDaniel, N.D. Olson, J. Wagner, H. Parikh, H. Heaton, et al. (2019). An open resource for accurately benchmarking small variant and reference calls. Nature Biotechnology. 37(5): 561–566.

Zook, J.M., N.F. Hansen, N.D. Olson, L.M. Chapman, J.C. Mullikin, C. Xiao, et al. (2020). A robust benchmark for detection of germline large deletions and insertions. Nat. Biotechnol. 38: 1347–1355.

CHAPTER 7

Bioinformatics for Whole Exome Studies

Manojkumar Kumaran and Bharanidharan Devarajan*

Department of Bioinformatics, Aravind Medical Research Foundation, Madurai

1 INTRODUCTION

Next-generation sequencing technologies employ different sequencing approaches, they share a common feature that is massively parallel sequencing of clonally amplified or single DNA molecules that are spatially separated in a flow cell. Recently, it has improved immensely capable of producing hundreds of megabases to gigabases per run. Thus, it enables the comprehensive genetic sequencing of all (Whole genome sequencing) or part (Whole-exome sequencing), i.e. sequencing the protein-coding regions of the human genome. WES has been a successful cost-effective tool for the discovery of disease-causing variants. Whereas, though with recent advancements, WGS is still expensive in terms of data storage and analysis. Nevertheless, recent developments are accelerating these technologies to advance the discovery of novel variant/gene and therapeutic interventions.

WES, only covers 1–1.5% of the human genome and houses approximately 85% of the known disease-causing variants, which is a feasible method for the immediate implementation in the clinical arena. Although it poses several challenges that certain regions in the genome are difficult to sequence include GC-rich regions, repeat expansions (interspersed or tandem repeat), and regions of high sequence homology (from pseudogenes or gene families), the current bottleneck moved to towards bioinformatics analysis to identify true positive clinically-relevant variants.

Bioinformatics challenges concerned with quality control; short read-mapping (Langmead et al., 2009; Li and Durbin, 2009), variant calling (Albers et al., 2011; Li et al., 2009; McKenna et al., 2010), and variant annotation (Jager et al., 2014; Liu et al., 2013; Ng et al., 2009; Yang and Wang, 2015), have now been tackled by various bioinformatics tools (DePristo et al., 2011; Pabinger et al., 2014). Several benchmarking studies have been performed to evaluate the

---
*Corresponding author: *bharani@aravind.org*

different variant calling pipelines, and they reported discordance among variant calls (Liu et al., 2013; Pirooznia et al., 2014; Kumaran et al., 2019). In this review, we first present an evaluation of the major aligners and variant caller tools and based on that we provide our recommendations for the selection of variant analysis tools for WES.

In the context of WES in the clinical setup, multiple assumptions regarding the filtering and prioritizing disease-causing variants were made. For instance, any given individual's exome contains many protein sequence–altering inherited genetic variations and de novo mutations, but only a small fraction of these can be expected to impact protein function (e.g., nonsense mutations that result in a truncated protein). Moreover, a smaller number of these mutations are likely to be deleterious or relevant to a disease study, even if they significantly alter protein function or expression levels, due to incomplete or non-penetrance. Several bioinformatics tools are currently being used to predict the functional impact of genetic variants. Further, these variants require filtering and prioritization to the establishment of their relevance with human disease (MacArthur et al., 2012; Richards et al., 2015). The ExAC consortium recently published data and findings based on the sequencing of nearly 65,000 human exomes that can be valuable in the development of rules and protocols for the efficient filtering of candidate disease-causing variants (Lek et al., 2016). Here, we will also review various variant filtering strategies and prioritization tools to identify variants relevant to human disease.

2 BIOINFORMATICS ANALYSIS FOR WES

Several open-source bioinformatics algorithms and commercial software exist to analyze WES large data files and process into variant call files (VCF) with high-quality variants, which require substantial computational resource and bioinformatics expertise. Each lab has a unique pipeline made up of open-source, in-house developed, and/or commercial software, the WES pipeline we use is shown in Fig. 1. The bioinformatics analysis, although there are variations in the protocol, is a common multistep process for WES. The primary analysis starts with the processes of initial alignment and mapping of sequence reads to the human genome reference in order to generate a binary alignment and mapping file after the quality control analysis of NGS data (Fig. 1). The secondary analysis is the variant preparation, involving variant calling and

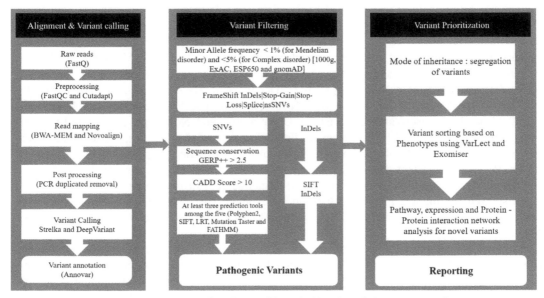

Figure 1 Work flow of variant calling pipeline for whole-exome studies.

annotations, for the downstream clinical interpretation (tertiary analysis). The tertiary analysis includes variant incidence, prioritization, classification, and integration with the clinical features. Several reviews are referred to here (Lelieveld et al., 2015; Lelieveld et al., 2016; Bao et al., 2014) for the primary and secondary analyses of WES and WGS data, have emphasized the sensitivity and accuracy of different algorithms in the identification of variants. The tertiary analysis, a complex process, requires a customized data-mining process for the identification of a disease-causing or associated variant, which is depending on the phenotype.

3   PERFORMANCE ASSESSMENT OF VARIANT CALLING PIPELINES USING HUMAN WHOLE EXOME SEQUENCING AND SIMULATED DATA

The whole-exome sequencing (WES) is a time-consuming technology for the identification of clinical variants, and it demands accurate variant caller tools. The currently available tools compromise accuracy in predicting the specific types of variants. Thus, it is essential to find out the possible combination of best aligner-variant caller tools for detecting SNVs and InDels separately.

For benchmarking of variant calling pipelines, many studies used a set of high confident variant calls for one individual (NA12878), published by the Genome in a Bottle (GiaB) consortium as a gold standard reference set, which can be extended to individual sequence data for clinical genomics (Cornish and Guda 2015; Highnam et al., 2015; Hwang et al., 2015; Li et al., 2018; Zook et al., 2014). Recently, we reported several performance metrics with respect to F-score aimed to build an extensive benchmark for studying the performance of pipelines with current well-known tools in detecting SNVs and InDels Also, we addressed how these different tools performed with the improved version of the human reference genome (GRCh38) and how was the current well-known tools work in identifying accurate variant call set (Kumaran et al., 2019). Here, we report with an assessment of different variant calling pipelines with updated and newly improved tools such as Strelka for variant calling.

To assess the performance of variant (especially InDels) caller in combination with different aligners, we developed 25 automated pipelines and evaluated using gold reference variant dataset (NA12878) from Genome in a Bottle (GiaB) consortium of human whole-exome sequencing. Additionally, the simulated exome data from human reference genome sequences (GRCh38) were used to compare the performance of the pipelines. To access the performance of pipelines, we calculated true positive (TP), false positive (FP) and false-negative (FN) variants using GiaB variant call set as standards. It contains 23,686 SNVs and 1,258 InDels for NA12878 exome. We used F-score as the function of performance assessment. In all the exome datasets, BWA_DeepVariant, Novoalign_DeepVariant, BWA_Strelka, Novoalign_Strelka were the top-performing pipelines for the SNVs detection. The F-score of the top 4 pipelines were 0.97 on BWA_DeepVariant, Novoalign_DeepVariant, and Novoalign_Strelka and 0.96 on BWA_Strelka on NA12878 SNVs detection. Following these four pipelines, we obtained better results from BWA_SAMtools, Novoalign_SAMtools, and Bowtie_DeepVariant. In the case of InDels, BWA_DeepVariant, Novoalign_DeepVariant scored best followed by BWA_Strelka and Novoalign_Strelks. Of these, DeepVariant based pipelines performed better than Strelka based, which showed the highest F-score of 0.99 on all exomes. Also, we reported that DeepVariant based pipeline performed better than other pipelines based on the various performance matrices (Kumaran et al., 2019).

In order to compare the performance of variant calling pipelines with different human datasets with GRCh38 reference, we have included the recently added human whole exome datasets NA24385 and NA24631. The average performance (F-score) of the pipelines with all three datasets including NA12878 and simulated Exome (Fig. 2) showed that there were no changes in the top-performing pipelines. In particular, we found that DeepVariant performed best invariably with all data sets. However, the aligners BWA and Novoalign both performed equally well on the new datasets compared with NA12878. Further, we improved the accurate variant call set by merging the top-performing pipelines. Collectively, this would help the investigators to improve the sensitivity and accuracy in detecting specific variants effectively. However, the users should be aware that the pipelines may fail to detect ~1% to ~2% of true variants.

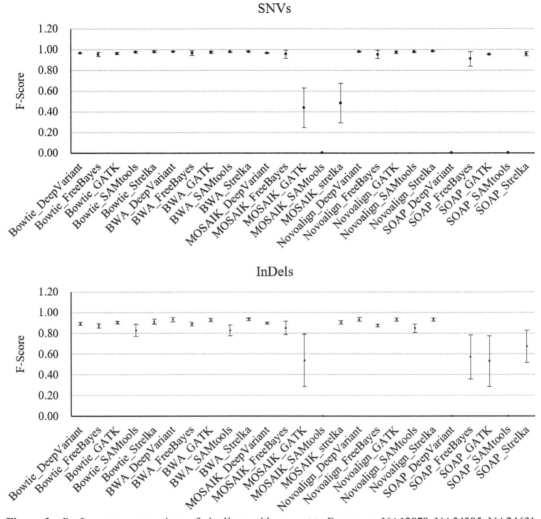

Figure 2 Performance comparison of pipelines with respect to F-score on NA12878, NA24385, NA24631 and simulated exome. The values and the error bars represent the average and standard deviation respectively of F-score obtained from all four datasets. Performance comparison of pipelines in SNVs and InDels detection for GRCh38.

4 COMPARISON OF BEST-PERFORMING PIPELINE

To improve accurate call detection, we compared the GiaB call set against the variants detected by the top four pipelines (mentioned earlier) BWA_DeepVariant, Novoalign_DeepVariant, BWA_Strelka2, and Novoalign_Strelka2 for SNVs and InDels. All four merged pipelines on all exomes improved the concordance of variants with GiaB call set (Fig. 3). It improved the accuracy in calling true positive SNVs to ~99% on Simulated Exome, and ~98% on NA12878. In the case of InDels, we observed ~96% on NA12878 and ~98% on simulated exome. Further, we evaluated best performing caller DeepVariant by merging its call set from BWA and Novoalign alignments. This merged call set showed ~98% and ~96% TP for SNVs and InDels respectively on all the exomes. Altogether, merged pipelines showed better performance, despite the increased FDR.

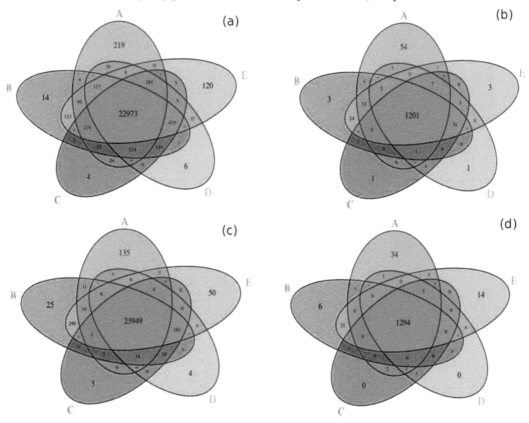

Figure 3 Venn diagram depicting the comparison of top 4 pipelines. GiaB variants (A) compared against the top 4 performing pipelines, (B) BWA_Strelka2, (C) BWA_DeepVariant, (D) Novoalign_DeepVariant, (E) Novoalign_Strelka2, for SNVs (a, c) and InDels (b, d) on NA12878 (top row) and Simulated exome (bottom row).

5   VARIANT ANNOTATION

All the selected variants based on the targeted regions of whole-exome sequencing kits require annotations, a critical step for further filtering and prioritization for the identification of disease-causing variants. The annotation tools aim to annotate variants functional effects/consequences, including but not limited to (i) list of gene(s)/transcript(s) that are affected, (ii) the consequence on protein sequence, (iii) annotating the variant with known genomic locations (e.g., coding sequence, intronic sequence, noncoding RNA, regulatory regions, etc.), and (iv) matching known variants in the various databases (e.g., dbSNP (Sherry et al., 2001), 1000 Genomes Project (Auton et al., 2015), ExAc (Lek et al., 2016), gnomAD (Karczewski et al., 2020), ClinVar (Landrum et al., 2014), etc.). The consequence of each variant is expressed through Sequence Ontology (SO) terms and severity qualifiers. The most widely used annotation tools include but are not limited to ANNOVAR (Wang et al., 2010), SeattleSeq (Ng et al., 2009), SnpEff (Cingolani et al., 2012) Variant Effect Predictor (VEP) (Mclaren et al., 2016), GEMINI (Paila et al., 2013),

VAAST (Hu et al., 2013). Studies have benchmarked the performance of various annotation tools. McCarthy et al., 2014 have compared VEP and ANNOVAR with respect to transcript available from Ensembl and RefSeq. The study concluded that 65% concordance between annotation for Loss of Function (LoF) variants produced using VEP and ANNOVAR using the same transcript set. While using different transcript ANNOVAR reported 44% concordance among the putative variants (McCarthy et al., 2014). Based on the publication search on WES, ANNOVAR is the most commonly used variant annotation tool which provides three annotation modes, gene-based, region-based, and filter-based, with a collection of over 4,000 public databases for annotation. Thus, we recommend ANNOVAR and also one can use online version of ANNOVAR or SeattleSeq.

6 VARIANT FILTERING AND PRIORITIZATION

The exome sequencing is estimated to provide more than 30000 to 50000 variants depending on the exome capturing kit, and thus, the number is reduced to generate a short list of variants that could impact the protein function and cause disease. First, several metrics provided by the variant callers is used to reduce the numbers such as low coverage, low quality, strand biased etc. Variants with base quality of ≥ 20 and depth of ≥ 30 were preferred for the clinical setup (Li et al., 2014). Next, all common variants are avoided, assuming that only rare variants cause disease. This step may differ based on the individual patients, disease model of the studies and laboratories. In common, variants with high minor allele frequency (MAF) equal to or greater than 1% in public databases will be omitted (Cooper et al., 2013). GWAS has been widely used for investigating the genetic architecture of complex diseases by the following common variant filter cutoff of greater than or equal to 5% in public databases (Manolio et al., 2009). ANNOVAR consists of several public databases include the 1000 Genomes Project (http://www.1000genomes.org/), ESP6500 (http://evs.gs.washington.edu/EVS/), dbSNP (http://www.ncbi.nlm.nih.gov/SNP/), ExAC (http://exac.broadinstitute.org/) and GenomeAD (http://gnomad.broadinstitute.org) are used for MAF estimations. MAF cutoff around 1% and 0.5% or less may be used for rare recessive disorders and a dominant or X-linked disorder respectively.

Next, the remaining variants are filtered using the functional impact of the variant.The truncating variants (stop gain/loss, start loss, or frameshift), missense variants, canonical splice-site variants are considered first as protein-function altering variants, followed by silent and +in-frame indels affecting protein-coding regions. Missense variants are further prioritized by their functional impact on the protein using in silico tools such as SIFT (http://sift.jcvi.org/) and Polyphen2 (http://genetics.bwh.harvard.edu/pph2/), and others (Table 1).

Chengliang et al., 2015 have compared the predictive performance of all prediction methods (Table 2). Despite their differences in the use of prediction features, training data and statistical models, most of the algorithms assumed that variants are evolutionary conserved and/or affect protein structure and function, are most likely deleterious (Chengliang et al., 2015). We recommend starting with a conservation score at least ≥ 2.5 (GERP score) and further filtering with a CADD score of ≥ 10 and any three variant effect prediction tools among the five (SIFT, Polyphen-2, FATHMM, MutationTaster and LRT) should evaluate the variant as the deleterious.

Although WES methods have mostly been used for the diagnosis and personalized treatment of human diseases, it is still challenging to identify disease-causing variants from the potential candidate list filtered through various functional annotation tools. Yet, there are standardized guidelines from the American College of Medical Genetics and Genomics (ACMG) (Rehm et al., 2013), EuroGentest, and the European Society of Human Genetics guidelines (Matthijs et al., 2015) for interpretation of clinically-relevant variants. A growing number of *in silico*

Bioinformatics and Human Genomics Research

phenotype-driven tools have been developed to select and prioritize the disease-causing variants. These tools majorly rank the candidate variants with the use of the Human Phenotype Ontology (HPO) database, which aims to provide a computable representation of the clinical abnormalities observed in human disease (Köhler et al., 2014). Additionally, these tools integrate several other databases with the patient's phenotypic information (Table 2).

Table 1 List of tools used for predicting the severity of the variants with qualifiers (e.g., benign/mild, probably damaging/moderate, damaging/deleterious)

Tools	Category	Deleterious threshold/ qualifier	Features
SIFT	Function prediction	>0.95	Protein sequence conservation among homologs
PolyPhen-2	Function prediction	>0.5	Eight protein sequence features, three protein structure features
LRT	Function prediction	P	DNA sequence evolutionary model
MutationTaster	Function prediction	>0.5	DNA sequence conservation, splice site prediction, mRNA stability prediction and protein feature annotations
Mutation Assessor	Function prediction	>0.65	Sequence homology of protein families and sub-families within and between species
FATHMM	Function prediction	≥ 0.45	Sequence homology
GERP++ RS	Conservation score	≥ 4.4	DNA sequence conservation
PhyloP	Conservation score	>1.6	DNA sequence conservation
SiPhy	Conservation score	>12.17	Inferred nucleotide substitution pattern per site
PON-P	Ensemble score	P	Random forest methodology-based pipeline integrating five predictors
PANTHER	Function prediction	P	Phylogenetic trees based on protein sequences
PhD-SNP	Function prediction	P	SVM-based method using protein sequence and profile information
SNAP	Function prediction	P	Neural network-based method using DNA sequence information as well as functional and structural annotations
SNPsandGO	Function prediction	P	SVM-based method using information from protein sequence, protein sequence profile and protein function
MutPred	Function prediction	>0.5	Protein sequence-based model using SIFT and a gain/loss of 14 different structural and functional properties
KGGSeq	Ensemble score	P	Filtration and prioritization framework using information from three levels: genetic level, variant-gene level and knowledge level
CONDEL	Ensemble score	>0.49	Weighted average of the normalized scores of five methods
SIFT_InDel	Function prediction	>0.95	Decision tree for the insertion/Deletion of amino acid based on Protein sequence conservation among homologs
CADD	Ensemble score	≥ 15	63 distinct variant annotation retrieved from Ensembl Variant Effect Predictor (VEP), data from the ENCODE project and information from UCSC genome browser tracks

Table 2 List of prioritizing variants software

Software	Availability	Population, Disease-specific, and sequence databases	In silico algorithms
eXtasy	Online and Standalone	1000 Genomes Project dbNSFP database HGMD	Polyphen2 SIFT MutationTaster CAROL LRT PhastCons Phylop
Phen-Gen	Online and Standalone	HGMD	Polyphen2 SIFT
PhenIX	Online and Standalone	1000 Genomes Project ESP 6500	Polyphen2 SIFT MutationTaster
hiPHIVE	Online and Standalone	1000 Genomes Project ESP 6500 MGD IMPC	Polyphen2 SIFT MutationTaster
Exome Walker	Online	1000 Genomes Project String dbSNP OMIM	CADD SIFT Mutation Taster DbNSFP
Phenolyzer	Online	OMIM clinVar KEGG Reactome Pathway	—
Phevor	Online	1000 Genomes Project dbSNP	SIFT, PhastCons and VAAST
VarElect	Online	GeneCards MalaCards PathCards	—
Ifish	Online	1000 Genomes Project dbSNP HGMD	SIFT Polyphen2 MutationAssessor
Exomiser	Standalone	1000 Genomes Project ESP EXAC dbNSFP	Polyphen2 SIFT MutationTaster LRT Phylop

CAROL, Calculated Combined Annotation Scoring Tools; dbNSFP, database for nonsynonymous SNPs' functional predictions; ESP 6500, Exome Server Project; HGMD, Human Gene Mutation Database; IMPC, International Mouse Phenotyping Consortium; LRT, Likelihood-Ratio Test; MGD, Mouse Genome Database; SIFT, Sorting Intolerant from Tolerant. Software version: eXtasy (Sifrim et al., 2013) ver.0.1, Phen-Gen (Javed et al., 2014) ver.1.0, PhenIX and hiPHIVE (Smedley et al., 2015) ver.10.0.1.

Despite the above, a careful examination is required for the filtered and prioritized variants prior to confirm their significance in the clinical practice, since a number of variants could be prioritized as causative variants through the above described methods. In presumed monogenic-disease cases, first one must use the above phenotype-based tools to evaluate genes and variant previously reported in disease phenotypes. For novel variants, the new gene can be implicated only when variants in the same gene and similar clinical features have been implicated in multiple individuals, along with unaffected controls, which requires considerable expertise and collaborative input from physician and geneticin. Further functional studies are required to validate experimentally the predicted disease-causing variants. Prioritization of variants in a complex disease is very difficult and is reviewed elsewhere (Bharanidharan et al., 2019).

In summary, this chapter provides widely used bioinformatics tools for whole exome data analysis, including data preprocessing, alignment, variant calling, annotation, and variant prioritization. In this study, we compared the performance of various aligner and variant callers using standard human reference whole-exome and simulated data, and provided recommendation of tools for whole exome studies. Additionally, we highlighted the several considerations using variant filtering and prioritization tools for the identification of disease-causing variants.

REFERENCES

Albers, C.A., G. Lunter, D.G. MacArthur, G. McVean, W.H. Ouwehand and R. Durbin (2011). Dindel: accurate indel calls from short-read data. Genome Res. 21: 961–973.

Auton, A., L.D. Brooks, R.M. Durbin, E.P. Garrison, H.M. Kang, J.O. Korbel, et al. (2015). A global reference for human genetic variation. Nature. 526(7571): 68–74.

Bao, R., L. Huang, J. Andrade, W. Tan, W.A. Kibbe, H. Jiang, et al. (2014). Review of current methods, applications, and data management for the bioinformatics analysis of whole exome sequencing. Cancer Inform. 13(suppl 2): 67–82.

Cingolani, P., A. Platts, L.L. Wang, M. Coon, T. Nguyen, L. Wang, et al. (2012). A program for annotating and predicting the effects of single nucleotide polymorphisms, SnpEff: SNPs in the genome of Drosophila melanogaster strain w1118; iso-2; iso-3. Fly (Austin). 6(2): 80–92.

Cooper, D.N., M. Krawczak, C. Polychronakos, C. Tyler-Smith and H. Kehrer-Sawatzki (2013). Where genotype is not predictive of phenotype: Towards an understanding of the molecular basis of reduced penetrance in human inherited disease. Hum. Genet. 132: 1077–1130.

Cornish, A. and C. Guda. (2015). A Comparison of variant calling pipelines using genome in a bottle as a reference. Biomed. Res. Int. 2015: 456479.

DePristo, M.A., E. Banks, R. Poplin, K.V. Garimella, J.R. Maguire, C. Hartl, et al. (2011) A framework for variation discovery and genotyping using next-generation DNA sequencing data. Nat. Genet. 43: 491–498.

Devarajan B., Vanniarajan A., Sundaresan P. (2019) Genomic approaches to eye diseases: An asian perspective. pp. 403–415. *In*: G. Prakash and T. Iwata (eds). Advances in Vision Research, Volume II. Essentials in Ophthalmology. Springer, Singapore. https://doi.org/10.1007/978-981-13-0884-0_33.

Dong, C., P. Wei, X. Jian, R. Gibbs, E. Boerwinkle, K. Wang, et al. (2015). Comparison and integration of deleteriousness prediction methods for nonsynonymous SNVs in whole exome sequencing studies. Hum. Mol. Genet. 24(8): 2125–2137.

Highnam, G., J.J. Wang, D. Kusler, J. Zook, V. Vijayan, N. Leibovich, et al. (2015). An analytical framework for optimizing variant discovery from personal genomes. Nat. Commun. 6: 62–75.

Hu, H., C.D. Huff, B. Moore, S. Flygare, M.G. Reese and M. Yandell (2013). VAAST 2.0: Improved variant classification and disease-gene identification using a conservation-controlled amino acid substitution matrix. Genetic Epidemiology. 37(6): 622–634.

Hwang, S., E. Kim, I. Lee and E.M. Marcotte (2015). Systematic comparison of variant calling pipelines using gold standard personal exome variants. Sci Rep. 5: 17875.

Jager, M., K. Wang, S. Bauer, D. Smedley, P. Krawitz and P.N. Robinson (2014). JANNOVAR: A java library for exome annotation. Hum. Mutat. 35: 548–555.

Javed, A., S. Agrawal and P.C. Ng (2014). Phen-Gen: Combining phenotype and genotype to analyze rare disorders. Nat. Methods. 11: 935–937. 10.1038/nmeth.3046.

Karczewski, K.J., L.C. Francioli and G. Tiao, B.B. Cummings, J. Alföldi, Q. Wang, et al. (2020). The mutational constraint spectrum quantified from variation in 141,456 humans. Nature. 581: 434–443.

Köhler, S., S.C. Doelken, C.J. Mungall, S. Bauer, H.V. Firth, I. Bailleul-Forestier, et al. (2014). The human phenotype ontology project: Linking molecular biology and disease through phenotype data. Nucleic Acids Res. 42: D966–74.

Kumaran, M., U. Subramanian and B. Devarajan (2019). Performance assessment of variant calling pipelines using human whole exome sequencing and simulated data. BMC Bioinformatics. 20: 342.

Landrum, M.J., J.M. Lee, G.R. Riley, W. Jang, W.S. Rubinstein, D.M. Church, et al. (2014). ClinVar: Public archive of relationships among sequence variation and human phenotype. Nucleic Acids Research. 42(Database issue): D980–D985.

Langmead, B., C. Trapnell, M. Pop and S.L. Salzberg (2009). Ultrafast and memory-efficient alignment of short DNA sequences to the human genome. Genome Biol. 10: R25.

Lek, M., K.J. Karczewski, E.V. Minikel, K.E. Samocha, E. Banks, T. Fennell, et al. (2016). Analysis of protein-coding genetic variation in 60,706 humans. Nature. 536(7616): 285–291.

Lelieveld, S.H., M. Spielmann, S. Mundlos, J.A. Veltman and C. Gilissen (2015). Comparison of exome and genome sequencing technologies for the complete capture of protein-coding regions. Hum Mutat. 36 (8): 815–822.

Lelieveld, S.H., J.A. Veltman and C. Gilissen (2016). Novel bioinformatic developments for exome sequencing. Hum Genet. 135(6): 603–614.

Li, H., J. Ruan and R. Durbin (2008). Mapping short DNA sequencing reads and calling variants using mapping quality scores. Genome Res. 18: 1851–1858.

Li, H. and R. Durbin (2009). Fast and accurate short read alignment with Burrows–Wheeler transform. Bioinformatics. 25: 1754–1760.

Li, H., B. Handsaker, A. Wysoker, T. Fennell, J. Ruan, N. Homer, et al. (2009). The sequence alignment/ map format and SAMtools. Bioinformatics. 25: 2078–2079.

Li, H. (2014). Toward better understanding of artifacts in variant calling from high-coverage samples. Bioinformatics. 30(20): 2843–2851

Li, Z., Y. Wang and F. Wang (2018). A study on fast calling variants from next-generation sequencing data using decision tree. BMC Bioinformatics. 19(1): 145.

Liu, X., S. Han, Z. Wang, J. Gelernter and B.Z. Yang (2013a). Variant callers for next-generation sequencing data: A comparison study. PloS One. 8: e75619.

Liu, X., X. Jian and E. Boerwinkle (2013b). dbNSFP v2.0: A database of human non-synonymous SNVs and their functional predictions and annotations. Hum. Mutat. 34: E2393–E2402.

MacArthur, D.G., S. Balasubramanian, A. Frankish, N. Huang, J. Morris, K. Walter, et al. (2012). A systematic survey of loss-of-function variants in human protein-coding genes. Science. 335: 823–828.

Manolio, T.A., F.S. Collins and N.J. Cox, D.B. Goldstein, L.A. Hindorff, D.J. Hunter, et al. (2009). Finding the missing heritability of complex diseases. Nature 461(7265): 747–753.

Matthijs, G., E. Souche, M. Alders, A. Corveleyn, S. Eck and I. Feenstra, et al. (2015). Guidelines for diagnostic next-generation sequencing. Eur J Hum Genet. 24: 2–5.

McCarthy, D.J., P. Humburg, A. Kanapin, M.A. Rivas, K. Gaulton, J.-B. Cazier, et al. (2014). Choice of transcripts and software has a large effect on variant annotation. Genome. Med. 6: 26.

McKenna, A., M. Hanna, E. Banks, A. Sivachenko, K. Cibulskis, A. Kernytsky, et al. (2010). The genome analysis toolkit: a MapReduce framework for analyzing nextgeneration DNA sequencing data. Genome Res. 20: 1297–1303.

Mclaren, W., L. Gil and S.E. Hunt, H.S. Riat, G.R.S. Ritchie, A. Thormann, et al. (2016). The Ensembl variant effect predictor. Genome Biol. 17(1): 122.

Ng, S.B., E.H. Turner, and P.D. Robertson, S.D. Flygare, A.W. Bigham, C. Lee, et al. (2009). Targeted capture and massively parallel sequencing of 12 human exomes. Nature. 461(7261): 272–276.

Pabinger, S., et al. (2014). A survey of tools for variant analysis of next-generation genome sequencing data. Brief. Bioinf. 15: 256–278.

Paila, U., B.A. Chapman, R. Kirchner and A.R. Quinlan (2013). GEMINI: Integrative exploration of genetic variation and genome annotations. PLoS Computational Biology. 9(7): e1003153.

Pirooznia, M., M. Kramer, J. Parla, F.S. Goes, J.B. Potash and W.R. McCombie, et al. (2014). Validation and assessment of variant calling pipelines for next-generation sequencing. Hum. Genomics. 8:14.

Rehm, H.L, S.J. Bale, P. Bayrak-Toydemir, J.S. Berg, K.K. Brown, J.L. Deignan, et al. (2013). ACMG clinical laboratory standards for next-generation sequencing. Genet. Med. 15(9): 733–747. doi:10.1038/ gim.2013.92.

Richards, S., N. Aziz, S. Bale, D. Bick, S. Das, J.W. Gastier-Foster, et al. (2015). Standards and guidelines for the interpretation of sequence variants: a joint consensus recommendation of the american college of medical genetics and genomics and the association for molecular pathology. Genet. Med. 17: 405–424.

Sherry, S.T., M.H. Ward and M. Kholodov, J. Baker, L. Phan, E.M. Smigielski, et al. (2001). dbSNP: The NCBI database of genetic variation. Nucleic Acids Research. 29(1): 308–311.

Sifrim, A., D. Popovic, L.C. Tranchevent, A. Ardeshirdavani, R. Sakai, P. Konings, et al. (2013). eXtasy: variant prioritization by genomic data fusioneXtasy: variant prioritization by genomic data fusion. Nat Methods. 10(11): 1083–1084.

Smedley, D., J.O.B. Jacobsen, M. Jäger, S. Köhler, M. Holtgrewe, M. Schubach, et al. (2015). Next-generation diagnostics and disease-gene discovery with the Exomiser. Nat. Protoc. 10: 2004–2015. 10.1038/nprot.2015.124.

Wang, K., M. Li and H. Hakonarson (2010). ANNOVAR: Functional annotation of genetic variants from next-generation sequencing data. Nucleic Acids Research. 38: e164.

Yang, H. and K. Wang (2015). Genomic variant annotation and prioritization with ANNOVAR and wANNOVAR. Nat. Protoc. 10: 1556–1566.

Zook, J.M., B. Chapman, J. Wang, D. Mittelman, O. Hofmann, W. Hide, et al. (2014). Integrating human sequence data sets provides a resource of benchmark SNV and indel genotype calls. Nat. Biotechnol. 32: 246–251.

CHAPTER 8

Bioinformatics of Variant Effect Prediction

Ariel José Berenstein[*][1], **Franco Gino Brunello**[*][2],
Adrian Turjanski[2] **and Marcelo A. Marti**[**][2]

[1]Instituto Multidisciplinario de Investigaciones en Patologías Pediátricas (IMIPP),
CONICET-GCBA, Laboratorio de Biología Molecular, División Patología, Hospital de Niños
Ricardo Gutiérrez, Buenos Aires, Argentina

[2]Departamento de Química Biológica, Facultad de Ciencias Exactas y Naturales,
Universidad de Buenos Aires (FCEyN-UBA) e Instituto de Química Biológica de la Facultad
de Ciencias Exactas y Naturales (IQUIBICEN) CONICET, Pabellòn 2 de Ciudad Universitaria,
Ciudad de Buenos Aires C1428EHA, Argentina

1 INTRODUCTION

1.1 NGS Revolution and Its Application to Human Health

One of the early and major areas adopting Next Generation Sequencing (NGS) in relation
to human health, is the molecular diagnosis of genetic (usually Mendelian) disorders. In its
mainstream application, patients with a clinical diagnosis of a suspected genetic disease are
sequenced to look for the disease-causative variant(s). If the disease is clearly monogenic,
such as cystic fibrosis, usually only the relevant gene is sequenced, for other diseases like
autoinflammatory conditions, small (10) to medium (up to 50) gene panels are used, and finally
whole exome sequencing (WES, around 20 k genes), or whole genome sequencing (WGS) can be
performed. The number of variants to be analyzed, and clinically interpreted, increases linearly
with the number of genes sequenced, ranging from a few to about 50–100k for a typical WES,
and over a million in WGS. Given the magnitude, relevance and complexity of this task, it is

*Equally contributed
**Corresponding author: *marti.marcelo@gmail.com*

hardly surprising that the development and application of bioinformatic tools that contribute to its successful achievement is an active research field.

1.2   The Problem of Variant Interpretation

Variant analysis and clinical interpretation are usually performed in two steps. The first consists of the variant annotation process, where several layers of information are added to each variant. Mainly, "mandatory" properties are: (i) variant molecular effect (the gene where it belongs, coding, non-coding, missense, nonsense, affecting splicing, intronic, etc.), (ii) population allele frequency, and (iii) clinical information (links to OMIM, ClinVar, etc.). The second is the clinical classification and interpretation. Classification should be made according to the recommended guidelines of the American College of Medical Genetics (ACMG) which is based on five categories: Pathogenic (P), Likely Pathogenic (LP), Variant of Uncertain Significance (VUS), Likely Benign (LB) and Benign (B) (Richards et al., 2015). In any given case, most variants are LBB, and only 1 or 2 are P or LP, and can thus be considered a proper diagnostic. Moreover, in many cases, no P/LP variant can be found, and several VUS must be analyzed in detail as potential candidates.

In order to classify variants according to ACMG rules, each of them is first analyzed according to 28 different evidence criteria, such as population frequency, type of variant (nonsense, missense), previous reports, etc. Each evidence criteria provides (if fulfilled) an alphanumeric score to the variant. Scores are divided between those contributing to the variant pathogenicity, starting with Pathogenic Very Strong (PVS) up to Pathogenic Supporting (PP); and those contributing to its benignity, ranging from Benign Stand-alone (BA) to Benign Supporting (BS). To be classified as LP a variant must have at least one Pathogenic Moderate (PM) and four or more PP, while to be classified as P it needs the presence of an additional Pathogenic Strong (PS) evidence. The presence of VUS arises from two possibilities, either the variant has not enough evidence to be classified as pathogenic (or benign), or there is contradictory evidence (i.e., some evidence supporting pathogenicity and others supporting its benignity). In those "borderline" cases, each small bit of evidence becomes relevant to assist in the variant classification (and interpretation) criteria, and therefore, to finally reach a positive or negative diagnosis.

The evidence criteria that we will discuss in deep correspond to what is known as "Bioinformatic Pathogenicity Prediction". According to ACMG, a variant will display PP3 if several lines of computational evidence support its pathogenicity, while it will display BP4 if several lines support its benign character. In practice, bioinformatic analysis considers the prediction of different programs and/or algorithms (usually 3 to 5), and if all (or most) of them point in the same direction, the variant is assigned the corresponding score. Thus the question, what is conceptually a bioinformatic pathogenicity predictor?

1.3   Bioinformatic Variant Pathogenicity Predictors

Conceptually, a bioinformatic variant pathogenicity predictor is an algorithm and its implementation, that given as input one (or a list) of variants will yield as result a prediction, usually in terms of a score and a recommended cut-off value, of its likeness to be pathogenic. As will be described below, these programs rely on different underlying biological information (sequence, structure, clinical), theoretical frameworks (evolutionary, statistical, physicochemical etc.) and algorithmic implementation. Finally, it is important to mention that prediction can be performed on different levels ranging from a prediction of the variant effect on gene (or protein) function to high level phenotypic outcome prediction. Here, we will focus mostly on those methods that try to predict and understand the variant effect at the molecular level, leaving its clinical interpretation to be performed by the physician in the context of other information related to each particular case.

2 FOUNDATIONS OF BIOINFORMATIC APPROACHES

2.1 Sequence-based Approaches

An indirect approach to infer the functional impact of a variant is to consider the level of genomic sequence conservation across a selected group of divergent species (or sequences). The underlying idea is that conservation across evolution is a good proxy of functional relevance, and could therefore be used to identify functional elements across the genome. A primary advantage of this approach is the broad application scope, namely, these scores are usually available for evaluation of coding as well as non-coding regions, missense or silent variants, splicing sites, regulatory sites, etc.

The central idea about all conservation algorithms, is that some genomic regions are less susceptible to experiment substitutions than others and that reluctance to change is what makes us think that they may be biologically important. This is what we call "negative selection" in evolution. The key question that arises from this reasoning is "less susceptible compared to what?". The consensus about this topic is that we might think the genome as having a "neutral rate of substitution" through time, and that regions functionally active at biological level would exhibit a lower observed rate of substitution as compared to the general background. This kind of analysis is achieved by making nucleotide multiple-sequence alignments (nMSA) among many species with variable divergence level at the phylogenetic level, and applying different strategies for further analysis.

In this context, sequence regions (or individual positions) under negative selection and enriched in biological meaning, should be less tolerant to mutations (since they are expected-on average- to reduce fitness), which will therefore be pruned by natural selection, leading to higher observed conservation in the nMSA. To utilize this idea to predict a novel variant effect, we therefore look at the variant position conservation scores as derived from the MSA. If the variant falls in a very conserved position, then it is more likely to affect gene/protein negatively and thus being characterized as pathogenic, while if the variant falls in a very degenerated loci (highly variable position in the MSA), we would assign it as likely benign.

From a more technical, or bioinformatic point of view, when talking about conservation algorithms, we may start by dividing them into two different approaches to the problem. On the one hand, we have the bottom-up approach, as represented by GERP++ (Davydov et al., 2010), which intends to quantify position-specific constraints in terms of rejected substitutions (RS), the difference between the neutral rate of substitution and the observed rate as estimated by maximum likelihood. Other algorithms, such as MCS (Margulies and Blanchette, 2003), also follow this bottom-up approach.

On the other hand, we find those generative model-based approaches, which attempt to explicitly model the quantity and distribution of constraint within a nMSA. With this aim, they utilize a phylo-Hidden Markov Model (HMM), a type of statistical model that considers both the process by which nucleotide substitutions occur at each site in a genome and how this process changes from one site to the next, to find the most likely parse of the alignment into constrained and neutral hidden states. One of the most cited conservation tools is PhastCons, which applies phylo-HMM in an easy and more friendly manner that allows not only to identify conserved sequences but also generate a continuous-valued "conservation score" for each base of the reference genome Siepel et al., 2005. In addition, other tools like phyloP prioritize some variables like the evolutionary distance between species inside a branch of the tree, giving place to lineage-specific conserved sequences (Siepel et al., 2006). Another scope is given by SiPhy (Garber et al., 2009), who moved away from the idea of a rate-based substitution method and went towards the analysis of substitution patterns at every site and singling out those that are biased.

Due to their relative early development (in the context of NGS based diagnostic), all these algorithms have been widely used yielding meaningful results, particularly when used to predict the effect in coding regions and other known functional elements. It is important nonetheless to mention some of their critical assumptions and caveats, such as the phylogenetic distance between the species being used in the MSA. If this distance is big enough, we might be introducing some errors by not considering the occurrence of compensatory mutations that may offset the deleterious effect of other ones. This problem may be addressed by considering shorter evolutionary time scales, at the expense of restricting the amount of data exploited.

2.2   Coding Regions: The Protein Evolution Approach

Protein-coding regions represent just a small fraction of the genome (1–2%) (Consortium, 2002). However, they host the lion's share of the known pathogenic variants and clinical sequencing efforts. Amino acid sequences constitute a critical input at determining variants' functional effects, since proteins are the ultimate biological effectors of genes. By applying amino acid multiple sequence alignments (aaMSA) across homologous sequences, residue positions might be analyzed as conserved or not, and indirectly predict the functional effect of an amino acid substitution in a similar way as described above for nucleotide sequences. SIFT (Kumar et al., 2009), for example, assumes that important positions in a protein sequence have been conserved throughout evolution and therefore substitutions at these positions may affect protein function negatively.

An alternative to a "simple" aaMSA is given by PROVEAN (Choi et al., 2012), which carries on a succession of pairwise-alignments between all the homologous sequences against the wild-type and mutated human sequences where the mutation is being tested, respectively. The aim is to obtain a difference in alignment scores for both situations that correlates with the functional impact of non-synonymous amino acid substitutions.

Going beyond pure sequence conservation, some algorithms have enriched their predictions with information from a diverse nature. Polyphen-2 (Adzhubei et al., 2010), for example, not only makes use of aaMSA to capture evolutionary conservation, but also includes other features in the analysis such as sequence annotations from Uniprot, as well as 3-D structures when available. Mapping of an amino acid replacement to the known 3-D structure reveals whether the replacement is likely to destroy the hydrophobic core of a protein, electrostatic interactions, interactions with ligands, or other important features of a protein (More details about the structural approach for variant interpretation is presented in next section). Taking it to another level, we could mention LRT (Chun and Fey, 2009) that despite not strictly analyzing amino acid positions at the aaMSA, it carries on its analysis on nucleotide sequences by comparing a null model that each codon is evolving neutrally (with no difference in the rate of nonsynonymous to synonymous substitution) to the alternative model that the codon has evolved under negative selection and there is therefore an enrichment in synonymous substitutions against non-synonymous ones.

Finally, another interesting approach that adds to sequence approach is nicely described by fitCons (Gulko et al., 2015), which used functional genomic data (such as DNase-seq, RNA-seq and histone modification data) from three cell types, to generate "clusters of genome positions", characterize them, and that way predict consequences from variants on protein fitness.

In summary, sequence-based algorithms (of either nucleotides or amino acids) use pairwise or multiple alignments to infer evolutionary conserved regions which thus are predicted to be pathogenic when mutated. Those using protein sequences are more accurate but restricted to coding regions, while, as expected, those based on nucleotide sequences work better for known functional elements. Also, they are mostly restricted to single nucleotide or single amino acid substitutions or very small (2–5) inframe insertions and deletions. The analysis of more complex traits, such as out-of-frame indels, splice site variants and others requires more complex strategies that utilize sequence annotations to train more sophisticated—usually Machine learning based—algorithms in order to predict changes on protein functionality, as will be described in later sections.

2.3 Beyond Sequence Data 1: Structure

There are two main strategies to go beyond sequence data to predict the effect of a given variant. One is to add—as briefly mentioned for Polyphen-2—other features and combine them in some predictive model, as will be discussed in the next section. The other, which works for coding variants that correspond to Single (or multiple) amino acid Substitutions (SAS), is to analyze the protein itself, using as starting point its structure.

To take advantage of structural information there are also two main possible strategies. The first one corresponds to a simple lookup table of structurally identified functional sites (which interestingly can also be coded in a sequence-only approach once the sites are known). In this approach, active, allosteric, structure-defining and protein-protein interaction (among other) residue sites are first identified and listed. Second, the impact of possible (or previously known) SAS on these sites can be evaluated using residue similarity scores.

In the second one, a physicochemical-based approach, the impact of the SAS is evaluated using some thermodynamic force field model which, for example, estimates the change in the protein folding free energy due to the SAS. Those changes that result in large free energy differences are thought to destabilize the protein, leading to non or misfolded proteins, which are non-functional, and thus disease-causing. Further refinement of this structure-based approach is performed when also determining free energy change associated to protein-ligand and/or protein-protein interactions. In other words, thermodynamic models evaluate whether the SAS is likely (or not) to result in a non-functional protein and is therefore pathogenic.

2.4 Beyond Sequence Data 2: Machine Learning Approaches

The ultimate goal of a variant effect prediction model, as already mentioned, is to infer in some degree the functional impact of a given variant, in order to use it as a proxy of their pathogenicity condition (Benign/Pathogenic). In this context, Machine Learning approaches have been applied as part of an automated integration process that includes and processes a broad spectrum of biological information. The applied strategies vary from unsupervised approaches, to binary classification strategies, like generalized linear models, boosting and bagging methods, random forests, support vector machines, or even more, deep neural networks. Finally, the so-called ensemble techniques are based on meta-predictors that take advantage of previously trained tools.

In general, the binary classification strategies follow a very similar work path. They use a big fraction of data as a training set (usually 50–80%) to actually train the algorithm, and they preserve a small one (50–20%) as a blinded test set to evaluate the performance of the results thrown by the predictor. To further compare their performance against other predictors (usually by comparing the Area Under a Receiver Operating Characteristic Curve, i.e. AUC-ROC or in short, AUC), they must be careful that test sets must not have been included previously (direct or indirectly) in the training set of none of them, or otherwise results would be biased.

2.4.1 The learning process

In the context of variant effect prediction, the most usually considered strategy for building predictive tools based on machine-learning (ML) is the supervised binary classification. This approach is based on previously labelled known variants as benign or pathogenic, and aims to predict the most probable class (P or B) for new "unknown" cases. For this purpose and based on the labelled variants, algorithms need to build a decision boundary function (the function that better separates benign and pathogenic classes) in order to be used for pondering novel unknown variants. As an easy and concrete example of decision boundary, you can think about the sigmoid function used by a logistic regression. Different ML algorithms vary essentially in the family of boundary decision functions that they build, as well as the way and strategy in which they optimize it. Some classical examples involved in the context of variant effect prediction are Logistic Regression, ensemble tree-based models like Random Forest and XGBoost, Support Vector Machines, and lastly, in sintony with the AI trends, also powerful approaches based on Deep Neural Network (for a complete detail about the adopted strategy used by different existing tools survey in this manuscript, refer to Table 1).

In spite of the big conceptual differences among these ML algorithms, there exist some technical concepts that cross all of them and are worth mentioning before moving forward. First, all these ML methods need to estimate their predictive and generalization power in an unbiased way. To that end, an usual strategy is to split the available labelled data into a training and a blinded evaluation set. While the first one is used to find the optimal model, the last one (usually smaller) allows to evaluate the performance and generalization power. A good practice for that, is to extract random but balanced versions of train and evaluation sets, that is, ensuring that the proportions of pathogenic and benign data remains equal in both sets. In order to avoid overfitting (that is, a model that works greatly with our training set but poorly at the moment of the evaluation), the blinded evaluation set would never be used as part of the model training, neither in the building of features used as part of the training process (type 1 circularity (Grimm et al., 2015).

Taking advantage of the training set, all ML models will need to fit the parameters of their decision boundary function in order to find an optimal solution to the separability problem (remember that at the end of the day we want to find the function that better separates benign and pathogenic classes). This process is usually tackled by optimizing some cost function, like the Likelihood function, but it may actually vary from model to model. The obtained parameters are those that our decision boundary function will use in order to predict new unclassified variants.

2.4.2 Model performance and transferability

Training the model implies both finding optimal parameters as well as the hyperparameters themselves. The last ones could be thought of as extra parameters that must be optimized independently of the model parameters. Once finished, the predictive power must be reported by applying the model on the blinded evaluation set. Also, the generalization power must be estimated by comparing differences between the mean performance among the trained process and the obtained in the blinded test. That is, small differences between the training and blinded evaluation performance tell us that our model is generalizing well. On the other hand, obtaining higher performance metrics on the training sets accompanied by lower ones on the evaluation would represent overfitting risk.

At this point we must describe some key issues that are a general concern of any ML algorithm. There always exists a trade-off between complexity and generalization power of a model (the bias-variance trade-off). That is to say, the more complex a model becomes (for example, as the number of input features or the number of model's hyperparameters increases), the more risk of losing generalization power, i.e., to overfit our model to specific training data used to build the boundary function. There are several ways for which a model could get more complex appart to the number of features. For example, in a tree-based model the complexity could be increased by admitting deeper trees, or by increasing the number of leaves, while in other models like neural networks, the complexity increases typically with the number of involved hidden layers. The standard way to deal with this bias-variance trade-off is by adding a regularization term in the cost function that we use to optimize the model parameters. For example, in the case of Logistic Regression, there exist different regularized versions of the Likelihood function namely, the Ridge and the Lasso methods. Dealing with the bias-variance trade-off, and surfing among different regularization strategies is a key part of any good training process in supervised ML models.

On the other hand, the degree of explainability (or interpretability) of the different existing algorithms has a trade-off with the algorithm complexity. For example, a Logistic Regression has the goodness of being easily interpretable in terms of the weight and importance of the utilized features to build the decision boundary, and at the end of the day, we can learn something about our data after running this multivariate model in terms of what features were more or less relevant for making predictions. Also, the scores that this model produces are directly interpretable as probabilities of belonging to one or other class (benign-pathogenic). In contrast, given the linearity nature of the model (strictly speaking this is a kind of generalized linear model), their predictive power is limited when it is compared with more sophisticated approaches. On the other side, we can think in deep neural networks as a model having a high complexity that usually offers a high predictive power but little about interpretability of the predicted results. Nevertheless, it is worth mentioning that given the demonstrated power in other fields of that kind of model, there is a marked tendency in recent years on the use of Deep Neural Networks as the ML tool by excellence.

2.4.3 Data sources and ground truth for supervised analysis

As expected, the validity and performance of any *in silico* model depends entirely on the nature and quality of the used data source. For example, it is a very hard task to achieve a good generalization behaviour in a model when training data sources are intrinsically biased, or to reach good performance levels when the ground truth is actually built on the basis of noise data, lacking of standardized quality checks or even more if its mined of subjective as well as erroneous classifications. Also the size of these data sets (i.e., the number items that you have classified and characterized) usually will affect the final quality of your model.

For that reason, the starting point of any ML tool is to define the dataset on which the model will be developed. In the case of ML supervised approach, on the selected dataset, variants must be labeled according to this pathogenicity level. A common strategy to deal with this problem is directly to take advantage of publicly available sources like ClinVar database (Landrum et al., 2014), SwissProt (Famiglietti et al., 2014), or even private ones, typically HGMD (Stenson et al., 2003). These databases contain variants labeled with different pathogenicity criteria, that is, for example ClinVar uses the ACMG (Richards et al., 2015), criteria, whereas HGMD adopt an entirely different criteria, based on 6 categories among *Disease Mutations* and *Polymorphisms*, that are not directly interchangeably with the ACMG criteria. Whereas ACMG criteria is designed for minimizing false positives in a clinical setting, HGMD states that their classification system is based *"on the cogency and credibility of the associated literature"*, prioritizing the minimization of false negatives and warning about the chance of finding false positive variants. Also it is worth mentioning that the HGMD database, at the moment of its publication (Stenson et al., 2017) had a 4-fold increment of Disease-Causing Mutations over the number of pathogenic/likely pathogenic variants found in ClinVar.

As a main drawback, ClinVar is mined of misclassified variants, annotations without provided criteria and even more with conflicts of interpretation. Luckily it also has a five-tier

Table 1 Characterization of variant effect prediction tools. This table shows a detailed description of the kind of data, approach and scope used for different algorithms. For those machine learning-based algorithms, a description of the kind of features, training and test data are provided. (+): pathogenic variants; (–): neutral/benign variants. Last columns show the total number of citations of the original work and those obtained since 2016

Algorithm name	Year	Family	Level/unit	Approach	Scope	Features	Training data (n)	Test data	Total cites	Cites since 2014
phasCons	2005	Conservation	DNA	Generative (phylo-HMM)/rate-based	Genome-wide/General	–	–	–	3175	1070
GERP++	2010	Conservation	DNA	Button-up/rate-based	Genome-wide/General	–	–	–	1026	659
SiPhy	2009	Conservation	DNA	Generative (phylo-HMM)/substitution patterns	Genome-wide/General	–	–	–	258	148
phyloP	2006	Conservation	DNA	Generative (phylo-HMM)/rate-based	Genome-wide/General	–	–	–	226	68
MCS	2003	Conservation	DNA	Button-up	Genome-wide/General	–	–	–	388	25
SIFT (Sorting Tolerant From Intolerant)	2009	Function prediction of missense variants	AA	Evolutionary conserved residues, aaMSA	Coding regions				5398	3070
PROVEAN (Protein Variation Effect Analyzer)	2012	Function prediction of missense variants, in-frame insertions and deletions and multiple substitutions	AA	Evolutionary conserved residues, pair-wise alignments	Coding regions				1747	1250

Algorithm name	Year	Family	Level/ unit	Approach	Scope	Features	Training data (n)	Test data	Total cites	Cites since 2014
Polyphen-2 (Polymorphism Phenotyping v2)	2010	Function prediction of missense variants	AA	Evolutionary conserved residues, aaMSA/ Structural	Coding regions				9379	5140
LRT (Likelihood Ratio Test)	2009	Function prediction of missense variants	DNA	Related proteins, aaMSA probabilistic framework	Coding regions				671	417
Mutation Assessor	2011	Function prediction of missense variants	AA	Evolutionary conserved residues	Switch-of-function/ Coding regions/ Cancer		COSMIC		1253	793
fitCons (Fitness Consequence)	2015	Function prediction in a broad sense	DNA RNA-Seq Chip-Seq	Conservation-generative probabilistic model-(INSIGHT; [https://www.ncbi.nlm.nih.gov/pmc/articles/PMC3697874/])	Genome-wide/ General		HUVEC, H1 hESC, and GM12878 (UCS). Array Express, 25–state ChromHMM, [Hoffman MM 2013], etc.		152	131
VEST3 (Variant Effect Scoring Tool)	2013	Function prediction of missense variants	AA	Machine learning, Random Forest	Coding regions		HGMD (+), ESP (−)		204	171
COSSMO (Competitive Splice Site Model)	2018	Function prediction of splicing variants	DNA	Machine learning, Neural Networks	Genes		Gencode v19 (annotations), GTEx (RNA–Seq data)		15	15

Table 1 Contd....

Table 1 Characterization of variant effect prediction tools. This table shows a detailed description of the kind of data, approach and scope used for different algorithms. For those machine learning-based algorithms, a description of the kind of features, training and test data are provided. (+): pathogenic variants; (–): neutral/benign variants. Last columns show the total number of citations of the original work and those obtained since 2016. (Contd....)

Algorithm name	Year	Family	Level/ unit	Approach	Scope	Features	Training data (n)	Test data	Total cites	Cites since 2014
ALoFT (Annotation of Loss-of-Function Transcripts)	2017	Function prediction of pLoF variants	DNA	Machine learning, Random Forest	Genes		HGMD (+), ESP (–), ExAC (–)		16	16
Mutation Taster 2	2014	Function prediction of intragenic variants	DNA	Machine Learning, Bayes classifier.	Intragenic variants	DNA conservation, ENCODE, JASPAR, regulatory features,	Clinvar-HGMD	Clinvar-HGMD	2195	1130
CADD (Combined Annotation Dependent Depletion)	2014	Prediction of deleteriousness	DNA AA	Machine Learning, SVM Linear Kernel	Genome-wide	GERP, phastCons, phyloP, regulatory information like genomic regions of DNase hypersensitivity and transcription factor binding, transcript information like distance to exon-intron boundaries or expression levels in commonly studied cell lines, and protein-level scores like Grantham, SIFT, PolyPhen	Differences between human genomes and the inferred human-chimpanzee ancestral genome where humans carry a derived allele with a frequency of at least 95% for benign variants. Simulated variants from an empirical model of sequence evolution for pathogenic variants.	*De novo* exome variants (SNVs and indels) identified in children with autism spectrum disorders and intellectual disability, ClinVar, GWAS	3381	2910

Algorithm name	Year	Family	Level/ unit	Approach	Scope	Features	Training data (n)	Test data	Total cites	Cites since 2014
DANN (deleterious annotation of genetic variants using neural networks)	2015	Prediction of deleteriousness	DNA AA	Machine Learning, Deep Neural Network	Genome-wide	GERP, phastCons, phyloP, regulatory information like DNase hypersensitivity and transcription factor binding, transcript information like distance to exon-intron boundaries or expression levels in commonly studied cell lines, and protein-level scores like Grantham, SIFT, PolyPhen	Differences between human genomes and the inferred human-chimpanzee ancestral genome where humans carry a derived allele with a frequency of at least 95% for benign variants. Simulated variants from an empirical model of sequence evolution for pathogenic variants.	*De novo* exome variants (SNVs and indels) identified in children with autism spectrum disorders and intellectual disability, ClinVar, GWAS	376	376
Eigen	2016	Prediction of functionality	DNA AA	Machine Learning, Unsupervised spectral approach	Genome-wide	SIFT, PolyPhen, Mutation Assessor, GERP, phyloP, PhastCons, 1000 Genomes project, ENCODE histone modification, transcription factor binding and open chromatin data	dbNSFP (Non-synonimous variants), 1000 Genomes Project (Noncoding and Synonimous Coding Variants)	ClinVar, GWAS, COSMIC, eQTLs, de novo mutations reported in autism, schizophrenia, epileptic encephalopathies and intellectual disability	256	248

Table 1 Contd.....

Table 1 Characterization of variant effect prediction tools. This table shows a detailed description of the kind of data, approach and scope used for different algorithms. For those machine learning-based algorithms, a description of the kind of features, training and test data are provided. (+): pathogenic variants; (−): neutral/benign variants. Last columns show the total number of citations of the original work and those obtained since 2016. (Contd....)

Algorithm name	Year	Family	Level/ unit	Approach	Scope	Features	Training data (n)	Test data	Total cites	Cites since 2014
FATHMM-MKL	2015	Prediction of functional consequences	DNA AA	Machine Learning, Multiple Kernel Learning	Genome-wide	46-Way Sequence Conservation, Histone Modifications (ChIP-Seq), Transcription Factor Binding Sites (TFBS PeakSeq), Open Chromatin (DNase-Seq), 100-Way Sequence Conservation, GC Content, Open Chromatin (FAIRE), Transcription Factor Binding Sites (TFBS SPP), Genome Segmentation, Footprints	HGMD (+), 1000 Genomes Project (−)	HGMD (+), 1000 Genomes Project (−)	286	254
GenoCanyon	2015	Prediction of functionality	DNA	Machine Learning, Unsupervised Statistical Learning	Genome-wide	GERP, phyloP, DNase I (open chromatin), FAIRE (histone modifications), and TFBS (Transcription Factor Binding Sites)	Cis-regulatory Modules in the HBB Gene Complex, ZRS (an enhancer of the SHH gene), Functional Elements in the Human X-inactivation Center, ClinVar	72	70

Algorithm name	Year	Family	Level/ unit	Approach	Scope	Features	Training data (n)	Test data	Total cites	Cites since 2014
M-CAP (Mendelian Clinically Applicable Pathogenicity)	2016	Prediction of pathogenicity of missense variants	DNA AA	Machine Learning, Gradient Boosting Tree	Coding regions	SIFT, PolyPhen-2, CADD, MutationTaster, MutationAssessor, FATHMM, LRT, MetaLR, MetaSVM, RVIS, PhyloP, PhastCons, PAM250, BLOSUM62, SIPHY, GERP	HGMD (+), ExAC (−)	HGMD (+), ExAC (−)	292	284
MetaLR	2015	Prediction of deleteriousness of missense variants	DNA AA	Machine Learning, Support Vector Machine	Coding regions	PolyPhen-2, SIFT, MutationTaster, Mutation Assessor, FATHMM, LRT, PANTHER, PhD-SNP, SNAP, SNPs&GO, MutPred, CADD, PON-P, KGGSeq, CONDEL, GERP++, SiPhy, PhyloP	Uniprot	Variants reported to cause Mendelian diseases from the journal Nature Genetics (+), ARIC study via the CHARGE sequencing project (−), VariBench	477	445
MetaSVM	2015	Prediction of deleteriousness of missense variants	DNA AA	Machine Learning, Logistic Regression	Coding regions	PolyPhen-2, SIFT, MutationTaster, Mutation Assessor, FATHMM, LRT, PANTHER, PhD-SNP, SNAP, SNPs&GO, MutPred, CADD, PON-P, KGGSeq, CONDEL, GERP++, SiPhy, PhyloP	Uniprot	Variants reported to cause Mendelian diseases from the journal Nature Genetics (+), ARIC study via the CHARGE sequencing project (−), VariBench	477	445

Table 1 Contd....

Table 1 Characterization of variant effect prediction tools. This table shows a detailed description of the kind of data, approach and scope used for different algorithms. For those machine learning-based algorithms, a description of the kind of features, training and test data are provided. (+): pathogenic variants; (−): neutral/benign variants. Last columns show the total number of citations of the original work and those obtained since 2016. (Contd....)

Algorithm name	Year	Family	Level/ unit	Approach	Scope	Features	Training data (n)	Test data	Total cites	Cites since 2014
REVEL (Rare Exome Variant Ensemble Learner)	2016	Prediction of pathogenicity of missense variants	DNA AA	Machine Learning, Random Forest	Coding regions	MutPred, FATHMM, VEST, PolyPhen, SIFT, PROVEAN, MutationAssessor, MutationTaster, LRT, GERP, SiPhy, phyloP, and phastCons	HGMD (+), ESP (−), ARIC (−), 1000 Genomes Project (−)	SwissVar (+), ESP (−), ARIC (−), 1000 Genomes Project (−), ClinVar(+/−)	337	321
ClinPred	2018	Prediction of disease-relevant non-synonymous variants	DNA AA	Machine Learning, Random Forest and Gradient Boosting Tree	Coding regions	gnomAD, SIFT, PolyPhen-2 HDIV, PolyPhen-2 HVAR, LRT, MutationAssessor, PROVEAN, CADD, GERP, DANN, PhastCons, fitCons, PhyloP, SiPhy	ClinVar	ClinVar, mutagenetix, DoCM, 31 exome case subjects with rare disease (obtained from the FORGE Canada, Care4Rare Canada Consortia, and collaborators), "A Database of Functional Classifications of BRCA1 Variants based on Saturation Genome Editing"	18	18

confidence criteria (the five starts). Therefore, a database cleaning (that is, retaining only high confidence annotations, removing variants with conflicting interpretations) is advised before you start using it as your ground truth of pathogenic or disease-associated variants for training ML models. On the other hand, the use of HGMD (or any other commercial database) as a source of pathogenic variants is at the expense of reproducibility, since researchers are not allowed to provide the variant identifiers used as a training or evaluation set. Wherever the case, a matching with population frequency databases based in consortium large projects like *gnomAD* (Karczewski et al., 2019) is advisable for discarding false positives (i.e., frequent variants incorrectly labelled as pathogenic ones).

Another key point (but not consensuated among literature) is the selection of variants used as benign class. If you consider the benign and/or likely benign classes reported in ClinVar, you will notice that you were working with a huge proportion of highly frequent polymorphisms. Therefore, you run the risk of training (or evaluating) your prediction model to distinguish between pathogenic (typically infrequent) from high frequent polymorphisms. The bad news is that this is not the most interesting problem to be solved: the interesting and complex dilemma in clinical practice, lies where frequent variants are discarded at the very beginning of the analysis, and thus being able to detect potentially pathogenic variants among benign rare (infrequent) ones.

Among the literature, a major consensus is observed on the use of HGMD as a source of pathogenic variants for training purposes (VEST, FATHMM-MKL, M-CAP, REVEL, ALoFT), only MetaLR/SVM, ClinPred and MPC (Samocha et al., 2017; Qi et al., 2018) were trained with UniProt or ClinVar. On the other hand, no consensus was observed on the determination of benign variants. Whereas some works consider frequent polymorphisms with Allele Frequency greater than 1% (VEST, FATHMM-MKL, MetaLR/SVM), others address the challenge of distinguishing it from rare benign cases (M-CAP and REVEL). In contrast, MetaLR/SVM takes both, rare and common variants as benign in pursuit of a better generalization.

A few additional comments could be said about the used metrics and datasets for performance evaluation. There is a broad consensus that Area Under ROC Curves (AUC_{ROC}) must be used as the way of measuring and comparing algorithms. Nevertheless, since it is a good way of evaluating and comparing algorithms, the reader should remain cautious about interpretation of the reported AUC in literature. The point here is that these performance values were generally evaluated over balanced datasets (i.e., with the same proportions of Benign and Pathogenic variants), rather than across extremely unbalanced sets as we must handle in the clinical practice. For further details on the right way of training and evaluating a model, the reader should refer to VariBench paper (Sarkar et al., 2020).

2.4.4 Methods based on simulated data and unsupervised approaches

A common denominator across all previously mentioned approaches is that they need high quality labeled data to perform the training process. This requirement biases the tools to regions where the variant effect is better understood, namely, the coding regions. This is the reason for which the vast majority of the algorithms based on ML supervised approaches are typically focused on missense variants. Nevertheless, an alternative approach is to build simulated datasets, or mixes between simulated and observed variants to get its plausible pathogenicity condition (i.e., its binary label). Algorithms like CADD and DANN take advantage of this kind of approach to train its predictors (Kircher et al., 2014; Quang et al., 2015). They have the ability to cover broad regions along the genome, i.e., coding, non-coding, splicing sites, regulatory regions, synonymous SNVs, etc. In a similar fashion, unsupervised approaches that essentially do not require a training stage nor labeled data, and are based essentially on different clustering techniques were implemented and also became of broad usage among different genomic regions, like Eigen or GenoCanyon (Ionita-Laza et al., 2016; Lu et al., 2015).

2.4.5 Ensemble models

A well-known and used learning technique in the field of ML is the Ensemble approach. Here, the general idea is to take advantage of multiple predictors to generate a new more powerful one. In the context of variant effect prediction, several tools based on this technique have been developed. These tools take into consideration available predictors as features and ensemble them with some ML model, like Random Forest, XGBoost or any other. One major challenge when you train an Ensemble model, is avoiding a type 1 circularity, i.e., the fact that a set of variants that have been used to train a given feature, will be used to evaluate the Ensemble-based predictor. Such risk is increased by the lack of an exhaustive detail in literature about variant identifiers used to train models (as part of supplementary materials). Authors usually tackle this problem by (i) including all those predictors developed under an unsupervised ML methodology or those models that do not utilize any ML approach) or (ii) limiting the training dataset to variants reported after some specific date.

Another challenge when you train an ensemble method is the data collection process, since you will need all the predictors computed on the same variant set. The feature normalization could also be a critical step, depending on the algorithm you apply to the ensemble. For example, if you use a Logistic Regression as a meta-predictor, keeping features in comparable scales is mandatory. On the other hand, if you adopt a tree-based method, the results would be invariant regarding the feature scales, and a renormalization process becomes unnecessary.

Since 2011, Boerwinkle et al. have developed and maintained dbNSFP, an invaluable database of missense variant characterization. This integrative database contains not only the results of more than 29 predictors for more than 87×10^6 missense and splice variants, but also their allele frequency along multiple projects, as well as ClinVar and OMIM identifiers, among others. Moreover, each predictor contains its raw data value score as well as a normalized version which facilitates the feature integration and building of new Ensemble models. As a huge depository of an unimaginable amount of biological, algorithmical and genetical data, this makes dbNSFP an invaluable tool for his application on the variant effect prediction research field and the clinical exome routine.

As a closing remark, it is worth mentioning that while there are multiple machine learning-based tools for variant effect prediction, there are also significant overlaps in the basic principles they use. The reader must be familiar with those principles, the features and strategies applied for each algorithm. First, the idea is to avoid an overestimation of importance when several predictors, redundant in their principles, coincide in the level of pathogenicity (or score) assigned to a variant. Second, understanding the principles on which each predictor is based, allows for better interpretation of discordant predictions between models based on different principles. In other words, taking into account the level of redundancy among different predictors helps to have a better interpretation of these *in silico* results.

3 DISCUSSION

3.1 Overall Comparison of the Presented Methods

So far we have presented the basic ideas behind bioinformatic algorithms for variant effect prediction. There exists a broad and diverse spectrum of approaches in literature, from algorithms analyzing sequence of amino acid conservation, to those employing complex data mining techniques for elucidating functional consequences, or their putative damaging effect (Table 1). Although it is very difficult to perform an exhaustive comparison (for the problems already mentioned above), we can easily look at their popularity. According to the total number of citations and its age, the most popular used algorithms were Polyphen-2 (9379 cites from

2010), SIFT (5398 cites from 2009), PhastCons (3175 cites from 2005) and CADD (3381 cites from 2014). Interestingly, the big amount of citations of CADD far exceeds the citation scores in even older publications. Its great impact could be attributed perhaps to the fact that this work was one of the first algorithms in applying powerful Machine Learning techniques, as well as for doing it in a broad purpose sense (it is suitable for estimating deleteriousness of coding, non-coding, splice sites, intronic or intergenic variants). All this despite its pathogenic variants being simulated from an empirical model of sequence evolution, a very original and unique way of approaching the subject among its peers.

Another interesting observation derived from Table 1 is that there is a major predominance of predictors working over missense (SAS producing) variants. Despite non-synonymous substitutions being one of the most frequent causes of cancer and Mendelian genetic disease, and therefore one of the most studied targets among these algorithms, we must realize that other events could be responsible for patients' phenotype, as splice site or premature stop-causing variants. For this reason we shall highlight the usefulness of approaches designed for a broad-spectrum scope like those based on genomic conservation, or specific algorithms like fitCons, CADD, DANN, EIGEN, FATHMM-MKL and GenoCanyon.

Also interesting to highlight are those algorithms that take advantage of integrative methodologies, incorporating not only information about DNA changes, but also post-traductional consequences or transcriptional profiles based on RNA-Seq data. This is the case of COSSMO, an algorithm that having genome annotations and large-scale RNA-Seq datasets as input, manages to capture the competence existing between splice sites, which can be extended to predict in the field how genomic variation affects splice site choice through mechanisms like splice site variants or cryptic splice site activation (Bretschneider et. al, 2018). Another recent example is represented by ALoFT, which intends to model the impact of putative loss of function (pLoF) variants, including within this group stop-causing single nucleotide polymorphisms (SNPs), frameshift-causing indels and variants affecting canonical splice sites. This kind of variants implying the loss of many times long protein segments requires significant attention on issues as cigosity, allele frequency and conservation in the really hard job of determining the potential phenotypic effect of novel variants, as many of them promote disease development not only on a recessive model of inheritance, but also in a dominant one. This implies not only training algorithms with large datasets, including numerous features (ALoFT includes 108 features), but also incurring in some cases in utilizing the output of other predictors as GERP to approach specific problems, such as evolutionary conservation.

3.2 Performance Comparison

Although performing an exhaustive comparison of all methods performance is out of the scope of the present work [for this purpose see reviews (Li et al., 2018; Zeng and Bromberg 2019) we performed a preliminary analysis by comparing the results—mainly AUCs of the ROC curves—presented by different authors (Table 2). We prioritized those results that came from ROC curves determined by using datasets built from well-known and commonly used variant databases. Not surprisingly, in all cases the algorithm presented in the corresponding work is top-ranked, the best in many of them, as shown by red and yellow cells in Table 2. However, cross-confirmation in other works, where two algorithms are presented as other methods for comparison purposes, usually shows a different result. The reason behind this observation, could be an inherent bias towards type 1 circularity when the authors test their algorithm against other alternatives. Another source of biasis a better tuning of each algorithm parameters by its authors compared to those used for alternative methods, which are usually set as defaults.

This observation leads us to conclude that in order to select good performing algorithms, we should look not for those being the best in any particular study, but for those showing

Table 2 Performance comparison table. Cells depict the ranking according to AUC metric reported in each paper (columns). Papers which do not utilize AUC metrics were disgarder. Red cells represent cases where testing revealed its own algorithm as first-ranked, while yellow ones represent the same but for second place. Mean ranking is computed taking into consideration all values reported. Mean ranking (2) is computed in the same way but excluding red and yellow cells to avoid self-over appreciation.

Algorithm name	CADD	Eigen	FATHMM-MKL	M-CAP	MetaLR/SVM	REVEL	Clin-Pred	PROVEAN	VEST3	Jinchen Li 2018	Zishuo Zeng 2019	Mean ranking	Mean ranking (2)
CADD	1	3	2	6	4	5	8			3	1	3.67	4.00
DANN						6				14	2	7.33	7.33
Eigen		2		3		4	9			5		4.60	5.25
FATHMM-MKL			1		3		11			12	3	6.00	7.25
M-CAP				1			3			13		5.67	8.00
MetaLR				2	1	2	5			4		2.80	3.25
MetaSVM					2	3	6			9		5.00	6.00
REVEL					1	1	2			2		1.67	2.00
ClinPred							1					1.00	No comparison
SIFT Sorting Tolerant From Intolerant	2			4	9		10	1	3	7		5.14	5.14
PROVEAN Protein Variation Effect Analyzer							7	2		8		5.67	7.50
Polyphen-2 Polymorphism Phenotyping v2	3	1		5	6		12	3	2	6		4.75	4.75
MutationAssessor					5			2		10		5.67	5.67
VEST Variant Effect Scoring Tool							4		1	1		2.00	2.50
GERP++	4				8					16		9.33	9.33
phasCons	5									15		10.00	10.00
phyloP	6				10					11		9.00	9.00
SiPhy					7					14		10.50	10.50

consistently good performance over time in different studies (e.g., being always on top 3). As deduced from Table 2, we could cite as examples Revel, Vest3, Polyphen-2, CADD or Eigen, which performance has been shown to be consistent across studies and generally well-ranked, even when setting aside their own self-consideration. It is also important to mention that even if an algorithm performs extremely well for a given test set, it does not guarantee that its performance will be the same in a real world scenario (i.e., clinical practice).

3.3 Variant Effect Interpretation

In this final section we want to go back to the use of variant effect predictors in the context of the clinical practice. As was pointed out in the Introduction, the first step in the clinical interpretation process is the functional annotation of the variant profile (usually in a VCF format). This annotation includes different layers of information for each detected variant, including frequency across different populations, functional, structural and physicochemical features, as well as protein family specific annotations. Additionally, it is usual to include the *in-silico* predictions of several variant effect predictors. Several widely used variant annotation software (and pipelines) such as VEP (McLaren et al., 2016), SNPEFF/SnpSift (Cingolani et al., 2012) and ANNOVAR (Wang et al., 2010) include in their annotations several predictive methods. However, the integration of this information in the clinical practice is far from straightforward.

The first problem is how to properly scoreaccording to ACMG criteria the results of the variant effect predictors. ACMG PP3 criteria reads "Multiple lines of computational evidence support a deleterious effect on the gene or gene product (conservation, evolutionary, splicing impact, etc.)", while BP4 reads "Multiple lines of computational evidence suggest no impact on gene or gene product". The problem lies in what we interpret by the word multiple and the fact that despite some cases, where a predictor is not needed, methods may differ in their prediction. Usually, 4–5 different methods are used and if all predict the variant as pathogenic, then the variant is assigned PP3, while if all predict is benign, it is assigned BP4. The problem arises when the results are contradictory. Moreover, the multiple lines should be based on different approaches (or underlying theories) but as methods become more complex and incorporate in the prediction several lines of evidence, or are ML methods trained on the same (or similar) variant sets, or are meta-predictors based on the same methods, how can the multiple lines be taken as independent?

In this context, we believe that correct assignment of a variant as PP3 (pathogenic) or BP4 (bening) based on computational prediction, requires a careful analysis of why the "different" predictors have reached their corresponding verdict. In other words, what are the reasons that justify a given variant pathogenic or benign prediction and how can we rationalize it. With this idea in mind, we recently developed a novel tool named VarQ (Radusky et al., 2018), which incorporates detailed information related to a variant effect on protein function (conservation, structural impact, frequency, presence in active and/or protein-protein interaction sites etc.) and presents the result in a user-friendly manner, that allows the researcher to analyze the information and judge the variant as either pathogenic or benign. In this sense, the aim of VarQ is not to predict whether a variant is pathogenic/benign but to provide healthcare professionals with a tool they might use to understand why "different" predictors assigned the variant in either category.

4 FINAL REMARK

As a final remark, we go back to some important warnings that the reader must always keep in mind. Almost all methods discussed in this review were designed for research purposes, and not for the direct application into clinical practice. Nevertheless, they can be used not only as an ACMG scoring evidence level, but also as a filter for selecting those variants more likely to be pathogenic and thus merit deeper analysis. In other words, these tools are very powerful to assist in the arduous task of prioritizing and sorting a long list of variants in a large panel, whole exome or whole genome context, where Uncertain Significant Variants are usually predominant.

Given the enormous amount of available algorithms and its growing tendency, it is not a trivial task to select one (or a few) for its regular use in clinical practice. In this review, we are not favoring this or that method, although some general guidelines are given in Table 1 and along the work. A few good rules of thumb are: (i) use what you know well, or if you don't know any, learn about the one you are going to use; (ii) use what your colleagues use (so you can consult and compare results), (iii) Try to understand why a given variant is predicted to be pathogenic/benign, and if you cannot rationalize it, do not trust the prediction.

REFERENCES

Adzhubei, I.A., S. Schmidt, L. Peshkin, V.E. Ramensky, A. Gerasimova, P. Bork, et al. (2010). A method and server for predicting damaging missense mutations. Nat. Methods. 7: 248–249.

Bretschneider, H., S. Gandhi, A.G. Deshwar, K. Zuberi and B.J. Frey (2018). COSSMO: Predicting competitive alternative splice site selection using deep learning. Bioinformatics. 34: i429–i437. doi:10.1093/bioinformatics/bty244.

Choi, Y., G.E. Sims, S. Murphy, J.R. Miller and A.P. Chan (2012). Predicting the functional effect of amino acid substitutions and indels. PLoS One. 7: e46688.

Chun, S. and J.C. Fay (2009). Identification of deleterious mutations within three human genomes. Genome Res. 19: 1553–1561.

Cingolani, P., A. Platts, L.L. Wang, M. Coon, T. Nguyen, L. Wang, et al. (2012). A program for annotating and predicting the effects of single nucleotide polymorphisms, SnpEff: SNPs in the genome of Drosophila melanogaster strain w1118; iso-2; iso-3. Fly. 6: 80–92.

Consortium, M.G.S. (2002). Mouse genome sequencing consortium. Initial sequencing and comparative analysis of the mouse genome. Nature. 420: 520–562. doi:10.1038/nature01262.

Davydov, E.V., D.L. Goode, M. Sirota, G.M. Cooper, A. Sidow and S. Batzoglou (2010). Identifying a high fraction of the human genome to be under selective constraint using GERP++. PLoS Comput Biol. 6: e1001025.

Famiglietti, M.L., A. Estreicher, A. Gos, J. Bolleman, S. Géhant, L. Breuza, et al. (2014). Genetic variations and diseases in UniProtKB/Swiss-Prot: the ins and outs of expert manual curation. Hum Mutat. 35: 927–935.

Garber, M., M. Guttman, M. Clamp, M.C. Zody, N. Friedman and X. Xie (2009). Identifying novel constrained elements by exploiting biased substitution patterns. Bioinformatics. 25: i54–i62.

Grimm, D.G., C.A. Azencott, F. Aicheler, U. Gieraths, D.G. MacArthur, K.E. Samocha, et al. (2015). The evaluation of tools used to predict the impact of missense variants is hindered by two types of circularity. Hum Mutat. 36: 513–523.

Gulko, B., M.J. Hubisz, I. Gronau and A. Siepel (2015). A method for calculating probabilities of fitness consequences for point mutations across the human genome. Nat. Genet. 47: 276–283.

Ionita-Laza, I., K. McCallum, B. Xu and J.D. Buxbaum (2016). A spectral approach integrating functional genomic annotations for coding and noncoding variants. Nat. Genet. 48: 214–220.

Karczewski, K.J., L.C. Francioli, G. Tiao, B.B. Cummings, J. Alföldi, Q. Wang, et al. (2019). The mutational constraint spectrum quantified from variation in 141,456 humans. Genomics. bioRxiv. 806.

Kircher, M., D.M. Witten, P. Jain, B.J. O'Roak, G.M. Cooper and J. Shendure (2014). A general framework for estimating the relative pathogenicity of human genetic variants. Nat. Genet. 46: 310–315.

Kumar, P., S. Henikoff and P.C. Ng (2009). Predicting the effects of coding non-synonymous variants on protein function using the SIFT algorithm. Nat. Protoc. 4: 1073–1081.

Landrum, M.J., J.M. Lee, G.R. Riley, W. Jang, W.S. Rubinstein, D.M. Church, et al. (2014). ClinVar: Public archive of relationships among sequence variation and human phenotype. Nucleic Acids Res. 42: D980–D985.

Li, J., T. Zhao, Y. Zhang, K. Zhang, L. Shi, Y. Chen, et al. (2018). Performance evaluation of pathogenicity-computation methods for missense variants. Nucleic Acids Res. 46: 7793–7804.

Lu, Q., Y. Hu, J. Sun, Y. Cheng, K.-H. Cheung and H. Zhao (2015). A statistical framework to predict functional non-coding regions in the human genome through integrated analysis of annotation data. bioRxiv 018093; doi: https://doi.org/10.1101/018093.

Margulies, E.H. and M. Blanchette, NISC Comparative Sequencing Program; D. Haussler and E.D. Green (2003). Identification and characterization of multi-species conserved sequences. Genome Res. 13: 2507–2518.

McLaren, W., L. Gil, S.E. Hunt, H.S. Riat, G.R.S. Ritchie, A. Thormann, et al. (2016). The ensembl variant effect predictor. Genome Biol. 17: 122.

Qi, H., C. Chen, H. Zhang, J.J. Long, W.K. Chung and Y. Guan, et al. (2018). MVP: Predicting pathogenicity of missense variants by deep learning. bioRxiv 259390. doi: https://doi.org/10.1101/259390.

Quang, D., Y. Chen and X. Xie (2015). DANN: A deep learning approach for annotating the pathogenicity of genetic variants. Bioinformatics. 31: 761–763. doi:10.1093/bioinformatics/btu703.

Radusky, L., C. Modenutti, J. Delgado, J.P. Bustamante, S. Vishnopolska, C. Kiel, et al. (2018). VarQ: A Tool for the Structural and Functional Analysis of Human Protein Variants. Front Genet. 9: 620.

Richards, S., N. Aziz, S. Bale, D. Bick, S. Das, J. Gastier-Foster, et al. (2015). Standards and guidelines for the interpretation of sequence variants: A joint consensus recommendation of the American College of Medical Genetics and Genomics and the Association for Molecular Pathology. Genet. Med. 17: 405–424.

Samocha, K.E., J.A. Kosmicki, K.J. Karczewski, A.H. O'Donnell-Luria, E. Pierce-Hoffman, D.G. MacArthur, et al. (2017). Regional missense constraint improves variant deleteriousness prediction. bioRxiv 148353; doi: https://doi.org/10.1101/148353.

Sarkar, A., Y. Yang and M. Vihinen (2020). Variation benchmark datasets: Update, criteria, quality and applications. Database. 2020. doi: 10.1093/database/baz117.

Siepel, A., G. Bejerano, J.S. Pedersen, A.S. Hinrichs, M. Hou, K. Rosenbloom, et al. (2005). Evutionarily conserved elements in vertebrate, insect, worm, and yeast genomes. Genome Res. 15: 1034–1050.

Siepel, A., K.S. Pollard and D. Haussler (2006). New methods for detecting lineage-specific selection. pp. 190–205. *In*: A. Apostolico, C. Guerra, S. Istrail, P.A. Pevzner and M. Waterman (eds). Research in Computational Molecular Biology. RECOMB 2006. Lecture Notes in Computer Science, vol 3909. Springer, Berlin, Heidelberg. https://doi.org/10.1007/11732990_17.

Stenson, P.D., E.V. Ball, M. Mort, A.D. Phillips, J.A. Shiel, N.S.T. Thomas, et al. (2003). Human Gene Mutation Database (HGMD): 2003 update. Hum. Mutat. 21: 577–581.

Stenson, P.D., M. Mort, E.V. Ball, K. Evans, M. Hayden, S. Heywood, et al. (2017). The Human Gene Mutation Database: towards a comprehensive repository of inherited mutation data for medical research, genetic diagnosis and next-generation sequencing studies. Hum Genet. 136: 665–677.

Wang, K., M. Li and H. Hakonarson (2010). ANNOVAR: Functional annotation of genetic variants from high-throughput sequencing data. Nucleic Acids Res. 38: e164.

Zeng, Z. and Y. Bromberg (2019). Predicting functional effects of synonymous variants: A systematic review and perspectives. Front Genet. 10: 914.

CHAPTER 9

Bioinformatics of Genome-wide DNA Methylation Studies

Neeti Sharma* and Anshika N. Singh

School of Engineering, Ajeenkya DY Patil University (ADYPU)
Charholi Budruk, Pune 412105

1 BACKGROUND

The initiation and progression of several diseases, including cancer, is usually the consequence of both genetic and epigenetic aberrations. The term 'Epigenetics' coined by Waddington can be defined as the study of both mitotic and meiotic changes in gene functions that are heritable in nature without any changes in the DNA sequence. Epigenetics deals with the encoding of genetic information in the DNA and also the packaging of DNA inside the nucleus and consequently gene expression. The mechanisms of epigenetics can be studied under (i) DNA methylation, (ii) modifications in histone proteins and (iii) binding of non-histone proteins (Chen et al., 2014).

1.1 DNA Methylation

One of the most important and frequently reported epigenetic deregulation is DNA methylation in the promoter region of genes. The event of DNA methylation occurs at the cytosine base of DNA, which then gets converted into 5-Methylcytosine (5mC), facilitated by the DNA methyltransferase enzymes (Fig. 1). 5-mC has been identified to be essential for mammalian development and was first recognized to serve as an epigenetic marker in the 1970s. Previously, 5-Methylcytosine was thought to exist primarily in the CpG nucleotides, however, recently the presence of 5-mC has been observed in CpNpG (N: A, T or C) islands in human tissues also. CpG islands are approximately 200 bp—several kB in length and are richer in GC%. The islands are located in the promoter regions of genes and are scattered all over the human genome (Chen et al., 2014; Lee et al., 2010).

---

*Corresponding author: *neetimohan27@gmail.com*

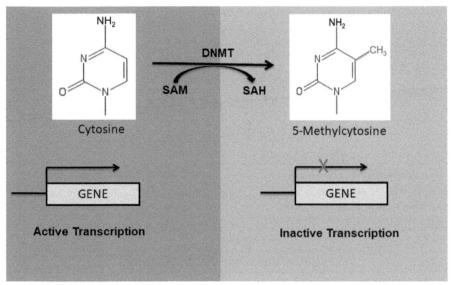

Figure 1 Effect of DNA methylation on gene transcription (Adapted from Zhong et al., 2016).

In diseases such as neurodegenerative disorders, cardiovascular diseases, and cancers, several CpG islands exhibit differential methylation patterns in the form of hypomethylation or hypermethylation often resulting in gene silencing or overexpression. Similar patterns of aberrant methylation pattern in promoters of deregulated tumor suppressor genes and overexpressed oncogenes have often been observed in tumor tissues thereby suggesting that epigenetic alterations in the form of DNA methylation are an indication of significant association of differential methylation of these genes with initiation and progression of diseases like cancer (Chen et al., 2014; Lee et al., 2010; Zhong et al., 2016)

Based on the research expanding for several decades we have acquired vast knowledge about the impact of epigenetic alterations in the etiology of different diseases. However, there are several aspects associated with the analysis of epigenetic alterations that still present potential problems. For example, first, the tissue from which DNA is extracted for methylation analysis is representative of the nature of the disease and hence may influence the analytical methods being used for analysis. Second, depending on the variation in the disease nature, the analysis will have to be genome-wide or region-specific. Epigenetic variations among cases are also observed in several diseases including cancer (Watanbe and Maekawa, 2018).

With the advancement in technology, several of these epigenetic issues have been resolved to some extent, however, need of the hour demands for more high throughput research to achieve better results during analysis. Various international projects have been initiated to meet such issues such as Epigenomics NCI browser, The Cancer Genome Project, the NIH Roadmap Epigenomics Program, the ENCODE project, and the AHEAD project. Such databases provide detailed epigenetic maps, which will provide more insight during basic and applied research and enabling more promising epigenetic biomarkers (Watanbe and Maekawa, 2018)

This chapter aims to review relevant computational tools and databases available for analysis and interpretation of DNA methylation data. The first section discusses various technologies available for retrieving DNA methylation data from samples. In the next section, we have focused on essential steps and tools available for processing of the data and also for quality control of the methylation data. This section also highlights tools involved in the transformation of raw DNA methylation sequencing data into accurate methylation-specific maps. The third section sheds light on the computational tools available for visualization of DNA methylation data and also for statistical calculations for the identification of sample-specific methylation data. Lastly, we have summarized computational tools available for the interpretation of methylation data into a wider biological context. The chapter is based on a typical DNA methylation mapping workflow as shown in Fig. 2 and the list of relevant tools and databases have been described in Table 1.

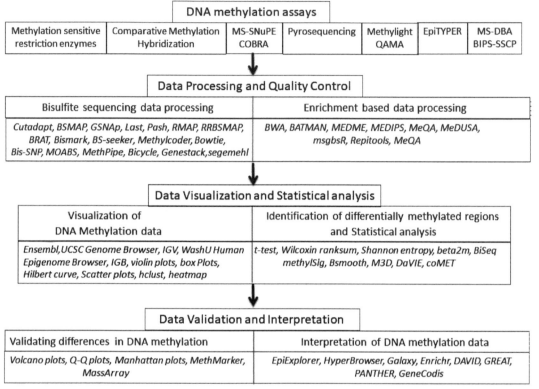

Figure 2 Workflow for DNA methylation whole-genome sequencing analysis.

1.2   DNA Methylation Analysis

The advancement in technology has led to the evolution of several techniques for DNA methylation analysis wherein initially the analysis was limited to be loci-specific. However, nowadays analysis on a genome-wide scale for characterization of entire methylome with the single base-pair resolution is possible, although the availability of several techniques leads to the researcher's challenge to decide the best technique for the best experimental results (Ongenaerta, 2010).

1.2.1   Methylation-sensitive restriction enzymes (MSREs)

The requirement for this technique involves high molecular weight DNA for identification of the methylation status of cytosine residues in the sequence and is limited according to the target of the methylation-sensitive restriction enzyme. These MSREs are unable to cleave methylated cytosine residues and hence the methylated DNA remains intact. Although using enzymes that are sensitive to CpG sites is a low-resolution technique, but it has proven to be very useful when used in combination with genomic microarrays (Hashimoto, 2007).

1.2.2   Bisulfite conversion

This the most widely used "gold standard" technique for the identification of methylation sites at single pair residues. In bisulfite conversion, the genomic DNA is denatured and then treated

Table 1 Tools and databases for DNA methylation analysis

Name	Description	Hyperlink	Reference
Bisulfite sequencing data processing			
Cutadapt	Cutadapt allows users to locate and removes adapter sequences, primers, poly-A tails from sequencing data.	https://cutadapt.readthedocs.io/en/stable/installation.html	Martin, 2011
BSMAP	BSMAP is a whole genome bisulfite whole-genome mapping program.	http://code.google.com/p/bsmap/	Xi and Li, 2009
GSNAp	Genomic Short-read Nucleotide Alignment Program can be used for alignment of bisulfite sequencing data.	http://research-pub.gene.com/gmap/src/gmap-gsnap-2020-03-12.tar.gz	Wu and Nacu, 2010
Last	LAST can be used for alignment of reads from bisulfite-converted DNA to a genome.	http://last.cbrc.jp/doc/bisulfite.html	Shreshta and Frith, 2013
Pash	PASH enables users to read, map and perform integrative analysis of genomic and epigenomic variation using massively parallel DNA sequencing.	http://www.brl.bcm.tmc.edu/pash/pashDownload.rhtml	Coarfa et al., 2010
WALT	The Wildcard ALignment Tool (WALT) allows fast and accurate mapping of bisulfite sequencing reads.	https://github.com/smithlabcode/walt	Chen et al., 2016b
RRBSMAP	RRBSMAP, a version of BSMAP can be used on reduced representation bisulfite sequencing (RRBS) data.	http://rrbsmap.computational-epigenetics.org/	Xi et al., 2012
segemehl	Segemehl is a mapping tool that can be used on short sequencer reads to map with reference genomes.	https://www.bioinf.uni-leipzig.de/Software/segemehl/	Hoffman et al., 2009
BRAT	BRAT can be specifically use to map short bisulfite-treated reads retrieved from from the Solexa-Illumina Genome Analyzer.	http://compbio.cs.ucr.edu/brat/downloads/index.html	Harris et al., 2016
Bismark	BISMARK enables mapping of bisulfite converted sequence reads and also determination of cytosine methylation states.	https://www.bioinformatics.babraham.ac.uk/projects/bismark/	Krueger and Andrews, 2011
BS-Seeker	BS-SEEKER is another mapping tool for bisulfite sequencing data.	https://github.com/khuang28jhu/bs3/	Huang et al., 2018
Methylcoder	Methylcoder uses bisulfite-treated reads as inputs and returns per-base methylation data information.	https://github.com/brentp/methylcode/	Pederson, 2011
Bowtie	BOWTIE has been developed as an ultrafast, short read aligner which can align short DNA sequences (reads) to the human genome at a rate of over 25 million 35-bp reads per hour.	http://bowtie-bio.sourceforge.net/index.shtml	Langmead et al., 2009
Bis-SNP	Bis-SNP can combine DNA methylation and SNP calling on Bisulfite-sequencing data.	http://people.csail.mit.edu/dnaase/bissnp2011/	Liu et al., 2012

Table 1 Contd....

Table 1 Tools and databases for DNA methylation analysis (Contd....)

Name	Description	Hyperlink	Reference
	Enrichment based data processing		
BWA	The Burrows-Wheeler Aligner (BWA) can be used to map low-divergent sequences against a large reference genome.	http://bio-bwa.sourceforge.net	Li and Durbin, 2009
BATMAN	This bayesian tool for methylation analysis has been developed as a statistical tool for analysis of MeDIP profiles.	http://td-blade.gurdon.cam.ac.uk/software/batman/	Down et al., 2008
MEDME	MEDME can be used to estimate DNA methylation levels specifically from microarray derived MeDIP-enrichment data.	http://bioconductor.org/packages/release/bioc/manuals/MEDME/man/MEDME.pdf	Pelizzola et al., 2008
MEDIPS	MEDIPS can be used for analysis of sequences obtained from MeDIP sequencing experiments.	https://bioconductor.org/packages/release/bioc/html/MEDIPS.html	Lienhard et al., 2014
MeQA	MeQA can be used for analysis and quality assessment for MeDIP-seq data.	http://life.tongji.edu.cn/meqa/	Huang et al., 2012
MeDUSA	MeDUSA allows sequence alignment, quality control (QC), and determination and annotation of DMRs in MeDIP sequencing data.	https://www.ucl.ac.uk/cancer/research/department-cancer-biology/medical-genomics/medical-genomics-past-projects/medusa/medusa	Wilson et al., 2012
msgbsR	msgbsR is an R package to analyze methylation sensitive genotyping by sequencing (MS-GBS).	https://www.bioconductor.org/packages/release/bioc/html/msgbsR.html	Mayne et al., 2018
Repitools	Repitools can be used to summarize and visualize epigenomic data across promoters, identify DMRs and also for methylation quantification.	https://www.bioconductor.org/packages/release/bioc/html/Repitools.html	Statham et al., 2010
	Data visualization tools		
UCSC Genome Browser	USCS Genome Browser is an interactive website that offers access to genome sequence data and is also integrated with several aligned annotations.	https://genome.ucsc.edu	Fujita et al., 2010
Ensembl	Ensembl is a genome browser for gene annotations, multiple alignments, also prediction of regulatory functions.	https://asia.ensembl.org/index.html	Fernández and Birney, 2010
WashU Human Epigenome Browser	The WashU Human Epigenome Browser can be used for visualizing and interacting with whole-genome datasets.	http://epigenomegateway.wustl.edu/info/	Zhou et al., 2011
IGV	The Integrative Genomics Viewer is a visualization tool for interactive exploration of genomic datasets.	http://software.broadinstitute.org/software/igv	Thorvaldsdóttir et al., 2013

Name	Description	Hyperlink	Reference
IGB	The Integrated Genome Browser can be used for visualization and exploration of large genomic datasets.	https://bioviz.org	Nicol et al., 2009
Hclust	Hclust allows hierarchical cluster analysis on genomic datasets.	https://uc-r.github.io/hc_clustering	Oksanen, 2014
Heatmap3	Heatmap3 is an R package that enables users for clustering and developing heat maps.	https://github.com/slzhao/heatmap3	Zhao et al., 2014
Statistical analysis tools			
Q-value	The Q-value is an R-package that can be used for estimation of false discovery rates.	https://www.bioconductor.org/packages/release/bioc/html/qvalue.html	Dabney et al., 2010
BSmooth	BSmooth can be employed for alignment, quality control and analysis of methylation data even in cases of low coverage data.	https://www.bioconductor.org/packages/release/bioc/html/bsseq.html	Hansen et al., 2012
methylSig	methylSig is a package for analysis of whole-genome bisulfite sequencing (bis-seq), reduced representation bisulfite sequencing (RRBS), or enhanced RRBS experiments and also for identification of DMRs.	https://github.com/sartorlab/methylSig	Park et al., 2014
BiSeq	BiSeq allows detection of DMRs in targeted bisulfite sequencing (BS) data.	https://www.bioconductor.org/packages/release/bioc/html/BiSeq.html	Hebestreit et al., 2013
MethylPipe	MethylPipe is a memory efficient tool for base resolution of DNA methylation data.	http://bioconductor.org/packages/release/bioc/html/methylPipe.html	Kishore et al., 2015
MethMarker	MethMarker can be used for design and optimization of gene-specific DNA methylation assays.	https://methmarker.mpi-inf.mpg.de	Schüffler et al., 2009
MassArray	MassArray enables users to import, perform quality control, analyze and visualize methylation data retrieved from Sequenom's MassArray platform.	https://bioconductor.org/packages/release/bioc/html/MassArray.html	Thompson and Greally, 2019
Tools for Interpretation of DNA methylation data			
EpiExplorer	EpiExplorer allows global analysis of large epigenomic datasets.	http://epiexplorer.mpi-inf.mpg.de	Halachev et al., 2012
HyperBrowser	HyperBrowser allows users to analyze large collection of genomic datasets.	http://hyperbrowser.uio.no	Sandve et al., 2013
Galaxy	Galaxy is a Web-based tool for analysis of genome wide datasets.	http://g2.bx.psu.edu	Giardine et al., 2005
Enrichr	Enrichr is an interactive web tool for enrichment analysis.	http://amp.pharm.mssm.edu/Enrichr	Kuleshov et al., 2016
DAVID	The Database for Annotation, Visualization and Integrated Discovery (DAVID) is widely used tool for functional annotation of large list of genes.	https://david.ncifcrf.gov	Dennis et al., 2003

Table 1 Contd....

Table 1 Tools and databases for DNA methylation analysis (Contd....)

Name	Description	Hyperlink	Reference
PANTHER	The PANTHER (Protein ANalysis THrough Evolutionary Relationships) Classification System can classify proteins (and their respective genes) in several biological and functional annotations.	http://pantherdb.org/about.jsp	Mi et al., 2017
GeneCodis	GeneCodis is another web-based tool for developed for identifying significant concurrent annotations in large gene sets.	https://genecodis.genyo.es	Nogales-Cadenas et al., 2009
GREAT	The Genomic Regions Enrichment of Annotations Tool (GREAT) can be used for analysis of functional significance of cis-regulatory regions identified by localized measurements of DNA binding events across an entire genome.	http://great.stanford.edu/public/html/	McLean et al., 2010
GBSA	The Genome Bisulfite Sequencing Analyser (GBSA) is an open-source software for analysis of bisulfite sequencing data.	https://bioinfo-csi.nus.edu.sg/gbsa/	Benoukraf et al., 2013
MOABS	The MOdel based Analysis of Bisulfite Sequencing data allows users to analyze large-scale base-resolution DNA methylation data.	https://github.com/sunnyisgalaxy/moabs	Sun et al, 2014
methpipe	methpipe is a tool used for analysis of bisulfite sequencing data (WGBS and RRBS).	http://smithlabresearch.org/software/methpipe/	Song et al., 2013
Bicycle	The BICYCLE (bisulfite-based methylcytosine caller) is another NGS pipeline used for analysis of whole genome bisulfite sequencing data.	https://www.sing-group.org/bicycle/index.html	Graña et al., 2018
Genestack	Genestack can be used to manage, process and visualize biological data especially NGS and bisulfite sequencing data.	https://www.genestack.com	Genestack, 2020
Tools for CpG Islands detection			
CpGIS	The CpG island searcher is based on Gardiner-Garden and Frommer (GGF) principle for CpG island identification.	http://www.cpgislands.com	Takai and Jones, 2003
CpGProD	CpGProD can be used for prediction of promoters associated with CpG islands (CGIs) in mammalian genomic sequences.	http://doua.prabi.fr/software/cpgprod	Ponger and Mouchiroud, 2002
CpGIF	CpGIF's is another tool for prediction of CpG islands (CGIs) in DNA sequences.	http://www.usd.edu/~sye/cpgisland/CpGIF.htm.	Sujuan et al., 2008
CpG_MPs	CpG_MPs allows identification of CpG methylation patterns of genomic regions from bisulfite sequencing data.	http://bioinfo.hrbmu.edu.cn/CpG_MPs	Su et al., 2013
WordCluster	WordCluster can detect clusters of DNA words and genomic elements in large sets of genomic data.	https://bioinfo2.ugr.es/ceUGR/wordcluster/	Hackenberg et al., 2011

Name	Description	Hyperlink	Reference
CpG_MI	The CpG_MIs can be used for identification of functional CpG islands in mammalian genomes.	http://bioinfo.hrbmu.edu.cn/cpgmi/	Su et al., 2010
CpGCluster	The CpGCluster is developed on a distance based algorithm for CpG-island detection.	http://bioinfo2.ugr.es/CpGcluster	Hackenberg et al., 2006
GenomicRange	GenomicRange is widely used for genomic annotations and alignments of genomic datasets.	https://bioconductor.org/packages/release/bioc/html/GenomicRanges.html	Aboyoun et al., 2010
GenomicFeature	GenomicFeatures can be used for computing and analyzing transcript centric annotations.	https://bioconductor.org/packages/release/bioc/html/GenomicFeatures.html	Lawrence et al., 2013
Genomation	Genomation is a widely employed toolkit package that enables users to summarize, annotate and view genomic data.	https://www.bioconductor.org/packages/release/bioc/html/genomation.html	Akalin et al., 2015
Bioconductor packages for DNA methylation analysis			
Bsseq	Bsseq can be used for analysis, management and storage of bisulfite sequencing data.	https://www.bioconductor.org/packages/release/bioc/html/bsseq.html	Hansen et al., 2012
M3D	M3D is kernel-based test for identification of spatially correlated changes in methylation profiles.	http://www.bioconductor.org/packages/release/bioc/html/M3D.html	Mayo et al., 2015
DMAP	DMAP is a differential methylation analysis package designed for analysis of RRBS and WGBS data.	http://biochem.otago.ac.nz/research/databases-software/	Stockwell et al., 2014
DMRcate	DMRcate is a bioconductor package for identification of DMRs in Methylation array and also sequencing spatial analysis.	https://bioconductor.org/packages/release/bioc/html/DMRcate.html	Peters et al., 2015
RnBeads	RnBeads allows a comprehensive investigation of DNA methylation data.	https://rnbeads.org/	Assenov et al., 2014
Minfi	Minfi is a bioconductor package that can be used for analysis of methylation data generated from Illumina Infinium DNA methylation arrays.	https://bioconductor.org/packages/release/bioc/html/minfi.html	Aryee et al., 2014
ChAMP	The Chip Analysis Methylation Pipeline (ChAMP) is another widely used bioconductor pakage for analysis of methylation data retrieved from Illumina HumanMethylation450 and EPIC	https://bioconductor.org/packages/release/bioc/html/ChAMP.html	Morris et al., 2014
coMET	The comet allows users to visualize regional epigenome-wide association scan results and also DNA co-methylation patterns.	http://epigen.kcl.ac.uk/comet	Martin et al., 2015

Table 1 Contd....

Bioinformatics and Human Genomics Research

Table 1 Tools and databases for DNA methylation analysis (Contd....)

Name	Description	Hyperlink	Reference
	Databases for DNA methylation data		
DaVIE	The Database for the Visualization and Integration of Epigenetic (DaVIE) data provides vast amount of epigenetic related information to its users.	http://echelon.cmmt.ubc.ca/dbaccess/	Fejes et al., 2014
TCGA	The Cancer Genome Atlas (TCGA) contains information of molecularly characterized more than 20,000 primary cancer and matched normal samples spanning 33 cancer types. The TCGA large data pertaining to genomic, epigenomic, transcriptomic, and proteomic data.	https://portal.gdc.cancer.gov	Silva et al., 2016
MethHC	MethHC is a widely used database providing information about DNA methylation patterns and gene expression in human cancer.	http://methhc.mbc.nctu.edu.tw	Huang et al., 2015
DiseaseMeth	DiseaseMeth is an interactive methylation database that provides annotation of aberrant DNA methylation patterns in several human diseases.	http://bioinfo.hrbmu.edu.cn/diseasemeth/	Lv et al., 2012
NGSmethDB	NGSmethDB provides high-quality information regarding methylomes and also differential methylation patterns.	https://bioinfo2.ugr.es/NGSmethDB/	Hackenberg et al., 2010
MethBase	MethBase is a central reference methylome database developed from public Bisulfite sequencing datasets.	https://smithlabresearch.org/software/methbase/	Song et al., 2013
Wanderer	Wanderer allows an interactive exploration of DNA methylation and gene expression data in human cancer.	http://maplab.imppc.org/wanderer/	Diez-Villanueva et al., 2015
MethyCancer	MethyCancer database is widely used to examine CpG islands and other related methylation information from integrated DNA methylation datasets, and also cancer-related information such as mutations derived from large scale sequencing data.	http://methycancer.psych.ac.cn	He et al., 2007

with sodium bisulfite that consequently leads to the deamination of unmethylated cytosines into uracils while the methylated cytosine (5-mC) remains intact. The most common downstream strategies for DNA methylation analysis followed by bisulfite treatment include bisulfite sequencing, methylation-specific PCR amplification, and also methylation-based microarrays (Li and Tollefsbol, 2011). Although these techniques are labor-intensive but still it has proven to yield reliable and high-quality data to the research fraternity.

1.2.3 Comparative methylation hybridization

Another emerging technique involves a genomic clone-based hybridization approach with microarray technology to assay the methylation status of the genome. The methylated DNA fragments once affinity purified by using the DNA binding domain of methylated CpG binding protein or anti-5-mC antibody are then used as probes for genomic microarrays (Nelson, 2008).

1.2.4 MS-SNuPE and COBRA

The Methylation-Sensitive Single Nucleotide Primer Extension technique (MS-SNuPE) based on the bisulfite conversion strategy is widely used for the rapid quantification of methylation at individual CpG sites. This is followed by strand-specific PCR to generate a DNA template for quantitative methylation evaluation using MS-SNuPE. The next step involves performing MS-SNuPE with oligonucleotides, which are designed to hybridize upstream to the CpG site of interest. The reaction products are then electrophoresed for visualization and phosphorimage analysis. This analysis when carried out using multiplex PCR can enable simultaneous quantification of multiple CpG sites (Gonzalgo and Liang, 2007).

Similar to MS-SNuPE, the Combined Bisulfite Restriction Analysis (COBRA) assay allows for analysis of Locus-Specific changes in methylation patterns by involving restriction enzymes for analysis. This technique allows bisulfite conversion of non-methylated cytosines to uracils, the locus-specific PCR amplification of converted DNA, restriction digestion, the analysis of restriction patterns on the gel, and the quantification of these restriction patterns using ImageJ or a similar program (Bilichak and Kovalchuk, 2017).

1.2.5 Pyrosequencing

Pyrosequencing is a replication-based sequencing-by synthesis based method that allows quantitative real-time monitoring of incorporation of nucleotides through enzymatic conversion of released pyrophosphate signaled by the photometrically detectable reaction. During DNA methylation analysis, post bisulfite treatment the ratio of Thymine and Cytosine residues are used for quantification of methylated CpG sites. This technique offers high resolution and reliable quantitative measurements of closely positioned methylated CpG sites (Delaney et al., 2015).

1.2.6 Methylight and QAMA

Methylight allows sensitive detection and quantification of DNA methylation using a fluorescent-based sodium bisulfite dependent PCR strategy. This technique involves combining methylation-specific PCR with methylation-specific probing leading to a high methylation-specific detection technology capable of detecting very low frequencies of hypermethylated alleles also (Eads et al., 2000).

The quantitative analysis of methylated alleles (QAMA) is an improvement in the Methylight technology involving usage of TaqMan probes based on minor groove binder (MGB) technology. QAMA allows relative quantification of both methylated and unmethylated alleles amplified in a single tube (Zeschhigk et al., 2004).

1.2.7   EpiTYPER

EpiTYPER is a MALDI-TOF spectrometry-based bisulfite sequencing method that involves gene-specific amplification of bisulfite-treated DNA, which is followed by *in vitro* transcription. This technique is particularly for large-scale research focused on identifying candidate regions or for validation of potential methylated regions from the entire genome (Suchiman et al., 2015)

1.2.8   Other strategies

Several other techniques which are commonly used during methylation analysis include methylation-sensitive dot blot assay—MS-DBA which combines bisulfite modification (Clement and Benhattar, 2005), **PCR amplification** and **dot blot analysis** with two probes for both methylated and unmethylated DNA and **BIPS-SSCP**, which involves the combination of bisulfite treatment with PCR-based single-strand DNA conformation polymorphism (Maekawa et al., 2001).

1.3   Computational Analysis of DNA Methylation Data

The three main approaches for computational analysis of DNA methylation data include: (i) data processing and quality control, (ii) data visualization and statistical analysis and (iii) validation and interpretation of methylation data (Rauluseviciute et al., 2011).

1.3.1   Data processing and quality control

For post-experimental analysis for restriction enzyme and enzyme-based approaches the methylation data is analyzed by comparing the relative abundance of the fragments, whereas for bisulfite sequencing, the methylation is evaluated at individual cytosine residues and these differentially methylated regions are then statistically tested.

1.3.1.1   Bisulfite sequencing data processing

The majority of unmethylated cytosines are converted into thymines in the sequence read and the methylated cytosines (5mC) are protected due to bisulfite-induced treatment. Therefore it becomes crucial to have high-quality sequencing reads to achieve good alignment and consequently accurate methylation scores (Bock, 2012; Rauluseviciute et al., 2019). Therefore, before initiating alignment the incorrectly converted reads need to be discarded as part of quality control, and reads with adapter sequences should be identified and then trimmed with tools such as **Cutadapt** (Martin, 2011).

In the next step, the trimmed sequence reads are aligned with the reference genome and locations of methylation are identified. These aligners for methylation sequencing data are based on either the wild-card algorithm or the three-letter algorithm. In the scenario of Wild card aligners [**BSMAP** (Xi and Li, 2009), **GSNAp** (Wu and Nacu, 2010), **Last** (Shrestha and Frith, 2013), **Pash** (Coarfa et al., 2010), **WALT** (Chen et al., 2016b), **RRBSMAP** (Xi et al., 2012), and **segemehl** (Hoffman et al., 2009)], the cytosines (Cs) in the DNA sequence are replaced by the wild card letter 'Y' which matches both cytosines (Cs) and thymines (Ts) in the sequence read. In some cases, the alignment-scoring matrix is modified to adjust mismatches among the cytosines in the genomic DNA sequence and thymines in the read sequence are not penalized.

The three-letter algorithms such as **BRAT** (Harris et al., 2016), **Bismark** (Krueger and Andrews, 2011), **BS-seeker** (Huang et al., 2018), and **Methylcoder** (Pederson, 2011) allow conversion of cytosines into thymines both in the reference genome and read sequence. By this approach, the algorithm can align exclusively on three-letter alphabets viz., A, G, and T using a standard aligner tool such as **Bowtie** (Langmead et al., 2009).

Once the bisulfite alignment step is completed, the absolute DNA methylation values are calculated from the frequency of cytosines (Cs) and thymines (Ts) in the read sequence, which aligns with each cytosine in the reference genomic DNA sequence. In common practice, researchers divide the number of observed cytosines by the total number of cytosines and thymines for inferring the absolute methylation score. However during this inference, usage of several other tools as precautions is advised to achieve more reliable and accurate results by steps such as local realignment, sequence quality score analysis, and also statistical modeling of allele distributions (Bock, 2012). Tools such as **Bis-SNP** (Liu et al., 2012) can be used to distinguish bisulfite-induced changes from genetic variants during methylation score analysis. Similarly, tools such as M bias plot can be used to locate and discard unmethylated cytosines added at the ends of both fragments during end repair step of restoration of double-stranded DNA post fragmentation which may represent globally biased DNA methylation levels.

1.3.1.2 Enrichment-based data processing

Methylation levels in enrichment-based approaches viz., MRE-seq, and MeDIP-seq are achieved by comparing the relative abundance of fragments, i.e., the enrichment or depletion in the sequencing reads. During methylation sequencing, the frequency of specific DNA fragments, i.e., methylated and unmethylated fragments are counted in each library as raw data from which methylation levels can be inferred. The fluctuations in DNA sequencing due to batch effects need to be addressed during this process.

In the initial steps, the MeDIP-seq data is processed with the standard aligners such as **Bowtie** (Langmead et al., 2009) and **BWA** (Li and Durban, 2009). The enrichment scores are calculated by first extending the sequencing reads to the estimated size of DNA fragment and then counting the unique reads overlapping with each CpG or genomic regions of interest usually in the form of tilling map of the reference genome. However, this step requires normalization for correcting uneven CpG distribution in the genome. Tools such as **BATMAN** (Down et al., 2008) and **MEDME** (Pelizzola et al., 2008) or **MEDIPS** (Lienhard et al., 2014) algorithm that combines both are most commonly used for data normalization. Researchers have developed **MeQA** (Huang et al., 2012) and **MeDUSA** (Wilson et al., 2012) that include tools for both alignment (BWA) and normalization (MEDIPS) hence providing complete packages for MeDIP-seq data analysis.

During the analysis of the MRE-seq data, the sequencing reads are aligned to reference genomes using an aligner followed by checking and matching the restriction sites of the enzymes used during the experiment. The methylation scores are evaluated by analyzing the read coverage by tools such as **msgbsR** (Mayne et al., 2018) from the R package. Another package from R namely **Repitools** (Statham et al., 2010) is widely used for quality control of enrichmentbased datasets.

1.4 Data Visualization and Statistical Analysis

After the initial DNA methylation analysis, it is essential to visualize the identified genomic regions in a genome browser. For the preparation of visualization files, the CpG methylation tables identified from initial data processing are then converted into suitable file formats, which enable dynamic visualization of these methylation datasets. The methylation tables achieved from databases in BED or bedGraph formats are then converted into bigBed or bigWig formats. These file formats allow visualization of the methylation databases in genome browsers such as **UCSC Genome Browser** (Fujita et al., 2010), **Ensembl** (Fernández and E. Birney, 2010) and **WashU Human Epigenome browser** (Zhou et al., 2011). Other available desktop browsers for visualization include **Integrative Genomics Viewer (IGV)** (Thorvaldsdóttir et al., 2013) and **Integrated Genome Browser (IGB)** (Nicol et al., 2009).

Besides, region-specific visualization several other diagrammatic representations can be employed for a more global view of DNA methylation status. **Violin plots** and *box plots* can be used for identifying global changes in the methylated sequence by visualization of the distribution of methylation across the genome (Bock, 2012). Similarly, the **Hilbert curve** method can be used for the detection of spatial patterns in the distribution of DNA methylation. The tree-like diagrams of DNA are representatives of repeat elements in the reference genome and thus represent the global trends in methylation of repetitive DNA. **Scatter plots** are most frequently used to demonstrate the similarities and differences in sample pairs. All of these plots can be easily generated from R/Bioconductor. Hierarchical clustering using R packages such as 'hclust' (Oksanen, 2014) and 'heatmap3' (Zhao et al., 2014) enables users to identify systematic differences and similarities in DNA methylation maps of sample groups (for example, control and tumor samples), which can then be represented by clustering trees.

1.4.1 Identification of differentially methylated regions (DMRs)

After viewing the DNA methylation in the read sequence, the next step is the identification of differentially methylated regions, which represent consistently different methylation levels in samples (for example control and tumor samples). The actual size of these DMRs can vary from single cytosine residues to entire gene loci since this assay independent strategy is dependent on the biological question and also on the bioinformatics analysis pipeline used for identification. In the case of bisulfite sequencing pipelines, DMRs are detected from methylation tables, and count data in enrichment-based sequencing.

t-test or **Wilcoxin ranksum** tests which compare the DNA methylation levels of each cytosine in the sample groups are the most commonly used algorithms for the identification of DMRs. Other strategies for DMR identification include Shannon entropy, mixture models, aggregation of genomic regions, mixture models, logistic M values, or linear regression with peak detection and removal of batch effects (Bock, 2012; Omics, 2020; Rauluseviciute et al., 2019).

1.4.2 Statistical analysis

Accurate determination of DMRs is dependent on the computational power and also statistical verification. The algorithms for most of the tools for the identification of DMRs are based on a sliding window approach across the genome. Statistical correction for hypothesis testing allows the testing of multiple sites simultaneously. This correction is exclusively carried out by controlling the false discovery rate (FDR). The inference of FDR for each identified differentially methylated region is achieved by approaches such as the **q-value** (Dabney et al., 2010) method available in R/Bioconductor. The identified DMRs are then ranked according to their statistical significance and effect size (t-score from t-test or p-values and methylation difference). The most commonly used tools for the detection of DMR include **BSmooth** (Hansen et al., 2012), **methylSig** (Park et al., 2014), **BiSeq** (Hebestreit et al., 2013), and **methylPipe** (Kishore et al., 2015).

1.5 Validation and Interpretation

The statistical comparison between sample groups leads to the identification of several differentially methylated regions of interest, which can provide crucial information for biological interpretation. It should be noted that the statistical interpretation does not provide any information that could be biologically significant hence before validation and interpretation the identified DMRs are ranked according to the strength of association. The DMRs are ranked by *p*-values but relative and absolute differences in DNA methylation are also considered while ranking.

1.5.1 Validating differences in DNA methylation

Once the identified DMRs are identified and ranked, the accuracy and reproducibility of the results should be confirmed via several computational and experimental algorithms. Among the first steps for validation, the highest-ranked DMRs are reviewed manually in the genome browser to avoid any technical errors. The manual inspection should be accompanied by quality control checks for visualization of the global properties of shortlisted DMRs. As mentioned above, the volcano plots demonstrate the association between statistical significance and methylation differences between sample groups. Similarly, Q-Q plots can be used for the identification of technical artifacts and global biases that can lead to elevated P values and Manhattan plots are the representation of DMRs distribution across the genome (Bock, 2012; Rauluseviciute et al., 2019).

The verification of the identified DMRs is conducted by experimental measurements of DNA methylation on the same set of samples using different assays for detection of the technical accuracy of the DMRs. Similarly, the validation is achieved by experimental verification on a new sample cohort with similar characteristics to establish the biological reproducibility of identified DMRs. Locus specific DNA methylation assays are used for the verification and validation of DMRs to avoid the cost of validation on large cohorts. Numerous software and tools are available to support the most widely used DNA methylation protocols. Tools such as *MethMarker* (Schüffler et al., 2009) allow a graphical interface for designing and validating locus-specific DNA methylation assays such as COBRA, MSP, and MethyLight. Similarly, *MassArray* in R package enables assay design and validation for EpiTYPER assay providing support for bisulfite sequencing of selected loci which is the most commonly used and quantitatively accurate strategy for DMR identification (Thompson and Greally, 2019).

1.5.2   Interpretation of DNA methylation data

The accuracy of the biological interpretation drawn from the methylation data set is dependent on the phenotype being investigated and the algorithms for data processing and interpretation, which can be enhanced by the use of computational tools. Web-based software such as *EpiExplorer* allows exploration and interactive analysis of differentially methylated regions from the epigenomic public reference datasets (Halachev et al., 2012). Similarly, *Genomic HyperBrowser* (Sandve et al., 2013) and *Galaxy* (Giardine et al., 2005) enable the researchers to compare the identified DMR data with other available genomic datasets. Further gene set enrichment and functional annotation can be performed to gain further insights into the identified DMRs by computational tools such as *Enrichr* (Kuleshov et al. 2016), *DAVID* (Dennis et al., 2003), *PANTHER* (Mi et al., 2017), and *Genecodis* (Nagales-Cadenas et al., 2009). Another web server, *GREAT* (Genomic Regions Enrichment of Annotation Tool) can internally map the genomic regions and further statistically control the difference in gene size and the relative distance between them (McLean et al., 2010). Below are some more approaches to computationally infer biological functions of identified differentially methylated loci.

1.5.3   Enhancer gene association

Although enhancers are known to be distant from their target genes however, recent research has shown that methylated enhancers can also regulate the expressions of any associate genes. A newly developed approach based on *CAGE* (Cap Analysis of Gene Expressions) allows users to correlate a promoter with an enhancer based on their expression profiles (Kodzius et al., 2006; Medvedeva and Shershebnev, 2018).

1.5.4   3D chromatin structure

The association between Topologically associated domains (TADs) with CG-rich regions has been frequently reported. The existence of genes and DMRs in the same TAD regions can shed light on the function association (Babenko et al., 2017).

1.5.5   Transcriptomics

Sometimes the correlation of DNA methylation with the gene expression may not be very strong but in those cases, testing the same samples for transcriptomics data may help in interpreting methylation data and establishing a particular epigenetic mark (Chen et al., 2016a).

However, integration of biological interpretation of DNA methylation changes with omics data is quite complicated due to biological variations and demands for further standardization of algorithms.

1.6   Roadblocks in DNA Methylation Analysis

1.6.1   Cell population variability

Variation in DNA methylation can also lead to tumor heterogeneity that is considered to be a major obstacle in cancer treatment. Therefore, looking for these regions of variations in methylation levels within a group or tumor stage in a specific population may lead to a better understanding of the treatment regimen for therapy of specific disease types (Islam et al., 2019).

1.6.2   Single-cell methylation variability

So far research has shown that epigenetic modifications can be based on correlations obtained from a bulk cell population. However, research in the last decade has depicted that single-cell epigenomics can be used to assess disease heterogeneity and also for the assessment of heterogeneous responses to drugs (Qu et al., 2016).

1.6.3   Non-CpG methylation

Sometimes bisulfite reads can also detect non-CpG methylation sites but these non-CpG-methylation sites are filtered out during sequencing. However, these methylation sites are also known to be crucial for the regulation of transcription factors (TF) GR, ER, and BMAL1 binding. Several of these transcription factors binding to unmethylated CpGs can also bind to methylated CpGs (Jin et al., 2016).

1.6.4   5-Hydroxymethylcytosine

High methylation variability is also an indication of active demethylation in a region of interest. This can be investigated by measuring 5hmC, which is the first active demethylation product. However, techniques such as Bisulfite sequencing which is the gold standard for detection of DNA methylation does not discriminate between 5mC and 5hmC. Hence, the need of the hour demands for development of more strategies such as oxBS-Seq (distinguishes between 5mC and 5hmC) for getting better insights into the dynamics of DNA methylation (Booth et al., 2013).

1.7   Specific Computational Tools and Databases for DNA Methylation

In this section, we have described some of the most commonly used tools and databases for DNA methylation analysis (Table 1).

1.7.1   Tools for bisulfite sequencing data analysis

Tools such as **BS Seeker** (Huang et al., 2018), **Bismark** (Krueger and Andrews, 2011), and **BSMAP** (Xi and Li, 2009) are most often used for reading alignment in bisulfite sequencing data. Similarly, **GBSA** (Benoukraf et al., 2013) and **BSmooth** (Hansen et al., 2012) are recommended to be used for specific downstream analysis. **BS Seeker** is another tool that can perform alignment and also call methylation but does not calculate methylation scores. **BSMAP** can also be considered for RRBS methylation data analysis wherein it focuses on reference preparation to the identification of SNPs and DMRs and also allele-specific methylation. **BSmooth** specifically is one tool that considers biological variability while searching for DMRs and also performs read alignment and calculates methylation scores.

Another frequently used tool is a command-line based **MOABS** (Model-based Analysis of Bisulfite Sequencing data) which can perform alignment, call methylation, identify DMRs and also perform differential methylation analysis across several platforms, viz. WGBS, RRBS, and 5hmC (Sun et al., 2014). **MethPipe** is based on a similar pipeline to MOABS and can perform a similar analysis by integrating various tools (Song et al., 2013).

Bicycle is a crucial tool for methylation data analysis since it is universal to all platforms and also allows both single-end and paired-end reads. This algorithm integrates all necessary steps ranging from conversion and indexing of the reference genome to differential methylation analysis. Bicycle can accurately estimate the efficiency of bisulfite conversion that is critical for correct calculation of methylation scores. The statistical analysis of the Bicycle is regulated by **MethylSig** (Park et al., 2014) protocol. Contrary to the above-mentioned command line algorithms, **Genestack** is an online web server that enables users to analyze various data types including WGBS and RRBS (Genestack, 2020).

1.7.2 MeDIP-Seq data processing and analysis

The most frequently used tools for MeDIP-Seq data analysis include *BATMAN* (Down et al., 2008) and *MEDIPS* (Lienhard et al., 2014) however both of these tools do not perform quality control or even mapping of the reads. *MeDUSA* (Methylated DNA Utility for Sequence Analysis) focuses on accurate DMR detection from MeDIP-Seq data (Wilson et al., 2012). The algorithm consists of several packages for complete data analysis, viz., BWA for read alignment, SAMtools for filtering, FastQC to perform quality control, and also integrates with MEDIPS fir methylation analysis. Another preferred tool for MeDIP Seq data analysis is *MeQA* which can pre-process data, assess data quality, and also estimate DNA methylation levels (Huang et al., 2012).

1.7.3 Other computational tools

1.7.3.1 Detection of *CpG islands*

Several algorithms have been developed both command-line and online web servers based on different algorithms including window-based, Hidden Markov Model, density-based, and distance-based that allows users to identify CpG islands computationally (Tahir et al., 2019). Tools such as *CpGIS* (Taki and Jones, 2003) and *CpGProD* (Ponger and Mouchiroud, 2002) use a sliding window-based approach for CGI detection and also CGI features including length, GC content, and O/E ratio. *CpGIF* is a PERL based tool that uses a density-based approach to detect the CpG dinucleotides in the sequence from 5′ to 3′ direction (Sujuan et al., 2008). CpG_MPs can also be used for the characterization of CpG islands from bisulfite sequencing data (Su et al., 2013). Some commonly used CpG detection tools based on distance-based algorithms include *WordCluster* (Hackenberg et al., 2006), *CpG_MI* (Su et al., 2010), and *CpGcluster* (Hackenberg et al., 2006).

1.7.3.2 Detection of DNMT-Enriched sites and Binding coordinates

The binning and identification of genomic intervals can be achieved by *GenomicRange* package in R. The package can also be used for storing sequencing data along with the defined annotations (Aboyoun et al., 2010).

Further, the identification of correct genomic coordinates is crucial for the analysis of DNMT binding sites at promoters or CpG islands. *GenomicFeature* package in R can be used to retrieve regions of interest in proximity to transcriptional start sites (TSS) (Lawrence et al., 2013). In addition to command-line tools, the UCSC table browser can be used to directly download TSS regions and promoters.

For visualization of DNMT protein localization, the **Genomation** package in R allows the depiction of coverage of DNMT proteins around all proteins of CpG islands using heat map profiles (Akalin et al., 2015).

1.8   Bioconductor Packages for Analysis

Bsseq is a bioconductor package that provides several tools for analysis and visualization of WGBS data for the identification of DMRs (Hansen et al., 2012). **M3D** uses a kernel-based approach for DMR identification (Mayo et al., 2014). **DMAP** is a C-based tool that includes statistical tools for analysis of RRBS and WGBS methylation data (Stockwell et al., 2014). Single-cell Bisulfite sequencing data can be retrieved from BEAT package. Besides **DMRcate** (Peters et al., 2015) and **RnBeads** (Assenov et al., 2014), another Bioconductor package **Minfi** can be used for the analysis of Illumina Infinium array that also considers cellular heterogeneity during analysis (Aryee et al., 2014). **ChAMP** offers QC/QA metrics along with several normalization methods for the identification of DMRs and also copy number variations in Illumina 450K methylation and EPIC array datasets (Morris et al., 2014). Researchers also employ **coMET** for Epigenome-wide association scans and also the generation of plots from DNA co-methylation patterns (Martin et al., 2015). The **DaVIE** (Database for the Visualization and Integration of Epigenetics data) enables identification of DNA methylation patterns, and also cross-checking of identified DMRs across several methylation samples available online (Fejes et al., 2014).

1.9   Databases for DNA Methylation Data

The emergence of several high throughput tools for DNA methylation sequencing and analysis based on NGS and microarray, have led to the development of DNA methylation-specific databases which provide information related to both methylation levels and also their respective gene information. The most common resource for DNA methylation is **TCGA**—The Cancer Genome Atlas launched in 2006 by the National Cancer Institute and the National Genome Research Institute (Silva et al., 2016). TCGA contains methylation data obtained from several array-based DNA methylation platform data viz., Illumina DNA Methylation Cancer Panel I, Illumina HumanMethylation27 BeadChip, and Illumina HumanMethylation450K BeadChip. Several other databases have been developed which integrate several interpretation databases with methylation data. **MethHC** (database of DNA methylation and gene expression in human cancer) is a web-based database known to integrate DNA methylation data with gene expression, miRNA methylation, miRNA expression, and also the correlation of methylation data with gene expression retrieved from TCGA (Huang et al., 2015). Another commonly used interactive methylation database is **DiseaseMeth**, which contains information on aberrant methylomes of human diseases (Lv et al., 2012). **NGSmethDB** is a methylation-specific database for whole-genome methylation maps (Hackenberg et al., 2010). **MethBase** is a DNA methylation database that contains methylomes from several organisms and allows visualization of bisulfite sequencing experiments retrieved from UCSC Genome Browser (Song et al., 2013). **Wanderer** also provides an interactive view of DNA methylation and gene expression data in human cancers (Diez-Villnueva et al., 2015). **MethyCancer** is an integrated database that provides annotation of aberrant DNA methylation, cancer-related genes, mutations and also CpG islands information retrieved from large-scale sequencing (He et al., 2007).

1.10 Conclusion and Future Prospects

DNA methylation is known to play regulatory roles during transcription, embryonic development, genomic imprinting, inactivation of X-chromosome, and chromosomal stability. The hypermethylation and hypomethylation also affect gene expression of crucial cell cycle genes, apoptosis-related genes, metabolism-related genes, and metastasis-related genes during initiation and progression of several diseases including neurodegenerative disorders and cancer. Various techniques and technologies nowadays have allowed researchers to determine DNA methylation levels of single nucleotides, their genomic positions, the transcription start sites, positions of CpG islands and also frequencies of C+G% thus leading to the generation of huge amounts of data providing better insights into mechanisms at DNA levels for different cells in different organisms. The computational prediction of methylation levels can boost genome-wide methylation profiling and thereby contribute to the identification of various methylation patterns in several diseases (Singh and Sharma, 2017). The algorithms for these bioinformatics tools are built on different principles, which can provide results with high accuracy, and sensitivity and are specific for different analysis parameters. In this chapter, we have tried to review the concepts of DNA methylation, various techniques available for analysis of DNA methylation, and also the bioinformatics techniques widely used for interpretation of generated DNA methylation data. Our aim behind this chapter remains to discuss the steps associated with DNA methylation analysis and the best tools and techniques available to interpret the data in the best manner possible. We further would like to emphasize on the critical steps of selecting the best technique for DNA methylation analysis which would answer your questions, quality control for generated data to reduce chances of omission of important data which might be filtered out and also to ensure minimum redundancy of data and thirdly, inference of biological functions from identified differentially methylated loci. The comparative analysis of methylation data can help in the identification of parameters and limitations of each tool, and thus allows users to prioritize and select the best detection algorithms for targeting epigenome.

However, there still exists a need for advanced and more sensitive detection algorithms, which can provide more accurate whole-genome methylation data. Also with the generation of large-scale whole-genome methylation sequencing data the need for the hour demands for more specific integrative databases specific to DNA methylation allowing public access to general whole-genome methylation sequencing data and its related biological and epigenomic inferences. The advancement in computational techniques for prediction of methylation status and also CpG islands offers great possibilities of unraveling more discoveries in epigenetics and gene regulations which can lead to a significant breakthrough in understanding epigenetic mechanisms and potential biomarkers involved in disease progression and their respective treatments in near future.

REFERENCES

Aboyoun, P., H. Pages and M. Lawrence (2010). GenomicRanges: Representation and manipulation of genomic intervals. R package version. 1(7).

Akalin, A., V. Franke, K. Vlahoviček, C.E. Mason and D. Schübeler (2015). Genomation: A toolkit to summarize, annotate and visualize genomic intervals. Bioinformatics. 31(7): 1127–1129.

Aryee, M.J., A.E. Jaffe, H. Corrada-Bravo, C. Ladd-Acosta, et al. (2014). Minfi: A flexible and comprehensive ioconductor package for the analysis of Infinium DNA methylation microarrays. Bioinformatics. 30(10): 1363–1369.

Assenov, Y., F. Müller, P. Lutsik, J. Walter, T. Lengauer and C. Bock (2014). Comprehensive analysis of DNA methylation data with RnBeads. Nature Methods. 11(11): 1138.

Babenko, V.N., I.V. Chadaeva and Y.L. Orlov (2017). Genomic landscape of CpG rich elements in human. BMC Evolutionary Biology. 17(1): 19.

Benoukraf, T., S. Wongphayak, L.H. Hadi, M. Wu and R. Soong (2013). GBSA: A comprehensive software for analysing whole genome bisulfite sequencing data. Nucleic Acids Research. 41(4): e55.

Bilichak, A. and I. Kovalchuk (2017). The combined bisulfite restriction analysis (COBRA) assay for the analysis of locus-specific changes in methylation patterns. pp. 63–71. *In*: Plant Epigenetics. Humana Press, Boston, MA.

Bock, C. (2012). Analysing and interpreting DNA methylation data. Nature Reviews Genetics. 13(10): 705–719.

Booth, M.J., T.W.B. Ost, D. Beraldi, N.M. Bell, M.R. Branco, W. Reik, et al. (2013). Oxidative bisulfite sequencing of 5-methylcytosine and 5-hydroxymethylcytosine. Nature Protocols. 8(10): 1841–1851.

Chen, Q., X.Y. Zhu, Y.Y. Li and Z.Q. Meng (2014). Epigenetic regulation and cancer. Oncology Reports. 31(2): 523–532.

Chen, D.P., Y.C. Lin and C.S. Fann (2016a). Methods for identifying differentially methylated regions for sequence-and array-based data. Briefings In Functional Genomics. 15(6): 485–490.

Chen, H., A.D. Smith and T. Chen (2016b). WALT: Fast and accurate read mapping for bisulfite sequencing. Bioinformatics. 32(22): 3507–3509.

Clement, G. and J. Benhattar (2005). A methylation sensitive dot blot assay (MS-DBA) for the quantitative analysis of DNA methylation in clinical samples. Journal of Clinical Pathology. 58(2): 155–158.

Coarfa, C., F. Yu, C.A. Miller, Z. Chen, R.A. Harris and A. Milosavljevic (2010). Pash 3.0: A versatile software package for read mapping and integrative analysis of genomic and epigenomic variation using massively parallel DNA sequencing. BMC Bioinformatics. 11(1): 572.

Dabney, A., J.D. Storey and G.R. Warnes (2010). Qvalue: Q-value estimation for false discovery rate control. R package version. 1(0).

Delaney, C., S.K. Garg and R. Yung (2015). Analysis of DNA methylation by pyrosequencing. pp. 249–264. *In*: Immunosenescence. Humana Press, New York, NY.

Dennis, G., B.T. Sherman, D.A. Hosack, J. Yang, W. Gao, H.C. Lane, et al. (2003). DAVID: Database for annotation, visualization, and integrated discovery. Genome biology. 4(9): R60.

Díez-Villanueva, A., I. Mallona and M.A. Peinado (2015). Wanderer, an interactive viewer to explore DNA methylation and gene expression data in human cancer. Epigenetics and Chromatin. 8(1): 22.

Down, T.A., V.K. Rakyan, D.J. Turner, P. Flicek, H. Li, E. Kulesha, et al. (2008). A Bayesian deconvolution strategy for immunoprecipitation-based DNA methylome analysis. Nature Biotechnology. 26(7): 779–785.

Eads, C.A., K.D. Danenberg, K. Kawakami, L.B. Saltz, C. Blake, D. Shibata, et al. (2000). MethyLight: A high-throughput assay to measure DNA methylation. Nucleic Acids Research. 28(8): e32.

Fejes, A.P., M.J. Jones and M.S. Kobor (2014). DaVIE: Database for the visualization and integration of epigenetic data. Front Genet. 5: 325.

Fernández, X.M. and E. Birney (2010). Ensembl genome browser. pp. 923–939. *In*: Vogel and Motulsky's Human Genetics. Springer, Berlin, Heidelberg.

Fujita, P.A., B. Rhead, A.S. Zweig, A.S. Hinrichs, D. Karolchik, M.S. Cline, M. Goldman, G.P. Barber, et al. (2010). The UCSC genome browser database: update 2011. Nucleic acids research. 39(suppl_1): D876–D882.

Genestack, (Internet). (Cited on 20 April 2020). Available from: https://www.genestack.com

Giardine, B., C. Riemer, R.C. Hardison, R. Burhans, L. Elnitski, et al. (2005). Galaxy: a platform for interactive large-scale genome analysis. Genome Research. 2005, Oct 1; 15(10): 1451–5.

Gonzalgo, M.L. and G. Liang, (2007). Methylation-sensitive single-nucleotide primer extension (Ms-SNuPE) for quantitative measurement of DNA methylation. Nature Protocols. 2007, Aug.; 2(8): 1931–6.

Graña, O., H. López-Fernández, F. Fdez-Riverola, D. González Pisano and D. Glez-Peña (2018). Bicycle: a bioinformatics pipeline to analyze bisulfite sequencing data. Bioinformatics. 2018, Apr 15; 34(8):1414–5.

Hackenberg, M., C. Previti, P.L. Luque-Escamilla, P. Carpena, J. Martínez-Aroza and J.L. Oliver (2006). CpGcluster: A distance-based algorithm for CpG-island detection. BMC Bioinformatics. 7(1): 446.

Hackenberg, M., G. Barturen and J.L. Oliver (2010). NGSmethDB: A database for next-generation sequencing single-cytosine-resolution DNA methylation data. Nucleic Acids Research. 39(suppl_1): D75–79.

Hackenberg, M., P. Carpena, P. Bernaola-Galván, G. Barturen, A.M. Alganza and J.L. Oliver (2011). WordCluster: Detecting clusters of DNA words and genomic elements. Algorithms for Molecular Biology. 6(1): 2.

Halachev, K., H. Bast, F. Albrecht, T. Lengauer and C. Bock (2012). EpiExplorer: Live exploration and global analysis of large epigenomic datasets. Genome Biology. (10): R96.

Hansen, K.D., B. Langmead and R.A. Irizarry (2012). BSmooth: From whole genome bisulfite sequencing reads to differentially methylated regions. Genome biology. 13(10): R83.

Harris, E.Y., R. Ounit and S. Lonardi (2016). BRAT-nova: Fast and accurate mapping of bisulfite-treated reads. Bioinformatics. 32(17): 2696–2698.

Hashimoto, K., S. Kokubun, E. Itoi and H.I. Roach (2007). Improved quantification of DNA methylation using methylation-sensitive restriction enzymes and real-time PCR. Epigenetics. 2(2): 86–91.

He, X., S. Chang, J. Zhang, Q. Zhao, H. Xiang, et al. (2007). MethyCancer: The database of human DNA methylation and cancer. Nucleic Acids Research. 36(suppl_1): D836–D841.

Hebestreit, K., M. Dugas and H.U. Klein (2013). Detection of significantly differentially methylated regions in targeted bisulfite sequencing data. Bioinformatics. 29(13): 1647–1653.

Hoffmann, S., C. Otto, S. Kurtz, C.M. Sharma, P. Khaitovich, J. Vogel, et al. (2009). Fast mapping of short sequences with mismatches, insertions and deletions using index structures. PLoS Computational Biology. 5(9): e1000502.

Huang, J., V. Renault, J. Sengenes, N. Touleimat, S. Michel, M. Lathrop, et al. (2012). MeQA: A pipeline for MeDIP-seq data quality assessment and analysis. Bioinformatics. 28(4): 587–588.

Huang, W.-Y., S.-D. Hsu, H.-Y. Huang, Y.-M. Sun, C.-H. Chou, S.-L. Weng, et al. (2015). MethHC: A database of DNA methylation and gene expression in human cancer. Nucleic Acids Res. 43(D1): D856–861.

Huang, K.Y., Y.J. Huang and P.Y. Chen (2018). BS-Seeker3: Ultrafast pipeline for bisulfite sequencing. BMC Bioinformatics. 19(1): 111.

Islam, S.A., S.J. Goodman, J.L. MacIsaac, J. Obradović, R.G. Barr, W.T. Boyce, et al. (2019). Integration of DNA methylation patterns and genetic variation in human pediatric tissues help inform EWAS design and interpretation. Epigenetics and Chromatin. 12(1): 1–8.

Jin, J., T. Lian, C. Gu, K. Yu, Y.Q. Gao and X.D. Su (2016). The effects of cytosine methylation on general transcription factors. Sci. Rep. 6(1): 1–3.

Kishore, K., S. de Pretis, R. Lister, M.J. Morelli, V. Bianchi, B. Amati, et al. (2015). MethylPipe and compEpiTools: A suite of R packages for the integrative analysis of epigenomics data. BMC Bioinformatics. 16(1): 313.

Kodzius, R., M. Kojima, H. Nishiyori, M. Nakamura, S. Fukuda, M. Tagami, et al. (2006). CAGE: Cap analysis of gene expression. Nature Methods. 3(3): 211–222.

Krueger, F. and S.R. Andrews (2011). Bismark: A flexible aligner and methylation caller for Bisulfite-Seq applications. Bioinformatics. 27(11): 1571–1572.

Kuleshov, M.V., M.R. Jones, A.D. Rouillard, N.F. Fernandez, Q. Duan, Z, Koplev, et al. (2016). Enrichr: A comprehensive gene set enrichment analysis web server 2016 update. Nucleic Acids Research. 44(W1): W90–W97.

Langmead, B., C. Trapnell, M. Pop and S.L. Salzberg (2009). Ultrafast and memory-efficient alignment of short DNA sequences to the human genome. Genome Biology. 10(3): R25.

Lawrence, M., W. Huber, H. Pages, P. Aboyoun, M. Carlson, R. Gentleman, et al. (2013). Software for computing and annotating genomic ranges. PLoS Computational Biology. 9(8).

Lee, J., S.J. Jang, N. Benoit, M.O. Hoque, J.A. Califano, B. Trink, et al. (2010). Presence of 5-methylcytosine in CpNpG trinucleotides in the human genome. Genomics. 96(2): 67–72.

Li, H. and R. Durbin (2009). Fast and accurate short read alignment with Burrows–Wheeler transform. Bioinformatics. 25(14): 1754–1760.

Li, Y. and T.O. Tollefsbol (2011). DNA methylation detection: Bisulfite genomic sequencing analysis. pp. 11–21. *In*: Epigenetics Protocols. Humana Press.

Lienhard, M., C. Grimm, M. Morkel, R. Herwig and L. Chavez (2014). MEDIPS: Genome-wide differential coverage analysis of sequencing data derived from DNA enrichment experiments. Bioinformatics. 30(2): 284–286.

Liu, Y., K.D. Siegmund, P.W. Laird and B.P. Berman (2012). Bis-SNP: Combined DNA methylation and SNP calling for Bisulfite-seq data. Genome Biology. 13(7): R61.

Lv, J., H. Liu, J. Su, X. Wu, B. Li, X. Xiao, et al. (2012). DiseaseMeth: A human disease methylation database. Nucleic Acids Research. 40(D1): D1030–D1035.

Maekawa, M., M. Ushiama, N. Fukayama, K. Nomoto, H. Kashiwabara, S. Fujita, et al. (2001). Heterogeneity of DNA methylation status analyzed by bisulfite-PCR-SSCP and correlation with clinico-pathological characteristics in colorectal cancer. Clinical Chemistry qnd Laboratory Medicine. 39(2): 121–128.

Martin, M. (2011). Cutadapt removes adapter sequences from high-throughput sequencing reads. EMBnet. Journal. 17(1): 10–12.

Martin, T.C., I. Yet, P.C. Tsai and J.T. Bell (2015). coMET: Visualisation of regional epigenome-wide association scan results and DNA co-methylation patterns. BMC Bioinformatic. 16(1): 131.

Mayne, B.T., S.Y. Leemaqz, S. Buckberry, C.M. Rodriguez Lopez, C.T. Roberts, T. Bianco-Miotto, et al. (2018). msgbsR: An R package to analyse methylation sensitive genotyping by sequencing (MS-GBS) data. Sci. Rep. 8: 2190.

Mayo, T.R., G. Schweikert and G. Sanguinetti (2015). M3D: A kernel-based test for spatially correlated changes in methylation profiles. Bioinformatics. 31(6): 809–816.

McLean, C.Y., D. Bristor, M. Hiller, S.L. Clarke, B.T. Schaar, C.B. Lowe, et al. (2010). GREAT improves functional interpretation of cis-regulatory regions. Nature Biotechnology. 28(5): 495.

Medvedeva, Y. and A. Shershebnev (2018). Experimental design and bioinformatic analysis of DNA methylation data. pp. 175–194. *In*: CpG Islands. Humana Press, New York, NY.

Mi, H., X. Huang, A. Muruganujan, H. Tang, C. Mills, D. Kang, et al. (2017). PANTHER version 11: Expanded annotation data from gene ontology and reactome pathways, and data analysis tool enhancements. Nucleic Acids Research. 45(D1): D183–D189.

Morris, T.J., L.M. Butcher, A. Feber, A.E. Teschendorff, A.R. Chakravarthy, T.K. Wojdacz, et al. (2014). ChAMP: 450k chip analysis methylation pipeline. Bioinformatics. 30(3): 428–430.

Nelson, S. (2008). Comparative methylation hybridization. Nature Education. 1(1): 55.

Nicol, J.W., G.A. Helt, S.G. Blanchard Jr., A. Raja and A.E. Loraine (2009). The Integrated Genome Browser: Free software for distribution and exploration of genome-scale datasets. Bioinformatics. 25(20): 2730–2731.

Nogales-Cadenas, R., P. Carmona-Saez, M. Vazquez, C. Vicente, X. Yang, F. Tirado, et al. (2009). GeneCodis: Interpreting gene lists through enrichment analysis and integration of diverse biological information. Nucleic Acids Research. 37(suppl_2): W317–W322.

Oksanen, J. (2014). Cluster analysis: Tutorial with R. University of Oulu. Oulu. pp. 1–13.

Omics, aX. Differentially methylated region identification software tools (Internet). (Cited on 20 April 2020). Available from: https://omictools.com/differentially-methylated-region-detection-category

Ongenaert, M. (2010). Epigenetic databases and computational methodologies in the analysis of epigenetic datasets. pp. 259–295. *In*: Advancesin Genetics, (Vol. 71). Academic Press.

Park, Y., M.E. Figueroa, L.S. Rozek and M.A. Sartor (2014). MethylSig: A whole genome DNA methylation analysis pipeline. Bioinformatics. 30(17): 2414–2422.

Pedersen, B., T.F. Hsieh, C. Ibarra and R.L. Fischer (2011). MethylCoder: Software pipeline for bisulfite-treated sequences. Bioinformatics. 27(17): 2435–2436.

Pelizzola, M., Y. Koga, A.E. Urban, M. Krauthammer, S. Weissman, R. Halaban, et al. (2008). MEDME: An experimental and analytical methodology for the estimation of DNA methylation levels based on microarray derived MeDIP-enrichment. Genome Research. 18(10): 1652–1659.

Peters, T.J., M.J. Buckley, A.L. Statham, R. Pidsley, K. Samaras, R.V. Lord, et al. (2015). *De novo* identification of differentially methylated regions in the human genome. Epigenetics and Chromatin. 8(1): 6.

Ponger, L. and D. Mouchiroud (2002). CpGProD: Identifying CpG islands associated with transcription start sites in large genomic mammalian sequences. Bioinformatics. 18(4): 631–633.

Qu, W., T. Tsukahara, R. Nakamura, H. Yurino, S.I. Hashimoto, S. Tsuji, et al. (2016). Assessing cell-to-cell DNA methylation variability on individual long reads. Sci. Rep. 6(1): 1–7.

Rauluseviciute, I., F. Drabløs and M.B. Rye (2019). DNA methylation data by sequencing: Experimental approaches and recommendations for tools and pipelines for data analysis. Clin. Epigenetics. 11(1): 1–3.

Sandve, G.K., S. Gundersen, M. Johansen, I.K. Glad, K. Gunathasan, L. Holden, et al. (2013). The genomic HyperBrowser: An analysis web server for genome-scale data. Nucleic Acids Research. 41(W1): W133–W141.

Schüffler, P., T. Mikeska, A. Waha, T. Lengauer and C. Bock (2009). MethMarker: User-friendly design and optimization of gene-specific DNA methylation assays. Genome Biology. 10(10): R105.

Shrestha, A.M. and M.C. Frith (2013). An approximate Bayesian approach for mapping paired-end DNA reads to a reference genome. Bioinformatics. 29(8): 965–972.

Silva, T.C., A. Colaprico, C. Olsen, F. D'Angelo, G. Bontempi, M. Ceccarelli, et al. (2016). TCGA workflow: Analyze cancer genomics and epigenomics data using bioconductor packages. F1000Research. 5.

Singh, A.N. and N. Sharma (2017). Identification of key pathways and genes with aberrant methylation in prostate cancer using bioinformatics analysis. OncoTargets and Therapy. 10: 4925–4933.

Song, Q., B. Decato, M. Kessler, F. Fang, J. Qu, T. Garvin, et al. (2013). A reference methylome database and analysis pipeline to facilitate integrative and comparative epigenomic. PLoS One. 8(12): e81148.

Statham, A.L., D. Strbenac, M.W. Coolen, C. Stirzaker, S.J. Clark and M.D. Robinson (2010). Repitools: An R package for the analysis of enrichment-based epigenomic data. Bioinformatics. 26(13): 1662–1663.

Stockwell, P.A., A. Chatterjee, E.J. Rodger and I.M. Morison (2014). DMAP: Differential methylation analysis package for RRBS and WGBS data. Bioinformatics. 30(13): 1814–1822.

Su, J., Y. Zhang, J. Lv, H. Liu, X. Tang, F. Wang, et al. (2010). CpG_MI: A novel approach for identifying functional CpG islands in mammalian genomes. Nucleic Acids Research. 38(1): e6.

Su, J., H. Yan, Y. Wei, H. Liu, F. Wang, J. Lv, et al. (2013). CpG_MPs: Identification of CpG methylation patterns of genomic regions from high-throughput bisulfite sequencing data. Nucleic Acids Research. 41(1): e4.

Suchiman, H.E., R.C. Slieker, D. Kremer, P.E. Slagboom, B.T. Heijmans and E.W. Tobi (2015). Design, measurement and processing of region-specific DNA methylation assays: the mass spectrometry-based method EpiTYPER. Frontiers in Genetics. 6: 287.

Sujuan, Y., A. Asaithambi and Y. Liu (2008). CpGIF: An algorithm for the identification of CpG islands. Bioinformation. 2(8): 335.

Sun, D., Y. Xi, B. Rodriguez, H.J. Park, P. Tong, M. Meong, et al. (2014). MOABS: Model based analysis of bisulfite sequencing data. Genome Biology. 15(2): R38.

Tahir, R.A., D. Zheng, A. Nazir and H. Qing (2019). A review of computational algorithms for CpG islands detection. Journal of Biosciences. 44(6): 143.

Takai, D. and P.A. Jones (2003). The CpG island searcher: A new WWW resource. In Silico Biol. 3(3): 235–240.

Thompson, R.F. and J.M. Greally (2019). MassArray: Analytical tools for MassArray data. R package version. 1. 38.0.

Thorvaldsdóttir, H., J.T. Robinson and J.P. Mesirov (2013). Integrative Genomics Viewer (IGV): High-performance genomics data visualization and exploration. Briefings in Bioinformatics. 14(2): 178–192.

Watanabe, Y. and M. Maekawa (2018). Methods and strategies to determine epigenetic variation in human disease. pp. 13–37. *In*: T.O. Tollefsbol (ed.). Epigenetics in Human Disease. Academic Press.

Wilson, G.A., P. Dhami, A. Feber, D. Cortázar, Y. Suzuki, R. Schulz, et al. (2012). Resources for methylome analysis suitable for gene knockout studies of potential epigenome modifiers. GigaScience. 1(1): 2047-217X-1-3. doi: 10.1186/2047-217X-1-3

Wu, T.D. and S. Nacu (2010). Fast and SNP-tolerant detection of complex variants and splicing in short reads. Bioinformatics. 26(7): 873–881.

Xi, Y. and W. Li (2009). BSMAP: Whole genome bisulfite sequence MAPping program. BMC Bioinformatics. 10(1): 232.

Xi, Y., C. Bock, F. Müller, D. Sun, A. Meissner and W. Li (2012). RRBSMAP: A fast, accurate and user-friendly alignment tool for reduced representation bisulfite sequencing. Bioinformatics. 28(3): 430–432.

Zeschnigk, M., S. Böhringer, E.A. Price, Z. Onadim, L. Maßhöfer and D.R. Lohmann (2004). A novel real-time PCR assay for quantitative analysis of methylated alleles (QAMA): Analysis of the retinoblastoma locus. Nucleic Acids Research. 32(16): e125.

Zhao, S., Y. Guo, Q. Sheng and Y. Shyr (2014). Heatmap3: An improved heatmap package with more powerful and convenient features. BMC Bioinformatics. 15(10): 16.

Zhong, J., G. Agha and A.A. Baccarelli (2016). The role of DNA methylation in cardiovascular risk and disease: Methodological aspects, study design, and data analysis for epidemiological studies. Circulation Research. 118(1): 119–131.

Zhou, X., B. Maricque, M. Xie, D. Li, V. Sundaram, E.A. Martin, et al. (2011). The human epigenome browser at Washington University. Nature Methods. 8(12): 989–990.

CHAPTER 10

Bioinformatics of Transcription Factor Binding Prediction

**Erick I. Navarro-Delgado[1,*], Marisol Salgado-Albarrán[2,3,*],
Karla Torres-Arciga[1], Nicolas Alcaraz[4], Ernesto Soto-Reyes[2],
Luis A. Herrera[1,5] and Rodrigo González-Barrios[1†]**

[1]Unidad de Investigación Biomédica en Cáncer,
Instituto Nacional de Cancerología-Instituto de Investigaciones Biomédicas,
UNAM, Avenida San Fernando No. 22,
Colonia Sección XVI, Tlalpan, CP 14080, Mexico City, Mexico

[2]Natural Sciences Department,
Universidad Autónoma Metropolitana-Cuajimalpa (UAM-C), Mexico City, 05300, Mexico

[3]Chair of Experimental Bioinformatics, TUM School of Life Sciences,
Technical University of Munich

[4]The Bioinformatics Centre, Department of Biology,
University of Copenhagen, 2200 Copenhagen

[5]Instituto Nacional de Medicina Genómica, Periférico Sur 4809,
Arenal Tepepan, Tlalpan, CP 14610, Mexico City, Mexico

1 INTRODUCTION

Transcription Factors (TFs) are proteins directly involved in interpreting the genome. These proteins are crucial to the cell, performing the first step in decoding the DNA sequence, which leads to chromatin remodeling and ultimately transcription. TFs belong to a wide number of proteins that are involved in different molecular machineries that regulate the transcriptional control of the cell. The diverse functions of TFs regulate the language of the cell, which directs the development, differentiation, specialization, and response to the environment.

[†]Corresponding author: *rodrigop@ciencias.unam.mx*
*These authors contributed equally to this work.

Historically, the term TF has been applied to describe any protein involved in transcription and/or capable of altering gene-expression levels. However, nowadays the term is applied to proteins that directly perform transcriptional control. The key components to understand such transcriptional control were established by Jacob and Monod, more than half a century ago (1961), with their groundbreaking genetic and biochemical experiments in bacterial systems. Their findings shed light to two major concepts in gene regulation: a) protein-binding regulatory sequences are present in the DNA and b) proteins bind to such DNA sequences to activate or repress transcription. Through their pioneering work and many subsequent studies, it was established that TFs recognize and occupy those specific DNA sequences, regulating the transcriptional machinery and the outcome of genes (Fulton et al., 2009; Lee and Young, 2013; Vaquerizas et al., 2009). Due to the importance that TFs exert to the control of gene expression; an intense study has been carried out for decades to understand their functions. This led to the discovery of many general TFs and cofactors in eukaryotic organisms, as well as various chromatin regulators and the mechanisms by which they control gene expression (Jolma et al., 2013; Lambert et al., 2018).

Since TFs depend on DNA sequences and its specific location on chromosomes to carry out their function, it is important to emphasize that these proteins cannot be functionally understood without a detailed knowledge of the DNA sequences to which they bind. These specific TF DNA binding sites (TFBSs) are often referred to as "motifs", which are templates representing the set of related short DNA sequences which are recognized by a given TF (Bejerano et al., 2004; Cusanovich et al., 2014). These sequences can be used to scan longer sequences, such as genetic promoters and enhancers in order to identify possible binding sites (BS). Identifying a DNA binding motif is often the first step towards a detailed understanding of the function of a given TF; knowing the possible BS of a protein provides a gateway for further analysis.

Due to recent advances in biotechnology and especially after the advent of DNA massive sequencing, our knowledge of the mammal regulatory elements, as well as the transcription and chromatin regulators that operate at these sites, has increased considerably in the last decade. Currently there are enormous amounts of data of TFs and the sequences they are associated to. However, being able to predict the expression pattern of a gene based only on its regulatory sequence, turns out to be more complicated when studying the cell; it is generally highly context-specific, depending on the cell type and intracellular factors (ENCODE PROJECT CONSORTIUM, 2012; Vaquerizas et al., 2009) . Also, the regulatory regions are not necessarily organized in discrete, easily identifiable regions of the genome and can exert their influence on genes at great genomic distances (Nobrega et al., 2003). Furthermore, even experimentally determined BSs are relatively poor predictors of genes that the TF actually regulates (Cusanovich et al., 2014).

To date, genomic studies are trying to elucidate regulatory elements, as well as to identify and/or predict the regulatory sequences of the TFs in different species. They have taken two main paths: a) those studies that identify specific TF binding sites using experimental techniques such as ChIP-seq, SELEX-seq, ChIP-on-chip, CUT&RUN or CUT&Tag; or b) those studies focused on predicting the possible regulatory elements and their sites in the genome through computational reconstructions and genetic regulatory networks (Degner et al., 2012; ENCODE PROJECT CONSORTIUM, 2012; Fulton et al., 2009; Jolma et al., 2013; Kellis et al., 2014; Matys et al., 2006; Song and Crawford, 2010; Vaquerizas et al., 2009).

Due to the biological importance and implications of understanding gene regulatory machinery, many groups have dedicated themselves to develop various catalogs of TFs, their binding sites and their associated gene elements, as well as various tools for their analysis, visualization, and prediction. Knowing these elements will have important implications for understanding the cell, its development and differentiation, as well as their implications in human medicine. In this chapter, the two different approaches to TF binding analysis will be reviewed.

We will also show an overview of the different tools used and their pros and cons in practice in order to understand the general workflow of TFBS studies, as well as the experimental basis, which are necessary to identify the limitations of the field.

1.1 High-throughput Experimental Approaches to detect TF-DNA Interactions

The study of TFBS has been approached by multiple methodologies through time, each of them with particular advantages and disadvantages. The experimental methodologies can be divided into low and high throughput methods. In this chapter, we will focus on high throughput methodologies, which include Systematic Evolution of Ligands by EXponential enrichment-sequencing (SELEX-seq), Chromatin Immunoprecipitation and DNA microarrays (ChIP-on-chip), Chromatin Immunoprecipitation and sequencing (ChIP-seq and ChIP-exo), and Cleavage Under Targets (CUT&RUN and CUT&Tag). Their basis is briefly explained in the following paragraphs.

Systematic Evolution of Ligands by EXponential enrichment (SELEX, Fig. 1A) consists of finding the TFBS by creating a pool of random double-stranded DNA sequences (or aptamers) and incubating it with the TF of interest. Following, an immunoprecipitation against this protein is performed, resulting in a selection of DNA fragments containing potential TFBS. The aptamers usually have adapters in the 5' and 3' ends to allow primer hybridization (Smaczniak et al., 2017), which makes them suitable for amplification and sequencing (SELEX-seq). The main limitation of SELEX is the fact that it is performed completely *in vitro*; thus, several factors that can be important for a TF binding in a living cell, such as transcriptional co-factors, epigenetic modifications or DNA accessibility are absent (Park, 2009).

Chromatin Immunoprecipitation (ChIP) allows the identification of DNA fragments bound to a TF. The first step in ChIP is the fixation of DNA-protein complexes with formaldehyde, followed by fragmentation of the DNA. Next, only the DNA bound to the TF of interest is immunoprecipitated using specific antibodies and isolated. The advantage of ChIP is that it captures the DNA-protein interaction *in vivo*; however, it depends on the formaldehyde fixation and the efficiency of the antibody used to immunoprecipitate. The DNA obtained from ChIP can be evaluated by multiple methods to identify the DNA fragments that contain a TFBS; for instance, it can be evaluated by DNA microarrays (ChIP-on-chip) or by high throughput sequencing (ChIP-seq, Fig. 1B) (Park, 2009; Collas, 2010). ChIP-exo is a variant of ChIP-seq which uses exonucleases to reduce the length of the DNA fragments used for sequencing, which improves resolution and the identification of TFBSs (Rhee and Pugh, 2011). These methods offer several advantages, such as the low number of cells needed, the high amount of information generated, the reliability and the higher signal to noise ratio (Fattori et al., 2014).

Cleavage Under Targets and Release Using Nuclease (CUT&RUN, Fig. 1C) is a strategy that utilizes TF-specific antibodies and a micrococcal nuclease (MNase) to produce and select the specific DNA fragments bound to the TF *in situ*. Briefly, in this approach, TFs of interest are recognized by a specific antibody coupled with the MNase, which then cleaves the DNA in the surrounding nucleotides of the TFBS, releasing the TF-DNA complexes. Finally, DNA is extracted, amplified and used for high throughput sequencing (Skene and Henikoff, 2017). Cleavage Under Targets and Tagmentation (CUT&Tag) is an *in situ* methodology derived from CUT&RUN. Instead of MNase, it utilizes a transposase that cleaves the DNA and integrates sequencing adapters at the same time. DNA fragments bound to TFs are purified and sequenced (Kaya-Okur et al., 2019). The advantages of these methodologies are the absence of crosslinking, the reduction of background noise, cost and time compared to ChIP-seq, the low number of required starting cells and the improved resolution of TFBSs identification. Due to all of their advantages, CUT protocols are quickly establishing themselves over ChIP-seq as the standard methods for obtaining genome-wide TFBS.

Finally, data obtained from all the methodologies described above require specific pre-processing to generate a set of selected sequences that contain a potential TFBS that one aims to identify. These final sequences are used as input in the *de novo* motif discovery tools (*Section 3*).

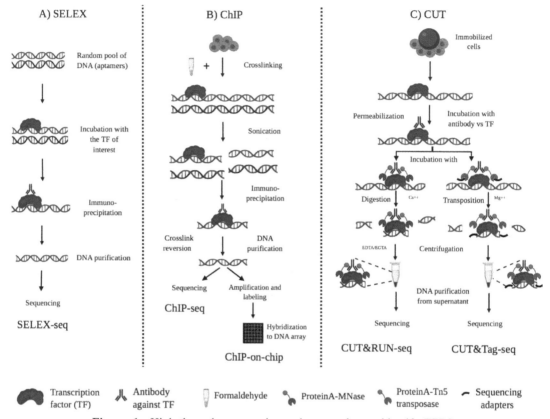

Figure 1   High-throughput experimental approaches to identify TFBSs.

(A) SELEX-seq: A random pool of DNA fragments are incubated with a TF of interest *in vitro*, the DNA-TF complexes are immunoprecipitated and sequenced. (B) ChIP: the DNA-TF interactions in a cell are fixated with formaldehyde and sonicated to break the strands, then TF-DNA complexes are immunoprecipitated and the DNA fragments are evaluated through DNA microarrays (ChIP-on-chip) or sequenced (ChIP-seq). (C) CUT: cells are permeabilized to allow the entrance of the reagents and immobilized on magnetic beads, then the antibody binds to the TF and is recognized by an A-MNase (CUT&RUN) or by a transposase (CUT&Tag), which break the surrounding DNA and allow the isolation of the DNA-TF complexes, finally isolated DNA is sequenced.

2   TF BINDING MOTIF REPRESENTATIONS

TFBS can be represented (or modeled) in different ways, which provide different levels of information about the motif recognized by the TF. For instance, the consensus string is the most basic and simple representation, since it depicts the most frequent nucleotide in a motif (i.e., CTCF binding motif 5'-TGGCCACCAGGGGGCGCTA-3') (Matrix Profile, 2020; Stormo, 2000; Schneider, 2002). Other simple representations exist, such as mismatch strings (MM) and IUPAC strings, which are consensus representations that permit mismatches or include IUPAC degenerate base symbols, respectively (Sandve et al., 2007).

However, TFs do not recognize fixed and invariable sequences; instead, the nucleotides in each position of a binding site are variable to some extent and the consensus representation does not capture the complexity of TFBS recognition. To address these issues, other representations have been proposed, such as Position Weight Matrix (PWM) (Stormo, 2013), Dinucleotide Weight Matrix (DWM) (Siddharthan, 2010) and Transcription Factor Flexible Models (TFFM) (Mathelier and Wasserman, 2013). In this section, we will describe the different representation models for TFBSs, focusing on PWMs since their use in the study of TFs is widespread.

2.1 Position Weight Matrix

A Position Weight Matrix (PWM), also referred by some authors as Position Specific Scoring Matrix (PSSM), is the most common representation of TFBS. It is constructed from a group of aligned sequences recognized by a TF (Fig. 2A). It consists of a matrix where the probability of appearance of the bases at each position is given, taking into account the background genome frequencies (Jayaram et al., 2016). A PWM is defined as a matrix of numbers ($M(b,i)$) for each base ($b = A, C, G, T$) in any position ($i = 1$ to l) of a TFBS of length L. It provides an additive score system that reflects the contribution of each position to the TF binding (Fig. 2B). PWMs offer the following advantages (Stormo, 2013):

1. It depicts the nucleotide frequencies in each position in the motif, which could reflect their importance for the TF binding.
2. It includes position-specific penalties for a mismatch; thus, mismatches at different positions are not treated equally.
3. It employs a logical, easy to understand mathematical model.
4. It is flexible, since it can be modified to incorporate additional characteristics in order to improve the representation accuracy.

The most common visualization of a PWM is via a logo representation, which shows the contribution of each position to the binding of the TF, as well as the base frequency associated with each of them. In a typical logo representation, the x-axis shows each position of the motif, and the y-axis the information content (IC) measured in bits (Fig. 2C). When the frequency of each nucleotide at a given position is random (taking into account the specific composition of each base in the genome), the IC equals 0. In the opposite case, if a particular nucleotide is found in that position in 100% of the sequences, the IC at that position would be 2. This measure indicates the importance of that position to the specificity of the TF. Consequently, positions with the highest IC are the most critical to the binding, while the ones with the lowest values can have variations without having big effects on the binding (Stormo, 2013). Further information on the computation of the IC, as well as the equations and concepts, can be found in Stormo, 2013.

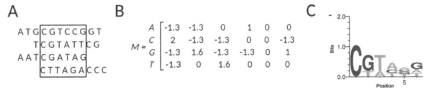

Figure 2 PWM and its representation.
(A) Aligned sequences containing the 6 nucleotides where a hypothetical TF binds. (B) PWM of the TFBS; each element in the matrix represents the score of every base at any position of the motif. (C) Logo representation of the hypothetical TFBS.

Even though this model is the most used nowadays, it is important to remember that it is just a way to approximate and represent the real specificity of a protein, and it has limitations as any model. First, this model assumes that each position contributes independently and additively to the binding of the TF, which is not always true (Man, 2001). This simplification is preferred because a complete dependence model would require to estimate a joint distribution that grows exponentially with the size of the motif and becomes computationally intractable (Hannenhalli, 2008). Also, when trying to scan PWM to the genome, in order to find new TFBS, the false-positive rate is usually high. This could happen because some TFBS might be in a non-permissive locus, being inaccessible to the TF (Stormo, 2000). Finally, it is worth mentioning that the representation accuracy of the TFBS is highly dependent on the algorithms that generate the PWM, as well as the parameters that they use. Therefore, they can lead to poor models that result from the limitations of the tools, not from the PWM approach *per se* (Stormo, 2013). Nevertheless, due to their simplicity and interpretability PWMs remain a popular and standard representation of TFBS.

2.2   Other Representations

Given the limitations of PWMs, which assume independence among nucleotides in a TFBS, there have been several efforts to develop alternative representations capable of incorporating additional information that allow the improvement of TFBS predictions in new locations.

As an example, one way to improve the consensus and PWM representations is by incorporating the inter-position dependence between the nucleotides in a motif. As an example, given a group of sequences known to be recognized by a TF, Osada et al., 2004 also considered the number of shared bases and the pairwise nucleotide dependencies within the sequence to construct their model. The work of Osada et al., along with other studies, show that the incorporation of the inter-position dependencies improves the prediction of new sites in the genome (Barash et al., 2003; Bulyk et al., 2002; King and Roth, 2002).

Another approach was proposed by Hannenhalli and Wang, who used mixture models to search for subclasses of a given TFBS. The rationale behind this approach is that one TF can have different binding preferences depending on the biological context (i.e., cell type or high and low-affinity sites); thus, classifying one PWM into subclasses of PWMs can provide better TFBS predictions (Hannenhalli and Wang, 2005).

Finally, an important representation model is the one introduced by Mathelier and Wasserman, named Transcription Factor Flexible Model (TFFM), which is based on Hidden Markov Models. The main advantage of this model is its capacity to capture nucleotide inter-position dependencies and variable lengths in a motif, which has led this model to outperform PWMs in several contexts. Furthermore, the TFBS database Jaspar (*Section 4*) contains TFFM in addition to the PWMs (Fornes et al., 2020; Mathelier and Wasserman, 2013).

3   *De novo* MOTIF DISCOVERY: OBTAINING TFBSS FROM A SET OF SEQUENCES

A number of methods with different approaches have been developed to find the optimal model with accurate weights to generate the best representation of the TFBS. The problem of *de novo* motif discovery can be stated as following: given a group of sequences, one must infer both the binding motif and the position (which can be different for each sequence) at the same time. Solving this problem involves applying some form of algorithm to find the most likely TFBS motif and constructing its corresponding PWM or another representation model. Finally, the resultant motifs can be evaluated with different tools (Section 4) to filter the best TFBS candidates that could play a potential biological role.

The main challenges in *de novo* motif discovery are that, given a set of sequences with different lengths and unknown motifs at unknown positions, we have to obtain an accurate motif representation. Furthermore, the motifs are usually not identical to each other, since some nucleotide positions might not be critical for the binding of the TF (Hashim et al., 2019). With over a hundred publications to date and countless software tools, *de novo* motif discovery has been one of the oldest core computational problems tackled in the field of bioinformatics. They can be classified according to the approach of their algorithms in enumerative, probabilistic, nature-inspired, deep learning-based and ensemble (Fig. 3). For the purposes of this book, only the most representative and widely used methods will be described (Table 1).

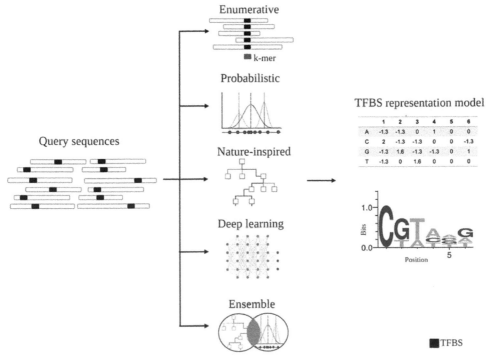

Figure 3 *De novo* motif discovery.
Sequences with a potential TFBS are used to perform the *de novo* motif discovery analysis, which can be done with enumerative (simple-word enumeration), probabilistic (EM), nature-inspired (GA), deep learning-based (CNN) or ensembl approaches. After this step, a TFBS representation is obtained, such as a PWM, which can be represented as a sequence logo.

3.1 Enumerative Approaches

Enumerative approaches perform an exhaustive search for a consensus motif by the comparison and computation of the similarity between oligonucleotides. Therefore, this method is more likely to find the global optimum (i.e., the best solution in the whole search space). It works well for short motifs, as the ones found in eukaryotes, and is suitable for finding totally constrained motifs (i.e., where all the instances are identical) (Bailey, 2011). Some of the programs that use this approach are DREME (Bailey, 2011) and CisFinder (Sharov and Ko, 2009).

Since this approach analyzes the frequencies of all the DNA strings in order to generate a PWM from the overrepresented oligonucleotides identified (Jayaram et al., 2016), it has an exponential time complexity. Thus, it has problems handling big data or finding long motifs. Also, it needs a high amount of parameters specified by the user, such as motif length, mismatches allowed and a certain number of sequences where the motif appears. In addition, because most of the TF in eukaryotes have weak constrained positions, the results of this approach can be problematic, so they need to be post-processed with clustering systems (Hashim et al., 2019).

In order to adapt these methods to high-throughput sequencing data, parallel processing and optimized data structures have been implemented to accelerate the algorithms.

DREME is a simple word enumeration method developed to find multiple short, non-redundant and statistically significant eukaryotic motifs in an optimized way using regular expression words. The speed is achieved in part by limiting the search to short motifs (4–8 bp). Also, it is exhaustive for exact words and heuristic for words with wildcards. The general algorithm workflow starts with generating a set of short oligonucleotides, which are tested with Fisher's exact test using a threshold to calculate the significance of each k-mer. This test looks for an overrepresentation of the sequence identified as a motif in the data. To perform it, two datasets are used: the enriched regions obtained from an experimental technique (Section 2) and unrelated regions, which could be shuffled sequences produced from the same dataset (Bailey, 2011). The most significant motif is used in an inner loop, where it becomes a seed regular expression to conduct a beam search that identifies the most significant generalization (Hannenhalli, 2008). Then, a PWM is created by aligning the sequences that match with the suggested motif. Finally, the best motif is erased in order to find multiple non-redundant motifs, and the previous steps are repeated iteratively until there are no more motifs found with an E-value less than the specified significance threshold (Bailey, 2011).

An alternative approach is CisFinder, a word clustering-based method that detects short motifs as well, but with a more efficient processing speed. This method is based on clustering short Position Frequency Matrices (PFMs) that are overrepresented in the dataset using a hypergeometric probability distribution, similar to the method described above. Briefly, PFMs are estimated from 8 base pairs sequences with and without gaps. Then, the flanking regions of the overrepresented motifs are extended, generating PFM for the sequences in the gaps and on the sides. If these regions are not informative, they are trimmed. Then, these matrices are clustered based on their similarity using Pearson correlations. After single-linkage clustering, each group is evaluated for homogeneity and separated if they are not similar enough. Separated motifs are used as seeds for adding more motifs, which are later evaluated. These processes are repeated iteratively until all the motifs are separated in homogeneous groups. Finally, the PWM of each entire cluster is estimated, giving as result several non-redundant TF binding motifs. The advantage of this method is its capacity to discover multiple and weak motifs in a single run, even with a low level of enrichment and the ability to process large sequences (Sharov and Ko, 2009).

3.2   Probabilistic Approaches

Probabilistic approaches are the most used currently. They test PWM parameters with probabilistic methods while doing multiple local sequence alignment (Narlikar and Ovcharenko, 2009). These algorithms have some improvements in comparison to the enumeration ones: they are faster, require fewer parameters, remain unaffected by motif length, can handle big datasets and are able to find weak constrained motifs (i.e., motifs where not all the instances are identical). Nevertheless, these algorithms scale poorly with dataset size and converge to a locally optimal solution (Hashim et al., 2019). These methods typically use Expectation Maximization (EM), like MEME, and Gibbs sampling, like Align ACE (Hughes et al., 2000).

EM is a deterministic approach that works under the assumption that each sequence of the data has at least one common motif. It works in two phases: the expectation and the maximization. During the expectation phase, the score for different motifs in all the sequences is estimated based on the entries in the PWM and the base pair composition of the genome (which reflects the background probability of each nucleotide). In the second step, those estimated values are used to refine the PWM through several iterations (Hashim et al., 2019). This approach uses oligonucleotides from the data as starting points to increase the probability of getting to a global optimum (Storm, 2000). In other words, the goal in this method is to find an initial motif and then use the described phases to improve it until it converges to a locally optimal solution. This approach has been widely used in various software tools, being MEME (Multiple EM for Motif Elicitation) (Bailey and Elkan, 1994) the most popular. The main disadvantages are that this algorithm is very sensitive to the initial conditions and it assumes only one TF binding motif per sequence (Hashim et al., 2019). Also, it is very time consuming, so a usual strategy when using this algorithm in large datasets is to run it on a small subset of the data.

Another algorithm that is widely used is Gibbs sampling. This is a Markov Chain Monte Carlo (MCMC) approach, where the results of every step depend only on the immediately previous state. This is rather a stochastic model since each step is based on random sampling. In this approach, the mutual segments within the sequences are analyzed. The goal is to find the best common pattern, which is obtained by localizing the alignment with the highest ratio of pattern probability to background one (Das and Dai, 2007). It is less dependent on the initial conditions, but more dependent on the input sequences. Align ACE (Hughes et al., 2000) is a program that uses Gibbs sampling. This program evaluates the motifs with the MAP (maximum *a priori* log-likelihood) score, which judges the motifs that are obtained through the course of the program. Briefly, this score takes into account the direct relationship between the number of aligned sites and the degree of overrepresentation of the TF binding motif in the input data (Hannenhalli, 2008). Some of Align ACE's advantages are that the base frequencies are fixed according to the source genome, both strands of the input sequence are considered without allowing overlaps and multiple motifs can be found by masking iteratively single motifs (Hughes et al., 2000).

3.3 Nature-inspired Approaches

This category includes algorithms that have been inspired by natural phenomena. They are typically based on swarm intelligence, as well as biological, chemical and physical systems. Some of them have been created to solve complex and dynamic problems, offering low-time and optimal-cost solutions. Even though not all of them are very efficient or widely used, some have offered new approaches to the field with different advantages over the other categories. However, approaches solely based on these algorithms are rare; they are more frequently used in this field in combination with other methods. Popular algorithms used in *de novo* motif discovery include Genetic Algorithms (GA), Particle Swarm Optimization (PSO), Ant Colony Optimization (ACO) (Dorigo et al., 2004) and Artificial Bee Colony (ABC) (Hashim et al., 2019).

Genetic Algorithms are optimization procedures that iteratively improve a set of solutions (population). The main goal of these types of algorithms is the production of "offspring" results by mutation and recombination. The starting point is a set of random individuals, which are used to produce offspring. After each step, a set of new solutions is generated and evaluated, keeping only the ones with the best fitness for further exploration (i.e., the ones with the highest score). Throughout several generations, local optimum solutions are found (Hashim et al., 2019). Some methods, like rGADEM (Mercier et al., 2011), which will be explained in a following subsection, use this algorithm.

Alternative methods that have been explored in the field encompass PSO, which simulates the behavior of social animals like birds to find resources. This algorithm consists in a population of candidate solutions that keep moving in the search space. Each solution can communicate with the other ones to influence their movement toward the best positions, so that the swarm can explore and find local optimal solutions. This algorithm has been used to generate seeds that are used afterward by the EM method (Hashim et al., 2019). In a similar way, both ACO and ABC algorithms simulate the social behavior of ants and bees respectively when trying to find food. In the case of ACO, artificial ants randomly search the solution space and leave "pheromone" over their search paths for other ants to use as "memory" of good solutions and moving towards better ones. In the case of ABC, three roles of artificial bees exist: employees, onlookers and scouts. The candidate solutions can communicate as well and inform the other ones about the best positions to explore these search spaces. The evaluation of the new possible solutions are done based on the similarity values of the consensus sequences (Hashim et al., 2019).

3.4   Deep Learning

Artificial Neural Networks (ANN) are mathematical models that attempt to mimic how the biological brain learns to solve problems by training on a set of examples. In ANNs, artificial neurons are interconnected in sets of at least three layers: the input layer, one or more intermediate (hidden) layers that learn the features driving the prediction, and an output layer providing the final predicted value or values. When presented with an input example, each neuron can activate and "fire" a value to its output connections in the next layer if a certain threshold is reached. The value compared to this threshold is the weighted sum function of the values of their firing input connections in the previous layer. On each training phase, the weights for each connection are updated by backpropagating the error from the final predicted value compared to the actual value; these networks are iteratively trained until convergence to a minimum error.

Although the origin of ANNs can be traced back to the 1950s with the perceptron model (Freund and Schapire, 1999), until recently, several challenges made them difficult to apply to complex problems: large computational requirements, need for very large datasets to train with and low performance due to numerical optimization problems in the backpropagation step. However, the last two decades have seen major algorithmic breakthroughs and technological advancements that have enabled to train "deep" ANNs with many layers and millions of neurons. This new Deep Learning paradigm has enabled researchers to solve complex problems and greatly outperform conventional algorithms in a wide range of fields.

One of the first models used to predict TFBS from sequence was DeepBind (Freund and Schapire, 1999), which predicted *in vivo* and *in vitro* binding affinities of various proteins. Other methods soon followed, such as DeepSea (Zhou and Troyanska, 2015) and Basset (Goodfellow et al., 2016) which in addition to TFBS predict other features such as histone modifications and chromatin accessibility, DeepSite (Shrikumar et al., 2017) which uses protein structure in addition to sequence, DESSO (Mercier et al., 2011) that incorporates DNA shape, and many others. The success of the first Deep Learning methods have inspired a growing number of models that try to improve them in different ways, such as using more complex architectures (e.g. combining other types of networks with CNNs), solving other problems (e.g., enhancer prediction, Protein-RNA binding site prediction) or using other types of information as input in addition to the sequences (e.g., DNA methylation, phylogenetic conservation).

Although Deep Learning is making substantial gains in the genomics fields and is quickly outperforming traditional methods for TFBS, it is still considered to need some time until it reaches a mature state where non-expert users are able to make use of them on a daily basis. A standardized protocol to develop, train, report, validate and share the models has yet to be defined by the scientific community, making most models difficult to use or adapt to other more specific problems. Some challenges also remain to be tackled, such as training with a low number of examples, improving the interpretability of more complex architectures and defining good sets of "negative" examples to train with. Nevertheless, given their superior performance and multi-tasking capabilities it is just a matter of time until these drawbacks are surpassed and Deep Learning becomes the standard method for TFBS prediction.

3.5   Ensemble Approaches

The programs described here combine different approaches from the above-described algorithms. Therefore, there is not an established algorithm or a set of characteristics for the methods here mentioned. Rather, their strengths and limitations depend on the hybrid algorithm that results from the integration of other approaches. Examples of this type of methods are MEME-ChIP

(Ma et al., 2014), HOMER (Heinz et al., 2010), rGADEM (Mercier et al., 2011) and DeepFinder (Lee et al., 2018).

MEME-ChIP (Ma et al., 2014) is a web-based tool that mixes 4 algorithms for *de novo* motif discovery, comparison and visualization. This tool mixes the advantages of two already explained approaches; the probabilistic algorithm MEME (Bailey and Elkan, 1994) and the enumerative one DREME (Bailey, 2011). After using both approaches, CentriMo (Bailey and Machanick, 2012) evaluates the enrichment of the candidate motifs in the input data. The last component of this tool is Tomtom (Gupta et al., 2007) which helps to identify TFs that could mediate an indirect and cooperative binding in the source protein (Ma et al., 2014).

HOMER (Hypergeometric Optimization of Motif EnRichment) (Heinz et al., 2010) is a tool that combines enumeration and probabilistic approaches. The algorithm is composed of 2 stages: the first one is an exhaustive search for overrepresented putative motifs, which correspond to the enumerative stage. To speed this process, a sequence tree is used to optimize the comparison between words and the consensus motif. Then, a modified version of the Fisher exact test is used to identify the enriched motifs. Afterward, the top results are converted into probability matrices to start the probabilistic step, where the putative motifs are refined using a local hill-climbing approach, an iterative local optimization algorithm. Whenever the local optimization algorithm finds a solution, the motif is reported and the matching sequences are removed. This step is then repeated in order to find multiple motifs. In the end, the best threshold and probability matrices are reported (Heinz et al., 2010).

Table 1 Non-exhaustive list of tools used for *de novo* motif discovery

Tool	Main method(s)	Reference
Enumerative		
DREME	Simple-word enumeration	(Bailey, 2011)
CisFinder	Word-clustering based method	(Sharov and Ko, 2009)
Probabilistic		
MEME	Expectation Maximization	(Bailey and Elkan, 1994)
Align ACE	Gibbs sampling	(Hughes et al., 2000)
Deep learning-based		
DESSO	Convolutional Neural Networks	(Yang et al., 2019)
DeepBind	Convolutional Neural Networks	(Alipanahi et al., 2015)
DeepSite	Convolutional Neural Networks	(Zhang et al., 2020)
Basset	Convolutional Neural Networks	(Kelley et al., 2016)
Combinatorial		
MEME-ChIP	Expectation Maximization and simple-word enumeration	(Ma et al., 2014)
HOMER	Enumeration and hill-climbing approach	(Heinz et al., 2010)
rGADEM	Genetic Algorithm and Expectation Maximization	(Mercier et al., 2011)
DeepFinder	Probabilistic algorithms and neural networks	(Lee et al., 2018)

Alternatively, rGADEM (Mercier et al., 2011) is an R package that combines GA with EM. Briefly, short candidate words of 4–6 nucleotides are used to construct spaced dyads (i.e., motifs with gaps in between). These spaced dyads are sorted according to their enrichment in the input dataset, followed by a conversion to PWM. The matrices are then optimized with EM and passed to the GA as starting points in order to increase the probability of finding the best local optimums. Afterward, the GA runs with the generated population, where the fitness score is based on the logarithm of the E-value. The motif with a fitness value less or equal to a specified cutoff value is reported, followed by the mask of its binding sites in the input dataset. This step is repeated iteratively to find multiple motifs until no new ones with the required fitness value are found. This tool can process big datasets, identifies multiple dimer and monomer motifs and adjusts motif widths, offering a fast and efficient framework (Mercier et al., 2011).

Finally, DeepFinder (Lee et al., 2018) utilizes other tools for identification of initial candidate motifs (MEME, MotifSampler, Bioprospector and MDSCAN), followed by a stacked-autoencoder neural network learning step which is used to predict the associated TFBS in the input sequences.

4   MOTIF PREDICTION: IDENTIFYING CANDIDATE TFBS IN THE GENOME

As mentioned in the previous sections, the approaches for *de novo* motif discovery yield a high number of false-positive sites because TFBS are short and variable (Bulyk, 2003). To address this problem, PWMs obtained from the discovery phase or from a database containing TFBS (Box A) can be further filtered to retain only the candidates with a potential biological function. Furthermore, we can use PWMs to know if a particular TFBS is contained in a sequence of interest, such as a promoter region. In this section, we refer as "prediction" to the process of scanning a region of interest for a TFBS.

Box A   Databases containing human PWM

There are different databases where PWMs can be obtained, being TRANSFAC (Matys et al, 2006) and JASPAR (Fornes et al., 2020) the most popular. However, other ones have information of human binding sites as well, like HOCOMOCO (Kulakovskiy et al., 2018), HOMER (Heinz et al., 2010) and CIS-BP (Weirauch et al., 2014) (Table 2).

Table 2   TFBS databases

Database	*Description*	*Link*
TRANSFAC (Matys et al., 2006)	Focused on model organisms > 67,000 manually annotated TF interactions ≈ 7000 TF binding profiles	http://genexplain.com/transfac/
JASPAR (Fornes et al., 2020)	Focused on 6 main taxonomic groups ≈ 1700 TF binding profiles	http://jaspar.genereg.net/
HOCOMOCO (Kulakovskiy et al., 2018)	Focused on mice and humans ≈ 680 human and 453 mouse TF binding profiles	https://hocomoco11.autosome.ru/
HOMER(Heinz et al., 2010)	Focused on humans ≈ 400 TF binding profiles	http://homer.ucsd.edu/homer/ motif/motifDatabase.html
CIS-BP (Weirauch et al., 2014)	Wide range of species (> 700 organisms) > 165,000 TF binding profiles Collects data from >70 sources	http://cisbp.ccbr.utoronto.ca/

TRANSFAC is a commercial database that contains TFBS of several species, with a focus on model organisms. It has more than 67,000 manually annotated TF site interactions, over 7,000 PWM derived from experimental evidence, and more than 2,000 TFBS ChIP-seq experiment reports. Additionally, it offers additional tools and data, like pathway visualization for regulatory networks, promoter reports and TF reports (Matys et al, 2006).

JASPAR is an open-access database of curated, non-redundant TF binding profiles derived from experimental evidence and ChIP-seq data. These representations are stored as PWMs and TFFMs and cover a wide range of species grouped in six main taxonomic groups (vertebrates, plants, insects, nematodes, fungi and Urochordata). It is the most complete free resource, collecting over 1,700 TF binding profiles (Fornes et al., 2020).

Finally, some research groups have made alternative databases with public data analyzed or curated in a different way, which is typically utilizing their own software tools. HOCOMOCO (Kulakovskiy et al., 2018) (Homo sapiens comprehensive Model Collection) provides TF binding models for 680 human and 453 mouse TFs. All of these models are generated with ChIPMunk, a probabilistic de novo motif discovery tool that mixes greedy optimization with bootstrapping (Kulkovskiy et al., 2010). On the other hand, HOMER is a database maintained as part of the HOMER software. It is based on the analysis of public datasets using their suggested approach, collecting over 400 TF binding representations (Heinz et al., 2010). Finally, CIS-BP is a public database that incorporates data of more than 390,000 TFs data from around 700 species. It collects data from other databases like TRANSFAC and JASPAR. The novelty of this database is that it includes inferred motifs, which are TF binding motifs that are inferred from related species with the known TFBS of the ortholog protein (Weirauch et al., 2014). It is important to mention that several other databases that focus on specific organisms exist. However, since they do not contain human-related content, they are not mentioned.

The first step of the prediction process is the search for occurrences of one or multiple PWMs in a sequence of interest (Fig. 4A) (Korhonen et al., 2017). Several tools are available for this purpose which can search for individual sites or for several TFBS (clusters) (Jayaram et al., 2016). For a detailed review on the topic, see Aerts, 2012, Hannenhalli, 2008, Das and Dai, 2007 and Bulyk, 2003. The principle behind the prediction of TFBS is the search for the number of occurrences (or matches) in a sequence of interest, given one PWM. Several tools are available for this purpose which rely on nucleotide sequence information only and use a pattern matching method to identify an occurrence. The degree of match can be represented in different ways (*p*-value, percentage, etc.), depending on the method used (Hannenhalli, 2008; Aerts, 2012). Some example tools are: FIMO (Grant et al., 2011), MATCH (Kel et al., 2003) and Matrix-Scan (Turatsinze et al., 2008).

Once the starting match-based search has been performed, tools are available for predicting and/or filtering potential false positive matches by incorporating extra layers of biological information, such as evolutionary conservation, gene expression or epigenetic data (Aerts, 2012), which will be briefly described in the following subsections.

4.1 TFBS Clusters

This approach is based on searching for clusters of TFBS in a region (Fig. 4B), instead of looking for individual TFBSs. The premise is that transcriptional regulation is not controlled by one TF, but by a combination of several ones and that regulatory regions with a higher density of TFBS (clusters) can be biologically relevant. Most of the tools developed, search for clusters of TFBS regardless of the order, strand or the separation between the sites (Aerts, 2012). Representative examples of tools are Cluster-Buster (Frith et al., 2003), MCast (Grant et al., 2016) and BayCis (Lin et al., 2008).

4.2 Phylogenetic Footprinting

The premise of phylogenetic footprinting is that TFBSs located in conserved regions among different species (orthologous) are more likely to be biologically relevant, in contrast to TFBSs located in non-conserved regions (Fig. 4C). Phylogenetic footprinting is capable of identifying potential TFBSs for a single region in the genome, provided that it is conserved across other species (orthologous). For a detailed description of phylogenetic footprinting see Hannenhalli, 2008.

Several tools have been developed and can significantly improve the discovery of relevant motifs (Das and Dai, 2007). These tools usually involve two phases: (1) global multiple alignment of the orthologous sequences and (2) identification of the conserved region in the alignment. Some tools also incorporate a third phase which includes the search for matching PWMs, only if the TF binding site is conserved (Das and Dai, 2007; Aerts, 2012). Some examples of tools are: TargetOrtho (Glenwinkel et al., 2014), rVISTA (Loots and Ovcharenko, 2004), MONKEY (Moses et al., 2004) and TFLOC (Fujita et al., 2011).

4.3 Co-expression

These approaches work under the assumption that genes with similar patterns of expression (co-regulated) can contain some similarities in their regulatory regions, including TFBSs (Fig. 4D). Thus, the purpose is to find PWM matches enriched or overrepresented in co-expressed genes (Das and Dai, 2007). This is usually done with the integration of RNA-seq or expression microarray data.

4.4 Multiple Evidence

These approaches take advantage of the high number of genome-wide data available, such as gene expression and epigenetic modifications, to identify combinatorial codes and to better predict TFBSs (Fig. 4E) (Aerts, 2012). As an example, PriorsEditor (Klepper and Drabløs, 2010) is a tool that can combine different data, such as phylogenetic conservation, DNA melting temperatures, nucleosome-positioning, GC content, DNA bendability and DNA duplex-free energy to better identify functional TFBS in a cell type of interest. Other examples are CHROMIA (Cheng et al., 2011), CENTIPEDE (Pique-Regi et al., 2011) and MotifLab (Klepper and Drabløs, 2013).

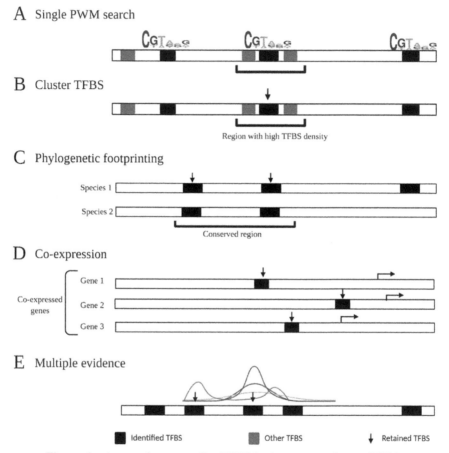

Figure 4 Approaches to predict TFBS in the genome from a PWM.

(A) Initial matching of a PWM in a region provides potential TFBSs. Further methods can be used to reduce the false-positives based on; (B) the density of TFBS (clusters); (C) conservation of the matching region across different species; (D) the presence of co-expressed genes in the sample; (E) integration of several layers of information such as phylogenetic conservation, GC content and physicochemical information of the protein, among others.

5 CONCLUDING REMARKS

Studies performing comparisons between methods for discovering TFBS have not had conclusive results (i.e., no method consistently outperforms the others in all data sets). Interestingly, most algorithms work better in simpler organisms' data, like yeasts, than in similarly created datasets from higher organisms, like mice and humans (Das and Dai, 2007). Therefore, no standard methodology exists; the accuracy and performance of the approaches change with different input data.

Additionally, it is very difficult to evaluate the performance of *de novo* motif discovery and PWM scanning tools. In order to do so, one should have complete annotations of precise validated sets of TFBS in the DNA for specific proteins, which would be used as a gold standard reference. This kind of information is usually missing or limited in the majority of situations. However, in human ChIP-seq data, rGADEM has shown to be one of the best-performing tools, outperforming HOMER and MEME-ChIP (Jayaram et al., 2016). Regarding PWM scanning tools, MCAST and FIMO perform better than some of its competitors (Jayaram et al., 2016).

It is worth to mention that some TFs interact with other partners in the cell, which might change their binding motif either by indirect binding (the partners are the ones that bind to the DNA) or cooperative binding (the protein binds to a different motif when interacting with its partner). Furthermore, we must remember that, in a cell, there are multiple factors that influence the specific binding of a TF. Just to mention some, the methylation status of a sequence can change the affinity of the binding of the protein, as well as the DNA shape, features of the sequence, the GC content of the surrounding regions, the concentration of other molecules and other context variables (Inukai et al., 2010). These factors add additional layers of complexity that are not being totally captured in the developed methods, and need to be taken into account when interpreting the motif discovery and prediction results.

By understanding the limitations of the protocols and tools, we can explore further hypotheses and build models that could explain the biological phenomenon we are interested in. Therefore, advances toward integrating different types of data offer very promising approaches that will very likely increase the accurateness of the current TFBS models.

Acknowledgements

We thank CONACyT FOSISS (290041) for their support in the present work. MSA is grateful for a PhD fellowship funding from CONACYT (CVU659273) and the German Academic Exchange Service, DAAD (ref. 91693321). KTA is thankful for a Masters scholarship from CONACYT (CVU1009360). NA would like to acknowledge the Independent Research Fund Denmark (6108-2700038B). ESR would like to acknowledge the CB-SEP-CONACyT (284748) grant, and Fondo desarrollo, tecnológico e innov. COVID-19 (312021).

REFERENCES

Aerts, S. (2012). Computational strategies for the genome-wide identification of cis-Regulatory elements and transcriptional targets. pp. 121–145. *In*: S. Plaza and F. Payre (eds). Current Topics in Developmental Biology. Academic Press.

Alipanahi, B., A. Delong, M.T. Weirauch and B.J. Frey (2015). Predicting the sequence specificities of DNA- and RNA-binding proteins by deep learning. Nat. Biotechnol. 33(8): 831–838.

Bailey, T.L. and C. Elkan (1994). Fitting a mixture model by expectation maximization to discover motifs in biopolymers. Proc. Int. Conf. Intell. Syst. Mol. Biol. 2: 28.

Bailey, T.L. (2011). DREME: Motif discovery in transcription factor ChIP-seq data. Bioinformatics. 27(12): 1653–1659.

Bailey, T.L. and P. Machanick (2012). Inferring direct DNA binding from ChIP-seq. Nucleic Acids Res. 40(17): e128.

Barash, Y., G. Elidan, N. Friedman and T. Kaplan (2003). Modeling dependencies in protein-DNA binding sites. pp. 28–37. In: Proceedings of the seventh annual international conference on Research in computational molecular biology. New York, NY, USA: Association for Computing Machinery; 2003. (RECOMB '03).

Bejerano, G., M. Pheasant, I. Makunin, S. Stephen, W.J. Kent, J.S. Mattick, et al. (2004). Ultraconserved elements in the human genome. Science. 304(5675): 1321–1325.

Bulyk, M.L., P.L.F. Johnson and G.M. Church (2002). Nucleotides of transcription factor binding sites exert interdependent effects on the binding affinities of transcription factors. Nucleic Acids Res. 30(5): 1255–1261.

Bulyk, M.L., (2003). Computational prediction of transcription-factor binding site locations. Genome Biol. 2003 Dec 23; 5(1): 201.

Cheng, C., C. Shou, K.Y. Yip and M.B. Gerstein (2011). Genome-wide analysis of chromatin features identifies histone modification sensitive and insensitive yeast transcription factors. Genome Biol.12(11): R111.

Collas, P. (2010). The current state of chromatin immunoprecipitation. Mol. Biotechnol. 45(1): 87–100.

Cusanovich, D.A., B. Pavlovic, J.K. Pritchard and Y. Gilad (2014). The functional consequences of variation in transcription factor binding. PLoS Genet. 10(3): e1004226.

Das, M.K. and H.K. Dai (2007). A survey of DNA motif finding algorithms. BMC Bioinformatics. 8(Suppl 7): S21.

Degner, J.F., A.A. Pai, R. Pique-Regi, J.B. Veyrieras, D.J. Gaffney, J.K. Pickrell, et al. (2012). DNase I sensitivity QTLs are a major determinant of human expression variation. Nature. 482(7385): 390–394.

Dorigo, M. (2009). Du Fnrs Marco Dorigo, D de R, and Stützle, T. Ant Colony Optimization. MIT Press; 2004. 305 p.

ENCODE Project Consortium. An integrated encyclopedia of DNA elements in the human genome. Nature. 489(7414): 57–74.

Fattori, J., N. de Carvalho Indolfo, J.C.L. de Oliveira Campos, N.B. Videira, A.V. Bridi, T.R. Doratioto, et al. (2014). Investigation of interactions between DNA and nuclear receptors: A review of the most used methods
. Nuclear Receptor Research. 1: 1–20.

Fornes, O., J.A. Castro-Mondragon, A. Khan, R. van der Lee, X. Zhang, P.A. Richmond, et al. (2020). JASPAR 2020: Update of the open-access database of transcription factor binding profiles. Nucleic Acids Res. 48(D1): D87–D92.

Freund, Y. and R.E. Schapire (1999). Large margin classification using the perceptron algorithm. Mach Learn. 37(3): 277–296.

Frith, M.C., M.C. Li and Z. Weng (2003). Cluster-Buster: Finding dense clusters of motifs in DNA sequences. Nucleic Acids Res. 31(13): 3666–3668.

Fujita, P.A., B. Rhead, A.S. Zweig, A.S. Hinrichs, D. Karolchik, M.S. Cline, et al. (2011). The UCSC genome browser database: Update 2011. Nucleic Acids Res. 39(Database issue): D876–D882.

Fulton, D.L., S. Sundararajan, G. Badis, T.R. Hughes, W.W. Wasserman, J.C. Roach, et al. (2009). TFCat: the curated catalog of mouse and human transcription factors. Genome Biol. 10(3): R29.

Glenwinkel, L., D. Wu, G. Minevich and O. Hobert (2014). TargetOrtho: A phylogenetic footprinting tool to identify transcription factor targets. Genetics. 197(1): 61–76.

Goodfellow, I., Y. Bengio and A. Courville (2016). Deep Learning. MIT Press. 800 p.

Grant, C.E., T.L. Bailey and W.S. Noble (2011). FIMO: Scanning for occurrences of a given motif. Bioinformatics. 27(7): 1017–1018.

Grant, C.E., J. Johnson, T.L. Bailey and W.S. Noble (2016). MCAST: Scanning for cis-Regulatory motif clusters. Bioinformatics. 32(8): 1217–1219.

Gupta, S., J.A. Stamatoyannopoulos, T.L. Bailey and W.S. Noble (2007). Quantifying similarity between motifs. Genome Biol. 8(2): R24.

Hannenhalli, S. and L.S. Wang (2005). Enhanced position weight matrices using mixture models. Bioinformatics. Suppl 1: i204–i212. doi: 10.1093/bioinformatics/bti1001.

Hannenhalli, S. (2008). Eukaryotic transcription factor binding sites–modeling and integrative search methods. Bioinformatics. 24(11): 1325–1331.

Hashim, F.A., M.S. Mabrouk and W. Al-Atabany (2019). Review of different sequence motif finding algorithms. Avicenna J. Med. Biotechnol. 11(2): 130–148.

Heinz, S., C. Benner, N. Spann, E. Bertolino, Y.C. Lin, P. Laslo, et al. (2010). Simple combinations of lineage-determining transcription factors prime cis-Regulatory elements required for macrophage and B cell identities. Mol. Cell. 38(4): 576–589.

Hughes, J.D., P.W. Estep, S. Tavazoie and G.M. Church (2000). Computational identification of cis-regulatory elements associated with groups of functionally related genes in Saccharomyces cerevisiae. J. Mol. Biol. 296(5): 1205–1214.

Inukai, S., K.H. Kock and M.L. Bulyk (2017). Transcription factor–DNA binding: Beyond binding site motifs. Curr. Opin. Genet. Dev. 43: 110–119.

Jayaram, N., D.R. Usvyat and A.C. Martin (2016). Evaluating tools for transcription factor binding site prediction. BMC Bioinformatics. 17(1): 547.

Jolma, A., J. Yan, T. Whitington, J. Toivonen, K.R. Nitta, P. Rastas, et al. (2013). DNA-binding specificities of human transcription factors. Cell. 152(1-2): 327–339.

Kaya-Okur, H.S., S.J. Wu, C.A. Codomo, E.S. Pledger, T.D. Bryson, J.G. Henikoff, et al. (2019). CUT&Tag for efficient epigenomic profiling of small samples and single cells. Nat. Commun. 10(1): 1930.

Kel, A.E., E. Gössling, I. Reuter, E. Cheremushkin, O.V. Kel-Margoulis and E. Wingender (2003). MATCH: A tool for searching transcription factor binding sites in DNA sequences. Nucleic Acids Res. 31(13): 3576–3579.

Kelley, D.R., J. Snoek and J.L. Rinn (2016). Basset: learning the regulatory code of the accessible genome with deep convolutional neural networks. Genome Res. 2016 Jul; 26(7): 990–9.

Kellis, M., B. Wold, M.P. Snyder, B.E. Bernstein, A. Kundaje, G.K. Marinov, et al. (2014). Defining functional DNA elements in the human genome. Proc. Natl. Acad. Sci. USA. 111(17): 6131–6138.

King, O.D. and F.P. Roth (2003). A non-parametric model for transcription factor binding sites. Nucleic Acids Res. 31(19): e116.

Klepper, K. and F. Drabløs (2010). PriorsEditor: A tool for the creation and use of positional priors in motif discovery. Bioinformatics. 26(17): 2195–2197.

Klepper, K. and F. Drabløs (2013). MotifLab: A tools and data integration workbench for motif discovery and regulatory sequence analysis. BMC Bioinformatics. 14: 9.

Korhonen, J.H., K. Palin, J. Taipale and E. Ukkonen (2017). Fast motif matching revisited: high-order PWMs, SNPs and indels. Bioinformatics. 2017 Feb 15; 33(4): 514–21.

Kulakovskiy, I.V., V.A. Boeva, A.V. Favorov and V.J. Makeev (2010). Deep and wide digging for binding motifs in ChIP-Seq data. Bioinformatics. 26(20): 2622–2623.

Kulakovskiy, I.V., I.E. Vorontsov, I.S. Yevshin, R.N. Sharipov, A.D. Fedorova, E.I. Rumynskiy, et al. (2018). HOCOMOCO: Towards a complete collection of transcription factor binding models for human and mouse via large-scale ChIP-Seq analysis. Nucleic Acids Res. 46(D1): D252–D259.

Lambert, S.A., A. Jolma, L.F. Campitelli, P.K. Das, Y. Yin, M. Albu, et al. (2018). The human transcription factors. Cell. 172(4): 650–665.

Lee, T.I. and R.A. Young (2013). Transcriptional regulation and its misregulation in disease. Cell. 152(6): 1237–1251.

Lee, N.K., F.L. Azizan, Y.S. Wong and N. Omar (2018). DeepFinder: An integration of feature-based and deep learning approach for DNA motif discovery. Biotechnol Biotechnol Equip. 32(3): 759–768.

Lin, T.H., P. Ray, G.K. Sandve, S. Uguroglu and E.P. Xing (2008). BayCis: A bayesian hierarchical HMM for cis-Regulatory module decoding in metazoan genomes. pp. 66–81. *In*: Research in Computational Molecular Biology. Springer, Berlin, Heidelberg.

Loots, G.G. and I. Ovcharenko (2004). rVISTA 2.0: Evolutionary analysis of transcription factor binding sites. Nucleic Acids Res. 32(Web Server issue): W217–W221.

Ma, W., W.S. Noble and T.L. Bailey (2014). Motif-based analysis of large nucleotide data sets using MEME-ChIP. Nat. Protoc. 9(6): 1428–1450.

Man, T.K. (2001). Non-independence of Mnt repressor-operator interaction determined by a new quantitative multiple fluorescence relative affinity (QuMFRA) assay. Nucleic Acids Res. 29(12): 2471–2478.

Mathelier, A. and W.W. Wasserman (2013). The next generation of transcription factor binding site prediction. PLoS Comput. Biol. 9(9): e1003214.

Matrix profile: CTCF – MA0139.1 – from JASPAR 2018 [Internet]. [cited 2020 May 12]. Available from: http://jaspar.genereg.net/matrix/MA0139.1/

Matys, V., O.V. Kel-Margoulis, E. Fricke, I. Liebich, S. Land, A. Barre-Dirrie, et al. (2006). TRANSFAC(R) and its module TRANSCompel(R): Transcriptional gene regulation in eukaryotes. Nucleic Acids Res. 34(Database issue): D108–D110.

Mercier, E., A. Droit, L. Li, G. Robertson, X. Zhang and R. Gottardo (2011). An integrated pipeline for the genome-wide analysis of transcription factor binding sites from ChIP-Seq. PLoS One. 6(2): e16432.

Moses, A.M., D.Y. Chiang, D.A. Pollard, V.N. Iyer and M.B. Eisen (2004). MONKEY: Identifying conserved transcription-factor binding sites in multiple alignments using a binding site-specific evolutionary model. Genome Biol. 5(12): R98.

Narlikar, L. and I. Ovcharenko (2009). Identifying regulatory elements in eukaryotic genomes. Brief. Funct. Genomic Proteomic. 8(4): 215–230.

Nobrega, M.A., I. Ovcharenko, V. Afzal and E.M. Rubin (2003). Scanning human gene deserts for long-range enhancers. Science. 302(5644): 413.

Osada, R., E. Zaslavsky and M. Singh (2004). Comparative analysis of methods for representing and searching for transcription factor binding sites. Bioinformatics. 20(18): 3516–3525.

Park, P.J. (2009) ChIP-seq: Advantages and challenges of a maturing technology. Nat. Rev. Genet. 10(10): 669–680.

Pique-Regi, R., J.F. Degner, P.A. Pai, D.J. Gaffney, Y. Gilad and J.K. Pritchard (2011). Accurate inference of transcription factor binding from DNA sequence and chromatin accessibility data. Genome Res. 21(3): 447–455.

Rhee, H.S. and B.F. Pugh (2011). Comprehensive genome-wide protein-DNA interactions detected at single-nucleotide resolution. Cell. 147(6): 1408–1419.

Sandve, G.K., O. Abul, V. Walseng and F. Drabløs (2007). Improved benchmarks for computational motif discovery. BMC Bioinformatics. 8: 193.

Schneider, T.D. (2002). Consensus sequence zen. Appl. Bioinformatics. 1(3): 111–119.

Sharov, A.A. and M.S.H. Ko (2009). Exhaustive search for over-represented DNA sequence motifs with CisFinder. DNA Res. 16(5): 261–273.

Shrikumar, A., P. Greenside and A. Kundaje (2017). Learning important features through propagating activation differences. pp. 3145–3153. In: Proceedings of the 34th International Conference on Machine Learning, Volume 70. JMLR.org. (ICML'17).

Siddharthan, R. (2010). Dinucleotide weight matrices for predicting transcription factor binding sites: Generalizing the position weight matrix. PLoS One. 5(3): e9722.

Skene, P.J. and S. Henikoff (2017). An efficient targeted nuclease strategy for high-resolution mapping of DNA binding sites. Elife [Internet]. 6. Available from: http://dx.doi.org/10.7554/eLife.21856

Smaczniak, C., G.C. Angenent and K. Kaufmann (2017). SELEX-Seq: A method to determine DNA binding specificities of plant transcription factors. Methods Mol. Biol. 1629: 67–82.

Song, L. and G.E. Crawford (2010). DNase-seq: A high-resolution technique for mapping active gene regulatory elements across the genome from mammalian cells. Cold Spring Harb Protoc. (2): db.prot5384.

Stormo, G.D. (2000). DNA binding sites: representation and discovery. Bioinformatics. 16(1): 16–23.

Stormo, G.D. (2013). Modeling the specificity of protein-DNA interactions. Quant. Biol. 1(2): 115–130.

Turatsinze, J.V., M. Thomas-Chollier, M. Defrance and J. van Helden (2008). Using RSAT to scan genome sequences for transcription factor binding sites and cis-regulatory modules. Nat. Protoc. 3(10): 1578–1588.

Vaquerizas, J.M., S.K. Kummerfeld, S.A. Teichmann and N.M. Luscombe (2009). A census of human transcription factors: Function, expression and evolution. Nat. Rev. Genet. 10(4): 252–263.

Weirauch, M.T., A. Yang, M. Albu, A.G. Cote, A. Montenegro-Montero, P. Drewe, et al. (2014). Determination and inference of eukaryotic transcription factor sequence specificity. Cell. 158(6): 1431–1443.

Yang, J., A. Ma, A.D. Hoppe, C. Wang, Y. Li, C. Zhang, et al. (2019). Prediction of regulatory motifs from human Chip-sequencing data using a deep learning framework. Nucleic Acids Res. 47(15): 7809–7824.

Zhang, Y., S. Qiao, S. Ji and Y. Li (2020). DeepSite: Bidirectional LSTM and CNN models for predicting DNA–protein binding. International Journal of Machine Learning and Cybernetics. 11(4): 841–851.

Zhou J. and O.G. Troyanskaya (2015). Predicting effects of noncoding variants with deep learning-based sequence model. Nat. Methods. 12(10): 931–934.

Chapter 11

Bioinformatics of Prediction of Secondary Structures of Non-coding RNAs

S.S. Vinod Chandra

Department of Computer Science, Kariavattom Campus,
University of Kerala Thiruvananthapurama, Kerala

The informational view of cellular processes at a molecular level is the significant scope of computational biology and bioinformatics. Most of the computational biology problems are related to evolutionary or molecular biology and focus on analyzing and comparing the composition of key biomolecules. The Deoxy-ribo Nucleic Acid (DNA), Ribo Nucleic Acid (RNA) and Protein sequence are significant molecular biology players. Friedrich Miescher isolated the DNA molecule in 1869. James D. Watson and Francis Crick discovered its secondary structure in 1953 (Watson and Crick, 1953). After discovering the double-helical structure of DNA, researchers had turnaround into the structure identification of ribonucleic acid. This was considered a critical puzzle that can solve the highway to thoughtful the molecular basis of life. Ribonucleic acid is a molecule that consists of a long chain of nucleotide units. This nucleotide consists of a ribose sugar, nitrogenous base and phosphate. In a most sense, similarities are between the RNA and DNA molecules, but they differ in a few important structural details. Usually, in living cells, DNA is double-stranded, but RNA is single-stranded.

1 RNA

DNA and RNA are a chain of molecules called nucleotides. A nucleotide consists of phosphoric acid, a pentose sugar and an amine base. In DNA, the amine bases are Adenine (A), Guanine (G), Cytosine (C) and Thymine (T). In RNA, the amine base Uracil (U) is seen instead of Thymine along with the other three amine bases. The two ends of the nucleotide sequence are conventionally denoted as the 5' end and the 3' end.

Corresponding author: *vinod@keralauniversity.ac.in*

DNA contains deoxyribose, which is a type of ribose that lacks one oxygen atom. But RNA nucleotides contain ribose. In DNA, thymine is present while RNA has the base uracil. Figure 1 gives the basic RNA structure. The presence of a hydroxyl group at the 2′ position of the ribose sugar is a fundamental difference between RNA and DNA. The 2′-hydroxyl group's presence is that in conformational flexible regions of an RNA molecule. It is not involved in forming a double helix and nearby phosphodiester bond to cleave the backbone is another difference. The difference between DNA and RNA chain is shown in Fig. 2.

1.1 Central Dogma of Molecular Biology

RNA plays an essential role in molecular biology's central dogma, namely, the transcription and translation process. DNA is transcribed into RNA by an enzyme called RNA polymerases and further processed by other enzymes. Generally, we can say that RNA is central to the synthesis of proteins. Messenger RNA (mRNA) is the player who carries information from DNA to ribosomes. The ribosome structures are made from proteins and ribosomal RNAs. It is a molecular machine that can read the mRNA's message and translate the information they carry into proteins.

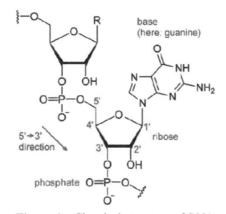

Figure 1   Chemical structure of RNA.

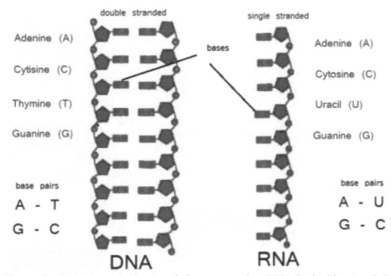

Figure 2   RNA is a single-stranded sequence, but DNA is double-stranded.

Some of the viruses have double-stranded RNA but most of the cellular RNAs are single-stranded. This is folded upon entirely or in certain regions. The majority of the bases are complementary and jointed by a hydrogen bond. The stability of the molecule is basically by this bond. There is no complement in the unfolded region because this RNA does not have the purine or pyrimidine equality found in DNA.

As accepted in the central dogma of molecular biology (Fig. 3), the flow of information from DNA to RNA to proteins has traditionally been less focused on RNA than in the other two. The attention received by genomics and proteomics as compared to transcriptomics is a pointer to this. Genomics is the study of the genomes of organisms. Proteomics is the large-scale study of proteins, particularly their structures and functions. The transcriptome is the set of all mRNA molecules, or "transcripts", produced in one or a population of cells. However, of late, RNA has been receiving much better attention as regards its direct and indirect roles in the basic cellular processes. RNA plays an essential role in molecular biology's central dogma, namely, the transcription and translation process (Novina and Sharp, 2004).

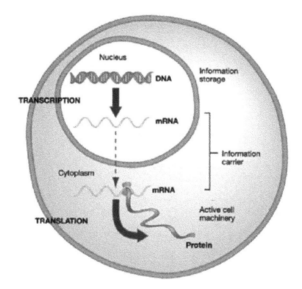

Figure 3   Central dogma of molecular biology.

1.2   The RNA Revolution

Studies under 'genome' in the early 1920 considered both DNA and RNA as mere genetic molecules that give birth to protein. In the 1960s, the importance of messenger RNA (mRNA) in the coding-decoding pathway of protein synthesis was revealed during the standard information flow and protein production sites were identified. Since RNA has proved its versatility in heredity flow than DNA molecules, it became certain that the first hereditary molecule aroused was RNA.

In the standard pathway of information flow, RNA was initially considered mainly a passive intermediate mechanism. Studies were carried out in enzymes and other biological catalysts, exclusively on proteins. In the 1980s, Cech discovered the enzyme activity of RNA (Zang and Cech, 1986). This discovery led to the view that the origin of life on the earth might come from RNA, with DNA and protein coming later. These studies are considered as the first RNA revolution.

The discovery of RNA interference (RNAi) and microRNAs is considered the second RNA revolution (Novina and Sharp, 2004). RNAi is the process of silencing of gene expression by double-stranded RNA. This discovery lead to a powerful experimental tool to decipher the functions of genes. The exogenous double-stranded RNA (dsRNA) is converted into 21–22 nucleotides RNA molecules (siRNA), which guide the cleavage and degradation of complementary mRNA targets. These are key findings of the biochemical mechanism of RNAi. microRNAs are small RNAs that play an essential role in gene regulation.

The search for active components of protein synthesis ended in identifying some non-coding small RNA's functional roles. This is considered to be the second RNA revolution. The discovery of transfer RNA (tRNA) and ribosomal RNA (rRNA) tremendously elucidated regulatorily as well as supporting roles of RNAs in protein-making. Discovery of RNA's catalytic functions, stable small RNAs in the eukaryotic nucleus and RNA induced (RNAi) silencing mechanism in the 1980s are considered to be benchmarks in RNA history.

Catalytic RNAs, termed as ribozymes, play significant roles in mRNA transcript editing to removing introns to produce mature mRNAs prior to translation. RNAi is the process of silencing gene expression by double-stranded RNA. Later, RNAi gave new molecular insights to the concept of small non-coding RNAs and their role in gene regulatory pathways and specific gene silencing. RNAi has unveiled RNAs' active participation in the quantity and quality of protein manufacturing depending on need, time, and location. This happened to radiate major clues on RNA's regulatory functions in multiple gene silencing and in chromatin re-modeling to enable transcriptional regulation. Current biology uses RNAi as a research tool to silence particular genes to study the cell responses and functions in the 'gene off' state (Meister and Tuschi, 2004).

The therapeutic aspects of RNAi have tremendously triggered gene therapy and have energized modern drug discovery research (Kim and Rossi, 2007). Silencing RNAs (siRNAs) synthesized using RNAi has enabled designing new drug molecules and paved the wayway forclinical trials against cancer, Alzheimer's disease, cardiac and neurogenesis disorders, and viral and bacterial infections. Another crucial breakthrough of the decade was discovering non-coding small RNAs that have later proved to exert controlled action in up-regulating or down-regulating a specific gene. microRNA (miRNA), small interfering RNA (siRNA), small nuclear RNA (snRNA), small nucleolar RNA (snoRNA) and piwi interacting RNA (piRNA) are few among the new form non-coding RNAs that have changed the pace of medical diagnosis and prognosis (Mochizuki et al., 2002) .

Clustered Regularly-Interspaced Short Palindromic Repeats (CRISPR) interference is a synthetically designed guide for RNA strand developed as one of the latest genetic engineering tools analogous to RNAi technology (Ledford, 2016). CRISPR functionally alters various organisms, genetically modified food crops, and produced modified yeasts to make biofuels commercially. RNA medicines developed using the hot technology of CRISPR are under clinical trials for many rare genetic diseases.

After coining the term 'genomics' by Tom Roderick in 1986, the journey of metagenomics through functional genomics, structural genomics and epigenetics has been far and wide. This has revolutionized RNA research.. RNA appeals to a perplex biomolecule that signatures various phases of heredity and metamorphic cellular life. Rapidly expanding cross-linked biological techniques has accelerated the RNA revolution to a greater extent and has helped to keep dozens of promises in designing precision medications and treatments.

1.3   RNA Classification

The gene expression information is stored in chromosomes in the form of compressed DNA. It is investigated that a DNA molecule does not leave the nucleus to participate directly in protein synthesis but employs different types of non-genetic RNA molecules for carrying the messages from the nucleus to the ribosome where it is converted to proteins. To accomplish a gene expression, DNA needs to be converted to RNA molecules (transcription) and RNA molecules to protein molecules (translation). However, only 2% of the transcribed RNA is converted to proteins, while the other 98% assist the transcribed RNAs in translational or post-translational processes. According to the specific functions during protein synthesis, RNAs are broadly grouped into two—protein-coding RNAs and non-protein-coding RNAs (Kim, 2005). Figure 4 shows the classification of RNAs.

1.3.1   Coding RNAs

Coding RNAs are RNAs transcribed from a large number of genes and codes for proteins. These are called messenger RNAs (mRNAs) that have base sequences complementary to DNA and are single-stranded. They copy the protein-coding information from genes for the assembly of amino acids into polypeptide chains (proteins) and carry it to the cytoplasmic ribosome where it is translated into proteins. In prokaryotes, mRNA transcription is simultaneous with translation since there is no distinct cellular organization. That is, as soon as RNA polymerases are transcribing the mRNA, the ribosomes initiate protein synthesis. In eukaryotes, RNA polymerase II enzyme initiates mRNA synthesis from the template DNA by catalyzing the formation of 5′ to 3′ phosphodiester bonds of the RNA by reading the DNA template in 3′ to 5′ direction. The developed mRNA is expelled to the cytoplasm, where it gets attached to ribosomes and eventually translated into corresponding proteins with the help of transfer RNAs (tRNAs). mRNA makes up only 5% of the total cellular RNA and has an average life span of 1–4 hours.

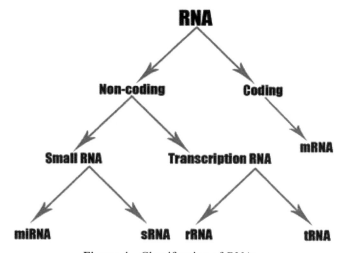

Figure 4   Classification of RNAs.

1.3.1.1   Messenger RNA

In 1961, Jacob and Monod proposed the name messenger RNA for the RNA carrying information for protein synthesis from the genes (DNA) to protein formation (ribosomes). Only 3 to 5% of the total cellular RNA resides in the mRNA of the whole cellular RNA.

Genetic information is transferred through a three-letter genetic code from DNA to RNA. In a cell, the information flow from DNA to a ribosome is performed by an RNA molecule for protein synthesis or translation. This RNA molecule is called messenger RNA. The coding sequence of the mRNA determines the amino acid sequence in the protein that is produced. All RNAs do not code to proteins. These non-coding RNAs can be encoded by their own genes called RNA genes. These genes can also derive from mRNA introns. Transfer RNA (tRNA) and ribosomal RNA(rRNA) are prominent examples of non-coding RNAs. These RNAs are involved in the process of translation. The non-coding RNA is involved in the gene regulation process. One other role of non-coding RNA is RNA processing, such as cutting and ligating other RNA molecules. Some of the RNA performs catalytic function of catalysing the peptide bond in the ribosome. These are called ribozymes, which has the ability to catalyze biochemical reactions such as RNA splicing in gene expression. Figure 5 gives a simple illustration of a pre-mRNA, with introns (on top). The introns are being removed via splicing and the mature mRNA sequence is ready for translation (bottom), The final stand is 5′ UTR at one end and 3′ UTR at the other end. UTR stands for Untranslated Region.

In a cell, ribosomes are protein synthesis factories. During the translation, messenger RNA carries protein sequence information to the ribosomes. A codon or three successive nucleotides in the sequence make it coded into one amino acid. Mature mRNA is formulated in eukaryotic cells by pre-mRNA or precursor mRNA transcribed from DNA. This removes its introns, the non-coding sections of the pre-mRNA (Fig. 4). The mRNA is then exported from the nucleus to the cytoplasm, where it is bound to ribosomes and translated into its corresponding protein form with tRNA. As we know, in a prokaryotic cell, nucleus and cytoplasm compartments are absent. So, the mRNA can bind to ribosomes while it is being transcribed from DNA. The ribonuclease helps the mRNA for its degradation into its components after a particular time.

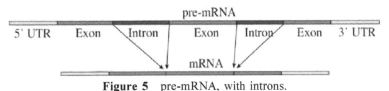

Figure 5 pre-mRNA, with introns.

The average size of mRNA molecules has a molecular weight of about 500,000, but mRNA varies greatly in length and molecular weight. Most of the proteins contain a hundred amino acid residues, three times nucleotides reside on the mRNA. Not large quantities of mRNAs are contained in a cell because it is a breakdown in time in a cell. Instead of the bases adenine, guanine, cytosine, and uracil in a mRNA, certain amounts of random coiling in extracted mRNA were not for base pairing. During biological activities, mRNA gets destroyed in the cell.

The mRNA molecules have the following structural features.

- **Cap:** A cap is usually seen in the 5′ end of the animal cells and virus's mRNA sequence. The protein synthesis rate is highly dependent on the presence of the cap. mRNA molecules bind very poorly to the ribosomes without the cap.
- **Nucleotides follow Non-coding region 1:** The non-coding region of mRNA is rich in A and U, not included in translation and the cap.
- **The initiation codon** is AUG in both prokaryotes and eukaryotes.
- **Coding region:** This is the protein translated region and consists of about 1,500 nucleotides m.
- **Transcription RNAs:** Two non-coding RNAs play an essential role in cell activities. Transcription RNAs are non-coding RNAs, divided into transfer RNA (tRNA) and ribosomal RNA (rRNA).

1.3.2 Non-coding RNAs

Non-coding RNAs (ncRNAs) never translate into proteins but perform diversified functions from mRNA splicing and RNA modification to translational regulation. These small metabolically stable untranslated transcripts are categorized as transcription RNAs or housekeeping RNAs and small regulatory RNAs based on functional importance. Housekeeping RNAs participate in the maintenance and active physiological functioning of the cell. These transcripts are major partners in primary transcript processing and quality or quantity control of translation, thereby occupying a direct role in translational functions.

1.3.2.1 Housekeeping RNAs

Housekeeping RNAs mainly constitute tRNA (transfer RNA) and rRNA (ribosomal RNA). Transfer RNA is a 75 to 95 nucleotides long transcript that connects mRNA to a protein molecule. Transfer RNA is transcribed from several particular sites on template DNA. It possesses a site for binding amino acids and sites for interacting with a ribosome along with an anticodon that must be exposed to the codons of mRNA. During the initiation step of translation, with the help of specific syntheses, enzyme tRNA recognizes the genetic code of mRNA codons using anticodon patterns and generates the particular amino acid. Each codon responds to specific tRNAs and a complete polypeptide protein chain is built after continuous codon recognition and corresponding amino acid transfer by different tRNAs.

Ribosomal RNAs (rRNAs) are insoluble and stable RNAs of ribosomes transcribed from one of the DNA strands of a gene and constitute 80% of the total cellular RNA. rRNAs provide structural support and catalyze the chemical reactions in which amino acids are covalently linked to one another during protein synthesis in the ribosomes. The eukaryotic cells have four kinds of rRNA, namely, 28S rRNA, 18S rRNA, 5.8S rRNA and 5S rRNA, where 28S rRNA, 5.8S rRNA and 5S rRNA occur in 60S ribosomal subunit and 18S rRNA occur in 40S subunit of 80S ribosomes. The prokaryotic cells have only three types of rRNAs, namely, 23S rRNA, 16S rRNA and 5S rRNA where 23S rRNA and 5S rRNA occur in 50S ribosomal subunit while 16S rRNA occurs in 30S ribosomal subunit of 70S prokaryotic ribosomes. In addition to its significant role in catalytic functions, rRNAs perform splicing activities inside the cell. rRNA is a potential, clinically targeted molecule in modern drug design. Phylogenetically, many rRNAs are now exploited to structurally analyze the relationship and divergence of different organisms' species.

1.3.2.2 Regulatory RNAs

Inside the cell, regulatory transcripts or ribo-regulators are directly involved in gene regulatory mechanisms (Erdmann et al., 2001). Transcription of these non-coding RNAs occurs only during certain cell differentiation phases and can further serve in a range of gene expression activities, from transcriptional and post-transcriptional regulation to translation control (Storz, 2002). Most regulatory RNAs are specific in sequence length with distinct functional and structural aspects. Hence, these are easily distinguishable except in the case of oligos.

Short non-coding regulatory RNA class constitutes mainly microRNAs (miRNAs), oligonucleotides, small nuclear RNAs (snRNAs), small nucleolar RNAs (snRNAs) and piwi interacting RNAs (piRNAs). microRNAs are highly conserved 18–25 nt long endogenously originated small RNAs that can up-regulate or down-regulate gene expression. Victor Ambrose discovered miRNAs for the first time in *C. elegans* complementary to target transcripts, lin-4 and let-7 genes and later were found to exist in diverse organisms ranging from worms to humans (Lee et al., 1993). These single-stranded RNAs are transcribed as precursors from non-coding DNAs and contain inverted repeats that form stem-loop structures. The precursors are then cleaved to yield mature miRNAs, short double-stranded RNAs of approximately 20–25 nucleotides. Mature miRNAs associate with RNA Induced Silencing Complex (RISC) and interact with target mRNAs at specific sites to either induce cleavage of the message or inhibit translation. The mRNA sequence's complementarity at 3′ Untranslated Regions (UTR) enables the gene expression suppression (Bartel, 2009). One miRNA may target more than one mRNA and many miRNAs may act on one mRNA so that gene expression intensity in various tissues and cells are synchronized. miRNA plays a vital role in the regulation of cellular differentiation, proliferation and apoptosis. It has been extensively implicated in several forms of cancer, neurological disorders, infectious diseases and other illness.

Oligonucleotides are short sequences with 7–30 nucleotides (nt) in length that binds to a specific region of a target messenger RNA (mRNA). Oligonucleotides inhibit a particular target mRNA expression by standard Watson-Crick base pair interaction through RNase-H enzyme-mediated cleavage (Wahlestedt, 1994). In addition, this helps to exploit the study of gene function and has been proposed as a strategy to design novel pathways and new gene-specific drugs in functional genomics (Huber et al., 2006).

Precisely, short antisense oligonucleotides are often referred to as small interfering RNAs (siRNAs) that individually perform translational arrests and interfere in gene expression or function. These are cleavage products of long double-stranded DNA molecules by the enzymatic activity of Dicer. Usually, due to the presence of RNA-DNA hybrids, oligonucleotides in the cells are easily attacked by RNA-degrading enzymes once it is formed. Antisense RNAs complementary to targeted genes can be introduced directly to the cell using electroporation or microinjection methods or cells can be transfected with vectors to express antisense RNA. Both antisense oligonucleotides are investigated as potential therapeutic agents (Opalinska and Gewirtz, 2002). Currently, scientists use antisense oligonucleotides as tools to identify novel genes and their related specific biological functions (Dean, 2001).

Small nuclear RNAs (snRNAs) are found in the cell nucleus of eukaryotes. snRNAs are initially transported from the nucleus to the cytoplasm and associate with specific proteins to form small nuclear ribonucleoproteins (snRNP), which are essential to remove introns from pre-mRNA. Later sequences present on snRNP proteins transport snRNP from the cytoplasm to the nucleus. These nuclear RNAs have secondary structures containing a stem-loop, internal loop, a stem-closing internal loop and the conserved protein binding site. The primary function of snRNAs includes splicing and telomere maintenance.

Small nucleolar RNAs (snoRNAs) are yet another class of regulatory RNAs that function within cell nucleus. snoRNAs actively involved in the pre-ribosomal RNA (pre-rRNA) processing in the nucleolus. Like snRNAs, snoRNAs binds with proteins forming snoRNPs that later on assembles on pre-rRNA to form processing complexes. During pre-rRNA synthesis, snoRNA act as guide RNAs that target the enzymes responsible for ribose methylation to the pre-rRNA molecule's correct site. Significant roles of snoRNA in ribosome synthesis include pre-rRNA folding, riborRNP substrate formation, RNA cleavage catalyzing, base modification, pre-ribosomal subunit assembly and rRNP export from the nucleus to the cytoplasm.

Piwi-interacting RNAs (piRNAs) are recently discovered endogenous small non-coding regulatory RNAs that regulate gene expression. They are found associated with the piwi domain of piwi protein belonging to the Argonaute family. These small RNAs were first discovered in the mammalian testis in 2006 while working on small RNA association in mouse testis. piRNAs are 26–32 nucleotides in length that reside both in nucleus and cytoplasm inside the cell. Gnomically, piRNAs are found in clusters with locations ranging from areas between protein-coding genes to areas that lack protein-coding genes. Each cluster accommodates ten to thousands of piRNA sequences and are conserved throughout different species while the sequences are not conserved. Characteristics of various regulatory non-coding RNAs are shown in Table 1.

Table 1 Characteristics of regulatory non-coding RNAs

Small non-coding RNAs	*Size* (nts)	*Functions/Roles*
miRNA	18–25	Post-transcriptional gene regulation
snRNA	80–350	Pre-mRNA splicing
snoRNA	80–1000	Pre-rRNA modification
Oligo	7–30	Translation regulation
piRNA	26–32	Germline transposon silencing

2 NON-CODING RNAS

The coding classes of RNAs are the messenger RNAs or mRNAs which copy the protein-coding information from the gene regions of the DNA (transcription process) and carry them outside the nucleus into the cytoplasm. Figure 6 shows an RNA sequence and its structure. The information is delivered to the ribosomal machinery (the protein synthesis factories in the cell) and is translated into amino-acid sequences, which make up the protein (translation process). In eukaryotic cells, mRNA is exported from the nucleus to the cytoplasm, where it is bound to ribosomes and translated into its corresponding protein. This process is associated with the help of the transfer RNA (tRNA). Ribosomes are molecular machines that make proteins out of amino acids. Prokaryotes are unicellular organisms that do not develop or differentiate into multicellular forms. Bacteria are a best example of known prokaryotic organisms. In prokaryotes, mRNA can bind to the ribosomes when it is transcribed from DNA. There is no nucleus and cytoplasm compartments in prokaryotes. The ribonuclease helps the mRNA for its degradation into its components.

The second classes of non-coding RNAs are small RNAs. microRNAs (miRNAs) are highly conserved, small, but endogenous non-coding regulatory RNAs that regulate gene expression (Salim et al., 2001). The microRNAs can interact with target mRNAs at specific sites to either induce cleavage of the message or inhibit translation (Reshmi et al., 2011). microRNAs were first identified in *C. elegans* as RNA molecules of 18 to 24 nucleotides that are complementary to the 3′ untranslated region (3′ UTR) of the target transcripts, including *lin-4* and *let-7* genes (Olsen and Ambros, 1999). These RNA genes regulate the development of worms. Later, most living cells were found microRNAs, meaning that these molecules denote a separate gene family. This family sequence is evolved from a small RNA (sRNA) gene system. Small interfering RNA (siRNA), sometimes known as short interfering RNA or silencing RNA, is a class of double-stranded RNA molecules that play a variety of roles in biology.

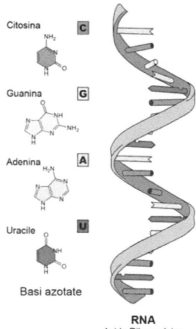

RNA
Acido Ribonucleico
Figure 6 RNA sequence.

MicroRNA is attached to a mRNA piece, which is the master template for building a protein in a non-coding part at one end of the molecule. This acts as a signal to prevent the translation of mRNA to protein. On the other hand, the siRNA is attached to a coding region of mRNA, so it physically blocks translation. Small interfering RNAs act through RNA interference in a fashion similar to microRNAs, including RNA activation.

2.1 tRNA

Transfer RNA helps the translation process by matching the three-letter RNA codes to the correct amino acid. Transfer RNA is a small RNA chain of 70 to 95 nucleotides (nt). In the translation time, tRNA transfers a precise amino acid to a polypeptide chain to the protein synthesis ribosomal site. The tRNA uses hydrogen bonding on the mRNA chain for codon recognition in amino acid attachment and anticodon region. Figure 7 shows the structure of tRNA.

2.2 rRNA

In the ribosome, RNAs play specific roles called ribosomal RNA (rRNA). In a cell, 80% of the total RNA are rRNA with complementary to that of the DNA region, where it is synthesized. In eukaryotes, ribosomes are formed on the nucleolus. No definite base relationship between rRNA and DNA because ribosomal RNA is formed from a small section of DNA molecule.

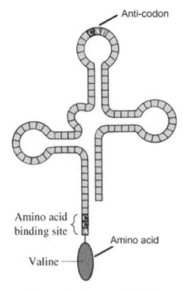

Figure 7 A sample tRNA.

rRNA has a singlestrand twisted upon itself in some intervening single-strand regions. The helical regions may show the presence or absence of positive interaction, and basest pairs are complementary with hydrogen bonds. The bases have no complementarities in the unfolded single-strand regions. The rRNA is different between species with relative proportions of bases. Single polynucleotide strand that is unbranched and flexible of its molecule.

A catalytic component of the ribosomes is called ribosomal RNA (rRNA). Eukaryotic ribosomes contain four different rRNA molecules such as 18S, 5.8S, 28S and 5S. Three rRNAs are synthesized in the nucleus. One of the rRNA molecules is synthesized outside the nucleus. Figure 8 shows the structure of an rRNA (23S rRNA). A ribosome in the cytoplasm is nothing but a combination of protein and ribosomal RNA. The protein synthesis is carried out through mRNA binding by ribosomes. During protein synthesis, one mRNA can attach several ribosomes. Certain RNAs can catalyze chemical reactions such as cutting and ligating other RNA molecules and catalyze peptide bond formation in the ribosome. These are known as ribozymes. Peptides are short polymers formed from the linking, in a defined order, of α-amino acids. The link between one amino acid residue and the next is known as an amide bond or a peptide bond.

Based on sedimentation and molecular weight, there are three types of ribosomal RNAs. Two of these classes are high molecular weight RNAs and one is a low molecular weight

RNA. That is, high molecular weight rRNA with a molecular weight of over a million (e.g., 21s–29s RNA), high molecular weight rRNA with a molecular weight below a million (e.g., 12–8–188 rRNA) and low molecular weight rRNA (e.g., 58 rRNA).

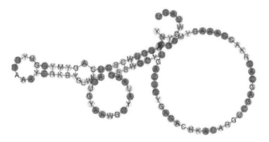

Figure 8   23S ribosomal RNA.

2.3   microRNAs

microRNAs (miRNAs) are a family of short non-proteincoding RNAs with diverse functions. The main functions of microRNA include regulation of cellular differentiation, proliferation and apoptosis. Many studies have been carried out on microRNA biogenesis and its functions.

The first microRNA (*lin-4*) was discovered in 1993 by three scientists: R.C. Lee, F.L. Feinbaum and V. Ambros (Lee et al., 2004; Olsen and Ambros, 1999). At the beginning stage, they were interested in *lin-4*, a worm mutant discovered in Sydney Brenner's laboratory in 1970. After a sequence of experiments, Ambros and his colleagues came to know that *lin-4* is a 22 nucleotides piece of RNA and could not encode a protein. At about the same time, a scientist, Ruvkun and his laboratory mapped the *lin-14* mutation to its 3′ UTR. Exchanging the sequence of *lin-4* and *lin-14*, Ambros and Ruvkum recognized a complementary site in the 3′ UTR of *lin-4* to *lin-14* (Lee et al., 2004; Olsen and Ambros, 1999). This result was published in 1993 in *Cell* journal. These results did nottrigger scientists to find new microRNAs till in 2000.

The term microRNA was introduced in an article titled "Molecular Biology: Glimpses of a Tiny RNA World", of *Science* published in 2001. The second microRNA, *let-7*, was identified in *C. elegans* in 2001. By homology search of *let-7* sequence against the whole genome of Drosophila and humans revealed that *let-7* conserved sequences could fold into stem-loop precursors as in *C. elegans*. The studies found that *let-7* is conserved in many species. The target of *let-7* (*lin-14*) is also conserved across species. Later, hundreds of microRNAs from *C. elegans* were identified. *lin-4* and *let-7* are the first named 'small temporal RNA (stRNA)', later re-designated as microRNAs.

A microRNA gene is first transcribed into a primary RNA (pri-miRNA) by Pol II enzyme. This primary microRNAs (pri-microRNAs) is a longer RNA sequence of nearly 1000 nucleotides (Fig. 9). Roughly 25% microRNAs are in introns and clusters while 15% of microRNAs are expressed (x14). The majority of the microRNA (around 60%) are expressed independently. The longer RNA molecules are processed in the nucleus into hairpin RNAs of 60–120 nucleotides by double-stranded RNA (dsRNA), specific ribonuclease *Drosha* enzyme and an RNA binding protein *Pasha* in animals. This hairpin RNA, known as pre-miRNA, is transported to the cytoplasm via *Exportin-5*-dependent mechanism. There it is digested by a dsRNA-specific ribonuclease called *Dicer* to form the mature microRNA (Only one of the two strands is microRNA; the counterpart is named microRNA*). Figure 10 shows a pre-miRNA hairpin with mature microRNA and its duplex. The resulting 18–24 mer microRNA is bound by a complex to the RNA-Induced Silencing Complex (RISC) that participates in RNA interference (RNAi). The strand with lower stability base pairing of the 24 nucleotides at the 5′ end of the duplex preferentially associates with RISC and thus becomes the active microRNA.

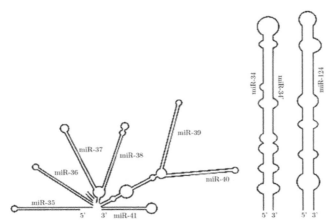

Figure 9 Transcription of microRNAs.

The mature microRNA makes base pairing with mRNA where complementarities exist between them. The mature microRNA can block mRNA translation by partial complementarities between microRNA and their targeted mRNA, mainly via base pairing with the 3′ UTR of the mRNA (Vinod Chandra et al., 2010). If there is perfect complementarity between the microRNA and their targeted mRNA, then degradation is similar to that mediated by siRNA. Auto-regulatory negative feedback via microRNA regulates some genes, including those involved in the RNA silencing mechanism itself. In animals, the complex-bound, single-stranded microRNA binds specific mRNAs through significant sequences, though not entirely, complementary to the mRNA. In general, microRNAs can regulate gene expression either by translational inhibition or mRNA destabilization.

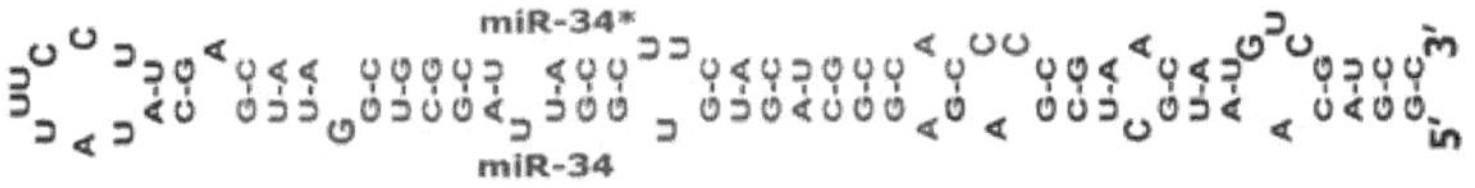

Figure 10 Pre-miRNA hairpin with mature microRNA and its duplex.

2.4 piRNA

piRNAs originate from clusters and repetitive elements localized in the genome. piRNAs are discovered in 2006 and the complete picture of piRNA biogenesis remains unknown even after ten years. piRNA researchers could not elucidate the biogenesis secrets due to its germline-specific orientation and diversified evolutionary pathway from miRNA and siRNA. There exist two widely accepted proposed piRNA biogenesis pathway. The first method is the primary processing pathway and the other is the secondary processing pathway or amplification loop pathway or ping-pong mechanism. Surprisingly, the antisense transcript strand from clusters and sense transcript strands from transposons is responsible for piRNAs' mass production.

The primary biogenesis pathway starts with the production of piRNA-like primitive transcripts from piRNA clusters. piRNA world is still arguing whether these piRNA-like molecules are the piRNA pre-cursors since there exist no supporting clues in this regard. Also, the knowledge on the promoting and controlling factors that cause piRNA cluster transcription still needs more research. However, once the antisense strand of piRNA precursor transcript is transported to the cytoplasm, they are attacked and cleaved by an endonuclease into small fragments.

Scientists believe that the nuclease in action during cleavage is a mitochondrial-associated enzyme called Zucchini. Zucchini loads these piRNA fragments with a 5′U into piwi or

Aubergine (Aub) present in the cytoplasm using Shutdown (Shu) and Heat shock proteins. After piwi association, the piRNA fragment undergoes two types of modifications such as 3′ trimming that gives mature piRNAs and later 3′ methylation that keeps the mature piRNAs stable. The trimming is done by an unknown nuclease to fit the piwi protein correctly and Hen1 proteins assist the methylation process.

3   SMALL RNA SECONDARY STRUCTURE PREDICTION

Secondary structure identification of RNA sequence is important in bioinformatics. RNA needs to perform its biological functions and give a lead for predicting the tertiary structure of RNA. The secondary structure of RNA sequence is used for the design and testing of pharmaceutical products (Vinod Chandra et al., 2008).

DNA/RNA bases' ability to form hydrogen bonding with complementary bases is known as base pairing. In an RNA sequence, Adenine (A) makes a bond with Uracil (U) and Cytosine (C) makes a bond with Guanine (G). These are called canonical Watson-Crick base pairing. Another weak pairing, Wobble Pair is formed between Guanine (G) and Uracil (U). The bond pairing between nucleotides are G-C and A-U form complementary hydrogen-bonded base pairs (canonical Watson-Crick). The G-C base pairs being more stable because there are three hydrogen bonds. The A-U base pairs less stable compared to G-C pair because there are two hydrogen bonds. G-U pair is a non-canonical pair that occurs in RNA. The resulting structure formed due to the base pairing of nucleotides is called Secondary Structure.

3.1   RNA Structure Energetics

The secondary structure is mainly composed of double-stranded RNA regions formed by folding the single-stranded RNA molecule. The number of G-C versus A-U and G-U base pairs determines the secondary structure. Higher energy bonds form more stable structures. The structure formation depends on several base pairs in a stem region and longer stems result in more bonds. The number of base pairs in a hairpin loop region with loops with more than 10 or less than 5 bases requires more energy. The inner loops or bulges are dependent on several unpaired bases. Unpaired bases decrease the stability of the structure. The main elements in secondary structure formation are stacked pair, hairpin loop, bulge loop, interior loop and multi-loop.

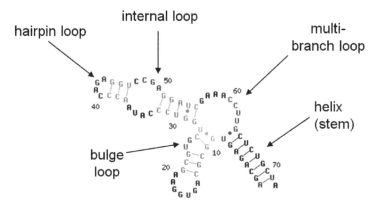

Figure 11   The secondary structure formed due to the base pairing of nucleotides of an RNA sequence.

A secondary structure formation need not have a perfectly complementary sequence-structure. Rather than, the missed pairing might result in loops, bulges, pseudoknots and stem-loops. Figure 11 shows a typical example of RNA secondary structure. A stem-loop structure has a long stretch of paired bases, followed by an unpaired loop. Pseudoknots contain at least two stem-loop structures, folded into a knot like shape and are connected by a single strand. Pseudo-knot represents a structurally diverse group due to varying lengths of stems and loops and variation in the interaction between them. Several algorithms have been proposed to predict the secondary structure of RNA sequence.

The following assumptions are made before predicting the secondary structure of a RNA sequence:

- Most likely, the structure is similar to the energetically most stable structure.
- The energy associated with any position is only influenced by local sequence and structure.
- The structure formed does not produce pseudoknots.

3.2 Base Pair Maximization Method

This is a comparative sequence analysis method that used sequence alignment to find conserved residues and covariant base pairs. The first and the most popular method was proposed by Ruth Nussinov, a dynamic programming approach that maximizes the number of base pairs in the resultant structure (Nussinov and Jacobson, 1980). Waterman and Smith proposed improving the Nussinov algorithm by providing a mechanism to handle stacking and destabilizing energies. But the size of the sequence that could be handled was less than 200 nucleotides. Zuker proposed optimal folding of large RNA sequences, which fold sequences up to 600 nucleotides. Many different representations are being used to represent RNA secondary structures, and the most widely used one is a dot-bracket representation, where each dot represents an unpaired base while a bracket represents a paired base. Figure 12 shows such a representation.

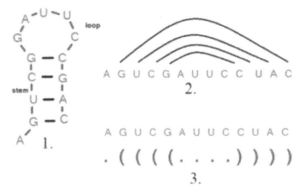

Figure 12   Different representations of an RNA secondary structure.

A single-stranded RNA sequence forms a secondary structure due to the hydrogen bonding of Watson-Crick pairs (A-U, G-C) and Wobble Pair (G-U). An RNA sequence's free energy is the total energy of the secondary structure that could be formed from a sequence. Lower free energy indicates more robust structural stability. There are different algorithmic approaches to find the possible RNA secondary structure. Nussinov proposed an algorithm that relies on maximizing base pairs in the structure, which in turn minimizes the free energy.

Figure 13 shows four possible ways to recursively add new bases to the best structure of smaller subsequence. The idea behind the algorithm is that when new bases are added, constraints are applied so that the structure remains optimal. There are four ways to get the best structure between position i and j from the best structures of the smaller subsequences

(1) Add i,j pair onto best structure found for subsequence $i + 1, j - 1$
(2) Add unpaired position i onto the best structure for subsequence $i + 1, j$

(3) Add unpaired position j onto the best structure for subsequence $i, j - 1$

(4) Combine two optimal structures i, k and $k + 1, j$

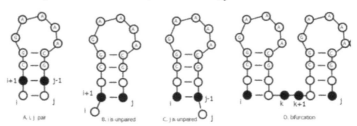

Figure 13 Nussinov Algorithm: Possible base pairing in an RNA secondary structure. (a) Nucleotides at position i and j forms stacked base pair to already formed the best structure. (b) The unpaired base at position i to best structure at $(i + 1)$ and j. (c) The unpaired base at position j to the best structure at (i) and $(j + 1)$. (d) Two separate structures are joined.

In algorithmic form, it is the computation of cell values of an (N × N) dynamic programming matrix. Each cell value is computed as the maximum among four quantities:

- A value in a column to the left of the current cell
- A value in a row above the cell
- Sum of values in the diagonal cell and a score value of the new pair
- Resultant value when two substructures are merged

Score values are assigned based on the strength of base pairing. For example, a (G-C) pair is assigned with the highest score value, (A-U) pair with the next lower value and (G-U) pair with the lowest value. A trace back starting from the upper right cell of the dynamic programming matrix, and following a path consisting of cells that had attributed a way to the current cell, gives the RNA secondary structure. The pseudo-code of Nussinov Algorithm is given below.

```
Initialization:
push (1, L) into the stack
Recursion:
Repeat until the stack is empty:
Pop (i,j)
if i ≥ j continue
else if γ(i+1,j) = γ(i,j) push(i+1,j)
else if γ(i,j-1) = γ(i,j) push(i,j-1)
else if γ(i+1,j-1) = γ(i,j)
record i,j base-pair
push(i+1, j-1)
else for k=i+1 to j-1
if γ(i,k)+ γ(k+1,j) = γ(i,j)
push(k+1,j)
push(i,k)
break
```

For example, consider a small RNA sequence GGGAAAUCC. First, initialize the matrix M for that score for matches along the main diagonal and diagonal just below it is set to zero (Fig. 14). Formally, the scoring matrix, M, is initialized:

$M[i][i] = 0$ for $i = 1$ to L (L is sequence length)

$M[i][i-1] = 0$ for $i = 2$ to L

In the next step, we need to fill the matrix M $[[i][j]$ with maximum value from the following:

1. $M[i+1][j] - i^{th}$ residue is hanging off by itself
2. $M[i][j-1] - j^{th}$ residue is hanging off by itself

3. $M[i+1][j-1] + S(x_i, x_j) - i^{th}$ and j^{th} residue are paired; if x_i = complement of x_j, then $S(x_i, x_j) = 1$; otherwise it is 0.

4. $M[i][j] = MAX_{i<k<j} (M[i][k] + M[k+1][j])$ – merging two substructures

After a complete cycle the final filled matrix is shown in Fig. 14.

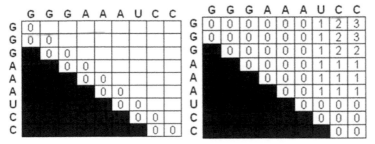

Figure 14   Scoring matrix M.

The trace backstage has O(L) in time. Sometimes, there are several structures with the same number of base pairs. However, this trace back algorithm only traces one of the best structures. The Nussinov algorithm does not deal with pseudoknots. Maximizing the number of base pairs is an overly simplistic criterion that cannot give an accurate prediction. But it is the first algorithm that shares the same idea with those more sophisticated energy minimizations and probabilistic based SCFG techniques.

The main drawback Nussinov algorithm is the non-realism of base-pair maximization. To overcome this, define an energy model for RNA that can be parameterized by experimentally measured energies. There is a scope of another algorithm that derives minimizes the free energy of RNA sequence.

3.3   Energy Minimization Method

This algorithm is based on the principle of energy minimization, using the energy terms' estimation to contribute to a secondary structure. This method is a dynamic programming approach that does not require prior sequence alignment.

Gibbs free energy (G) describes the energetics of biomolecules in an aqueous solution. The change in free energy, ΔG, for a chemical process, such as nucleic acid folding, can be used to determine the process's direction (Zuker and Stiegler, 1981). For an equilibrium process, $\Delta G = 0$, for an unfavorable process, $\Delta G > 0$ and for a favorable process, $\Delta G < 0$. To minimize free energy is the natural tendency of a biomolecule in a solvent. Gibbs free energy equation is $\Delta G = \Delta H - T\Delta S$. Here, ΔH is the enthalpy, ΔS is the entropy, and T is Kelvin's temperature. The hydrogen bond interactions, van der Waals and electrostatic interactions give to the ΔH term. Change of order of the system is described in ΔS. The direction of a chemical process is determined by molecular interactions and the system's order. It is very difficult to calculate free energy using the first principle for any nucleic acid solution. So, biophysical methods can be used to measure free energy changes.

Probability for a specific folding, s is calculated by

$$Q = \sum_{s \in S} e^{\frac{-\Delta Gs}{RT}}$$

S is the population of structures and Q is a partition function. This is a weighted counting of all structures. When the free energy becomes low weighting become higher.

Zuker algorithm can determine the free energy of an RNA secondary structure (Zuker, 1994). In this algorithm, the energy of stacked pairs and loops are added. Stacked pairs contribute negative (stabilizing) energy, while loops contribute positive (destabilizing) energy. The energy of each stacked pair depends on the base pair on which it is stacked. Turner's energy table specifies the stacked energy of all combinations of base pairs by statistical analysis. Consider an example of the structure as given in Fig. 15. Using free energy minimization technique, all possible choices of complementary sequences are considered. When RNA is folded, some bases are paired with others while others remain free. This will form "loops" in the molecule. It has been possible to estimate the free energy of some of the common types of loops that arise through thermodynamics experiments. The *RNA Folding Problem* predicts the secondary structure of an RNA sequence that minimizes the total free energy of the folded RNA molecule. The following assumptions are made for predicting minimum energy RNA secondary structure:

- The most likely structure is identical to the energetically preferable structure.
- Nearest-neighbor energy calculations give reliable estimates of experimentally achievable energy measurements.
- Usually, we can ignore pseudoknots.

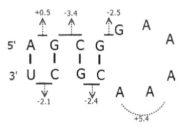

Figure 15   Free energy of RNA secondary structure.

The stacked energy of AU followed by GC is –2.1 kcal/mol, while the stacked energy of GC followed by CG is –3.4 kcal/mol. Thus, the total energy (ΔG) of this secondary structure is calculated as $0.5 + (-2.1) + (-3.4) + (-2.4) + (-2.5) + (+5.4) = -4.5$ kcal/mol. The free energy of mRNA sequence and concatenated microRNA, mRNA pair are included as feature vectors. The majority of features are obtained from the possible structure assembled due to microRNA binding to mRNA. A dynamic programming-based algorithm, the Smith-Waterman algorithm is used to obtain an optimal alignment between the sequences. A scoring matrix ($E_{i,j}$) is defined in this algorithm, with a score value for every possible base pairs. For alignment with complementary base pairing, score values are assigned as follows: G-C and A-U as 5, G-U as 2 and others as –3. Another matrix $V_{i,j}$, $0 \le i \le m$, $0 \le j \le n$, where m and n are the sequences' length to be aligned, computes the sequence alignment. Each $E_{i,j}$ value is computed using adjacent cell values, a score value $E_{i,j}$ and a gap penalty w. The free energy computation by Zuker energy minimization for the nucleotide sequence is given in Fig. 16.

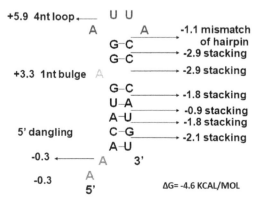

Figure 16   Free energy computation from the nucleotide sequence.

According to Zuker algorithm, a structure having minimum free energy value is taken as the biologically correct structure. Zuker uses a thermodynamic programming algorithm for RNA secondary structure formation. Zuker algorithm was developed from Nussinov RNA folding algorithm. It is a dynamic programming algorithm for finding the RNA secondary structure with maximum base pairs. There are two steps involved in secondary identification. First, to find auxiliary numbers $E_{i,j}$ of all RNA fragments and second, a folding of sequence with minimum energy, computed by traceback algorithm. For minimizing the energy, the following matrix is applied.

$$V_{i,j} = \min \{E(p)/p \text{ structure of } s_i,...,s_j \text{ and } (i, j) \in p\}$$

's' be a fixed sequence of RNA and 'p' be an RNA structure for 's'. Here V_i matrix is used to identify hairpin, stacked, internal loop or multi-loop structure. The auxiliary number calculation of RNA fragments can be done using recursion. A two-dimensional matrix is used for storing the energy values of various fragments of RNA. The minimum free energy value of RNA is found in the matrix. The energy matrix E is of size $n \times n$, where n is the length of input RNA sequence, which is used to store the energy of nucleotide pairs.

$$E_{i,j} = 0; \text{ if } j - i < 4;$$
$$= \min [E_{i+1,j}; E_{i,j-1}, e(I, j) + E_{i+1,j-1}, \min(E_{i,k} + E_{k+1,j})]$$

That is, fragments of length ≤ 4 have zero folding energy, since they cannot fold. Otherwise, s_i is unpaired or s_j is unpaired or s_i and s_j paired with each other, or s_i and s_j both paired, but not with each other. In this case, s_i paired with s_{k1} and s_j paired with s_{k2}, where $i < k_1 < k_2 < j$. The k in the recursion can be any integer satisfying $k_1 \leq k < k_2$.

Using the backtrace algorithm, we can identify the pairing status of each nucleotide in a sequence. This algorithm takes the time complexity of $O(N^2)$. A stack is used for storing the sequence index (start and end of a sequence or subsequence). The result is stored in a file, which consists of sequence positions in pairs. For example, for an RNA sequence, the first nucleotide is paired with the 95th nucleotide (A-U), the file contains {1, 95}. The second nucleotide is paired with the 92nd nucleotide (G-C), then the 2nd element in the file is {2, 92}. There is a bulge formed by the 93rd and 94th nucleotides.

Traceback algorithm

1. Initialize stack B by $(1, n)$. Set $i = 1$ and $j = n$.
2. If stack B is empty then stop, otherwise POP(i, j) from stack B
3. If $E_{i+1,j} = E_{i,j}$ then i is not paired
    If $(j - i) > 3$ then $i = i + 1$ and go to step 3
    If $(j - i) \leq 3$ then go to step 1
4. If $E_{i,j-1} = E_{i,j}$ then j is not paired
    If $(j - i) > 3$ then $j = j - 1$ and go to step 4
    If $(j - i) \leq 3$ then go to step 1
5. If $E_{i,j} = (e(i, j) + E_{i+1, i-1})$ then add (i, j) to list of base pairs
    $i = i + 1, j = j - 1$, go to step 2
6. Else
    find k, so that $E_{i,j} = E_{i,k} + E_{k-1,j}$
    PUSH $(k + 1, j)$ on to stack B
    $j = k$
    stop with error if no such k exists
    go to step 2

Traceback algorithm uses a two-dimensional matrix produced at the first step for finding a secondary structure. This algorithm extracts the base pairs contained in the structure. Using these base pairs, RNA structure can be depicted by appropriate secondary structure notations. There are four loop structures identified in the RNA secondary structure. They are bulge loop, stem-loop, interior loop and multi-loop. This algorithm fails Multi loops identification because the training dataset does not contain any multi-looped pre-miRNA hairpin structures.

For example, consider an RNA sequence GGGAAAUCC for a secondary structure prediction. First, initialize the matrix E using the equation. Figure 16 gives the values filled. The minimum free energy value is –7. The next step is the traceback procedure. The base pairs got are {(1,9), (2,8) and (3,7)}. Hence the corresponding bracket notation is (((. . .))). From this notation, the secondary structure is formed.

		1 G	2 G	3 G	4 A	5 A	6 A	7 U	8 C	9 C
1	G	0	0	0	0	0	0	-1	-4	-7
2	G	0	0	0	0	0	0	-1	-4	-6
3	G	0	0	0	0	0	0	-1	-3	-3
4	A	0	0	0	0	0	0	0	0	0
5	A	0	0	0	0	0	0	0	0	0
6	A	0	0	0	0	0	0	0	0	0
7	U	0	0	0	0	0	0	0	0	0
8	C	0	0	0	0	0	0	0	0	0
9	C	0	0	0	0	0	0	0	0	0

		1 G	2 G	3 G	4 A	5 A	6 A	7 U	8 C	9 C
1	G	0	0	0	0	0	0	-1	-4	-7
2	G	0	0	0	0	0	0	-1	-4	-6
3	G	0	0	0	0	0	0	-1	-3	-3
4	A	0	0	0	0	0	0	0	0	0
5	A	0	0	0	0	0	0	0	0	0
6	A	0	0	0	0	0	0	0	0	0
7	U	0	0	0	0	0	0	0	0	0
8	C	0	0	0	0	0	0	0	0	0
9	C	0	0	0	0	0	0	0	0	0

Figure 17 Matrix E, value-filled by Zuker algorithm.

MFOLD is a software that is used for secondary structure identification of an RNA sequence. Mike Zuker developed this software in 1989. It uses energy minimization to predict the folding of an RNA sequence into a secondary structure. The basic principle is a set of base-pairing rules (e.g. G-C, A-U, G-U only) to create "optimal" (lowest free energy) and "suboptimal" structures (within 12 kcal/mol of optimum). This software algorithm uses a dynamic programming alignment technique that attempts to maximize the score taking into account the thermodynamics. Figure 17 shows how the matrix is filled by Zuker Algorithm using energy minimization.

The major drawback of this technique is the prediction of only one optimal structure of a given sequence. Purely mathematical approaches are base principles behind this algorithm, which offers usual implementation drawbacks. To the above two techniques, the researcherswere designed some other RNA secondary structure prediction techniques. These techniques are somewhat improved methods of the existing algorithms.

REFERENCES

Bartel, D.P. (2009). microRNAs: Target recognition and regulatory functions. Cell. 136(2): 215–233.

Dean, N.M. (2001). Functional genomics and target validation approaches using antisense oligonucleotide technology. Curr. Opin. Biotechnol. 12: 622–625.

Erdmann, V.A., M.Z. Barciszewska, A. Hochberg, N. de Groot and J. Barciszewski (2001). Regulatory RNAs. Curr. Opin. Biotechnol. 58(7): 960–977.

Huber, L.C., O. Distler, R.E. Gay and S. Gay (2006). Antisense strategies in degenerative joint diseases: Sense or nonsense? Adv. Drug Deliv. Rev. 58: 285–289.

Kim, V.N. (2005). Small RNAs: Classification, biogenesis mechanism and function. Mol. Cell. 19: 1–15.

Kim, D.H. and J.J. Rossi (2007). Strategies for silencing human disease using RNA interference. Nat. Rev. Genet. 8(3): 173–184.

Ledford, H. (2016). CRISPR: Gene editing is just the beginning. Nature. 531(7593): 156–159.

Lee, R.C., R.L. Feinbaum and V. Ambros. (1993). The *C. elegans* heterochronic gene lin-4 encodes small RNAs with antisense complementarity to lin-14. Cell. 75(5): 843–854.

Lee, R., Feinbaum and V. Ambros, (2004). A short history of a short RNA. Cell. 116: S89–S92.

Meister, G. and T. Tuschl (2004). Mechanisms of gene silencing by double-stranded RNA. Nature. 431: 343–349.

Mochlzuki, K., N.A. Fine, T. Fujisawa and M.A. Gorovsky. (2002). Analysis of a piwi-related gene implicates small RNAs in genome rearrangement in tetrahymena. Cell. 110: 689–699.

Novina, C.D. and P.A. Sharp (2004). The RNA revolution. Nature. 430: 161–164.

Nussinov, R. and A.B. Jacobson (1980). Fast algorithm for predicting the secondary structure of single-stranded RNA. PNAS. 77(11): 6309–6313.

Olsen, P.H. and V. Ambros (1999). The lin-4 regulatory RNA controls developmental timing in *C. elegans* by blocking lin-14 protein synthesis after the initiation of translation. Dev. Biol. 216: 671–680.

Opalinska, J.B. and A.M. Gewirtz (2002). Nucleic-acid therapeutics: Basic principles and recent applications. Nat. Rev. Drug Discovery. 1: 503–514.

Reshmi, G., S.S. Vinod Chandra, V.J. Mohan Babu, P.S. Saneesh Babu, W.S. Santhi, Surya Ramachandran, et al. (2011). Identification and analysis of novel microRNAs from fragile sites of human cervical cancer: Computational and experimental approach. Genomics. 97(6): 333–340.

Salim, A., R. Amjesh and S.S. Vinod Chandra (2017). An approach to forecast human cancer by profiling microRNA expressions from NGS Data. BMC Cancer. 17(77): 1–9.

Storz, G. (2002). An expanding universe of noncoding RNAs. Science. 296(5571): 1260–1263.

Vinod Chandra, S.S., G. Gopakumar and A.S. Nair. (2008). Biolets: Statistical approach to biological random sequence generation. Malaysian Journal of Computer Science. 21(2): 116–121.

Vinod Chandra, S.S., R. Girijadevi, A.S. Nair, S.S. Pillai and R.M. Pillai. (2010). MTar: A Computational microRNA target prediction architecture for human transcriptome. BMC Bioinformatics. 10(S:1): 1–9.

Wahlestedt, C. (1994). Antisense oligonucleotide strategies in neuropharmacology. Trends Pharmacol. Sci. 15: 42–46.

Watson, J.D. and F.H.C. Crick (1953). Molecular structure of nucleic acids: A structure for deoxyribose nucleic acid. Nature. 171: 737–738.

Zang, A. and T. Cech (1986). The intervening sequences RNA of Tetrahymena is an enzyme. Science. 231: 470–475.

Zuker, M. and P. Stiegler (1981). Optimal computer folding of large RNA sequences using thermodynamics and auxiliary information. Nucleic Acids Res. 9(1): 133–148.

Zuker, M. (1994). Prediction of RNA secondary structure by energy minimization. Methods Mol. Biol. 25: 267–294.

CHAPTER 12

Bioinformatics of microRNA Target Prediction

**Abdul Rawoof, Aviral Kumar,
Shirish Tiwari and Lekha Dinesh Kumar***

CSIR-Centre for Cellular and Molecular Biology,
(CCMB) Uppal Road, Hyderabad, 500007, Telangana, India

1 INTRODUCTION

The post-genome era has seen new advancement in omics technologies that have provided deeper insights into the human genome, transcriptome and proteome. In this scenario, bioinformatics has become an intense area of research to analyse vast high throughput data generated to derive meaningful conclusions for medical research and its application. One of the most exciting findings of the human genome project was the discovery of a large number of non-coding RNAs known as microRNAs (miRNAs) that constitute 1% of human genome (Zhang et al., 2019). The importance of these small molecules was further corroborated when it was discovered initially that 30% of human genes are regulated by them (Li et al., 2009). However, recent studies estimate that around 84% of genes in genome are targeted by miRNA highlighting their significant role in gene regulation (Catalantto et al., 2016). Accumulating evidence suggests the involvement of microRNAs as modulators of gene expression in processes such as proliferation, differentiation, homeostasis, cell death, etc. and biological homeostasis (Wahid et al., 2010), and their aberrant expression is found to be associated with many human diseases (Bhaskaran and Mohan, 2014). For instance, in cancer, miRNA mediate both activation(oncogene) and inhibition (tumor suppressor gene) of transcription of gene (Peng and Croce, 2016). A better understanding of these dynamic molecules holds the key to unraveling the mechanism of disease which could help discover novel targets for therapeutic intervention. These small non coding (22 nt) single stranded RNA molecules bind to the complementary regions of the target mRNA leading to translational repression or its degradation (O'Brien et al., 2018). The development of bioinformatics tools for

*Corresponding author: lekha@ccmb.res.in

miRNA target prediction has brought a new era in RNA research, however existing algorithms still suffer from lack of optimal performance with frequent false positives (Liu and Wang, 2019). For any functional miRNA analysis, it is imperative to identify putative targets of the miRNA. The way to address this is by discerning the role of miRNA: mRNA interactions. However, because each miRNA has multiple targets with varied biological outcomes (Li and Zhang, 2013) the correct identification of an interaction remains challenging. Moreover, due to the high number of target sites, experimental validation becomes time consuming and costly. To this end, many computational tools have been developed, with gradual improvement on target prediction performance. The mechanism by which miRNAs post-transcriptionally hybridize to the target mRNAs have been studied at length (Riffo-Campos et al., 2016), thereby providing rules/features for development of computational tools. In most target prediction tools, 60–90% of protein coding genes are targeted by the conserved sequences near 5′ (seed region) and 3′ region (compensatory sites) of miRNAs (Vella et al., 2004). Recently, newer algorithms have been developed based on novel insights in miRNA interactions or through scientific breakthroughs in experimental methods such as low GC content, target site accessibility, binding of protein to RNA and methylation of RNA site (Ab Mutalib et al., 2019).

The scope of this chapter is to discuss updated information pertaining to computational tools involved in miRNA target prediction. We summarize the fundamental features of miRNA: mRNA interactions used by algorithms for sequence-based prediction of miRNA targets. We also describe frequently used bioinformatics tools explaining each parameter in the search results. Finally, we draw attention to general strategies commonly used in target analysis and present our approach for efficient target prediction.

2 SALIENT FEATURES OF MIRNA TARGET PREDICTION ALGORITHMS

Most microRNAs target several genes and at the same time a single target gene is regulated by multiple microRNAs. Therefore, computational prediction of miRNA: mRNA interaction network is very crucial for identifying targets for further experimental validation. This also helps to narrow down the targets for further functional analysis. A large number of computational tools are available for target prediction and their selection depends on the types of organism the user is dealing with (Chen et al., 2019). Animals and plants have different miRNA targeting patterns. In plants, there is a perfect hybridization/binding of miRNA to its target site. This near perfect binding makes target prediction relatively easy leading to less false positives and more accurate prediction (Dai et al., 2010; Rogers and Chen, 2013). This is in contrast with the animal system where partial pairing may also result in binding of miRNA with its targets. The seed region in 5′ region of miRNA mostly contains 2 to 8 nucleotides and is used for target prediction. However growing research integrates newer insights into miRNA target interactions increasing its complexity (Agarwal et al., 2015). Any algorithm that solely depends on base pairing will lack accuracy and produce false positives. Commonly used features in potential miRNA target prediction include seed region, conservation, free energy and site accessibility (Xia et. al., 2009). It is imperative to understand the basis of these features before using a prediction platform (Fig. 1). This chapter aims to provide a brief description about different algorithms available to aid the users in choosing the appropriate program.

2.1 Seed Region: A Base-pairing Pattern between miRNA and Target Sequence

The seed region is a region between 2 and 8 nucleotides from 5′ end of miRNA having a Watson-Crick (WC) pairing with 3′ UTR of target mRNA. It was first defined by

Lewis et al. (2005) as a basis of search in TargetScan algorithm (Lewis et al., 2005) and was further extended in the newer version TargetScanS (Friedman et al., 2009). Binding of miRNA with the target mRNA can be of three types which includes 5′ dominant canonical, 5′ canonical seed only and 3′ compensatory (Bartel, 2009). A perfect WC pairing occurs only when adenosine (A) pairs with uracil (U) and guanine (G) with cytosine (C) leaving no gaps in the alignment. As this region is highly conserved across species and specific across miRNAs, it also helps in classifying miRNAs into different families. Most miRNA target prediction software like Pic Tar (Krek et al., 2005), PITA (Kertesz et al., 2007), miRU (Zhang, 2005), RNA hybrid (Krüger and Rehmsmeir, 2006) use seed region as a key element in their target-based algorithm. Other algorithms like DIANA tools use miRNA recognition element (MERs) to predict the complementarity of miRNA: mRNA interactions. Notably, the presence of G:U wobble in the seed region may interfere with silencing capacity of miRNA (Doench and Sharp, 2004). Various algorithms have considered different kinds of seed matches. They are: 6mer: a perfect WC match between the miRNA and mRNA over 6 nucleotides; 7mer-m8: a perfect WC match for nucleotides 2–8 of miRNA seed; 7mer-A1: a perfect WC match for nucleotides 2–7 of miRNA seed and in addition to an A across for the miRNA nucleotide 1; 8-mer: a perfect WC match for nucleotides 2–8 of miRNA seed in addition to an A across from nucleotide 1 of miRNA (Brennecke et al., 2005; Krek et al., 2005).

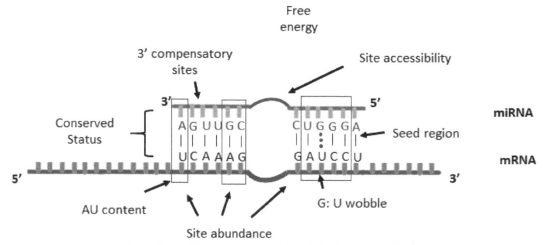

Figure 1   Salient features used in miRNA target prediction.
After miRNA biogenesis and maturation, it binds to the target mRNA leading to post-transcriptional gene silencing. Basic biological attributes like seed region, free energy, site accessibility, and conserved status are used by computational tools for target prediction. Other features such as 3′ compensatory sites, G:U wobble, and AU content can help in improving the accuracy of prediction.

2.2   Conservation of Target Site

When a miRNA binding site is preserved across species it is considered to be "conserved". Conserved regions can be present anywhere along the sequence but are mostly present at either the seed region or the 3′ end of miRNA or both (Riffo-Campos et al., 2016). The conservation at the 3′ end of the miRNA is referred to as compensatory sites, since they compensate for mismatches or gaps in the seed region (Bartel, 2009). Usually conservation in the 3′ UTR is considered but increasingly other regions of the gene, including the promoter and the protein-coding regions, are being explored (Elefant et al., 2011) Conservational analysis is performed by using either evolutionary distance or phylogenetic calculations. The degree of conservation is an important aspect that has been included in many target search algorithms like TargetScan

(Nam et al., 2014), DIANA-microT (Reczko et al., 2012), PicTar (Krek et al., 2005), miRanda (Enright et al., 2003), PITA (Kertesz et al., 2007) and EIMMO (Gaidatzis et al., 2007). Unlike aforementioned algorithms, RNA22 employs putative target sites which are different and do not have a conserved status (Miranda et al., 2006). A high conservation score results in better prediction of the targets. Though this approach helps in reducing false positives, it can lead to loss of less conserved targets or can identify regions that are conserved but are not miRNA targets. Experimental evidence suggests that at least 30% of the *in silico* validated sites are non-conserved implying that the functionality of target sites cannot be assessed by conservation status alone (Sethupathy et al., 2006a; Xu et al., 2013).

2.3 Minimum Free Energy: Thermodynamics Stability of miRNA: mRNA Duplex

According to thermodynamics, Gibbs free energy is used to measure the stability of any system. The binding efficiency of miRNA to the candidate target mRNA is estimated as the minimum free energy (MFE) of the putative binding. Since this is not directly measurable, we compute the change in free energy ΔG as the system goes from the unbound to bound state (Rehmsmeir et al., 2004). For the system to be more stable in the bound state compared to the unbound state ΔG has to be negative. Low values of free energy predict better hybridization and binding of miRNA to its targets making the duplex stable (Mathews et al., 1999). By predicting hybridization, regions of low and high energy within a miRNA can be inferred which along with other features can further help in determination of true targets (Yue et al., 2009). The effective and acceptable MFE value varies with algorithms and researcher's preferences. John et al. (2006) used a threshold of –17 kcal/mol as cut off (John et al., 2006); while the others set the maximum threshold of –8.5 kcal/mol for their study (Ragan et al., 2011). Different RNA folding algorithms like the Vienna RNA (Lorenz et al., 2011) packages uses RNA-RNA duplex prediction to estimate the energy value of the most suitable binding. Other programs like PITA (Probability of Interaction by Target Accessibility) (Kertesz et al., 2007) uses free energy to evaluate the accessibility in the 3′ UTR region assuming that the mRNA adopts a secondary structure and seed region is not easily accessible.

2.4 Accessibility of Target Site

Though MFE is a good criterion for selecting putative binding sites for miRNA, it is not the most efficient because of the mRNA structure (Martin and Vanicek, 2011). For miRNA to perform its regulatory function, it needs to bind and hybridize to the target mRNA. During hybridization, binding of miRNA to the accessible site results in unfolding of mRNA secondary structure (Mahen et al., 2010; Hofacker et al., 1994). Accessibility of target site refers to the ease by which the miRNA can locate and bind to the target. This feature is as important as seed matching in evaluating the efficacy of binding sites. PITA intensively uses this feature where it measures difference in energy gained from binding of miRNA to mRNA to energy cost in unpairing the mRNA secondary structure in the accessible site (Kertesz et al., 2007).

2.5 Other Features

With the advent of new algorithms and advances in characterization of miRNA: mRNA interaction, other distinct attributes of sites have been identified and incorporated for target prediction. These are either directly incorporated in target prediction tool or help to reflect the effectiveness of the putative targets. Local AU content denoted the number of A and U nucleotides flanking the seed regions of miRNA is one such feature (Betel, 2010;

Friedman et al., 2009). Microarray functional analysis of miRNA suggests that one can find target binding sites favourably in an AU rich region (Grimson et al., 2007). This also results in weaker mRNA secondary structure in the region, resulting in sites that are more accessible to the seed region hence facilitating better binding and translational suppression (Robins and Press, 2005). Recent studies are focussing their attention on conservation of genomic regions flanking the miRNA and its target genes.

G:U wobble refers to a situation when G pairs with U instead of C nucleotide. It is implicated in potential inhibition of miRNA transcriptional suppression (Doench and Sharp, 2004) There are lot of conflicting studies on the nature of G:U mismatch. Recent research suggests that the G:U mismatch in the seed region (G:U wobble) may still result in a functionally active miRNA (Wang, 2014). Target site abundance, another relevant feature, denotes the number of binding sites in a specific target mRNA (Garcia et al., 2011). Seed pairing stability is the free energy of the predicted duplex (Garcia et al., 2011). Position contribution looks at the position of the target site within the mRNA (Grimson et al., 2007). Increasingly machine-learning techniques are applied to predict miRNA-mRNA interactions. Since these techniques use experimental training dataset to learn to recognise miRNA-mRNA pairs, they use many more features with different weights to make their predictions (Sedaghat et al., 2018; Sydow et al., 2019). Many algorithms still consider site abundance in their sequence-based search as multiple target sites in the 3' UTR regions might increase transcriptional suppression (Brodersen and Voinnet, 2009). Recently, it has been suggested that a binding site is efficiently targeted if there is less abundance of target sites (Arvey et al., 2018). Other than 3' UTR a regular binding site, 5' UTR (Gu et al., 2014) introns, the coding sequence (CDS) (Guo et al., 2015), and open reading frames (ORFs) (Mandke et al., 2012) are also considered in target prediction (Hausser et al., 2013). Newer version of DIANA Tools uses miRNA recognition sites (MREs) which usually lie in the CDS regions (Reczko et al., 2012). Most of the bioinformatics tools use conserved seed region as the basis for their search but that approach is limited and can generate false positive. Machine learning employs trained models on multiple species without depending on evolutionary conservation status and seed region (Giansanti et al., 2019). Features used in different prediction tools are listed in Table 1.

3   PREDICTION TOOLS AND ALGORITHM

3.1   TargetScan

TargetScan is an algorithm that identifies targets for vertebrate miRNAs conserved across multiple species (Lewis et al., 2003). The algorithm implements thermodynamics-based modelling of duplex formed by miRNA-mRNA interactions along with comparative sequence analysis to identify potential targets conserved over genomes of human, mouse, rat and pufferfish. Considering that a conserved miRNA and a set of homologous 3' UTR sequences exist across different organism, the algorithm identifies 7 nucleotide long "miRNA seed" (from 2–8 bases from 5' end of miRNA) and its perfect Watson-crick complementary sequences in UTR region known as "seed match". Next, the search is extended to a longer site to miRNA, allowing only G:U wobble pair and the thermodynamics of duplex formed between miRNA seed and seed match to be calculated in term of free energy using RNAfold program (Hofacker, 2003). For each UTR sequence, a score (Z-score) is assigned which sorts and ranks the targets of UTRs from different organism.

Based on this score and ranking, putative targets are predicted for a given miRNA (Lewis et al., 2003, 2005) A simplified version of this algorithm known as TargetScanS was developed which depended on conserved miRNA seed with 6 nucleotide long (2–7 base position) flanked

Table 1 Computational Tools for miRNA targetprediction.

Tool	Description	Input	Output	Features	URL
TargetScan	A web-based tool that predicts targets based on conserved status and seed match	miRNA name, ID, family, or gene name	Ranks targets by probability of conserved target (PcT) scores	Seed match, Free energy, Conserved status, Site accessibility	http://www.targetscan.org/vert_71/ (Friedman, et al., 2009)
miRanda	An integrated system which predicts targets based on seed match alignments of miRNA and thermodynamic free energy	miRNA ID and UTR sequence for command line	A list of targets either by MirSVR score or presence of high multiple sites	Seed match, Free energy, Conserved status, G:U wobble	http://www.microrna.org/microrna/home.do (Enright, et al., 2003)
RNAhybrid	A web-based tool which calculate minimum free energy (MEF) of most favourable hybridization of miRNAs	miRNA or mRNA FASTA sequence	A list of miRNA target sites with MEF and p-values of pairs.	Pattern-based approach, G:U wobble, 3′ UTR compensatory sites, Seed match, Free energy	https://bibiserv.cebitec.uni-bielefeld.de/rnahybrid (Rehmsmeier, et al., 2004)
PicTar	A target prediction tool which uses multiple sites to access alignments across eight vertebrate species	miRNA ID, gene name, sequence data	Computes a Hidden Makarov Model (HMM) maximum likelihood score	Seed match, Free energy, Conserved status, Site accessibility, site abundance, G:U wobble	http://pictar.mdc-berlin.de/ (Kertesz et al., 2007)
RNA22	A pattern-based algorithm which identify miRNA/mRNA heteroduplex complexes in spite of cross species sequence conservation across genome	miRNA or mRNA FASTA sequence	Ranks pairs of miRNA: mRNA by p-value and folding energy	Pattern-based approach, G:U wobble, Seed match, Free energy	https://cm.jefferson.edu/rna22/ (Miranda et al., 2006)
PITA	A parameter-free approach which identify putative binding site based on the free energy acquired during miRNA-mRNA duplex formation and the free energy required for unpairing the target site	miRNA and UTR sequences in FASTA format	Tabulated list of miRNA: mRNA with minimum free energy score	Seed match, Free energy, Conserved status, Site accessibility, site abundance, 3′ UTR compensatory sites	https://genie.weizmann.ac.il/pubs/mir07/ (Zhang, 2005)
Diana Tools	A prediction tool which uses machine learning to identify miRNA recognition element (MERs) in 3′ UTR and other regions	miRNA name, ID, KEGG description, gene name	An integrated analysis results with miRNA target gene (miTG) prediction score	Seed match, Free energy, Conserved status, G:U wobble, AU content, 3′ UTR compensatory sites	http://diana.imis.athena-innovation.gr/DianaTools/index.php (Loher and Rigoutsos, 2012)

Table 1. Contd....

Table 1 Computational Tools for miRNA targetprediction (Contd....)

Tool	Description	Input	Output	Features	URL
miRSVR	A machine learning algorithm which ranks identified miRNA targets by support vector regression model	miRNA ID, family and gene name	Calculates the miRanda: miRSVR score for putative target sites	Seed match, Free energy, Conserved status, G:U wobble, AU content, 3' UTR compensatory sites, Machine learning	http://www.microrna.org/microrna/getDownloads.do (Betel et al., 2010)
mTar	A machine learning algorithm based on an artificial neural network (ANN) framework which incorporates 16 features for target prediction	miRNA ID, name, miRbase ID	Classifies potential miRNA target sites using a feed forward three-layer multilayer perceptron (MLP)	Seed match, Free energy, Conserved status, G:U wobble, AU content, 3' UTR compensatory sites, Site abundance, Site accessibility, Machine learning	https://doi.org/10.1186/1471-2105-11-S1-S2 (John, et al., 2004)
miRTar	A tool which facilitates potential miRNA-mRNA binding by providing regulatory information of their interactions	Single/ multiple miRNAs in FASTA format, miRbase ID, Ensembl ID	Calculates the free energy and alignment score of each set of miRNA: mRNA interaction	Seed match, Free energy, Conserved status, G:U wobble, AU content, 3' UTR compensatory sites, Site abundance	http://mirtar.mbc.nctu.edu.tw. (Chandra et al., 2010)
miRMap	A comprehensive tool which uses python libraries to predict miRNA targets based on four key features	miRNA name, miRbase ID, Ensembl ID	Ranks targets by a predictive miRMap score calculated from combining 11 features	Seed match, Free energy, Conserved status, AU content, Site abundance	https://mirmap.ezlab.org/ (Sayers et al., 2009)
miRTarCLIP	A target analysis and prediction platform solely based on crosslinking and immunoprecipitation (CLIP) and photoactivatable-ribonucleoside-enhanced (PAR-CLIP) sequencing data	Sequence file formats (.sra), FASTA file format	A list of predicted binding sites with scores integrated from TargetScan and miRTarBase	Seed match, Free energy, Conserved status, G:U wobble, AU content, 3' UTR compensatory sites, Site abundance	http://miRTarCLIP.mbc.nctu.edu.tw (Vejnar et al., 2013)
HomoTarget	A target prediction interface which incorporates pattern recognition neural network (PRNN) and principal component analysis (PCA) model	Single/ multiple miRNAs in FASTA format	Single/ Multiple set of mRNAs with predicted target sites	Pattern-based approach, AU content, Seed match, Free energy, Conserved status	lbb.ut.ac.ir/dynamic/uploads/soft/HomoTarget.rar (Langmead et al., 2009)

Tool	Description	Input	Output	Features	URL
SVMicrO	A machine learning platform which predicts targets by support vector machine (SVM) and UTR-SVM	miRNAs and UTR sequence in FASTA format	Ranks targets by a predictable F score	Machine learning, Seed match, Free energy, Conserved status, 3' UTR compensatory sites, Site abundance	http://compgenomics.utsa.edu/svmicro.html (Ahmadi et al., 2013)
mirMark	A machine learning based algorithm which applies random forest-based classifier to predicts potential target sites of miRNAs at site level and UTR-level	miRNA gene and UTR sequence in FASTA format	Considers >700 features with correlation-based feature selection to predict miRNA targets	Seed match, Free energy, Conserved status, G:U wobble, AU content, 3' UTR compensatory sites, Site abundance, Machine learning	https://github.com/lanagarmire/MirMark (Xiao et al., 2009)
TarpMiR	A supervised machine learning algorithm which implies on randomforest approach to discern putative target sites	miRNA/mR NA sequences in FASTA format	List of miRNA: mRNA predicted pair with seed region and p-value	Machine learning, Seed match, Free energy, Conserved status, 3' UTR compensatory sites	http://hulab.ucf.edu/research/projects/miRNA/TarPmiR/ (Hall et al., 2009)
DeepmiRTar	A machine-based algorithm which implement stacked denoising autoencoders (SdA) to identify human miRNA targets at site-level and UTR-level	miRNA/mR NA sequences in FASTA format	Predict potential or candidate target site of provided miRNA in a given 3' UTR sequences	Machine learning, Seed match, Free energy, Conserved status, 3' UTR compensatory sites,	https://github.com/Bjoux2/DeepMirTar_SdA (Chi et al., 2009)
FilTar	A web-based tool which incorporates RNA sequencing data to pre-existing miRNA target prediction algorithm in animals	Sequence file formats (.sra), (.ena), or users personal sequence files	Single/Multiple set of mRNAs with predicted target sites	Seed match, Free energy, Conserved status, 3' UTR compensatory sites	https://github.com/Tbradley27/FilTar (Wen et al., 2018)

with either t1A anchor or m8 match, to predict the potential miRNA target site (Lewis et al., 2005). The algorithm has been upgraded several times and additional target scoring parameters such as 3' pairing score to compensate for the low efficacy of 7–8 mer seed match sites (Grimson et al., 2007), probability of conserved targeting (P_{CT}) score (Friedman et al., 2009), context+ score based on the seed-pairing stability (SPS) and high target-site abundance (TA) of miRNAs (Garcia et al., 2011) has been incorporated to improve the performance. In its recent version, TargetScan (v7.2) provides identified targets for conserved or non-conserved mammalian miRNA families using a more refined model known as context++ model (Agarwal et al., 2015) for human, mouse, fly, worm, and zebrafish. TargetScan web interface provides user friendly, easy access to miRNA targeting a specific gene or mRNA. Also, users can find the target sites for broadly conserved or poorly conserved miRNA families belonging to species of interest. It does not accept any type of input or parameter adjustment from the user. The latest version of TargetScan can be accessed at URL http://www.targetscan. org/vert_72/.

3.2 miRanda

miRanda is a computational platform for the identification of potential miRNA binding sites in the genomic sequences based on sequence complementarity, free energy, and evolutionary conservation of the target site (Enright et al., 2003). Even though the algorithm is similar to Smith-Waterman algorithm (Smith and Waterman, 1981) it produces the alignment score based on sequence complementarity (A=U or G=C) instead of sequence similarity (A-A or G-G or U-U or C-C) and also allows identification of miRNA:mRNA duplex with G:U 'wobble' pairs. This algorithm performs miRNA target prediction in three different stages. At first step, it predicts sequences complementarity between mature miRNA sequences and mRNA sequences (such as UTRs) using dynamic local alignment programming with due consideration of several parameters such as G:U wobble pair, gap-opening, gap-extension and computes a complementarity score (S) between miRNA and matched target mRNA sequences. In the second step, the algorithm calculates the thermodynamic properties of each miRNA-mRNA complementarity match in terms of free energy using the Vienna package (Wuchty et al., 1999) In the final step, the algorithm inspects the evolutionary conservation of potential miRNA targets using genome sequences of *Drosophila melanogaster, D. pseudoobscura,* and *A. gambiae.* Sequences that are not conserved between these two species are filtered out and conserved sequences are sorted and ranked based on their score (S) and free-energy. After that, annotation and sorting of predicted miRNA targets are done using the FlyBase database (Gelbart et al., 1997).

The algorithm is available as open-source code written in C programming and can be run using the command line. It takes an input of two files; the first file should be mature miRNA sequences and the second file should be genomic DNA/RNA sequences. These files should be prepared in FASTA format. The command-line version allows the user to set the values for the parameters of his choice and output can be saved in a text file. These parameters includes −sc (alignment score), −en (energy threshold), −scale (scaling parameter applied to match/mismatch score), −strict (to strict alignment in seed region), −go (gap opening penalty), −ge (gap extension penalty) −out (print result in user define output file), etc. Users can see the manual for more details and executable the miRanda algorithm can be downloaded using URL http://www. microrna.org/microrna/getDownloads.do.

3.3 RNAhybrid

The RNAhybrid is a tool for identifying miRNA targets sites by calculating the minimum free energy (MFE) of the most favourable hybridization sites of miRNA in a large target mRNA sequence (Rehmsmeir et al., 2004). This tool is an extension of traditional RNA secondary structure prediction algorithms such as mfold and RNAfold (Hofacker, 2003; Zucker and Stegler, 1981). From single sequence folding to two sequences this tool identifies potential multiple hybridization sites on mRNA sequences which are energetically favourable in terms of MFE hybridizations while restricting various bulge loops, i.e., stretch of unpaired nucleotides, intramolecular base-pairing between miRNA or mRNA nucleotides and internal loop of unpaired nucleotide in both miRNA and mRNA sequences. It can take miRNA and mRNA FASTA sequence as two individual input sequences through the implementation of Algebraic Dynamic Programming (ADP) (Giegerich and Steffen, 2002) by an extension of ADP compiler into the C programming language, while for graphical output it utilizes Vienna RNA package in back-end interface (Hofacker, 2003).

Also, this tool provides various parameters under advance setting options such as hits per target, energy threshold, a parameter for helix constraints and loop constraints, p-value approximation based on binding sites within the 3′ UTRs, etc. The complete details of each parameter are available in the tool manual provided at the RNAhybrid website. RNAhybrid is available as a web tool on the Bielefeld University Bioinformatics Server and can be accessed and downloaded using URL https://bibiserv.cebitec.uni-bielefeld.de/rnahybrid.

3.4 PicTar

The Probabilistic Identification of Combination of Target sites (PicTar) is a probabilistic model that performs ranking of a target sequence (3′ UTR) for a group of miRNAs, using maximum likelihood score (Krek et al., 2005). To predict common targets for miRNAs, the multiple alignments of 3′ UTR sequences along with mature miRNA sequences as search sets were supplied as input and processed by PicTar. Using a program 'nuclMap', potential target site with a length of 7 nucleotides (starts from 1 or 2 base position of 5′ end of miRNA) will be identified and further filtered based on optimal free energy and underlying overlapping position of multiple alignments, to obtain anchors. The optimal free energy is calculated using RNAhybrid (Rehmsmeir et al., 2004). Further, 3′ UTR multiple alignments with a defined number of anchors are assigned a maximum likelihood score, i.e., PicTar scores and ranks the orthologous sets of transcripts targeted by a combination of miRNAs. To remove false positive, PicTar utilizes statistical test performed on cross-species comparisons using genome-wide 3′ UTR sequence multiple alignments of eight vertebrate genomes including human, rat, mouse, chimpanzee, dog, chicken, pufferfish and zebrafis (Krek et al., 2005). The algorithm provides pre-computed results and does not support user-provided input. Its web interface provides predicted targets for four different species, i.e., *Homo sapiens*, *Mus musculus*, *Drosophila melanogaster*, and *Caenorhabditis elegans*, and can be accessed using URL https://pictar.mdc-berlin.de/.

3.5 RNA22

For identification of miRNA target sites and their corresponding miRNA/mRNA heteroduplex complexes, a pattern-based algorithm known as "RNA22" was developed by Miranda et al., 2006 (Miranda et al., 2006). The algorithm does not rely on target site conservation across genomes of different species and hence provides more opportunity to discover the novel binding sites of miRNA which may not be available in the closely related species. Apart from that, well-known miRNAs have been used to train the algorithm. In addition to this, RNA22 provides a combination of G:U wobbles and bulges in the seed region of heteroduplex complexes for target site identification and it could predict both non-canonical and canonical target sites. Later, Loher and Rigoutsos (2012) developed a graphical user interface (GUI) of RNA22 which facilitates the user to select an organism available in the list namely *Homo sapiens*, *Mus musculus*,

Drosophila melanogaster and *Caenorhabditis elegans* (Loher and Rigoutsos, 2012). Using RNA22-GUI, the user can perform miRNA target prediction using a web-based server (http:// cm.jefferson.edu/rna22/Interactive/) or standalone java-based RNA22 batch submission tool which can run locally. The interactive prediction mode takes an input of miRNA and target sequence in FASTA format and provides a list of parameters such as sensitivity vs. specificity, seed region size, a minimum number of paired-up bases in heteroduplex, folding energy and allows number of G:U wobbles in the seed region. Further, the user can also check the pre-computed prediction (http://cm.jefferson.edu/rna22/Precomputed/) of miRNA targets available for *H. sapiens, M. musculus, D. melanogaster,* and *C. elegans.* The pre-computed prediction contains miRNA and target genes from three miRBase and Ensembl versions respectively and is also available for download. The RNA22-GUI is available at URL https://cm.jefferson.edu/rna22/.

3.6   PITA

The Probability of Interaction by Target Accessibility (PITA) is a parameter-free approach which identifies miRNA accessible site on mRNA based on the free energy acquired during miRNA-mRNA duplex formation and the free energy required for unpairing the target site to make it accessible to miRNA (Kertesz et al., 2007). To identify target sites or miRNA accessibility, the model scans the UTR sequences using seed match parameter for the potential site and then computes both free energy gained for miRNA-site duplex (deltaG$_{duplex}$ or dG$_{duplex}$) and required for the site open (deltaG$_{open}$ or dG$_{open}$) using modified RNAduplex and RNAfold (Hofacker, 2003). Further, site accessibility and interaction scores are calculated using the difference between dG$_{duplex}$ and dG$_{open}$ for the miRNA and its potential target site in UTRs. Overall, four features such as seed region (includes seed length of 6–8 bases with maximum one G:U pair permitted in 7-mer or 8-mers), free energy (includes dG$_{duplex}$ and dG$_{open}$), target site accessibility and abundance are incorporated in the algorithm of this tool to predict the putative targets.

The user-friendly web version of PITA is also available which allows users to identify site accessibility of miRNA related to four organisms, i.e., human, mouse, fly, and worm. In the web-interface users can provide miRNA and UTR sequences and can select parameters such as minimum seed size, allows single G:U, and single mismatch, minimum seed conservation, and flanking settings. Users can also perform PITA analysis on their Linux system using PITA executables wrapped in Perl scripts. The script accepts the UTR sequence files in FASTA format. The PITA web-interface and executable program can be accessed using the website https://genie.weizmann.ac.il/pubs/mir07/. The precomputed and predicted miRNA-target catalogues related to four species can be downloaded from the PITA website.

3.7   DIANA Tools

DIANA Tools is an integrated web server which provides access to various tools and database resources for miRNAs, their target mRNA, and their biological functions. Currently available tools for miRNA target prediction use the microT algorithm (Maragkakis et al., 2009; Reczo et al., 2011). At present, the microT-CDS v5.0 (Paraskevopoulou et al., 2013; Reczko et al., 2012), and microT-ANN v4 (Maragkakis et al., 2011; Reczko et al., 2011) algorithms are available for miRNA target prediction and can be accessed or downloaded using DIANA Tools web server (http://diana.imis.athena-innovation.gr/DianaTools/).

The DIANA microT-CDS algorithm is a machine learning-based approach which identifies the miRNA target site using parameters computed based on miRNA and miRNA recognition elements (MRE; sites with from 1 or 2 base position from 5′ end of miRNA), MRE binding and MRE conservation level. The identified features of miRNA MRE sites are combined into MRE score using a generalized linear model. The miRNA-target gene (miTG) interaction score of a gene is calculated using their weighted sum MREs score from both conserved and non-conserved MREs. The algorithm estimates the conservation of MREs from around 27 species. To remove false positives and to improve the precision of rate of miTG interaction prediction, signal-to-noise ratio (SNR) along with miTG score is implemented. The free energy of the duplex is calculated using the RNAhybrid program (Rehmsmeir et al., 2004). For both 3'UTR and CDS sequences, this algorithm implements a separate model for scoring the potential target site, and later this score is combined as a single score. This algorithm picks up relevant features using the datasets obtained from PAR-CLIP experiments, microarray expression data, etc. (Reczko et al., 2012). The web server of DIANA microT-CDS provides a user-friendly interface that can search for annotated miRNA sequences and their identified target genes (Paraskevopoulou et al., 2013). Users can provide input such as miRNA name, gene name or Ensembl gene ID, KEGG description, or part of them in double-quotes or a combination of these three terms. The result for input entry includes the target gene ID, miRNA, miTG score, the binding region on target, its location, target site conservation, chromosome position. In addition to this information, the web-server also provides miRNA related disease information, and the predicted target is experimentally verified in TarBase or also predicted a by TargetScan (Paraskevopoulou et al., 2013).

Another artificial neural network (ANN) based algorithm known as microT-ANN, predicts miRNA targets using a combination of several new target site features and is trained on high throughput data including HITS-CLIP dataset and pulsed stable isotope labelling with amino acids in cell culture (pSILAC) based proteomics dataset (Maragkakis et al., 2009). The miRNA recognition elements (MRE) are distinguished by features such as MRE binding structure, local AU composition, MRE conservation level, structural accessibility, location on the 3' UTR, and minimum thermodynamics free energy of the miRNA-target duplex. To identify targets, this algorithm aligns the miRNA extended seed sequences and a 9-nucleotide window (starts at 1 or 2 positions of extended seed) to the 3' UTR regions and identifies potential MRE sites using different MRE related features as mentioned above. Strong binding sites are considered as those having at least 4 successive Watson-crick (WC) binding nucleotides at start position 1 or 2 of miRNA extended seed or a single G:U wobble pair with >6 successive WC nucleotide or a single mismatch/bulge with 8 WC binding nucleotides. The remaining sites are considered as weak binding sites and are filtered by the ANN algorithm based on a free binding energy filter. Further, MRE score is calculated based on MRE conservation and binding which is ultimately used to calculate the final miTG score which combines all MRE features on the 3' UTR (Maragkakis et al., 2009).

The DIANA Tools also can be used and installed locally using DIANA-Taverna plug-in which provides ready to use miRNA target prediction and functional analysis. More professional users can also identify targets for miRNAs using Representational state transfer (REST) service which can access microT-CDS and microT-ANN web servers. For more details, utility, and usage, users can visit the DIANA Tools web server.

3.8 mirSVR

mirSVR, a machine learning algorithm based on the support vector regression model (Betel et al., 2010) provides downregulation score and ranking of miRNA targets identified using miRanda (John et al., 2004). Using supervised learning, the algorithm learns the prediction efficiency of a potential target site by training its regression model on mRNA expression data obtained from miRNA transfection experiments (Grimson et al., 2007). The model applies two different training mode, i.e., (i) canonical-only, where the model is trained on genes with a single canonical site in the 3' UTR regions and (ii) all-site mode, where a model is trained with either single canonical or non-canonical (single G:U pair or 1 mismatch in 6-mer seed region) sites.

Without incorporating the seed region and strict site conservancy, the mirSVR could effectively identify functional non-canonical and non-conserved or poorly conserved target sites, ultimately providing the regulatory effect of miRNA. To predict potential target site, the mirSVR model utilized a modified version of miRanda algorithm (John et al., 2004) which excludes the first and last two bases from 5′ and 3′ end of the miRNA from the alignment along with seed region restricted to single mismatch or G:U pair at 2–7 mer position. After that, the model applies a support vector regression model trained with a wide range of contextual features including AU composition, UTR length, site accessibility, target site position in 3′ UTR region. This tool is no longer maintained; however pre-computed results without user-based input data option are provided for model organism such as human, mouse, rat, fruit fly and nematode with miRanda-mirSVR score and are available at http://www.microrna.org/microrna/getDownloads.do.

3.9   MTar

MTar is a machine learning algorithm based on an artificial neural network (ANN) framework trained by wet-lab validated human miRNA targets (Chandra et al., 2011). Based on the experimentally validated training set, this algorithm distinguishes 16 different features including 8 structural (seed score, non-seed region score, WC and wobble pair, no. of mismatch in duplex, bulge length and number in duplex and A, G, C, U proportion in target sequence), 4 thermodynamic (free energy, hybridization energy of duplex, normalization free energy of duplex and difference in hybridization energy of miRNA : mRNA duplex), and 4 positional (positional pair score of G:C, A:U and G:U pair, matrix score of dynamic alignment, deviation matrix score, and deviation positional score) features of the potential miRNA target site. The model classifies potential miRNA target sites using a feed-forward three-layer multilayer perceptron (MLP) and predicts miRNA targets at 3′ canonical, 5′ dominant and 5′ seed only with high precision (92.8%), sensitivity (94.5%) and specificity (90.5%) with 9.5% false-positive rate for MFE < −17.0 kcal/mol. Overall, the MTar is a comprehensive algorithm that identifies all three potential (canonical and non-canonical) miRNA binding sites that can be utilized to predict targets for human transcriptome data also.

3.10   miRTar

The microRNA Target prediction (miRTar) (Hsu et al, 2011a) tool for human is an integrated web server which utilises well-known miRNA target prediction algorithms like TargetScan (Lewis et al., 2003), miRanda (Enright et al., 2003; John et al., 2004), PITA (Krek et al., 2005) and RNAhybrid (Rehmsmeir et al., 2004) to predict potential target sites against UTRs and coding regions. It is a user-friendly web tool that facilitates potential miRNA-mRNA interaction, their biological and regulatory function through gene set enrichment analysis (GSEA), and KEGG pathway analysis. Moreover, this tool also provides splicing information (alternative or constitutively spliced site) of the exons potentially targeted by miRNAs. At the back-end miRTar uses few popular data resources, for instance, it utilizes miRBase database (release 15) (Griffiths-Jones et al., 2008) as human miRNA source, ASTD database (release 1.1) (Koscielny et al., 2009) and Genbank (release 167) (Benson et al., 2009) as a source of gene annotation and their associated information, KEGG pathway database (Kanehisa et al., 2010) as a source of biological pathways and ASTD database (Koscielny et al., 2009), Genbank) (Benson et al., 2009) along with UniGene database (release 217) (Sayers et al., 2009) as a source of splicing events for transcripts.

For predicting potential miRNA target sites in humans, miRTar firstly utilizes TargetScan to detect perfect seed regions. Following seed region detection, miRanda identifies potential miRNA target sites using miRanda score cut-off of 120 with MFE <−12 kcal/mol, while potential targets within 3′ UTR regions are identified using PITA and RNAhybrid. On the webserver, miRTar has three main features which include firstly, the prediction system where multiple analyzing scenarios such as a single miRNA vs single gene or single miRNA vs multiple genes and vice versa combinations that can to predict miRNA and potential target sites in 3′ UTR, 5′ UTR and coding regions along with their regulatory relationship. Secondly, this tool can provide biological roles of miRNA by incorporating the KEGG pathways information of their important target. Third, miRTar could also facilitate the information regarding potential miRNA-mRNA target regions affected by any splicing events. MiRTar could be accessed through the URL http://mirtar.mbc.nctu.edu.tw.

3.11 miRmap

miRmap is an open-source comprehensive tool that integrates several python libraries utilized for the prediction of miRNA targets based on four key target site predictors such as thermodynamics, target site conservation, and probabilistic and target site sequences (Vejnar and Zdobnov, 2012). This tool implements linear model which identifies the repression power of miRNA on target mRNA based on 11 different features (such as ΔG duplex, ΔG binding, ΔG seed duplex, ΔG seed binding, ΔG open, ΔG total, Branch length score, PhyloP, P.over binomial, P.over exact, AU content, UTR position, and 3′ pairing) and is represented as miRMap score which is more predictive than a single feature. Most of the features incorporated in this model were from other tools such as PITA (Kertesz et al., 2007), TargetScan (Grimson et al., 2007), PACMIT (Martin and Vanicek, 2011) but only three, i.e., ΔG binding (based on ensemble free energy), PhyloP (significance test of the target region for evolutionary conservation) and P.over exact (probability of over-represented seed match or motif in 3′ UTR) were new features added in this algorithm. This model ranks miRNA targets based on the accuracy of these features and allows comparison of the predictive power of these features in identifying the miRNA-target mRNA repression strength in an impartial manner using a wide range of high-throughput experimental data such as transcriptomics, proteomics, immune-purification, and polysome fractionation and microarray experiments.

Users can also access miRmap through a user-friendly web interface that can predict and rank miRNA targets for sequences provided by users. Also, this web application allows users' precomputed and predicted targets for already annotated miRNAs (from miRbase 19 (Kozomara and Griffiths-Jones, 2011)) and genes (from Ensembl 69 (Flicek et al., 2012)) belonging to eight model organisms including Human, Mouse, Rat, Chimpanzee, Cow, Chicken, Zebrafish and Opossum (Vejnar et al., 2013). The miRmap web also allows users to perform different operations such as sorting, filtering, and downloading results for user-defined queries. The miRMap and its web application are available at https://mirmap.ezlab.org/.

3.12 miRTarCLIP

In 2013, Chou et al., developed miRTarCLIP, a first miRNA target analysis and prediction platform solely based on crosslinking and immunoprecipitation (CLIP) and photoactivatable-ribonucleoside-enhanced crosslinking and immunoprecipitation (PAR-CLIP) sequencing data (Chou et al., 2013). This platform locally runs on apache web server and provides an integrated user-friendly web-based graphical workflow of miRNA target identification and interaction analysis. It performs miRNA target identification in six steps. In the initial two steps, it removes adaptor sequences from sequencing read data and then subject them to quality check where reads with phred score <20 and read length <15 sequences are filtered out. The third step involves the conversion of cytosine (C) into thymine (T) as in PAR CLIP sequencing T to C transition occurs due to incorporation of 4-thiouridine (4SU) while for CLIP seq data no conversion is required. Further, at the fourth step, it aligns reads to 3′UTR sequences obtained from TargetScan (Garcia et al., 2011; Lewis et al., 2009) using bowtie. In the fifth step, reads with minimum overlap are clustered together and a cluster with more than 5 reads with 20% or more T to C conversion ratio is considered as valid. Moreover, sequences in a cluster are screened for possible miRNA seed regions obtained from miRbase. Finally, in the last step, the cluster is looked for potential miRNA target sites using TargetScan. Also, if any identified target site is available in the list of wet-lab proven targets supplied by miRTarBase (Hsu et al., 2011b), the system will keep it on the top of the result list. The miRTarCLIP is an integrated tool which was written in PHP script running in apache web server locally at the back-end with FASTX-Toolkit (http://hannonlab.cshl.edu/fastx_toolkit/), SRA-toolkit (Kodama et al., 2012), bowtie (Langmead et al., 2009), TargetScan (Lewis et al., 2005), and miRTarBase (Hsu et al., 2011b). It is freely available at http://miRTarCLIP.mbc.nctu.edu.tw.

3.13   HomoTarget

A combination of pattern recognition neural network (PRNN) and principal component analysis (PCA) model known as HomoTarget, was developed to identify targets for human miRNA (Ahmadi et al., 2013). This algorithm is more close to the MTar algorithm (Chandra et al., 2011), which utilizes an artificial neural network (ANN) for the identification of potential miRNA target sites. The PRNN, a feed-forward multilayer perceptron (MLP) classifies the potential target sites while target features selection is performed by PCA which ultimately lowers the complexity and increases the performance of HomoTarget. This model predicts target sites in 3′UTRs for predicted human miRNA available on miRbase (Griffiths-Jones et al., 2008) with high sensitivity (97.4%) and specificity (99.6%). This model utilizes 12 structural, thermodynamic and positional features such as total score calculated from a match, mismatch score, seed score, no. of Watson–Crick base pairs (G:C and A:U), wobble pairs, mismatches, bulges in duplex and proportion of A, C, G, U and A:U along with MFE in the miRNA:mRNA duplex for identification of potential miRNA target site. HomoTarget can also be run locally as a user-friendly standalone software tool that can be downloaded using URL lbb.ut.ac.ir/dynamic/uploads/soft/HomoTarget.rar. Users can perform single target prediction by providing the miRNA and mRNA sequences or can supply miRNA and mRNA sequence files in FASTA format to execute target prediction in batch form. The software also provides different parameters which could be defined to improve target prediction which are explained in help files of the software.

3.14   SVMicrO

Another SVM based tool, the algorithm was trained on a relatively large positive set from multiple species. Since experimentally validated negative set does not exist, the expression data has been used instead (Liu et al., 2009). It creates a training dataset from experimentally validated miRNAs in miRecords (Xiao et al., 2009) and its negative targets derived from 20 microarray data. By assuming two-stage structure system which is constructed on support vector machine (SVM) and UTR-SVM. The training resulted in 113 features on the miRNA along with 30 elements on the 3&39; UTR. On minimizing redundancy and maximizing relevance, the authors were left with 21 site-related and 18 UTR related features, which were used for prediction. Five elements were found to be most important, namely seed match, conservation, free energy, site accessibility, and target-site abundance. The major drawback of the algorithm is that it is standalone and there is no proper documentation for using it. Moreover, it runs on a 32-bit system and the source code needs to be modified to install it on a 64-bit machine. SVMicrO is available at http://compgenomics.utsa.edu/svmicro.html

3.15   mirMark

mirMark, a machine learning-based algorithm, developed by Menor et al. (2014), applies a random forest-based classifier that predicts potential target sites of miRNAs at site and UTR-level (Menor et al., 2014). The algorithm was trained using experimentally validated miRNA targets obtained from miRecords (Xiao et al., 2009) and miRTarBase (Hsu et al., 2014). For identifying targets, miRmark considered >700 features (151 site level and 624 UTR level features) and combined with correlation-based feature selection, it showed an improved prediction of miRNA target site both at sites and UTR level. Also, in consideration with PAR-CLIP data, it detects UTR targets with very high specificity and sensitivity. Further, miRMark showed a high number of true-positive target sites which is significantly higher (27%) than TargetScan, suggesting its better performance than TargetScan. It is available at URL https://github.com/lanagarmire/MirMark and is written in Perl script and uses RNAduplex, RNAfold, and RNAplfold (Lorenz et al., 2011) in Vienna RNA package for computing energy and accessibility of target site, Bioperl (Stajich et al., 2016) for nucleotide composition and Weka3 (Hall et al., 2009) for correlation-based feature selection. For site and UTR level, miRNA target predictions users can use Perl scripts "siteFeatures" ARFF.pl" and "utrFeaturesARFF.pl", respectively are available in the directory named 'core' of the miRMark program. These Perl scripts take miRNA and UTR sequences in FASTA format as input.

3.16   TarPmiR

For miRNA target prediction the machine learning-based random-forest approach known as Target Prediction for miRNA (TarPmiR) was developed by Ding et al. (Ding et al., 2016). Using the mammal CLASH (crosslinking ligation and sequencing of hybrids) dataset (Helwak et al., 2013), the approach uses 13 different features of a potential miRNA target site. Out of which, 6 of them such as (i) folding energy, (ii) seed match, (iii) target site accessibility, (iv) AU content, (v) stem conservation and (vi) flanking conservation were widely used features by other tools while remaining 7 features were newly identified features that include (i) m/e motif, (ii) the total number of paired position, (iii) the length of target mRNA region, (iv) the length of the largest consecutive pairings, (v) the position of the largest consecutive pairings relative to 5′ end of miRNA, (vi) the number of paired positions at the miRNA 3′ end and (vii) the difference between the number of paired positions in the seed region and the miRNA 3′ end. The prediction strength of this algorithm has been cross-validated on two human PAR-CLIP datasets (Hafner et al., 2010; Kishore et al., 2011), and one mouse HITS-CLIP dataset (Chi et al., 2009). With an average recall of 0.543 and with an accuracy of 0.181, the TarPmiR could successfully distinguish >74% of already known miRNA target sites in each dataset. Also, when compared with miRanda (Enright et al., 2003), TargetScan (Agarwal et al., 2009; Friedman et al., 2009), and miRMap (Vejnar et al., 2013), the TarPmiR showed 10% higher recall with 0.2% higher accuracy in identifying targets for miRNA.

TarPmiR accepts input of miRNA sequences and mRNA sequences separately in FASTA format and predicts the potential miRNA target sites in three steps which includes (i) screening of mRNA sequences to provide candidate target sites based on seed region and folding energy followed by (ii) evaluation and computing scores for 13 different features. Finally, at the last step (iii) the probability of the candidate target site being a true target site, is calculated by using a random-forest model based on the species. At present, TarPmiR can be applied to human and mouse miRNA and mRNA data. TarPmiR is available as a standalone python script and supported on both windows and Linux platform. It can be downloaded and accessed at URL http://hulab.ucf.edu/research/projects/miRNA/TarPmiR/.

3.17   DeepmiRTar

A deep-learning-based miRNA target prediction (DeepmiRTar) approach was developed by Wen et al. (2018), which implements stacked denoising auto-encoders (SdA) to identify human miRNA targets at site-level and UTR-level (Wen et al., 2018). This approach utilized wet-lab proven target sites of human miRNAs obtained from mirMark (Menor et al., 2014) and CLASH dataset (Helwak et al., 2013). The approach considered only miRNA target sites at 3'UTR and target sites with canonical and non-canonical seed (Helwak et al., 2013) were retained and filtered using miRanda (John et al., 2004). The negative dataset with both canonical and non-canonical seeds was also utilized and generated through a negative-data-generation approach. To represent potential targets or target sites for miRNAs, features were identified and calculated based on miRNA-mRNA duplex and their flanking regions. A total of 750 features were utilized and these were divided into 7 different categories belonging to three groups, i.e., (i) high-level expert-designed, (ii) Low level expert-designed and (iii) Raw data level. The categories under high-level group include seed match (26 features), free energy (5 features), sequence composition (98 features), and Site location (1 feature). The site conservation (160 features) and accessibility (370 features) comes under low-level group while hot-encoding with 90 features comes under raw data level group. These features were applied to build the DeepmiRTar model to predict potential or candidate target sites of provided miRNA in a given 3' UTR sequences. The source code of DeepmiRTar is freely available at github and can be downloaded through the URL https://github.com/Bjoux2/DeepMirTar_SdA.

3.18   FilTar

FilTar is a tool which incorporates context-specific (tissue or cell-line specific) RNA sequencing (RNAseq) expression data to pre-existing miRNA target prediction algorithm in animals (Bradley and Moxon, 2020). To increase the precision or correctness of miRNA target prediction in animals using RNAseq data, FilTar filter uses putative miRNA target transcripts based on their sample-specific read coverage or expression. Also, this tool provides annotation of a sample or context-specific 3'UTR of mRNA transcripts. This tool is implemented as a command-line tool under the GNU/Linux system and mainly written in python and R programming languages. All its dependencies are maintained and controlled using conda (v4.6.6; https://docs.conda.io/en/latest/), while it manages its analysis pipeline using Snakemake v5.4.0 (Köster and Rahmann, 2018). FilTar can be configured to process or handle different RNAseq data which are available on the public database such as Sequence Read Archive (Leinon et al., 2011) (SRA; https://ncbi.nlm.nih.gov/sra), European Nucleotide Archive (Harrison et al., 2018; Leinon et al., 2011) (ENA; https://www.ebi.ac.uk/ena) or user's personal sequencing data. The reannotation of 3'UTR sequences follows a series of steps which includes alignment of RNAseq reads to their respective genomes using splice aware aligner (e.g., Hisat2) following sorting and converting of aligned bam to bedgraph format. Then the mean of reading coverage value is calculated by FilTar. Further, the GTF annotation file converted into genePred format and ultimately into bed12 format using 'genePredToBed' binary (Kent et al., 2002). Then FilTar utilizes 3' UTR reannotation tool called APAtrap (Ye et al., 2018) on bed12 file and bedgraph file to refine the annotation. More details are available in the supporting document of FilTar available at https://tbradley27.github.io/FilTar/. For the prediction of miRNA targets, FilTar first converts the miRNA and 3'UTR sequences along with their identifier information into TargetScan v7 (Agarwal et al., 2015) format. Then miRNA target prediction is carried out using FilTar annotated 3'UTR annotation and existing annotations. The miRanda v3.3.a (Enright et al., 2003; John et al., 2004) can also be utilized with FilTar for the prediction of canonical and non-canonical miRNA. FilTar is freely available for download at github https://github.com/Tbradley27/FilTar.

3.19 R-packages

In recent years, several packages related to miRNA expression, their target prediction, and biological function analysis (see Table 2) have been developed as packages in the R statistical software (https://www.r-project.org/) and are integrated under Bioconductor (BioC), open-source software for bioinformatics. The BioC provides a vast number of packages for the analysis and understanding of high-throughput genomic, proteomics data.

The packages in R are available through BioC repository (https://www.bioconductor.org/) and to install any package, the core Bioconductor packages need to be installed first using following commands on R terminal.

if (!requireNamespace("BiocManager", quietly=TRUE))

install.packages("BiocManager")

After that any required package can be downloaded using the following command on R terminal:

BiocManager::install("Package_Name")

Here we are representing some of the R packages that are useful for miRNA-mRNA interaction studies using R statistical software tools.

3.19.1 miRNApath

The objective of miRNApath package was to identify and infer pathway enrichment of miRNAs using miRNA expression datasets (Cogswell et al., 2008). To operate on one to multi miRNA-mRNA targeting or multi to one miRNA-mRNA targeting situations, the package miRNApath provides different methods to identify miRNA:mRNA regulatory information. The input data includes tab-delimited text files of miRNAs differential expression data and miRNA target prediction data. Further, to analyze the pathway enrichment of miRNAs, users can supply a text file containing gene-path links information. The function "runEnrichment" performs hypergeometric tests to identify significantly enriched pathways and also performs random permutations to add confidence using the p-value. Finally, users can export results in a tabular summary format.

3.19.2 MiRaGE

The MiRNA Ranking by Gene Expression. (MiRaGE) package was developed by Yoshizawa et al. (2011) and it works on an algorithm reported earlier (Taguchi and Yasuda, 2010; Taguchi, 2013) which identifies miRNA-mRNA regulation based on gene expression data (Yoshizawa et al., 2011). MiRaGE does not depend on external programs for pre-computed miRNA targets rather it identifies miRNA targets using a simple seed match and calculates the probability (p-value) of mRNA as miRNA target performing multiple statistical tests such as Kolmogorov-Smirnov test, Wilcoxon rank-sum test, or Student t-test, etc. (Taguchi, 2013). Targets can be retrieved for conserved, weakly conserved or non-conserved miRNAs with higher efficiency and accuracy.

3.19.3 TargetScore

The package TargetScore in R is based on a probabilistic model to identify miRNA targets using miRNA overexpression data along with sequence information (Li et al., 2014). The package uses Variational Bayesian-Gaussian MixtureModel (VB-GMM) which considers and detects each score feature as an independent variable as input. This algorithm presumes the negative fold-change or sequence scores associated with miRNA targets and it is known as the target component. For each target, the TargetScore is computed using sigmoid transformed fold-change weighted by the mean posteriors of the miRNA targets over all of the target features. The package contains pre collated miRNA overexpression fold-changes from 84 Gene expression omnibus (GEO) dataset,

Table 2   Available R package related to miRNA and miRNA target interaction analysis

Package name	R version	Supported Organism	Input Data	Package availability/source
miRNApath	R >= 2.7.0	Any	miRNA expression data and miRNA-target data from RNAhybrid	https://bioconductor.org/packages/release/bioc/html/miRNApath.html; https://bioconductor.org/packages/miRNApath/ (Ye et al., 2018)
MiRaGE	R >= 3.1.0	*Homo sapiens, Mus musculus*	mRNA expression data	https://bioconductor.org/packages/release/bioc/html/MiRaGE.html (Taguchi and Yasuda, 2010)
TargetScore	R >= 3.0.0	*Homo sapiens*	miRNA expression data in term of fold-change values	https://bioconductor.org/packages/release/bioc/html/TargetScore.html (Taguchi, 2013)
multiMiR	R >= 3.4	*Homo sapiens, Mus musculus, Rattus norvegicus*	list of miRNA or gene or both	https://bioconductor.org/packages/release/bioc/html/multiMiR.html; https://github.com/KechrisLab/multiMiR (Li et al., 2014)
Roleswitch	R >= 2.1.0	*Homo sapiens, Mus musculus*	miRNA and mRNA expression data, expression data from The Cancer Genome Atlas (TCGA) along with miRNA-mRNA target seed-match matrix	https://bioconductor.org/packages/release/bioc/html/Roleswitch.html; http://www.cs.utoronto.ca/~yueli/roleswitch.html (Wang, 2008)
SpidermiR	R >= 3.0.0	*Homo sapiens, Mus musculus, Rattus norvegicus, Arabidopsis thaliana, C. elegans, Danio rerio, D. Melanogaster, Escherichia coli, and Saccharomyces cerevisiae*	miRNA or list of miRNAs	https://bioconductor.org/packages/release/bioc/html/SpidermiR.html; https://github.com/claudiacava/SpidermiR (Li et al., 2014)
miRLab	R >= 3.2.0	*Homo sapiens*	miRNA and mRNA expression profile data from TCGA	https://bioconductor.org/packages/release/bioc/html/miRLAB.html (Dweep et al., 2011)
miRComb	R >= 3.0.0	*Homo sapiens, Mus musculus*	MiRNA and mRNA expression data as normalized log2 intensity (from microarray) or log2 counts (from NGS) data	http://mircomb.sourceforge.net/; https://github.com/mariavica/mircomb (Le et al., 2015)

Package name	R version	Supported Organism	Input Data	Package availability/source
miRIntegrator	R >= 3.3.0	*Homo sapiens*	miRNA and mRNA expression data from GEO	https://bioconductor.org/packages/release/bioc/html/mirIntegrator.html; https://github.com/datad/mirIntegrator (Falcon and Gentleman, 2007)
anamiR	R >= 3.5.0	*Homo sapiens, Mus musculus*	miRNA and mRNA expression data along with phenotypic data	https://bioconductor.org/packages/3.8/bioc/html/anamiR.html (Diaz et al., 2017)
RmiR	R >= 2.7.0	*Homo sapiens*	miRNA and mRNA expression data	https://bioconductor.org/packages/release/bioc/html/RmiR.html (Evsikov et al., 2009)
miRNAtap	R >= 3.3.0	*Homo sapiens, Mus musculus, Rattus norvegicus*	miRNA identifiers or list of miRNAs	https://bioconductor.org/packages/release/bioc/html/miRNAtap.html; https://bioconductor.org/packages/miRNAtap/ (Favero, 2013)

77 human tissue or cells, and 112 distinct miRNAs. The package also included scores for target sequence features obtained from TargetScan Human (v6.1) as well as the context+ score and conserved target probability of each miRNA-target interaction (Lewis et al., 2005; Friedman et al., 2009; Grimson et al., 2007) The user can supply fold changes of miRNA with their ID, and can retrieve TargetScan context and P_{CT} score if available. After that, the validated targets can be retrieved from the local miRTarBase file and finally, TargetScore is computed. For more details, available functions, and parameter settings, users can follow the package manual.

3.19.4   multiMiR

multiMiR is an integrated R package and database of miRNA and target interaction related to humans and mouse (Ru et al., 2014). The database is hosted as a web-server at http://multimir.ucdenver.edu or http://www.multimir.org/ and can be accessed using RESTful service. The multiMiR database contains about 50 million records of miRNA and their predicted targets compiled using 14 different databases. The information obtained from these data was pre-processed and categorized into three groups, i.e., (i) validated miRNA targets, (ii) predicted miRNA targets, and (iii) drug or disease-related miRNAs which were loaded into MySQL databases. The validated miRNA targets entries are included from the databases namely miRecords (Xiao et al., 2009), miRTarBase (Hsu et al., 2011b) and TarBase (Vergoulis et al., 2012) while the predicted targets were included from DIANA-microT (Maragkakis et al., 2009), ElMMo (Gaidatzis et al., 2007), MicroCosm (Griffiths-Jones et al., 2008), miRanda (John et al., 2004), miRDB (Wang, 2008), PicTar (Krek et al., 2005), PITA (Kertesz et al., 2007) and TargetScan (Grimson et al., 2007). Using the multiMiR package in R, users can query the multiMiR database and can retrieve miRNA-mRNA target interaction and their disease association. The package provides several functions to query and access information from the databases such as "list.multimir" to list miRNAs, genes, diseases, and drug-related entries, "get.multimir" functions to get information for a provided list of miRNAs or genes. Input data includes mature miRNA IDs or their accession number, Entrez gene Ids or symbol or Ensembl gene Ids, disease or drug terms, or combination of these identifiers. Users can refer to the package vignettes and documentation available at http://multimir.ucdenver.edu/ for the usability of different functions available in this package.

3.19.5   Roleswitch

The Roleswitch package in R utilizes the probabilities of miRNA-mRNA Interaction Signature (ProMISe) model to identify miRNA targets on a paired expression data of a single sample (Li et al., 2014). Role switch package identifies miRNA targets in two steps including (i) the probability of mRNA as a potential target of miRNA predicted using seed match matrix which can be supplied by the user or can be retrieved from an existing database such as TargetScan and (ii) considering the expression of the mRNAs due to probable competition with other mRNAs being targeted by same miRNA. Overall, the ProMISe model facilitated by this package takes paired miRNA and mRNA expression data (microarray expression or RNA sequencing expression data) along with a seed match matrix to perform target prediction. For RNA sequencing data, mRNA expression represented as RPKM or FPKM (read or fragment per kilobase of exon per million mapped reads) values can be used while miRNA expression data represented as RPM (Reads per million), can be used as input.

3.19.6   SpidermiR

The package SpidermiR was developed by Cava et al. (2017) with the aim to provide miRNA regulatory network information, as well as miRNA target information in order to integrate miRNA data specific to the network belonging to 10 different species such as *Homo sapiens, Mus musculus, Rattus norvegicus, Arabidopsis thaliana, C. elegans, Danio rerio, D. Melanogaster, Escherichia coli,* and *Saccharomyces cerevisiae* (Cava et al., 2017). The package provides already predicted targets for miRNAs collected from four different algorithms including DIANA-microT 5.0 (Paraskevopoulou et al., 2013), miRanda (Enright et al., 2003), PicTar (Krek et al., 2005), and TargetScan v7.1 (Agarwal et al., 2015) combined in miRNAtap.db database. Moreover, user can also get information regarding the validated miRNA target information aggregated from miRTarBase release 7 (Chou et al., 2018) and miRwalk (Dweep et al., 2011) using the function "SpidermiRdownload_miRvalidate". Users can follow package vignettes for usage and functions information in detail. The package is also available on github https://github.com/claudiacava/SpidermiR.

3.19.7   miRLab

miRLab is an automated process for investigating the relationship between miRNA and mRNA and includes various computational methods as well as experimental methods for miRNA target prediction (Le et al., 2015) . This package works in three different parts, i.e., (i) Datasets and pre-processing which involves built-in miRNA and mRNA expression datasets, The Cancer Genome Atlas (TCGA) datasets retrieval pipeline, user-provided miRNA and mRNA expression datasets, (ii) Computational methods involve the identification of miRNA-mRNA relationship and target identification using experimentally validated datasets such as CLIP-seq or predicted miRNA target information from TargetScan and, (iii) Validation and post-processing of miRNA and mRNA interaction using experimentally confirmed datasets such as miRNA transfection studies. The package miRLab has implemented several methods that can be called using a simple one-liner code of functions. Each function returns a correlation coefficient score matrix of miRNA interaction on mRNAs. Also, different functions have been included in this package to validate the predicted miRNA-mRNA interaction through experimental data of mRNA as well as miRNA perturbation data and for miRNA target gene enrichment analysis. The input dataset can be provided in comma-separated value (csv) format. Users should follow the reference manual of the package to get more insight into the different functions and their input data types.

3.19.8   miRComb

miRComb is a package in R which provides an integrative platform to analyze miRNA-mRNA interaction through a combination of already normalized miRNA and mRNA expression datasets generated from various sources such as microarrays, quantitative real-time polymerase chain reaction (qRT-PCR) data or Next Generation Sequencing (NGS) data (Vila-Casadesús et al., 2016). Users can supply pre-normalized log2 intensity (from microarray) or log2 counts (from NGS) for miRNA and mRNA datasets separately. The package performs miRNA and mRNA differential expression analysis and then predicts the correlation between miRNA and mRNA expression datasets using Pearson correlation analysis. Further, the negatively correlated miRNA-mRNA interaction sets were examined for miRNA target genes using the database of the pre-computed or predicted miRNA targets known as miRData that integrate target information obtained from MicroCosm (Griffiths-Jones et al., 2006); Rehmsmeir et al. 2004) and TargetScan (Lewis et al., 2005) databases. The package also allows the user to provide custom miRNA-target information. After identifying targets, users can predict the biological functions of miRNA targets using GOstats package (Falcon and Gentleman, 2007). The package and its related documentation are available for download at sourceforge (http://mircomb.sourceforge.net/) and github (https://github.com/mariavica/mircomb).

3.19.9 miRIntegrator

This package is mainly used for visualizing and integrating miRNA into different signaling pathways available on KEGG using miRNA-target information (Diaz et al., 2017). It uses pre-computed computationally identified targets from TargetScan as well as experimentally validated targets of miRNAs from miRTarBase database. The miRIntegrator package provides an opportunityfor its user to visualize and integrated human miRNAs of their interest in the biological pathway through the cognate mRNA targets. Users can follow the package vignettes to work on different available functions. This package is also available on github and can be downloaded using URL https://github.com/datad/mirIntegrator.

3.19.10 anamiR

The R package anamiR (Wang et al., 2019) provides miRNA and target interaction information using a combination of miRNA and mRNA expression data. This package workflow includes data normalization, differential expression, correlation, and functional analysis based on pre-processed miRNA and mRNA expression data obtained from microarray or next-generation sequencing of humans or mice. Users can supply miRNA and mRNA expression data sheets where columns represent sample information while rows represent miRNAs or genes. For statistical analysis, along with expression data, the phenotypic data with sample group information should also be supplied where columns represent samples, and row names represent feature names as well as two groups, multi-groups or continuous data. The anamiR database includes miRNA target information integrated from various sources such as *in silico* predicted miRNA targets pairs from TargetScan (Lewis et al., 2005) and EIMMo (Gaidatzis et al., 2007). Moreover, it also includes thermodynamic free energy-based target site stability information from RNA22 (Loher and Rigoutsos, 2012), miRanda (Enright et al., 2003), MicroCosm (Griffiths-Jones et al., 2008), PITA (Kertesz et al., 2007), miRNA target predicted using machine learning approaches such as DIANA-microT-CDS (Paraskevopoulou et al., 2013), miRDB (Wang, 2008) and experimentally proved miRNA-targets information from miRecords (Xiao et al., 2009), and miRTarBase (Chou et al., 2016). Besides these, the database of this package also contains biological and pathway information of miRNAs and genes collected from KEGG (Kanehisa et al., 2008), Reactome (Croft et al., 2011), BioCarta, and MouseCyc (Evsikov et al., 2009). During each analysis step and statistical test, the package allows the user to change the input parameter and the generated results can be exported as output. The package performs permutation tests to identify significantly enriched functions or pathways. One can follow the user manual for a complete analysis pipeline and functions sourced at github (https://github.com/AllenTiTaiWang/anamiR). The package anamiR has some similarity in functions and utility with MiRComb (Vila-Casadesús et al., 2016), an already published R package.

3.19.11 RmiR

RmiR package was developed by Favero (2020) which is generally used for analyzing miRNA and mRNA expressions and their interaction. This package utilizes RmiR.Hs. miRNA package (Favero, 2013) which integrates several different databases of miRNA and their targets such as miRBase (Griffiths-Jones et al., 2006), TargetScan (Lewis et al., 2005), miRanda (Enright et al., 2003), TarBase (Vergoulis et al., 2012), miRTarget2 from miRDB, and PicTar, into a SQLite object. Users can supply a list of miRNA and genes separately along with their respective expression values as an input to RmiR. Users can also supply a different time series or treatment condition data of miRNA and mRNAs expression which can be used to analyze the correlation of miRNA and targets genes. The list of miRNAs or mRNAs can also be provided as input to this package.

3.19.12   miRNAtap

The package miRNAtap is a workflow to provide targets for user-defined miRNAs of human or mouse and recently it has been developed by Pajak and Simpson (Pajak and Simson, 2016). This package has accumulated the data related to miRNA targets into a database "miRNAtap. db" from 5 different prediction algorithms such as miRanda (Enright et al., 2003), PicTar (Krek et al., 2005), TargetScan (Friedman et al., 2009) and miRDB (Wong and Wang, 2015). To provide functional annotation, it utilizes GO and topGO package of R for predicting gene ontology (GO) annotation related to miRNA targets. The function "getPredictedTargets" takes the miRNA name as input and uses that to identify the ranked targets of that miRNAs in human or mouse if available. Currently, the package supports target prediction for three species, i.e., *Homo sapiens*, *Mus musculus*, and *Rattus norvegicus* (through homology with *M. musculus*).

Success in miRNA target prediction largely depends on the right selection of the available algorithm or program based on user needs. Due to increase in the development of pipeline tools with varied features, users are often confused in the selection of appropriate algorithms for their *in silico* analysis. By modelling the type of input data and combining the results obtained from different algorithms, one can predict and narrow down candidate targets for further experimental validation. This approach has been widely used to build up comprehensive database resources for miRNAs and their targets implicated in specific diseases or conditions. For instance, databases like miRWalk (Sticht et al., 2018), OncomiRdbB (Khurana et al., 2014), miR2Disease (Jiang et al., 2009), miRTarBase (Hsu et al., 2011b), LeukmiR (Rawoof et al., 2020), etc. have utilized several miRNA target prediction algorithms like miRanda, PITA, PicTar, TargetScan, etc. In the authors' lab, the two databases (Khurana et al., 2014; Rawoof et al., 2020) were developed after trying several available algorithms and the output files from these analyses were validated for providing a biological interpretation of the network changes predicted at the level of transcriptome as well (Nair et al., 2020). Such ready reckoner databases would come in handy for researchers who are not familiar with bioinformatics tools available for understanding the interplay between miRNA and their cognate target transcripts. Many of the databases are constantly updated with the information as and when available and thus will be quite useful for the experimenters. As the miRNA sequencing data is growing at unprecedented rate, the need for data integration by curating information becomes crucial for the development of a 'one-stop' tool in miRNA target prediction.

4   GENERAL STRATEGIES FOR MIRNA TARGET PREDICTION

Since the beginning of development of the target prediction tools, there exists a need to evaluate the authenticity of predicted target sites for their effectiveness. So far, there are around 60 prediction interfaces and all the tools use different combinations of features for prediction. For successful and efficient target prediction, one must be acquainted with detailed information about every distinct feature of available algorithms and platforms, their advantages, efficiency and performance. (Min and Yoon, 2010). Two statistical parameters are routinely employed to assess the efficacy of any computational tool namely sensitivity, percentage of correct prediction out of the total known targets and specificity, percentage of the correct targets predicted among all genes (Sydow et al., 2019). In the context of miRNA target prediction, sensitivity of an algorithm is its ability to correctly predict a known target and specificity is its ability to exclude a gene that is not its target. Tools4miR (Lukasik et al., 2016) is an integrative platform which collects and incorporates more than 170 different analysis tools for miRNA targets which could help to forge the path for better prediction.

Any approach in miRNA target prediction is dependent on the researcher and nature of the planned experiments. A basic researcher will always look into all the interactions within an mRNA, but a clinically oriented scientist will only see the best interactions among the pairs that could help in a therapeutic intervention. We present an illustrated flowchart that might help to frame appropriate steps for efficient target prediction (Fig. 2). The first step in any target prediction is to consider basic features like seed match, conserved status and free energy for analysis as it increases the sensitivity and precision of the sequence-based search (Witcos et al., 2011). Tools like TargetScan or PITA often rank the targets based on individual scores. Though they successfully predict targets with statistical support, it is always reliable to incorporate additional features for increasing the efficacy of prediction (Agarwal et al., 2015). The limitation of these algorithms is that they cannot be used for newly evolved genes or set of genes whose orthologs are not present in other species. The next step is to add other parameters like AU content, 3′ compenatory sites, site abundance, G:U wobbles to get a final score. These parameters are useful in cases of miRNA having fewer targets. After the prediction of targets, one can also check the expression pattern of the target gene of interest (Krek et al., 2005). miRGator a web-based interface can be used to access the physiological regulation of putative genes especially in a disease context (Cho et al., 2011). Selection of target sites is done which are close together as both experimental and genome wide analysis reports the importance of close proximity in improving the performance of prediction tools. (Saetrom et al., 2011). Combining results from different prediction tools should not be overlooked when performing target analysis. (Doran and Strauss, 2007).

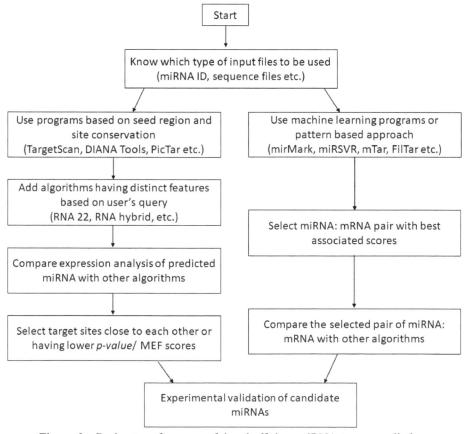

Figure 2   Basic steps for successful and efficient miRNA target prediction.
For any target prediction, the user should be well acquainted with the tool's interface. Based on the input file type, users can either go for traditional prediction algorithms like TargetScan, miRanda, DIANA tools, etc. or can use newer approaches like machine learning, pattern approach, etc. Combining and comparing different computational tools is anticipated to improve the performance and efficiency of miRNA target prediction.

Development of newer computational tools using machine learning approach such as support vector machine (SVM), Artificial neural network (ANN) and pattern-based approach has opened newer frontiers in miRNA target prediction (Pla et al., 2018; Sedaghat et al., 2018; Zheng et al., 2020). Machine learning algorithms use different datasets constructed from experimentally validated miRNA targets to extract features relevant for miRNA:mRNA interaction (Liu et al., 2008). Users can create a specified set of datasets for their search parameters after which distinct features are selected for implementation. Then pre-defined datasets are divided into training and test sets randomly. The parameters are first optimized on the training sets and later evaluated on the test set. The results are tabulated as pair of miRNA:mRNA with their score and accuracy. This approach helps in eliminating human bias, increasing accuracy and integrating multiple features on one user friendly integrative environment for understanding miRNA:mRNA interactions (Sturm et al., 2010). Based on the type of input, users can decide which computational tools that best serve their purpose, as some tools accept sequences of miRNA and 3' UTRs, while others work with gene name, miRNA name etc. For ease of understanding, a list of computational tools with input and output files has been provided in Fig. 3.

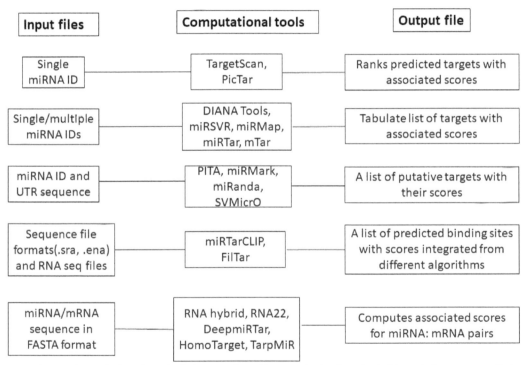

Figure 3 A schematic flowchart depicting user-based input and selection of suitable tools for target prediction. Different computational tools have distinct input types and varied back end output interface. Understanding the functions of each tool, its input file type, and how it works in interpreting results is essential for target prediction.

Once the miRNA targets are predicted with high accuracy and precision, there is a need for them to be experimentally verified since there is always a chance for them to be false positives (Pinzon et al., 2017). Earlier researchers have used experimental validation on miRNA datasets for accessing the specificity of computational tools (Sethupathy et al., 2006b). Selbach et al. employed modified SILAC (pulse labeling with two isotopes) with mass spectroscopy techniques to determine the efficacy of five different programs (TargetScan, TargetScanS, PicTar, DIANA-microT and EIMMO) (Selbach et al., 2008). Target validation is an inevitable step in miRNA target research. The most common method of validating a miRNA target is by transfecting cells with mimics/antimirs of miRNA followed by functional analysis at both transcript and proteome level (Liu et al., 2008; Thomson et al., 2011). For miRNA analysis, specific miRNA inhibitors can be used to silence the miRNA by complementary binding such as 2-O-methyl modified oligoribonucleotides (Davis et al., 2006), locked nucleic acids (LNA) (Ørom et al., 2006), antagomirs (cholesterol conjugated) (Krützfeldt et al., 2008), etc. Different experimental methods exist for verification of miRNA:mRNA interactions such as gene reporter assay, microarray and proteome analysis etc. (Kuhn et al., 2008). Various databases have been designed which incorporate experimentally validated miRNA:mRNA information and their fundamental interactions like TarBase (Papadopoulos et al., 2009), MiRecords (Xiao et al., 2009), miRNAMAP (Hsu et al., 2008) and Ago (Shahi et al., 2006), etc. A reporter assay is used to check the miRNA:mRNA interactions directly. A construct can be prepared by fusion of 3′ UTR target sites with a reporter system like luciferase, green fluorescent protein, etc. and its expression is analyzed by presence/absence of cognate mRNA (Kiriakidou et al., 2004; Jin et al., 2013). For negative controls, mutated target sites are used that are unable to bind to miRNA. Further confirmation can be done by transfecting the cells with miRNA inhibitors to check the interactions. This method is relatively simple and efficient but lacks high throughput identification of targets (Huang et al., 2010). Microarray is a high throughput technique which detects direct binding of miRNA to the target by measuring the levels of target genes (Wang and Wang, 2006). Analysis results in measurement of transcriptome levels of cells with miRNA overexpression/knockdown against untreated cells (Ovando-Vázquez et al., 2016). Similarly, proteomic approach measures the change in protein levels after the introduction of miRNA (Huang et al., 2013). This method uses stable isotope labeling with amino acids in cell culture (SILAC) followed by mass spectrometry (Vinther et al., 2006). Though both techniques can be used in large scale analysis, they share similar limitations like high dependency of transcriptome and proteome on cell type and behavior and some miRNAs can produce lower protein levels without change in transcript levels. Apart from commonly used experimental methods, recent methods employ co-immunoprecipitation as AGO proteins can bind to miRNA and mRNA, and when coupled with next generation sequencing, this technique can help in discovering novel interactions across the genome (Jin, et al., 2010; Beitzinger, et al., 2007). CLIP and PAR-CLIP (Photo-activatable-Ribonucleoside-Enhanced Crosslinking and Immunoprecipitation) use ultraviolet radiation to completely link RNA protein complexes in the cells (Hafner et al., 2012). Not only is this approach expensive and requires technical expertise, it also cannot distinguish the direct and indirect miRNA interactions (Lu and Leslie, 2016).

Collectively, the authenticity of miRNA:mRNA interactions can be checked (Elton and Yalowich, 2015) first by verifying the miRNA:mRNA interaction using an *in silico* approach. Next, both should be expressed in the cell. And most importantly, the miRNA should have a variable effect on protein expression levels, i.e., if miRNA is a true regulator of the target gene, its mimics should silence the gene and antimirs should increase the gene expression levels. Lastly, any miRNA: mRNA regulation should result in a valid biological outcome.

5 CONCLUSION AND FUTURE PERSPECTIVE

Though many computational tools have been developed for miRNA target prediction, there is not a single algorithm which can be routinely used for every analysis. As such there can be a growing confusion regarding the applicability and interface of these tools. In this chapter, we have tried to address this very issue by clearly explaining the biological and computational basis used to predict miRNA:mRNA interaction by various bioinformatics tools. This helps in understanding each tool, its origin, functioning, its prediction and interpretation of the results. Finally, we have discussed our approach in tackling miRNA target prediction.

It is very important to view miRNA regulation as an intricate and complex network of interactions leading to varied outcomes. Messenger RNAs and miRNAs from same source should be profiled simultaneously followed by integrated and correlation analysis which will assist in generating more reliable and statistically relevant results. Recently, newer features have come up that do not directly involve sequence-based pairing. Certain regulatory process like protein binding to RNA, methylation of RNA sites and long non-coding RNA (lcnRNAs) interactions with miRNA to act as inhibitors cannot be ignored in development of network-based modules. Biological systems always have a non-canonical regulation because any biological mechanism requires a different approach to compensate what normal physiological processes are unable to accomplish. These perturbations can be interpreted as evolutionary intermediates with different functions. However, it is necessary to incorporate these features into target prediction algorithms to obtain a true and reliable score. Combinatorial approach by integrating multiple platforms with varied features is anticipated to improve the performance, coverage and accuracy in near future.

Conflicts of Interest

Authors declare no competing interests

Acknowledgments

LDK was supported by CSIR-GENESIS funds and AR acknowledges Fellowship received from the same project. (AR is also affiliated to School of Life Sciences, Laboratory of Translational and Evolutionary Genomics, Jawaharlal Nehru University, New Delhi) AK was supported by MHRD fellowship. Authors would like to acknowledge Dr. V. Dinesh Kumar for his critical remarks, reviewing and editing this chapter.

REFERENCES

Ab Mutalib, N.S., S.A. Sulaiman and R. Jamal (2019). Computational tools for microRNA target prediction. pp. 79–105. *In*: L.K.BT.C.E. and D. Wei (ed.). Translational Epigenetics, vol. 9. Academic Press.

Agarwal, V., G.W. Bell, J.W. Nam and D.P. Bartel (2015). Predicting effective microRNA target sites in mammalian mRNAs. Elife. 4: e05005. doi: 10.7554/eLife.05005.

Ahmadi, H., A. Ahmadi, S. Azimzadeh-Jamalkandi, M.A. Shoorehdeli, A. Salehzadeh-Yazdi, G. Bidkhori, et al. (2013). HomoTarget: A new algorithm for prediction of microRNA targets in homo sapiens. Genomics. 101(2): 94–100.

Arvey, A., E. Larsson, C. Sander, C.S. Leslie and D.S. Marks (2010). Target mRNA abundance dilutes microRNA and siRNA activity. Mol. Syst. Biol. 6: 363.

Bartel, D.P. (2009) MicroRNAs: Target recognition and regulatory functions Cell. 136(2): 215–233.

Beitzinger, M., L. Peters, J.Y. Zhu, E. Kremmer and G. Meister (2007). Identification of human microRNA targets from isolated argonaute protein complexes. RNA Biol. 4(2): 76–84.

Benson, D.A., I. Karsch-Mizrachi, D.J. Lipman, J. Ostell and E.W. Sayers (2009). GenBank. Nucleic Acids Res. 37(D): D26–D31.

Betel, D., A. Koppal, P. Agius, C. Sander and C. Leslie (2010). Comprehensive modeling of microRNA targets predicts functional non-conserved and non-canonical sites. Genome Biol. 11(8): R90.

Bhaskaran, M. and M. Mohan (2014). MicroRNAs: History, biogenesis, and their evolving role in animal development and disease. Vet. Pathol. 51(4): 759–774.

Bradley, T. and S. Moxon (2020). FilTar: Using RNA-Seq data to improve microRNA target prediction accuracy in animals. Bioinformatics. 36(8): 2410–2416.

Brennecke, J., A. Stark, R.B. Russell and S.M. Cohen (2005). Principles of microRNA-target recognition. PLoS Biol. 3(3): e85.

Brodersen, P. and O. Voinnet (2009). Revisiting the principles of microRNA target recognition and mode of action. Nat. Rev. Mol. Cell Biol. 10(2) 141–148.

Catalanotto, C., C. Cogoni and G. Zardo (2016). MicroRNA in control of gene expression: An overview of nuclear functions. Int. J. Mol. Sci. 17(10): 1712.

Cava, C., A. Colaprico, G. Bertoli, A. Graudenzi, T.C. Silva, C. Olsen, et al. (2017). SpidermiR: An R/Bioconductor package for integrative analysis with miRNA data. Int. J. Mol. Sci. 18(2): 274.

Chandra, V., R. Girijadevi, A.S. Nair, S.S. Pillai and R.M. Pillai (2010). MTar: A computational microRNA target prediction architecture for human transcriptome. BMC Bioinformatics. 11(Suppl 1): p. S2.

Chen, L., L. Heikkinen, C. Wang, Y. Yang, H. Sun and G. Wong (2019). Trends in the development of miRNA bioinformatics tools. Brief. Bioinform. 20(5): 1836–1852.

Chi, S.W., J.B. Zang, A. Mele and R.B. Darnell (2009). Argonaute HITS-CLIP decodes microRNA-mRNA interaction maps. Nature. 460(7254): 479–486.

Cho, S., Y. Jun, S. Lee, H.S. Choi, S. Jung, Y. Jang, et al. (2011) miRGator v2.0: An integrated system for functional investigation of microRNAs. Nucleic Acids Res. 39(suppl_1): D158–D162.

Chou, C.H., F.M. Lin, M.T. Chou, S.D. Hsu, T.H. Chang, S.L. Weng, et al. (2013). A computational approach for identifying microRNA-target interactions using high-throughput CLIP and PAR-CLIP sequencing. BMC Genomics. 14(Suppl 1): S2.

Chou, C.H., N.W. Chang, S. Shrestha, S.D. Hsu, Y.L. Lin, W.H. Lee, et al. (2016). miRTarBase 2016: Updates to the experimentally validated miRNA-target interactions database. Nucleic Acids Res. 44(D1): D239–D247.

Chou, C.H., S. Shrestha, C.D. Yang, N.W. Chang, Y.L. Lin, K.W. Liao, et al. (2018). miRTarBase update 2018: A resource for experimentally validated microRNA-target interactions. Nucleic Acids Res. 46(D1): D296–D302.

Cogswell, J.P., J. Ward, I.A. Taylor, M. Waters, Y. Shi, B. Cannon, et al. (2008). Identification of miRNA changes in Alzheimer's disease brain and CSF yields putative biomarkers and insights into disease pathways. J. Alzheimers. Dis. 14(1): 27–41.

Croft, D., G. O'Kelly, G. Wu, R. Haw, M. Gillespie, L. Matthews, et al. (2011). Reactome: A database of reactions, pathways and biological processes. Nucleic Acids Res. 39(suppl_1): D691–697.

Dai, X., Z. Zhuang and P.X. Zhao (2010). Computational analysis of miRNA targets in plants: Current status and challenges. Brief. Bioinform. 12(2): 115–121.

Davis, S., B. Lollo, S. Freier and C. Esau (2006). Improved targeting of miRNA with antisense oligonucleotides. Nucleic Acids Res. 34(8): 2294–2304.

Diaz, D., M. Donato, T. Nguyen and S. Draghici (2017). Microrna-augmented pathways (mirAP) and their applications to pathway analysis and disease subtyping. Pac. Symp. Biocomput. 22: 390–401.

Ding, J., X. Li and H. Hu (2016). TarPmiR: A new approach for microRNA target site prediction. Bioinformatics. 32(18): 2768–2775.

Doench, J.G. and P.A. Sharp (2004). Specificity of microRNA target selection in translational repression. Genes Dev. 18(5): 504–511.

Doran, J. and W.M. Strauss (2007). Bio-informatic trends for the determination of miRNA-target interactions in mammals. DNA Cell Biol. 26(5): 353–360.

Dweep, H., C. Sticht, P. Pandey and N. Gretz (2011). miRWalk–database: Prediction of possible miRNA binding sites by 'walking' the genes of three genomes. J. Biomed. Inform. 44(5): 839–847.

Elefant, N., Y. Altuvia and H. Margalit (2011). A wide repertoire of miRNA binding sites: Prediction and functional implications. Bioinformatics. 27(22): 3093–3101.

Elton, T.S. and J.C. Yalowich (2015). Experimental procedures to identify and validate specific mRNA targets of miRNAs. EXCLI J. 14: 758–790.

Enright, A.J., B. John, U. Gaul, T. Tuschl, C. Sander and D.S. Marks (2003). MicroRNA targets in Drosophila. Genome Biol. 5(1): R1.

Evsikov, A.V., M.E. Dolan, M.P. Genrich, E. Patek and C.J. Bult (2009). MouseCyc: A curated biochemical pathways database for the laboratory mouse. Genome Biol. 10(8): R84.

Falcon, S. and R. Gentleman (2007). Using GOstats to test gene lists for GO term association. Bioinformatics. 23(2) 257–258.

Favero, F., (2013). RmiR package vignette.

Flicek, P., M.R. Amode, D. Barrell, K. Beal, S. Brent, D. Carvalho-Silva, et al. (2012). Ensembl 2012. Nucleic Acids Res. 40(D1): D84–D90.

Friedman, R.C., K.K.H. Farh, C.B. Burge and D.P. Bartel (2009). Most mammalian mRNAs are conserved targets of microRNAs. Genome Res. 19(1): 92–105.

Gaidatzis, D., E. van Nimwegen, J. Hausser and M. Zavolan (2007). Inference of miRNA targets using evolutionary conservation and pathway analysis. BMC Bioinformatics. 8: 69.

Garcia, D.M., D. Baek, C. Shin, G.W. Bell, A. Grimson and D.P. Bartel (2011). Weak seed-pairing stability and high target-site abundance decrease the proficiency of lsy-6 and other microRNAs. Nat. Struct. Mol. Biol. 18(10): 1139–1146.

Gelbart, W.M., M. Crosby, B. Matthews, W.P. Rindone, J. Chillemi, S.R. Twombly, et al. (1997). FlyBase: A *Drosophila* database. The FlyBase consortium. Nucleic Acids Res. 25(1): 63–66.

Giansanti, V., M. Castelli, S. Beretta and I. Merelli (2019). Comparing deep and machine learning approaches in bioinformatics: A miRNA-target prediction case study. pp. 31–44. In: J.M.F. Rodrigues, P.J.S. Cardoso, J. Monteiro, R. Lam, V.V. Krzhizhanovskaya, M.H. Lees, et al. (eds). Computational Science—ICCS 2019, 19th International Conference, Faro, Portugal, June 12–14, 2019, Proceedings, Part III. Springer International Publishing.

Giegerich, R. and P. Steffen (2002). Implementing algebraic dynamic programming in the functional and the imperative programming paradigm. pp. 1–20. In: E.A. Boiten and B. Möller (eds). Mathematics of Program Construction. MPC 2002. Lecture Notes in Computer Science, vol 2386. Springer, Berlin, Heidelberg. https://doi.org/10.1007/3-540-45442-X_1

Griffiths-Jones, S., R.J. Grocock, S. van Dongen, A. Bateman and A.J. Enright (2006). miRBase: microRNA sequences, targets and gene nomenclature. Nucleic Acids Res. 34D: D140–D144.

Griffiths-Jones, S., H.K. Saini, S. van Dongen and A.J. Enright (2008). miRBase: Tools for microRNA genomics. Nucleic Acids Res. 36D: D154–D158.

Grimson, A., K.K.H. Farh, W.K. Johnston, P. Garrett-Engele, L.P. Lim and D.P. Bartel (2007). MicroRNA targeting specificity in mammals: Determinants beyond seed pairing. Mol. Cell. 27(1): 91–105.

Gu, W., Y. Xu, X. Xie, T. Wang, J.H. Ko and T. Zhou (2014). The role of RNA structure at 5′ untranslated region in microRNA-mediated gene regulation. RNA. 20(9): 1369–1375.

Guo, Z.W., C. Xie, J.R. Yang, J.H. Li, J.H. Yang and L. Zheng (2015). MtiBase: A database for decoding microRNA target sites located within CDS and 5-UTR regions from CLIP-Seq and expression profile datasets. Database. bav102.

Hafner, M., M. Landthaler, L. Burger, M. Khorshid, J. Hausser, P. Berninger, et al. (2010). Transcriptome-wide identification of RNA-binding protein and microRNA target sites by PAR-CLIP. Cell. 141(1): 129–141.

Hafner, M., S. Lianoglou, T. Tuschl and D. Betel (2012). Genome-wide identification of miRNA targets by PAR-CLIP. Methods. 58(2): 94–105.

Hall, M., E. Frank, G. Holmes, B. Pfahringer, P. Reutemann and I.H. Witten (2009). The WEKA data mining software: An update. ACM SIGKDD Explor. Newsl. 11(1): 10–18.

Harrison, P.W., B. Alako, C. Amid, A. Cerdeño-Tárraga, I. Cleland, S. Holt, et al. (2019). The European Nucleotide Archive in 2018. Nucleic Acids Res. 47(D1): D84–D88.

Hausser, J., A.P. Syed, B. Bilen and M. Zavolan (2013). Analysis of CDS-located miRNA target sites suggests that they can effectively inhibit translation. Genome Res. 23(4): 604–615.

Helwak, A., G. Kudla, T. Dudnakova and D. Tollervey (2013). Mapping the human miRNA interactome by CLASH reveals frequent noncanonical binding. Cell. 153(3): 654–665.

Hofacker, I.L., W. Fontana, P.F. Stadler, L.S. Bonhoeffer, M. Tacker and P. Schuster (1994). Fast folding and comparison of RNA secondary structures. Monatshefte für Chemie/Chem. Mon. 125(2): 167–188.

Hofacker, I.L. (2003). Vienna RNA secondary structure server. Nucleic Acids Res. 31(13): 3429–3431.

Hsu, S.D., C.H. Chu, A.P. Tsou, S.J. Chen, H.C. Chen, P.W.. Hsu, et al. (2008). miRNAMap 2.0: Genomic maps of microRNAs in metazoan genomes. Nucleic Acids Res. 36(D): D165–D169.

Hsu, J.B.K., C.M. Chiu, S.D. Hsu, W.Y. Huang, C.H. Chien, T.Y. Lee, et al. (2011a). miRTar: An integrated system for identifying miRNA-target interactions in human. BMC Bioinformatics. 12: 300.

Hsu, S.D., F.M. Lin, W.Y. Wu, C. Liang, W.C. Huang, W.L. Chan, et al. (2011b). miRTarBase: A database curates experimentally validated microRNA-target interactions. Nucleic Acids Res. 39(D): D163–D169.

Hsu, S.D., Y.T. Tseng, S. Shrestha, Y.L. Lin, A. Khaleel, C.H. Chou, et al. (2014). miRTarBase update 2014: An information resource for experimentally validated miRNA-target interactions. Nucleic Acids Res. 42(D): D78–D85.

Huang, Y., Q. Zou, H. Song, F. Song, L. Wang, G. Zhang, et al. (2010). A study of miRNAs targets prediction and experimental validation. Protein Cell. 1(11): 979–986.

Huang, T.C., S.M. Pinto and A. Pandey (2013). Proteomics for understanding miRNA biology. Proteomics. 13(3-4): 558–567.

Jiang, Q., Y. Wang, Y. Hao, L. Juan, M. Teng, X. Zhang, et al. (2009). miR2Disease: A manually curated database for microRNA deregulation in human disease. Nucleic Acids Res. 37(D): D98–D104.

Jin, H., W. Tuo, H. Lian, Q. Liu, X.Q. Zhu and H. Gao (2010). Strategies to identify microRNA targets: New advances. N. Biotechnol. 27(6): 734–738.

Jin, Y., Z. Chen, X. Liu and X. Zhou (2013). Evaluating the microRNA targeting sites by luciferase reporter gene assay. Methods Mol. Biol. 936: 117–127.

John, B., A.J. Enright, A. Aravin, T. Tuschl, C. Sander and D.S. Marks (2004). Human MicroRNA targets. PLoS Biol. 2(11): e363.

John, B., C. Sander and D.S. Marks (2006). Prediction of human MicroRNA targets BT – MicroRNA protocols. pp. 101–113. *In*: S.Y. Ying (ed.). MicroRNA Protocols. Humana Press, Totowa, NJ.

Kanehisa, M., et al. (2008). KEGG for linking genomes to life and the environment. Nucleic Acids Res. 36(D): D480–484.

Kanehisa, M., S. Goto, M. Furumichi, M. Tanabe and M. Hirakawa (2010). KEGG for representation and analysis of molecular networks involving diseases and drugs. Nucleic Acids Res. 38(D): D355–D360.

Kent, W.J., C.W. Sugnet, T.S. Furey, K.M. Roskin, T.H. Pringle, A.M. Zahler, et al. (2002). The human genome browser at UCSC. Genome Res. 12(6): 996–1006.

Kertesz, M., N. Iovino, U. Unnerstall, U. Gaul and E. Segal (2007). The role of site accessibility in microRNA target recognition. Nat. Genet. 39(10): 1278–1284.

Khurana, R., V.K. Verma, A. Rawoof, S. Tiwari, R.A. Nair, G. Mahidhara, et al. (2014). OncomiRdbB: A comprehensive database of microRNAs and their targets in breast cancer. BMC Bioinformatics. 15: 15.

Kiriakidou, M., P.T. Nelson, A. Kouranov, P. Fitziev, C. Bouyioukos, Z. Mourelatos, et al. (2004). A combined computational-experimental approach predicts human microRNA targets. Genes Dev. 18(10): 1165–1178.

Kishore, S., L. Jaskiewicz, L. Burger, J. Hausser, M. Khorshid and M. Zavolan (2011). A quantitative analysis of CLIP methods for identifying binding sites of RNA-binding proteins. Nat. Methods. 8(7): 559–564.

Kodama, Y., M. Shumway and R. Leinonen (2012). The sequence read archive: Explosive growth of sequencing data. Nucleic Acids Res. 40(D): D54–D56.

Koscielny, G., V.L. Texier, C. Gopalakrishnan, V. Kumanduri, J.J. Riethoven, F. Nardone, et al. (2009). ASTD: The alternative splicing and transcript diversity database. Genomics. 93(3): 213–220.

Köster, J. and S. Rahmann (2018). Snakemake-a scalable bioinformatics workflow engine. Bioinformatics. 34(20): 3600.

Kozomara, A. and S. Griffiths-Jones (2011). miRBase: Integrating microRNA annotation and deep-sequencing data. Nucleic Acids Res. 39(D): D152–D157.

Krek, A., D. Grün, M.N. Poy, R. Wolf, L. Rosenberg, E.J. Epstein, et al. (2005). Combinatorial microRNA target predictions. Nat. Genet. 37(5): 495–500.

Krüger, J. and M. Rehmsmeier (2006). RNAhybrid: microRNA target prediction easy, fast and flexible. Nucleic Acids Res. 34(W): W451–W454.

Krützfeldt, J., N. Rajewsky, R. Braich, K.G. Rajeev, T. Tuschl, M. Manoharan, et al. (2005). Silencing of microRNAs in vivo with 'antagomirs'. Nature. 438(7068): 685–689.

Kuhn, D.E., M.M. Martin, D.S. Feldman, A.V Terry Jr, G.J. Nuovo and T.S. Elton (2008). Experimental validation of miRNA targets. Methods. 44(1): 47–54.

Langmead, B., C. Trapnell, M. Pop and S.L. Salzberg (2009). Ultrafast and memory-efficient alignment of short DNA sequences to the human genome. Genome Biol. 10(3): R25.

Le, T.D., J. Zhang, L. Liu, H. Liu and J. Li (2015). miRLAB: An R based dry lab for exploring miRNA-mRNA regulatory relationships. PLoS One. 10(12): e0145386.

Leinonen, R., H. Sugawara and M. Shumway (2011). The sequence read archive. Nucleic Acids Res. 39(D): D19–D21.

Leinonen, R., R. Akhtar, E. Birney, L. Bower, A. Cerdeno-Tárraga, Y. Cheng, et al. (2011). The european nucleotide archive. Nucleic Acids Res. 39(D): D28–D31.

Lewis, B.P., I. Shih, M.W. Jones-Rhoades, D.P. Bartel and C.B. Burge (2003). Prediction of mammalian microRNA targets. Cell. 115(7): 787–798.

Lewis, B.P., C.B. Burge and D.P. Bartel (2005). Conserved seed pairing, often flanked by adenosines, indicates that thousands of human genes are microRNA targets. Cell. 120(1): 15–20.

Li, M., C. Marin-Muller, U. Bharadwaj, K.H. Chow, Q. Yao and C. Chen (2009). MicroRNAs: Control and loss of control in human physiology and disease. World J. Surg. 33(4): 667–684.

Li, J. and Z. Zhang (2013). miRNA regulatory variation in human evolution. Trends Genet. 29(2): 116–124.

Li, Y., A. Goldenberg, K.C. Wong and Z. Zhang (2014a). A probabilistic approach to explore human miRNA targetome by integrating miRNA-overexpression data and sequence information. Bioinformatics. 30(5): 621–628.

Li, Y., C. Liang, K.C. Wong, K. Jin and Z. Zhang (2014b). Inferring probabilistic miRNA-mRNA interaction signatures in cancers: A role-switch approach. Nucleic Acids Res. 42(9): e76.

Liu, H., D. Yue, L. Zhang, S.J. Gao and Y. Huang (2008). A machine learning approach for miRNA target prediction. *In*: IEEE International Workshop on Genomic Signal Processing and Statistics 2008. IEEE Int Workshop Genomic Signal Process Stat. pp. 1–3.

Liu, Z., A. Sall and D. Yang (2008). MicroRNA: An emerging therapeutic target and intervention tool, Int. J. Mol. Sci. 9(6): 978–999.

Liu, H., D. Yue, Y. Chen, S.J. Gao and Y. Huang (2010). Improving performance of mammalian microRNA target prediction. BMC Bioinformatics. 11: 476.

Liu, W. and X. Wang (2019). Prediction of functional microRNA targets by integrative modeling of microRNA binding and target expression data. Genome Biol. 20(1): 18.

Loher, P. and I. Rigoutsos (2012). Interactive exploration of RNA22 microRNA target predictions. Bioinformatics. 28(24): 3322–3323.

Lorenz, R., S.H. Bernhart, C.H.Z. Siederdissen, H. Tafer, C. Flamm, P.F. Stadler, et al. (2011). ViennaRNA Package 2.0. Algorithms Mol. Biol. 6(1): 26.

Lu, Y. and C.S. Leslie (2016). Learning to predict miRNA-mRNA interactions from AGO CLIP sequencing and CLASH data. PLOS Comput. Biol. 12(7): e1005026.

Lukasik, A., M. Wójcikowski and P. Zielenkiewicz (2016). Tools4miRs – one place to gather all the tools for miRNA analysis. Bioinformatics. 32(17): 2722–2724.

Mahen, E.M., P.Y. Watson, J.W. Cottrell and M.J. Fedor (2010). mRNA secondary structures fold sequentially but exchange rapidly in vivo. PLoS Biol. 8(2): e1000307.

Mandke, P., N. Wyatt, J. Fraser, B. Bates, S.J. Berberich and M.P. Markey (2012). MicroRNA-34a modulates MDM4 expression via a target site in the open reading frame. PLoS One. 7(8): e42034.

Maragkakis, M., M. Reczko, V.A. Simossis, P. Alexiou, G.L. Papadopoulos, T. Dalamagas, et al. (2009). DIANA-microT web server: Elucidating microRNA functions through target prediction. Nucleic Acids Res. 37(W): W273–W276.

Maragkakis, M., T. Vergoulis, P. Alexiou, M. Reczko, K. Plomaritou, M. Gousis, et al. (2011). DIANA-microT web server upgrade supports fly and worm miRNA target prediction and bibliographic miRNA to disease association. Nucleic Acids Res. 39(W): W145–W148.

Marín, R.M. and J. Vanícek (2011). Efficient use of accessibility in microRNA target prediction. Nucleic Acids Res. 39(1): 19–29.

Mathews, D.H., J. Sabina, M. Zuker and D.H. Turner (1999). Expanded sequence dependence of thermodynamic parameters improves prediction of RNA secondary structure. J. Mol. Biol. 288(5): 911–940.

Menor, M., T. Ching, X. Zhu, D. Garmire and L.X. Garmire (2014). mirMark: A site-level and UTR-level classifier for miRNA target prediction. Genome Biol. 15(10): 500.

Min, H. and S. Yoon (2010). Got target? Computational methods for microRNA target prediction and their extension. Exp. Mol. Med. 42(4): 233–244.

Miranda, K.C., T. Huynh, Y. Tay, Y.S. Ang, W.L. Tam, A.M. Thomson, et al. (2006). A pattern-based method for the identification of MicroRNA binding sites and their corresponding heteroduplexes. Cell. 126(6): 1203–1217.

Nair, R.A., V.K. Verma, S.S. Beevi, A. Rawoof, L.E. Alexander, E.R. Prasad, et al. (2020). MicroRNA signatures in blood or bone marrow distinguish subtypes of pediatric acute lymphoblastic leukemia. Transl. Oncol. 13(9): 100800.

Nam, J.W., O.S Rissland, D. Koppstein, C. Abreu-Goodger, C.H. Jan, V. Agarwal, et al. (2014). Global analyses of the effect of different cellular contexts on microRNA targeting. Mol. Cell. 53(6): 1031–1043.

O'Brien, J., H. Hayder, Y. Zayed and C. Peng (2018). Overview of MicroRNA biogenesis, mechanisms of actions, and circulation. Frontiers in Endocrinology. 9: 402.

Ørom, U.A., S. Kauppinen and A.H. Lund (2006). LNA-modified oligonucleotides mediate specific inhibition of microRNA function. Gene. 372: 137–141.

Ovando-Vázquez, C., D. Lepe-Soltero and C. Abreu-Goodger (2016). Improving microRNA target prediction with gene expression profiles. BMC Genomics. 17(1): 364.

Pajak, M. and T.I. Simpson (2016). miRNAtap: miRNAtap: microRNA targets-aggregated predictions. R Packag. version, vol. 1, no. 0.

Papadopoulos, G.L., M. Reczko, V.A. Simossis, P. Sethupathy and A.G. Hatzigeorgiou (2009). The database of experimentally supported targets: A functional update of TarBase. Nucleic Acids Res. 37D: D155–D158.

Paraskevopoulou, M.D., G. Georgakilas, N. Kostoulas, I.S. Vlachos, T. Vergoulis, M. Reczko, et al. (2013). DIANA-microT web server v5.0: Service integration into miRNA functional analysis workflows. Nucleic Acids Res. 41W: W169–W173.

Peng, Y. and C.M. Croce (2016). The role of MicroRNAs in human cancer. Signal Transduct. Target. Ther. 1(1): 15004.

Pinzón, N., B. Li, L. Martinez, A. Sergeeva, J. Presumey, F. Apparailly, et al. (2017). microRNA target prediction programs predict many false positives. Genome Res. 27(2): 234–245.

Pla, A., X. Zhong and S. Rayner (2018). miRAW: A deep learning-based approach to predict microRNA targets by analyzing whole microRNA transcripts. PLOS Comput. Biol. 14(7): e1006185.

Ragan, C., M. Zuker and M.A. Ragan (2011). Quantitative prediction of miRNA-mRNA interaction based on equilibrium concentrations. PLOS Comput. Biol. 7(2): e1001090.

Rawoof, A., G. Swaminathan, S. Tiwari, R.A. Nair and L. Dinesh Kumar (2020). LeukmiR: A database for miRNAs and their targets in acute lymphoblastic leukemia. Database (Oxford). 2020: baz151.

Reczko, M., M. Maragkakis, P. Alexiou, G.L. Papadopoulos and A.G. Hatzigeorgiou (2011). Accurate microRNA target prediction using detailed binding site accessibility and machine learning on proteomics data. Front. Genet. 2: 103.

Reczko, M., M. Maragkakis, P. Alexiou, I. Grosse and A.G. Hatzigeorgiou (2012). Functional microRNA targets in protein coding sequences. Bioinformatics. 28(6): 771–776.

Rehmsmeier, M., P. Steffen, M. Hochsmann and R. Giegerich (2004). Fast and effective prediction of microRNA/target duplexes. RNA. 10(10): 1507–1517.

Riffo-Campos, Á.L., I. Riquelme and P. Brebi-Mieville (2016). Tools for sequence-based miRNA target prediction: What to choose? Int. J. Mol. Sci. 17(12): 1987.

Robins, H. and W.H. Press (2005). Human microRNAs target a functionally distinct population of genes with AT-rich 3-UTRs, Proc. Natl. Acad. Sci. U.S.A. 102(43): 15557–15562.

Rogers, K. and X. Chen (2013). Biogenesis, turnover, and mode of action of plant MicroRNAs. Plant Cell. 25(7): 2383 LP–2399.

Ru, Y., K.J. Kechris, B. Tabakoff, P. Hoffman, R.A. Radcliffe, R. Bowler, et al. (2014). The multiMiR R package and database: Integration of microRNA-target interactions along with their disease and drug associations. Nucleic Acids Res. 42(17): e133.

Saetrom, P., B.S.E. Heale, O. Snøve Jr, L. Aagaard, J. Alluin and J.J. Rossi (2007). Distance constraints between microRNA target sites dictate efficacy and cooperativity. Nucleic Acids Res. 35(7): 2333–2342.

Sayers, E.W., T. Barrett, D.A. Benson, E. Bolton, S.H. Bryant, K. Canese, et al. (2009). Database resources of the national center for biotechnology information. Nucleic Acids Res. 37(D): D5–D15.

Sedaghat, N., M. Fathy, M.H. Modarressi and A. Shojaie (2018). Combining supervised and unsupervised learning for improved miRNA target prediction. IEEE/ACM Trans. Comput. Biol. Bioinforma. 15(5): 1594–1604.

Selbach, M., B. Schwanhäusser, N. Thierfelder, Z. Fang, R. Khanin and N. Rajewsky (2008). Widespread changes in protein synthesis induced by microRNAs. Nature. 455(7209): 58–63.

Sethupathy, P., B. Corda and A.G. Hatzigeorgiou (2006a). TarBase: A comprehensive database of experimentally supported animal microRNA targets. RNA. 12(2): 192–197.

Sethupathy, P., M. Megraw and A.G. Hatzigeorgiou (2006b). A guide through present computational approaches for the identification of mammalian microRNA targets. Nat. Methods. 3(11): 881–886.

Shahi, P., et al. (2006). Argonaute–a database for gene regulation by mammalian microRNAs. Nucleic Acids Res. 34(D): D115–D118.

Smith, T.F. and M.S. Waterman (1981). Identification of common molecular subsequences. J. Mol. Biol. 147(1): 195–197.

Stajich, J.E., D. Block, K. Boulez, S.E. Brenner, S.A. Chervitz, C. Dagdigian, et al. (2002). The bioperl toolkit: Perl modules for the life sciences. Genome Res. 12(10): 1611–1618.

Sticht, C., C. De La Torre, A. Parveen and N. Gretz (2018). miRWalk: An online resource for prediction of microRNA binding sites. PLoS One. 13(10): e0206239.

Sturm, M., M. Hackenberg, D. Langenberger and D. Frishman (2010). TargetSpy: A supervised machine learning approach for microRNA target prediction. BMC Bioinformatics. 11(1) 292.

Sydow, D., L. Burggraaff, A. Szengel, H.W.T. van Vlijmen, A.P. IJzerman, G.J.P. van Westen, et al. (2019). Advances and challenges in computational target prediction. J. Chem. Inf. Model. 59(5): 1728–1742.

Taguchi, Y. and J. Yasuda (2010). Inference of gene expression regulation via microRNA transfection. pp. 672–679. *In*: D.S. Huang, Z. Zhao, V. Bevilacqua and J.C. Figueroa (eds). Advanced Intelligent Computing Theories and Applications. ICIC 2010. Lecture Notes in Computer Science, vol 6215. Springer, Berlin, Heidelberg.

Taguchi, Y.H., (2013). Inference of target gene regulation by miRNA via MiRaGE server. Aging Dis. 3(4): 301–306.

Thomson, D.W., C.P. Bracken and G.J. Goodall (2011). Experimental strategies for microRNA target identification. Nucleic Acids Res. 39(16): 6845–6853.

Vejnar, C.E. and E.M. Zdobnov (2012). MiRmap: Comprehensive prediction of microRNA target repression strength. Nucleic Acids Res. 40(22): 11673–11683.

Vejnar, C.E., M. Blum and E.M. Zdobnov (2013). miRmap web: Comprehensive microRNA target prediction online. Nucleic Acids Res. 41(W): W165–W168.

Vella, M.C., K. Reinert and F.J. Slack (2004). Architecture of a validated MicroRNA: Target interaction. Chem. Biol. 11(12): 1619–1623.

Vergoulis, T., I.S. Vlachos, P. Alexiou, G. Georgakilas, M. Maragkakis, M. Reczko, et al. (2012). TarBase 6.0: Capturing the exponential growth of miRNA targets with experimental support. Nucleic Acids Res. 40(D): D222–D229.

Vila-Casadesús, M., M. Gironella and J.J. Lozano (2016). MiRComb: An R package to analyse miRNA-mRNA interactions. Examples across five digestive cancers. PLoS One. 11(3) e0151127.

Vinther, J., M.M. Hedegaard, P.P. Gardner, J.S. Andersen and P. Arctander (2006). Identification of miRNA targets with stable isotope labeling by amino acids in cell culture. Nucleic Acids Res. 34(16): e107–e107.

Wahid, F., A. Shehzad, T. Khan and Y.Y. Kim (2010). MicroRNAs: Synthesis, mechanism, function, and recent clinical trials. Biochim. Biophys. Acta – Mol. Cell Res. 1803(11): 1231–1243.

Wang, X. and X. Wang (2006). Systematic identification of microRNA functions by combining target prediction and expression profiling. Nucleic Acids Res. 34(5): 1646–1652.

Wang, X., (2008). miRDB: A microRNA target prediction and functional annotation database with a wiki interface. RNA. 14(6): 1012–1017.

Wang, X. (2014). Composition of seed sequence is a major determinant of microRNA targeting patterns. Bioinformatics. 30(10): 1377–1383.

Wang, T.T., C.Y. Lee, L.C. Lai, M.H. Tsai, T.P. Lu and E.Y. Chuang (2019). anamiR: Integrated analysis of MicroRNA and gene expression profiling. BMC Bioinformatics. 20(1): 239.

Wen, M., P. Cong, Z. Zhang, H. Lu and T. Li (2018).. DeepMirTar: A deep-learning approach for predicting human miRNA targets. Bioinformatics. 34(22): 3781–3787.

Witkos, T.M., E. Koscianska and W.J. Krzyzosiak (2011). Practical aspects of microRNA target prediction. Curr. Mol. Med. 11(2): 93–109.

Wong, N. and X. Wang (2015). miRDB: An online resource for microRNA target prediction and functional annotations. Nucleic Acids Res. 43(D): D146–D152.

Wuchty, S., W. Fontana, I.L. Hofacker and P. Schuster (1999). Complete suboptimal folding of RNA and the stability of secondary structures. Biopolymers. 49(2): 145–165.

Xia, W., G. Cao and N. Shao (2009). Progress in miRNA target prediction and identification. Sci. China Ser. C Life Sci. 52(12): 1123–1130.

Xiao, F., Z. Zuo, G. Cai, S. Kang, X. Gao and T. Li (2009). miRecords: An integrated resource for microRNA-target interactions. Nucleic Acids Res. 37(D): D105–D110.

Xu, J., R. Zhang, Y. Shen, G. Liu, X. Lu and C.I. Wu (2013). The evolution of evolvability in microRNA target sites in vertebrates. Genome Res. 23(11): 1810–1816.

Ye, C., Y. Long, G. Ji, Q.Q. Li and X. Wu (2018). APAtrap: Identification and quantification of alternative polyadenylation sites from RNA-seq data. Bioinformatics. 34(11): 1841–1849.

Yoshizawa, M., Y.H. Taguchi and J. Yasuda (2011). Inference of gene regulation via miRNAs during ES cell differentiation using MiRaGE method. Int. J. Mol. Sci. 12(12): 9265–9276.

Yue, D., H. Liu and Y. Huang (2009). Survey of computational algorithms for MicroRNA target prediction. Curr. Genomics. 10(7): 478–492.

Zhang, Y. (2005). miRU: An automated plant miRNA target prediction server. Nucleic Acids Res. 33(W): W701–W704.

Zhang, P., W. Wu, Q. Chen and M. Chen (2019). Non-coding RNAs and their integrated networks. J. Integr. Bioinform. 16(3): 0027.

Zheng, X., L. Chen, X. Li, Y. Zhang, S. Xu and X. Huang (2020). Prediction of miRNA targets by learning from interaction sequences. PLoS One. 15(5): e0232578.

Zuker, M. and P. Stiegler (1981). Optimal computer folding of large RNA sequences using thermodynamics and auxiliary information. Nucleic Acids Res. 9(1): 133–148.

CHAPTER 13

Bioinformatics and Network Analysis of Biological Data

Enrique Hernández-Lemus[*,1,2], **Hugo Tovar**[1],
Laura Gómez-Romero[1] **and Mireya Martínez-García**[3]

[1]Computational Genomics Division, National Institute of Genomic Medicine, Mexico
[2]Center for Complexity Sciences, Universidad Nacional Autónoma de México, Mexico
[3]Sociomedical Research Unit, National Institute of Cardiology 'Ignacio Chávez', Mexico

1 INTRODUCTION

Life is a complex phenomenon. This complexity arises at multiple (often disparate) scales and as a consequence of a plethora of elements (genes, proteins, enzymes, metabolites, cells, tissues, organs, organisms, etc.) interacting on entangled and intertwined patterns. Said patterns are often concealed and may result extremely difficult to discern. With the advent of high-throughput, multidimensional experimental techniques in biology and biomedicine, it has been possible to probe simultaneously many (often *too many*) of these elements at the individual level. However, a theoretical framework is needed to conceptually accommodate and rationalize the deluge of data coming from such exquisite experimental sources (from molecular biology and omic experiments, to electronic health records, other types of clinical data and even social networks information).

In view of this, recent advances in network theory come in handy. Network science, was born two and a half decades ago (Barabási, 2003) as a contemporary interpretation (Barabási, 2016) of the well established ideas in mathematical graph theory (Bollabás and Béla, 2001) and its ideas have since then developed into subfields of network biology (Cagney and Emili, 2011; Cho et al., 2012) and network medicine (Loscalzo et al., 2017; Sonawane et al., 2019). Under this paradigm, it is possible to encompass the myriad of interactions behind biological function within a single (or a few) mathematical object with a well defined structure, namely a

*Corresponding author: *ehernandez@inmegen.gob.mx*

network. By analyzing biological networks with the tools of network science and graph theory, it is possible (yet still challenging, in many ways) to learn of the biological and biomedical systems behind the network. In this chapter, we will briefly introduce the network approach as it is understood in contemporary biological research and will present the bioinformatic tools and methods to implement network analysis in the context of biomolecular and clinical data.

2   FUNDAMENTALS OF NETWORK THEORY

2.1   Definitions

In order to establish the common ground language, useful for the rest of the chapter, in this subsection we will introduce some general definitions for concepts in network theory and biological network analysis. To exemplify some of these issues, a minimal *toy-network* is presented in Fig. 1.

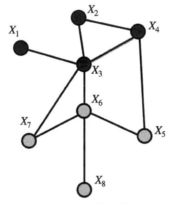

Figure 1   A toy-model of a network.

Degree, degree centrality.   Degree centrality or simply degree is defined as the number k_i of links incident on a node i (i.e., the number of ties that a node has). The degree measures the flow of information through this node in the network. In the case of a directed network two separate degree centralities are defined, in-degree k_i^{in} and out-degree k_i^{out}. Accordingly, in-degree is a measure of the number of links directed to the node and outdegree is the number of links that such node directs to others. The total number of links L of an undirected network is simply:

$$L = \frac{1}{2}\sum_{i=1}^{N} k_i \tag{1}$$

Hence the connectivity degree vector for the network in Fig. 1 is given as follows:

$$\vec{k} = k_i = \{1, 2, 5, 3, 2, 4, 2, 1\} \tag{2}$$

This means that the node X_1 has 1 link, the node X_2 has two links, X_3 has five links and so on.

The total number of links hence is given as:

$$L = \frac{1}{2}\sum_{i=1}^{8} k_i = \frac{1}{2}(1+2+5+3+2+4+2+1) = 10 \tag{3}$$

For a directed network, you may calculate the total number of incoming links L^{in} and the total number of outcoming links L^{out}, as follows:

$$L^{in} = \sum_{i=1}^{N} k_i^{in} \tag{4}$$

$$L^{out} = \sum_{i=1}^{N} k_i^{out} \tag{5}$$

The total number of links in the network will be simply given by:

$$L = L^{in} + L^{out} \tag{6}$$

Average degree. Average degree is simply the mean number of connections of the elements of a given network. It provides a sense of the typical connectivity of the network. It also allows the determination of families of network types via their degree distribution around the mean.

For the network in Fig. 1, this gives:

$$\langle k \rangle = \frac{1}{N} \sum_{i=1}^{N} k_i = \frac{2L}{N} \tag{7}$$

$$\langle k \rangle = \frac{1}{8} \sum_{i=1}^{8} k_i = \frac{2 \times 10}{8} = 2.5 \tag{8}$$

Degree distribution. It is the probability distribution of the number of connections per node in a given network. This is an extremely relevant mathematical object since different types of distributions will induce or represent different behaviors of the network.

For a network with N nodes the degree distribution is given by:

$$pk = \frac{N_k}{N}, \text{ subject to } \sum_{i=1}^{\infty} pk = 1 \tag{9}$$

With N_k, the number of nodes having exactly k links.
For the network in Fig. 1, the distribution is given as:

$$pk = \left\{ \frac{2}{8}, \frac{3}{8}, \frac{1}{8}, \frac{1}{8}, \frac{1}{8} \right\} \quad \text{for } k = 1, 2, 3, 4, 5 \text{ respectively} \tag{10}$$

From Eqn (9) it can be noticed that the average degree of a network is given by:

$$\langle k \rangle = \sum_{k=0}^{\infty} kp_k \tag{11}$$

Or, more commonly, in real networks with a maximum number of connections $k_{\max}$:

$$\langle k \rangle = \sum_{k=0}^{k_{\max}} kp_k \tag{12}$$

For our toy network in Fig. 1 this gives:

$$\langle k \rangle = \sum_{k=0}^{5} kp_k = \left(1 \times \frac{2}{8} + 2 \times \frac{3}{8} + 3 \times \frac{1}{8} + 4 \times \frac{1}{8} + 5 \times \frac{1}{8} \right) = \frac{20}{8} = 2.5 \tag{13}$$

as it was shown previously.

For instance, if the distribution is homogeneous (all nodes are equally connected) there is no relevant node, this is similar to having a random (e.g., normal) distribution in which *most* nodes are similarly connected. In contrast, in *long tail* distributions such as scale-free networks, there is a large difference among the connectivity of the least and most-connected nodes. Such highly-connected nodes, known as *hubs* will be quite relevant for the establishment of the main mathematical properties of the network, hence on their biological features.

Adjacency matrix. An adjacency matrix $\mathbb{A}_{ji}$ is one (of the many) useful mathematical representation of a network. It consists on a square matrix whose elements show whether pairs of nodes are connected by a link in the network or not. Often, the adjacency matrix has been written as a $(0, 1)$-matrix with zeros on its diagonal (indicating that a node is not connected to itself) and in the entries with no links, and ones if there is a connection between the row and column nodes. If the network is undirected, the adjacency matrix is symmetric, $A_{ji} = A_{ij}$. If the links are weighted the adjacency matrix may consists on zeros and relative weights, commonly but not necessarily, normalized. The degree k_i of a node can be computed directly from the adjacency matrix $\mathbb{A}_{ji}$ as follows:

$$k_i = \sum_{j=1}^{N} \mathbb{A}_{ji}, = \sum_{i=1}^{N} \mathbb{A}_{ji} \tag{14}$$

$$k_i^{in} = \sum_{j=1}^{N} \mathbb{A}_{ij}, \qquad k_i^{out} = \sum_{i=1}^{N} \mathbb{A}_{ji} \tag{15}$$

For example, the adjacency matrix of the toy network in Fig. 1 is as follows:

$$\mathbb{A}_{ij} = \begin{bmatrix} 0 & 0 & 1 & 0 & 0 & 0 & 0 & 0 \\ 0 & 0 & 1 & 1 & 0 & 0 & 0 & 0 \\ 1 & 1 & 0 & 1 & 0 & 1 & 1 & 0 \\ 0 & 1 & 1 & 0 & 1 & 0 & 0 & 0 \\ 0 & 0 & 0 & 1 & 0 & 1 & 0 & 0 \\ 0 & 0 & 1 & 0 & 1 & 0 & 1 & 1 \\ 0 & 0 & 1 & 0 & 0 & 1 & 0 & 0 \\ 0 & 0 & 0 & 0 & 0 & 1 & 0 & 0 \end{bmatrix}$$

Biological network. A **biological network** is formally defined as a graph $G(V, E)$ over a duplex formed by two sets, a set V of nodes or vertices ($v_i \in V$) given by **biomolecules,** and a set E of edges connecting such vertices ($e_i \in E$) representing **physical** or **chemical** interactions of several classes among such biomolecules. The connectivity rule is represented by the so-called **adjacency matrix** $A = A_{i,j}$, where $A_{i,j} \neq 0$ implies a non-null interaction between biomolecules v_i and v_j.

Shortest path. A shortest or geodesic path, between two nodes in a network is a trajectory with the minimum number of edges. If the network edges are weighted, it is a path with the minimum sum of edge weights. The length of a geodesic path is called geodesic distance or shortest distance. Geodesic paths are not necessarily unique, but the shortest path distance is well-defined since all shortest paths have the same length. The shortest path is often called the distance between nodes i and j, and is denoted by d_{ij}.

Connectedness. In graph and network theory, the concept of connectedness or *topological connectedness* is often used. In topology, a topological space is *connected* if it cannot be formed as the union of two disjoint nonempty open sets.

In terms of networks, a network is connected if every pair of nodes in the graph is joined by a path. A network is said to be fully connected if it consists in only one *island*. A network is connected if there is a path connecting every pair of nodes i and j, hence there is a finite d_{ij}. Two nodes are disconnected (thus disconnecting the whole network) if such a path does not exist, in which case we have $d_{ij} = \infty$.

Clustering coefficient. In network theory a measure of connectedness is the clustering coefficient that represents the degree to which nodes in a graph are clustered. For a node i with degree k_i the *local clustering coefficient* is given by:

$$C_i = \frac{2L_i}{k_i(k_i - 1)} \tag{16}$$

Here L_i is the number of links between the k_i neighbors of node i. C_i is normalized and thus can be interpreted as the average probability that two nodes, j and k, connected to node i are in turn directly connected to each other. The local clustering coefficient is thus a measure of link density. A densely connected neighborhood will have a larger clustering coefficient.

The global clustering coefficient is the average local clustering coefficient for all nodes in a network, i.e.:

$$\langle C \rangle = \frac{1}{N} \sum_{i=1}^{N} C_i \tag{17}$$

Random network. A random network is a collection of N nodes in which a link between two nodes exists with probability p. It can be defined in two mostly equivalent ways. N labeled nodes are connected with L randomly placed links, this is usually called a $G(N, L)$ model or Erdös and Rényi or fixed links model (Erdös and Rényi, 1959; 1961). You can also build a random network by having the N nodes connected with a constant probability p, called a $G(N, p)$ or Gilbert model (Gilbert, 1959).

The mean degree of a random network is given as:

$$\left\langle k^{random} \right\rangle = \frac{2\langle L \rangle}{N} = p(N - 1) \tag{18}$$

Notice that Eqn (18) as compared to Eqn (11) reveals the effect of the average probability p as representative for the distribution p_k. Careful analysis of most real networks has revealed however, that most of them do not actually follow such random behavior (that has been extremely useful both in the theoretical conceptualization and applications) but they present structural diversity. This fact leads to the proposal of a number of models, the most relevant of which is perhaps the so-called scale free networks.

Scale free networks. The analysis of the empirical degree distribution in a large number of naturally-occurring (as well as in social and technological) networks is, in a good approximation, described by a power-law equation (see Eqn 19) in which, the probability of nodes having more and more links become bounded, diminishing depending on the value of the exponent γ.

$$p_k = \alpha k^{-\gamma} \tag{19}$$

The constant α is determined via the normalization condition $\Sigma_k p_k = 1$, thus:

$$\alpha = \frac{1}{\displaystyle\sum_{k=1}^{\infty} k^{-\gamma}} = \frac{1}{\zeta(\gamma)} \tag{20}$$

Here ζ is Riemann's zeta function. In view of this, a major difference between a random and a scale-free network lies in the high k-value tail of the degree distribution p_k.

Degree correlations. An interesting phenomenon that arises in broad degree distributed networks such as scale-free networks lies in the way highly connected nodes, or hubs are connected in the network. These connectivity patterns induce the so-called degree correlations that in turn led to three different types of behaviors of networks. Networks are *assortative* whenever similarly connected nodes tend to connect with each other (hubs with other hubs and less-connected nodes among themselves). In the contrary case (hubs tend to link to less-connected nodes and viceversa) the networks are called *disassortative*. If none of these behaviors is *evident* (i.e., statistically significant), networks are called *neutral*.

Robustness.   Networks are known to play central roles in the development of robustness in biological systems. Cellular robustness for instance is currently understood to be encoded by an intricate tangle of regulatory, signaling and metabolic networks.

It is known, that the structure of the underlying network plays a role in a systems ability to survive attacks on the form of either random failures or specific *insults*. Networks are also involved in the emergence of cascading failures, that constitute a damage mechanism often found in actual biological systems.

Community structure.   A network community or module is defined as a set of nodes within a network that have a higher likelihood of (intra-) connection to each other than to (inter-) connection with nodes from other communities (see *Modules*).

Spreading phenomena.   A relevant application of the concepts of network science in biology is related to flow (of matter, energy or, more generally information) within a network. The mass and energy fluxes on a metabolic network or the spreading of disease in a networked population are both cases of spreading phenomena on a network. The recent rise of the COVID-19 pandemic has without doubt left a lasting impression upon most of us regarding the extraordinary efficiency of the world wide *network of human contacts* (even incidental ones) to act as chains of transmission. The concepts of *critical percolation limit* and *epidemic threshold* have been developed to analyze the phenomenon of information super-spreading on networks.

Bipartite graph.   A network with two different types of nodes. These nodes form a disjoint set and every edge (or link) of the network connects nodes from different type. A bipartite graph does not contain odd-length cycles.

Component.   A network component, often called a connected component or island, in an undirected network is a subgraph (a part of the network) in which any two nodes are connected to each other by one or more paths, and which is connected to no additional nodes in the supergraph (the full network).

Edge Betweenness.   or Edge Betweenness Centrality is a centrality measure for the links, it is defined as the number of shortest paths that go through a given link in a network.

Enzyme graph.   In the context of the present chapter an enzyme graph or enzyme network is an important biological network which relates enzyme, proteins and chemical compounds. It is the graph theoretical depiction of a metabolic pathway or a series of metabolic pathways.

Giant Connected Component (GCC).   A giant connected component is a connected component of a given network that contains a significant fraction (more than 50%) of the nodes of the network.

Hypergraph.   A hypergraph is a generalization of a network in which a link can connect an arbitrary number of nodes. In contrast, in an ordinary network, a link connects exactly two nodes.

Metabolite interactions graph.   In the context of KEGG, a metabolite interactions graph is different to an enzyme network in that it only contains metabolites as nodes.

Module.   Network modules (also called Communities) are understood as subnetworks formed by sets of nodes (or vertices) that are more densely connected among themselves than with the rest of the network. Modules are often viewed as semi-autonomous (but not independent) components of a network that are responsible for functionality in real networks.

Network modules play a relevant role in the way we understand specific biological functions as they are encoded in biomolecular networks. The modularity approach tries to analyze how biomolecules form functional modules specialized to perform specific cellular functions.

2.2 Network Analytics

The analysis of the structure and dynamics of networks at a deeper level, often depends on the specifics of the particular graphs under consideration that in turn depends on the nature of the elements and links that constitute them. It is in the choice of the type of network that one is able to capture the features of the system we are trying to model. Network features may sometimes reveal the true nature of our system, our choice in the modeling approach or even what we can do with the data available. In this subsection we will present some general principles behind the more common network types and features.

As we have already sketched, we can indeed consider directed networks as two sub-sets, the set of incoming links and that of outgoing links and calculate statistics and paths independently to later integrate the information, as we already did for the degree distributions and the number of links.

Directed and undirected networks. As we have already mentioned, networks can be either directed in which there is an unidirectional flow of information between the nodes or undirected in which the information flows bidirectionally. Transcriptional, signaling and metabolic networks are examples of the former, as we will abound later on this chapter, whereas co-expression, protein-protein and diseasome graphs are examples of the latter.

However, it is not always possible to experimentally measure the appropriate weights. In consequence, one often needs to approximate weighted graphs with an unweighted version. In general, this approximation affects less the structure of the network and more the information flow and the dynamic behavior.

Weighted and unweighted networks. Complex networks may be also categorized as being weighted and unweighted, based on the nature of the interactions they represent. It is safe to say that in most applications in biology, not all interactions in a network are alike, hence the vast majority of biological networks are indeed weighted graphs. In the case of weighted graphs, the elements of the adjacency matrix are not just zeros and ones but weights $A_{ij} = w_{ij}$.

However, it is not always possible to experimentally measure the appropriate weights. In consequence, one often needs to approximate weighted graphs with an unweighted version. In general, this approximation affects less the structure of the network and more the information flow and the dynamic behavior.

Deterministic and probabilistic networks. Another important distinction we need in biological networks resides on whether the links are given deterministically or if they obey a probabilistic depiction. For instance, transcriptional networks understood as those given by strong experimental evidence of transcription factor binding site analysis and accurate values of binding affinities are *deterministic*, whereas gene coexpression regulatory networks whose links are given by correlation measures are *probabilistic*. Another pair of examples will be deterministic metabolic networks as given by explicit chemical kinetics and cleavage experiments or rigorous docking calculations versus probabilistic graphs modeling epidemic spread as given by R_t dynamics.

Later on, when we consider inference and curation of real data biological networks, we will see that often we will consider networks curated from databases as *deterministic* and networks inferred from high throughput omic technologies as *probabilistic*, though this distinction is not always so simple to do.

For instance, some databases report *biomolecular interactions* (i.e., links) that have been explicitly measured in one context and one tries to use them to model other contexts. Say you have measured that proteins A and B form a complex in the healthy liver and you try to use this information to model a protein-protein network for tumors of the spleen, or more commonly, suppose you have measured the interaction between A and B homologue proteins in the mouse and use this fact to build a human protein-protein network. In these latter cases, even though the interactions have been explicitly measured *in a different setting* it is useful to consider them as probabilistic, an approach actually used by the STRING! database for instance (Franceschini, et al., 2016; Szklarczyk et al., 2016; Szklarczyk et al., 2019).

3   TYPES OF BIOLOGICAL NETWORKS

Now it is time to properly introduce (or in some cases re-introduce) the more common types of biological networks used within the biomedical research community. Some of the most common biomolecular interaction networks are depicted in Fig. 2.

3.1   Gene Regulatory and Transcriptional Networks

As it is well known, behind cell development, differentiation and phenotype establishment there is a complex web that controls gene expression. The integrated study of these regulatory processes, in particular in the eukaryotic cells is extremely relevant in todays biomedical research. There is a fine distinction between gene regulatory networks and transcriptional networks based on their original nature, but in most cases in biomedicine this distinction is somehow blurred. In general, gene regulatory networks (GRNs from now on) is a term that encompasses both deterministic TFBS-curated networks and omic-inferred gene correlations networks. This is perhaps one of the most prolific field in which the network science paradigm has permeated biomedical science.

In GRNs the nodes are *genes*: mostly mRNA, but increasingly including ncRNAs such as miRNAS and lncRNAs, as well as regulatory elements such as methylation sites and other epigenomic modifiers of gene expression. Interactions are either binding and activation signals or, more commonly association or correlation measures of co-expression or of activation/repression.

Applications of GRNs are vast and varied. Abedini and coworkers, for instance (Abedini, et al., 2019) have been using gene regulatory networks to study global regulatory processes related to hepatic lipid dysfunction with a view to implement pharmacological interventions to alleviate this dangerous systemic condition. They found that the mechanisms behind hepatic steatosis may be understood as an outcome of disruptions of lipid homeostasis in hepatocytes driven by a complex network of biological events that can be broadly categorized as hepatic fatty acid uptake, *de novo* fatty acid and lipid synthesis, fatty acid oxidation, and lipid efflux with the FOXM1 transcriptional network considered a set of key players.

The molecular mechanisms of anomalous gene expression in drug–treated breast cancers have been recently studied (Alshabi et al., 2019) by combining different biological network approaches aside from pure GRNs such as protein-protein interaction (PPI) networks, module decomposition analysis, construction of target genesmiRNA interaction networks and target genes-transcription factor (TF) interaction networks. With these studies they were able to discover and validate gene signatures related to lysine degradation II (pipecolate pathway), cholesterol biosynthesis pathway, cell cycle pathway, and response to cytokine pathway. Thus, aside from drug metabolism, network analyses revealed signaling and proliferative effects triggered by anti-cancer drugs. Some of these effects may be related to pharmacological resistance to therapy as it has been previously reported (de Anda-Jáuregui et al., 2015).

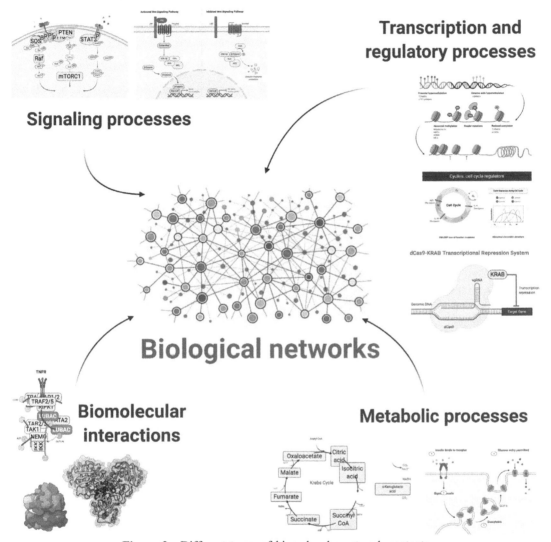

Figure 2 Different types of biomolecular network contexts.

Expression analysis via GRNs supplemented with pathway-based studies may also allow for toxicogenomics designs capable of elucidating toxicological mechanisms, building predictive models and improving diagnostics, as the manuscript by Barel and Herwig (Barel and Herwig, 2018) broadly discusses. The authors present a series of tools and approaches they consider relevant to integrate gene expression data with molecular interaction networks to uncover network modules related to drug toxicity. The study of the modules (much smaller than the whole GRNs) are though to be extremely useful for drug assessment.

GRNs can be also applied at improving diagnostics. Guan and co-workers, developed an approach in which by inferring the competing endogenous RNAs (ceRNAs) interaction network of differentially expressed genes were able to build a diagnostic tool for esophageal carcinoma (Guan et al., 2020). Thier study found four lncRNAs that showed an important effect on the survival and prognosis of esophageal carcinoma patients (RNF217-AS1, HCP5, ZFPM2-AS1 and HCG22) and hypothesized that their target genes may provide guidance on the molecular mechanism of esophageal carcinoma aimed at improved screening of molecular markers. Such candidate genes resulted significantly enriched in a number of pathways, mostly related to FoxO signaling and calcineurin cascading.

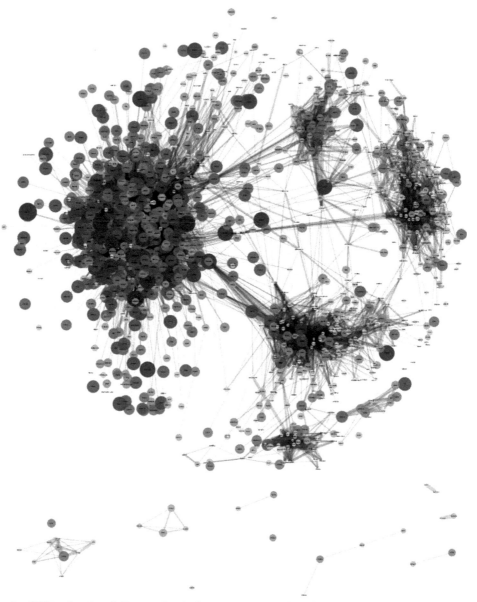

Figure 3   GRN related to inflammation in breast cancer. Node colors represent differential expression of tumors versus healthy adjacent tissue.

By combining gene expression profiling with protein-protein interaction (PPI) networks, the team led by Guo (Guo et al., 2019) unveiled some candidate mechanisms behind intracranial aneurysms aimed at providing a basis for further research and treatment of this high mortality cerebrovascular disease. By using a set of well known bioinformatic tools such as the Database for Annotation, Visualization, and Integrated Discovery (DAVID) (Dennis et al., 2003) and the

Kyoto Encyclopedia of Genes and Genomes (KEGG) (Kanehisa et al., 2019) the authors shown upregulated processes related to inflammatory response and the management of extracellular matrix, whereas downregulated ones were mostly involved in vascular smooth muscle contraction. In agreement with these gene expression results the PPI network pointed out to tumor necrosis factor (TNF), interleukin 8 and Tolllike receptor 4 as network hubs associated with inflammatory response.

A similar integrated network approach was followed by the team of He to investigate on potential biomarkers and central biological pathways for prostate cancer (He et al., 2019). In addition to KEGG and DAVID the authors used data from the cancer genome atlas collaboration (TCGA) via a web service tool (Tang et al., 2017) to identify abnormaly regulated processes such as oxidation-reduction, positive regulation of transcription from RNA polymerase II promoter, basal metabolism, protein digestion and absorption. These processes are likely deregulated by the concerted action of several key molecules such as KLK3, KLK2, CDH1 and FOXA1. All of them known as central regulators (hubs) in the associated molecular networks. Also using similar tools, supplemented with the STRING! database, Jiang and collaborators (Jiang and Yuan, 2019) identify competing endogenous RNAs in bladder cancer and found DNA replication and transcription processes such as strand displacement and homologous recombination as well as signaling processes guided by Fanconi anemia pathways as statistically significant players in bladder tumors.

A somehow different approach was used to investigate on RBM8A regulation in hepatocellular carcinoma by using data mining techniques in large experimental databases such as Oncomine (Rhodes et al., 2004). With this study, the authors were able to show that not only is RBM8A overexpressed and amplified in these tumors; it is also linked to functional networks involving the ribosome and RNA metabolic signaling pathways. This functional network analysis suggested that RBM8A regulates the spliceosome, ribosome, DNA replication and cell cycle signaling via pathways involving several cancer-related kinases, miRNAs and E2F1. The authors also present a novel kinase network approach known as LinkedOmics involving kinase activation of transcription factors and kinase interactions with regulatory microRNAs. In this way, they were able to find that the network of RBM8A alterations is associated to a post-transcriptional regulation cluster closely related to RNA splicing and protein translation. In agreement with the known physiological function of RBM8A.

GRNs have been revealed as extremely powerful tools to integrate detailed information of concurrent regulatory processes. Such is the case of studies involving not only transcription factor—mRNA regulation but also the effect of long non-coding RNAs, microRNAs, circular RNAs (cRNAs) and competitive endogenous RNAs (ceRNAs). Using an integrative network approach of this kind, Liu and coworkers (Liu et al., 2019) studied a ceRNA network to look up for prognostic cRNA biomarkers in bladder cancer. Hence, they were able to find that the associated ceRNA network consisted of 28 differentially-expressed RNAs, 12 miRNAs and 12 cRNAs. Prognostic assessment implied that a number of cRNA interacted with hsa-miR-106b, hsa-miR-145 and hsa-miR-214 and were associated with overall survival in patients with bladder cancer. Among these were hsa circ 0076704, hsa circ 0081963 and hsa circ 0001361 which resulted potential cRNAs related to the overall survival (OS) in bladder cancer and expressed in bladder cancer.

Spinal cord injury mechanisms were also investigated by using ceRNA-miRNA-mRNA networks (Wang et al., 2019) finding 3 lncRNA which were significantly clustered in the networks. Enrichment analyses showed that these were associated with biological functions such as autophagy, extracellular communication and transcription factor networks, respectively. The phosphoinositide 3kinase/protein kinase B/mammalian target of rapamycin signaling pathway response associated to XR 350851 indicates that these molecules may regulate autophagy in spinal cord injury. This possible role based on the regulatory mechanism of ceRNAs has uncovered a new repertoire of molecular factors with potential as novel biomarkers and therapeutic targets in this disease.

Gene regulatory network analysis was also used in connection with an approach to screening cRNAs associated to Gefitinib resistance in non-small cell lung cancer cell lines. Functional network and enrichment analyses of the associated cRNA regulatory clusters pointed out to deregulation of respiratory gaseous metabolism, as well as receptor complex, glutaminase activity, thyroid hormone transport and endopeptidase activity (Wen et al., 2020).

By applying deeper mathematical notions from network theory, Pouryahya and coworkers were able to implement a network-based analysis to generate novel insights about drug response and cancer biology in the NCI-60 dataset (Pouryahya et al., 2018). The use of the so-called Ricci curvature to measure the robustness of biological networks, via an association between Ricci curvature and network robustness, constructed with a pretreatment gene expression dataset and coupling the results with the GI50 response to the drugs by the NCI-60 cell lines. With this, they were able to assess the impact of genes associated with individual drug response and to look up for biological processes associated with drug response across cell lines and tissue types with a view to precision medicine. This was accomplished by finding the *average Ricci curvature* (ARC) (a network-derived mathematical parameter) of the genes whose expressions are significantly correlated to the response of a given drug, then proceed to identify which part of the network is most correlated to specific mechanisms. The ARC for this subnetwork may probe the relative sensitivity or resistance of cell lines to that therapy. In brief, subnetwork robustness implies resistance to the drug along the tested cell lines.

3.2   Metabolic and Pathway Networks

A metabolic network has been defined as the compendium of metabolic and physical processes behind the physiological and biochemical properties of a cell. This study of metabolic networks has been extremely important both in biotechnology and biomedical research (Dubitzky et al., 2013; Lee et al., 2008; Walhout et al., 2012).

Metabolic networks are complex mathematical objects comprising hundreds or even thousands of chemical reactions that are needed to sustain life. The vast majority of these reactions are in turn catalyzed by a collection of enzymes which are encoded finally by genes. A metabolic network then is able to extract mass and energy from the chemicals in the environment, and converts them (metabolize them) into forms that allow its use by the organisms (Wagner, 2012).

Indeed, the large scale structure of these metabolic networks has attracted a lot of attention due to its relevance to understand organismal robustness (Jeong et al., 2000). Aside from its known scale-free nature, metabolic networks are known to obey hierarchical modularity patterns, a fact that has been closely associated with biological robustness (Ravasz et al., 2002). Such structure has also profound implications for the control of metabolic fluxes, the ultimate response collection of switches, responsible for large scale regulatory principles that may be behind disease and that whose understanding will also allow for the design of engineering strategies at the interface of gene regulation, signaling, and metabolism in pharmacology and biotechnology (Basler et al., 2016). A recent application of these studies lies within the design of anti-microbial strategies (Shen et al., 2010) by combining system-level identification of drug targets with the atomistic modeling of small molecules capable of modulating their activity.

The impact of this research along with the development of studies of gene regulatory networks give rise to a whole new paradigm called *Network Biology* (Barabási et al., 2004).

Comprehensive approximations to model organismal level metabolism via the use of networks have been implemented looking for metabolic, signaling and regulatory integration. Some successful approaches were initially made in model organisms (Yilmaz and Walhout 2017), particularly in yeast and bacteria. Given that such organisms have relatively small genomes and are usually well-annotated this was an advantageous choice. One seminal study along these lines was conducted by the group of Palsson (Herrgård et al., 2006).

Their research consisted in a global analysis, integrating transcriptional regulatory and metabolic networks in *Saccharomyces cerevisiae*. Computational curation of the literature (or *bibliomics*) of the transcriptional regulatory network behind nutrient metabolism was analyzed in addition to a global scale metabolic network a fact that allowed the authors to predict how gene expression patterns change in response to perturbations. This in turn allow the identification of novel targets for transcription factors as well as to a better understanding of *growth phenotypes* (Stitt et al., 2000) driven by transcription factor knockout strains. These predictions were further verified by ChIP-chip and gene expression experiments.

The same lab published a landmark study with a full reconstruction of a human metabolic network (Duarte et al., 2007). Such comprehensive metabolic model was applied to derive detailed computational models making specific predictions for metabolic activity and gene expression. However, no detailed transcriptional regulatory network for human phenotypes was available at the time as human GRNs are extremely context dependent. The topological structure of their network, however helped to discover relevant processes behind intracellular compartmentalization and correlated with enzymatic reactions that may be used for drug target identification.

In a similar fashion, Covert et al. (Covert et al., 2008) introduced a comprehensive metabolic, transcriptional regulatory and signal transduction modeling scheme for the bacterium *E. coli*. Their analysis was founded upon flux balance analysis (a technique used in metabolic reconstruction to map the energy and mass balances to quasi-kinetic equations) (Beguerisse-Díaz et al., 2018), logic decision trees and ordinary differential equations. No attention was paid to the topological structural features of the underlying networks. Contemporary modeling approaches have used similar methods, such as the incorporation of computational intelligence algorithms such as Petri nets to integrate metabolic, transcriptional regulatory and signal transduction networks (Fisher et al., 2013) (all of them *directed graphs*) in specific contexts for some human cell types.

Regarding probabilistic approaches to model metabolic networks, Price and collaborators (Ma et al., 2015) analyzed the metabolic and gene regulatory networks in *M. tuberculosis*, with no explicit considerations on the role that signaling pathways or supramolecular protein-protein interaction networks may be playing.

A landmark development in the realm of metabolic reconstruction was published recently. Breuer et al., inferred the essential metabolic network for a minimal cell (Breuer et al., 2019), i.e., the full set of metabolic interactions in the synthetic bacterium **JCVI-syn3A** also known as *Mycoplasma laboratorium* (Gibson et al., 2010). They built an almost complete metabolic network, literally *from scratch*. With this information about a *minimal* organism whose genome is just 543 kbp distributed in a mere 493 genes that however fully supports its metabolism, it may become possible to answer what are the essential and redundant components and processes for life sustenance.

3.3 Signaling Networks

Signal transduction which occurs inside and across the cells, also known as cell signaling, is key to most biological functions and is ultimately related with both life and death of the organisms (Hernández-Lemus, 2012). The inference of cell signaling networks based on high-throughput data has become a challenging problem in systems biology. Cell signaling is known to play a relevant role in the way cellular processes adapt to constantly changing environments. Several cellular molecules (often hundreds, even thousands perhaps) interact to conform entangled signaling networks, a part of which form one or more signaling pathways, whose functions maintain both cellular tissue and organ health.

For these reasons signaling networks are not entirely predictable. In particular since information available is scarce and the phenomenon is highly non-linear (Hernández-Lemus, 2012). Statistical approaches then play a relevant role in network estimation and inference. Indeed, causal inference is an effective tool for signaling network reconstruction aimed at finding cause-effect relationships among biomolecules (Kontogeorgaki et al., 2017).

The study of signaling networks has been quite relevant for advances in the understanding of human development, response to infectious disease and drugs and immune responses in cancer and other chronic diseases. For instance, a detailed analysis of the hedgehog signaling network (Cohen, 2003) showed that alterations in its functioning result in various abnormal phenotypes, including holoprosencephaly, nevoid basal cell carcinoma syndrome, PallisterHall syndrome, Greig cephalopolysyndactyly, RubinsteinTaybi syndrome, isolated basal cell carcinoma, and medulloblastoma among others. The main balance mechanisms have been dissected by structural methods leading to conclude that such a balance is created by the antagonism of Hedgehog and Patched, whose relative concentrations alternate with respect to each other.

Analyzing the WNT signaling network, Katoh and coworkers (Katoh and Katoh 2007) discovered that since WNT signals are transduced to the canonical pathway for cell fate determination, and to the non-canonical pathway for control of cell movement and tissue polarity they may be involved as *switches* in the establishment of tumor phenotypes. Network analysis of the information flow of the kinase signals allow the researchers to disentangle the actual mechanisms for this switching. In brief, epigenetic silencing and loss-of-function mutation of negative regulators of the canonical WNT pathway are often present in human tumors.

The main hubs of this network which are WNT itself, FGF, Notch, Hedgehog, and TGF-β are implicated in the maintenance of tissue homeostasis by a series of regulatory loops behind self-renewal of normal stem cells, but also as regulators of proliferation or differentiation of progenitor (transit-amplifying) cells. Breakage of the stem cell signaling network then leads to carcinogenesis. These results are of relevance for the design of anti-cancer therapies: for instance non-steroidal anti-inflammatory drugs and PPAR-γ agonists able to inhibit the canonical WNT signaling pathway are being considered as candidate agents for chemoprevention. ZTM000990 and PKF118-310 are in turn, lead compounds targeting the canonical WNT signaling cascade. Anti-WNT1 and anti-WNT2 monoclonal antibodies have show in vitro effects in cancer treatment. Finally, derivatives of small-molecule compound and human monoclonal antibody targeting the WNT signaling pathway could be used as auxiliary biological drugs in cancer medicine.

The mTOR signaling network has also received attention in relation to its ability to form switches that when abnormally regulated are associated with disease (Martin and Hall, 2005) but at the same time are opening the way to discover important pharmacological targets (Chiang and Abraham, 2007; Meric-Bernstam et al., 2009). This is in part because mTOR works as a signal integrator. For instance, cell growth is known to be tightly co-regulated with nutrient availability, growth factors and cell energetics. Network analytics have shown that mTOR is indeed able to integrate all these inputs to control cell growth (Martin and Hall, 2005). However, there are challenges due to the complexity of both cancer as a disease target, and the mTOR signaling network, which contains two functionally distinct mTOR complexes, parallel regulatory pathways, and feedback loops that contribute to the variable cellular response to the current inhibitors (Chiang and Abraham, 2007).

Of special relevance to cancer biology is the ERBB signaling network (Olayioye et al., 2000). Cells are exposed to wide range of external stimuli from soluble endocrine and paracrine factors, also including signaling molecules coming from neighboring cells. Such extracellular signals need to be correctly *interpreted* to activate proper cellular responses, in order to set appropriate developmental or proliferative response. Tyrosine kinase receptor are key to this process. Specific peptide binding to their ligands enable them to integrate these external stimuli with a myriad internal signal transduction pathways, enhancing the ability of the cell to respond properly to its environment. Unveiling the actual mechanisms in which the ERBB network is systemically connected to other components of cell signaling and metabolism is of paramount importance in the development of targeted therapies against cancer. The cooperativity phenomena of cross-regulation between the ERBB1 and ERBB2 subnetworks have been found to play a concerting role in the mechanisms behind aberrant responses to stimuli, most noticeable those that turned out to be oncogenic by affecting the central PI3KAKT growth pathway.

Aside from driver-specific network approaches such as these, it is also relevant to study signaling networks with emphasis on their structural and dynamical features to see what are the biological consequences of these features. In this regard, the study by Barrios-Rodiles and collaborators results enlightening (Barrios-Rodiles et al., 2005). They developed and implemented a high-throughput mapping based on a large-scale dynamic signaling network in mammalian cells. Their developed a technique (LUMIER) for the automated high-throughput mapping of protein-protein interaction networks in a systematical manner in the context of mammalian cells. With this technique they showed how Occludin regulates TGFβ1R localization thus enhancing TGFβ-dependent dissolution of tight junctions during epithelial-to-mesenchymal transitions. These findings are relevant in the context of newborns developmental errors, of collagen-associated diseases and in metastatic cancers.

More general processes may be understood in terms of the structural and dynamical properties of signaling networks. That is the case of the complex phenomenon of oncogene induced senescence of enormous relevance in relation to tumor relapse after chemotherapy and radiotherapy. It has been shown that the control of oncogene-driven senescence can be traced back to a negative feedback circuit in the underlying signaling network (Courtois-Cox et al., 2006). In particular, network analysis showed how mutations affecting the NF1, Raf, and Ras genes are able to induce a global negative feedback response that suppresses Ras and its downstream effectors almost completely. Downstream Ras suppression promotes senescence by inhibiting the Ras/PI3K pathway, this in turn impacts on the senescence machinery via HDM2 and FOXO. This negative feedback program is regulated in part by RasGEFs, Sprouty proteins, RasGAPs, and MKPs. This is precisely the type of results that are almost impossible to fully grasp if one is not using a systemic network approach.

Using a similar approach Hitomi et al. (Hitomi et al., 2008) were able to identify a molecular signaling network that regulates a cellular necrotic cell death pathway. By applying a genome-wide siRNA screen to search for regulators of necroptosis. The authors identified a set of 432 genes able to regulate necroptosis. A subset of 32 genes that act either downstream and/or as regulators of RIP1 kinase, 32 genes required for death-receptor-mediated apoptosis, and 7 genes involved in both necroptosis and apoptosis. The expression of subsets of the 432 genes within this signaling network, is enriched in the immune and nervous systems, and cellular sensitivity to necroptosis is regulated by an extensive signaling network mediating innate immunity.

3.4 Molecular Interaction Networks

Molecular interaction graphs or protein-protein interaction (PPI) networks are becoming essential tools to understand cellular processes at different physiological levels, both in normal and disease phenotypes. PPI networks are also essential in drug development, since drugs can affect proteins and protein complexes. PPI networks are the mathematical representations of the physical contacts between proteins in the cell. These contacts are highly specific; have defined local contexts between defined binding regions in the proteins and serve a specific function or sets of functions.

PPI networks represent both transient and stable interactions. In this sense, we define *stable interaction*s as those formed in protein complexes like the ribosome, hemoglobin and *transient interactions* as temporary, unstable interactions with the ability to modify, transport or activate a protein, leading to further change (e.g., protein kinases, nuclear pore importins) in the downstream processes. Molecular interaction networks have been useful to assign candidate roles to previously uncharacterized proteins; but also to gain novel insights on signaling pathway mechanisms; and to understand what are the specific biochemical forces between proteins that form multi-molecular complexes like the proteasome.

Recent efforts to map molecular interaction networks in a comprehensive way from high throughput experiments are becoming more and more sophisticated. Vidal, Roth and their coworkers developed a systematic map of circa 14,000 high-quality human binary protein-protein interactions. Their research wanted to fill the gap since available information tended to be highly biased only covering a relatively small portion of the proteome. Their map also uncovered that there is a significant interconnectivity between known and candidate cancer gene products, thus providing unbiased evidence for an expanded functional cancer landscape (Rolland et al., 2014).

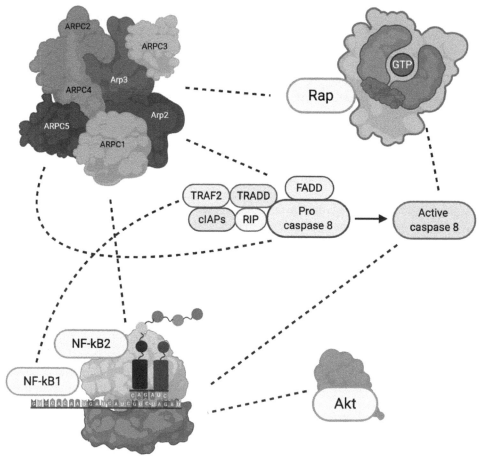

Figure 4 Protein-protein interaction network. Depending on the specific contexts and in the strength of the links (as given by physicochemical interactions) proteins and protein complexes may interact to enhance or block biomolecular processes.

Aside from the number of experimental high throughput techniques such as affinity assays, efforts have been made to map out the human interactome recently via network completion approaches. These studies have been developed to cope with data incompleteness that indeeds is limiting our understanding of the molecular origins of human disease (Menche et al., 2015). Computational tools offer new avenues to identify biologically significant, albeit unmapped, protein-protein interactions. These so-called link prediction methods are able to connect proteins based on biological or network-based similarity, there is still to be defined what to do in cases in which interacting proteins are not necessarily similar and similar proteins do not necessarily interact (Kovács et al., 2019).

Indeed, PPI networks such as the one depicted in Fig. 4, have also been useful for the large scale characterization of living organisms. Molecular interaction networks have been quite influential in revealing novel clues about mechanisms underlying disease phenotypes and the action of therapeutic strategies. For instance, the study of the molecular pathogenesis of non-small-cell lung cancer was analyzed by building up a PPI network and then performing modular decomposition and enrichment analysis on it (Wu et al., 2019).

The authors were able to find out 1283 interactions whose concerted biological functions were mainly responsible for wounding and cell adhesion. These modules were associated with shorter overall survival. By mapping these interactions to the CMap database of cancer therapeutics it was predicted that a set of 20 small molecules were promising therapies of which DL-thiorphan resulted the most promising. It was also found that PTTG1, TYMS, ECT2, COL1A1, SPP1 and CDCA5 may be considered novel diagnostic and therapeutic targets for non-small-cell lung tumors.

The PPI network in the work by Wu and coworkers was curated from data on the NCBI GEO (Barrett et al., 2009) and the STRING! public domain databases (Szklarczyk et al., 2019) and modular decomposition analyses were performed by using the MCODE algorithm (Saito et al., 2012; Wang et al., 2014) within the Cytoscape network analysis suite (Shannon et al., 2003). All of these standard resources in biological network analysis.

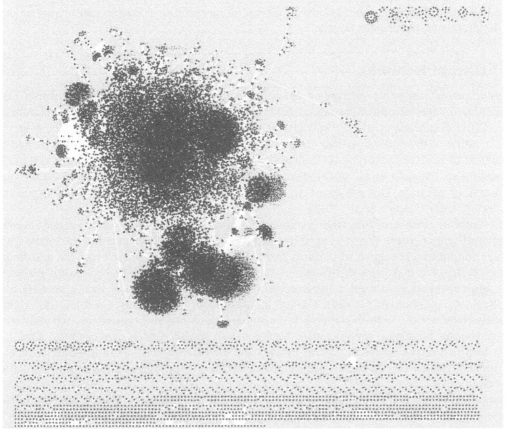

Figure 5 The complete human protein-protein interaction network. As reported in the BIND database.

Differential PPI network analysis as well as hub-outlier search were used to dissect kinase driven mechanisms involved in Glioma (Jean-Quartier et al., 2020). Cluster analysis from top hub nodes lists identified several glioma-associated gene products to function within protein complexes, including epidermal growth factors and cell cycle proteins or even proto-oncogenes of the RAS family. In this case the authors applied the combination of a number of bioinformatic tools such as NetworkAnalyst (Xia et al., 2015), Navigator (Brown et al., 2009), OmicsNet (Zhou and Xia, 2018), WebGestalt (Wang et al., 2017) and Cytoscape (Shannon et al., 2003). Among these, Cytoscape, NetworkAnalyst and OmcisNet were considered suitable tools for creating protein-coding gene networks based on gene lists. Whereas NetworkAnalyst and OmicsNet were web-based tools that were used to mine STRING! and Cytoscape was used to mine BioGRID (Oughtred et al., 2019) to build the PPI network.

In relation with the role that sex-specific features have in the pathophysiology of osteoarthritis as well as on its incidence and prevalence, a network based study was performed (Wang et al., 2019) to screen out key genes and pathways mediating biological differences between females after menopause and males, both affected with ostheoarthritis. By using public resources from NCBI GEO (Barrett et al., 2009) a PPI network was constructed to further analyze interactions between the overlapping set of differentially expressed genes. Enrichment analyses were separately performed using Gene Ontology and KEGG tools (Kanehisa et al., 2019). Seven hub genes were identified, including EGF, ERBB2, CDC42, PIK3R2, LCK, CBL, and STAT1.

Functional enrichment analysis revealed that these genes were mainly enriched in PI3K-Akt signaling pathway, osteoclast differentiation, and focal adhesion. The authors suggest that pathways of PI3K-Akt, osteoclast differen- tiation, and focal adhesion may play important roles in the development of Ostheoarthritis females after menopause. With EGFR, ERBB2, CDC42, and STAT1 being the key genes related to disease progression in postmenopausal women and may be promising therapeutic targets.

3.5   Disease Networks

Phenotype-endophenotype, phenotype-environment and phenotype-genotype networks also termed *disease networks* have become useful tools in the realms of network medicine (Loscalzo et al., 2017; Sonawane et al., 2019; Vidal et al., 2011; Barabási et al., 2011), aimed at the understanding of the differences and commonalities that groups of phenotypes (often treated in the context of relative phenotypes or contrasts) have in association with factors such as genetic predispositions (Menche et al., 2017), endophenotypes (Ghiassian et al., 2016), environmental conditions or lifestyle. Disease networks also include comorbidity networks and exposome networks (Gomez-Cabrero et al., 2016).

Connecting diseases that share associated clinical features in a so-called human symptomsdisease network (Zhou et al., 2014) was a strategy towards elucidating the relationship between the molecular origins of diseases and their resulting phenotypes. From the standpoint of clinical decision making and differential diagnostics is a crucial task for medical research. Zhou and coworkers have used a literature mining approach to construct such a network and investigate the connection between clinical manifestations of diseases and their underlying molecular interactions. With this approach the authors found that the symptom-based similarity of two diseases correlates strongly with the number of shared genetic associations. Also, the extent to which their associated proteins interact and the diversity of the clinical manifestations of a disease can be related to the connectivity patterns of the underlying protein interaction network.

Regarding molecular interaction networks, these can also become effective tools to model disease associated networks. Menche and collaborators from Barabasi lab (Menche et al., 2015) have used them to investigate how most diseases are not direct consequences of mutational abnormality in a single gene, rather malignant phenotypes are driven by the interplay of multiple molecular processes. They argue that the relationships among these processes are encoded in the *interactome*, i.e., the network that integrates all physical interactions within a cell, being protein-protein electrostatic interactions or complex biochemical regulatory proteinDNA and metabolic interactions.

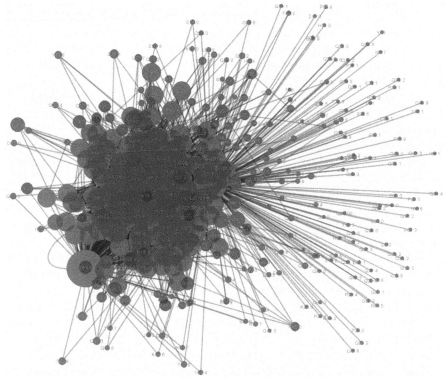

Figure 6 A comorbidity network for Q24.8 congenital malformations of the heart in a cohort of cardiovascular patients. Labels correspond to ICD10 codes for the different diseases. Node size and color are proportional to degree:from red/small to green/large. A cluster of tightly associated comorbidities may be noticed on the left side.

The identification of *disease modules* in the interactome is one initial step toward a systematic understanding of the molecular mechanisms underlying complex diseases. With this approach, the authors were able to derive mathematical conditions leading to the identifiability of disease modules and to show how the network-based location of each disease module determines its set of pathological relationships to other diseases. This allows the prediction of molecular commonalities between phenotypically related diseases, even if they do not share primary disease genes.

These models for disease-associated networks may also be supplemented with individualized gene expression profiles in order to construct personalized perturbation profiles for individual subjects. Doing this has allowed researchers to identify sets of genes that are significantly perturbed in each individual. It then becomes posible to characterize the heterogeneity of the molecular manifestations of complex diseases by quantifying the expression-level similarities and differences among patients with the same or similar phenotype (Menche et al., 2017). Despite the high heterogeneity of the so-called *personalized perturbation profiles*, it showed that patients with asthma, Parkinson and Huntingtons disease share a broad pool of sporadically disease-associated genes, and that individuals with statistically significant overlap within this pool have a 80100% chance of being diagnosed with the disease.

A related approach in which comorbidity networks were build to analyze sets of diseases commonly shared within the clinical setting (based on the automated data mining of around 13 million of electronic health records of patients in the Medicare database) (Gomez-Cabrero et al., 2016) lead the group of Gomez-Cabrero and coworkers to establish a model that goes from analyzing the comorbidities of chronic obstructive pulmonary disease to identifying shared molecular mechanisms. Network studies combined with rank-based statistics led to the discovery of the first set of COPD co-morbidity potential biomarkers, including IL15, TNF and JUP, and to characterize their association with aging and life-style conditions, such as smoking and physical activity. The rational behind this method is that it can be used to discover and decipher the molecular underpinning of other comorbidity relationships and to identify candidate co-morbidity biomarkers in diverse groups of diseases.

Thinking about the relationship between genetic origin, symptoms, comorbidities and their associated pathways led the team led by Barabási to think about the role that intermediate mesoscale processes play in the genesis and development of complex diseases. These common intermediate stages are known as endophenotypes (Ghiassian et al., 2016). Under their theoretical framework, it is possible to think about how the presence of a specific disease may be a consequence of the interplay between the relevant endophenotypes and their local, organ-based environment. Such endophenotypes may include inflammation, fibrosis, and thrombosis.

By a network approach, Ghiassian et al. (Ghiassian et al., 2016) developed the so-called Endophenotype Network Models to identify the subnetworks of the human inter-actome representing the *inflammasome, thrombosome*, and *fibrosome*. They find that these subnetworks are highly overlapping and significantly enriched with disease-associated genes. In particular they are also enriched with differentially expressed genes linked to cardiovascular disease risk, the primary cause of multimorbidity worldwide.

To identify these neighborhoods of endophenotype proteins, the authors made use of an algorithm developed within the same (large) research group: the DIseAse MOdule Detection (DIAMOnD) method (Ghiassian et al., 2016) which expands iteratively on a seed gene neighborhood by adding proteins with a significant number of connections to this *seed* gene pool. DIAMOnD is then devised as a systematic analysis of the connectivity patterns of disease proteins aimed at determining the most predictive topological property for their identification.

Further analysis have revealed that although human disease network modules are quite general, there is a subtle, yet important dependence on the type of tissue under consideration (Kitsak et al., 2016). This may be because for a disease to manifest itself in a particular tissue, a whole functional subnetwork of genes (the disease module itself) may need to be expressed in that tissue. By a systematic network analysis it has been possible to show that genes expressed in a specific tissue tend to be localized in the same *neighborhood* (in the graph-theoretical sense) of the interactome so that the integrity and completeness of the expression of the disease module determines whether or not that particular disease may manifest in a given tissue. Network modularity of interactome-disease networks has also use to explain heterogeneity in drug response, in the context of complex diseases such as the case of asthma, which results from chronic inflammation of the respiratory air ways (Sharma et al., 2015).

3.6   Drug-target Networks

A well known phenomenon in the design of therapeutic approaches to complex diseases is the fact that one has to consider that a single drug may have a number of molecular targets, also that a biomolecule may be targeted by different drugs and that complex diseases often need to be treated via polypharmacy, i.e., a combination of different drugs given concurrently or simultaneously to a single patient, either to treat one or more medical conditions.

A question arise about what may be the possible interactions among the sets of drugs, targets and conditions in the context of contemporary therapeutical approaches. One way to disentangle or at least analyze systematically this phenomenon is the use of drug-target networks. Some of these networks can be actually built upon molecular interaction networks by considering the relative binding affinities of drugs and targets. It has been devised that high-throughput analysis of drug-target interactions guided by PPI networks may allow the controllability of the sets of drugs and targets in the design of pharmacological therapy (Vinayagam et al., 2016).

A similar methodological approach may be used to design *in silico* drug efficacy screening assays (Guney et al., 2016) as well as to predict and validate novel drug-target interactions in a context guided by biological functional pathways aiming to design *in silico* drug repurposing strategies (Cheng et al., 2018). Drug-target network bioinformatic approaches can be applied even in the context of traditional therapies such as ethnobotanical methods (Wu et al., 2020).

3.7 Ecological and Epidemiological Networks

Also relevant in their own context, though perhaps not that common in the bioinformatics and biomedical settings, is the analysis of ecological networks. This is of course a well established field and has been for a long time. However, recent advances in the topological, functional and computational methods covered in this chapter have led to important advances in the field. Network topology studies of ecological networks have allowed researchers to understand the effects of the body size of the populations in their ecological networks (Woodward et al., 2005) and to map how these networks assemble and disassemble (Bascompte et al., 2009). But more importantly, in particular in the context of climate change and human-environmental interactions, these networks have allowed to understand the fragility and complexity of ecosystems (Montoya et al., 2006; Sole and Montoy, 2001) as well as their mechanisms of robustness and restoration (Pocock et al., 2012).

In a different context, more closer to our 2020 experience in the context of the COVID-19 pandemic is the study of epidemiological networks. Network epidemiology (for a simple example, see Fig. 7) is a branch of network science hat has existed for at least two decades. The first contemporary studies in network epidemiology arose in the context of the phenomenon of epidemic spreading in scale free-networks (Pastor-Satorras and Vespignani, 2001), a somehow theoretical question related to the phenomenon of percolation studied by statistical and condensed matter physicist. More recent network epidemiology issues have shown the effects that modern mobility patterns have in the spread of epidemics in human populations (Balcan et al., 2009). Our renewed understanding of epidemics has led to rethink classic paradigms such as the one of meta-populations (Ajelli et al., 2010). Data science and data based modeling have allowed to understanding all epidemics as potential pandemics due to global mobility patterns (Balcan et al., 2010).

Precisely, in the context of the COVID-19 international emergency, the combination of data mining on large scale epidemiological surveillance, mobility and healthcare data has led to sophisticated network epidemiological models put into action in record times (Vespignani et al., 2020), starting on the very early stages of the Wuhan outbreak (Zhang et al., 2020). Such early approaches have been steadily refined by the use of mobile phone data to infer disease lifecycle and have much better estimates of the basic reproduction rates almost in real time (Oliver et al., 2020). These efforts have allowed to take decisions based on the changes in the contact pattern matrices (Zhang et al., 2020) and even to assess the effects of policies like travel restrictions (Chinazzi et al., 2020). Impressive as these results are, we can expect that, after this pandemic, network epidemiology will become a more established tenet in the biomedical informatics arena.

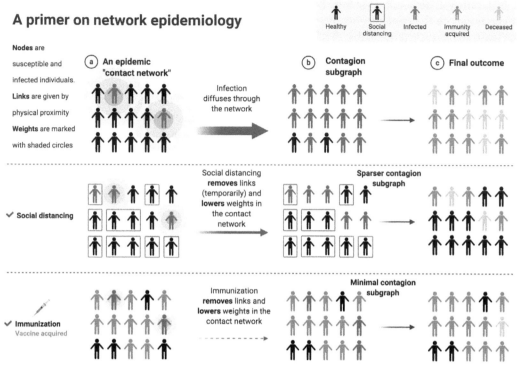

Figure 7 A simple epidemiological network model.

4   NETWORK INFERENCE AND CURATION

After a brief introduction to the thoery and methods of network science and a brief overview of their applications on the analysis of biological phenomena, we will present some of the main methods to reconstruct networks, either by modeling data via probabilistic and statistical approaches or by manual or automatic curation of databases.

4.1   Statistical Inference Methods for Biological Networks

The statistical inference of biological networks, often called *reverse engineering*, is the scientific process of using (low- and high-throughput) experimental data, statistical and computational techniques to reconstruct how the elements of the biological network (genes, proteins, signaling molecules, cells) interact and operate as a system (Tieri et al., 2019).

Mathematical methods to reverse engineer biological networks are highly dependent on the type of interaction that is captured in the networks. PPI networks, for instance are often better reconstructed by means of experimental approaches and database curation (see next subsection). It is however possible to generate statistical reconstruction schemes for PPI Networks, for instance the use of ortholog-based sequence approaches is grounded on the homologous nature of the query protein in the annotated protein databases using *pairwise local sequence alignment* algorithms. Other *in silico* approaches are based on protein sequences or protein structure, and still other are founded on gene fusion or gene expression, on chromosomal proximity, on phylogenetic trees or gene ontology. In all the cases, statistical over representation of patterns or motifs is the basis of the inference methods (Tieri et al., 2019).

In the case of GRNs, although in principle these are networks of causal interactions among transcription factors and downstream genes, and are usually understood as represented with directed graphs and inferred by gene expression data, a large number of methods to infer them are based on mutual information (MI), a probabilistically inferred measure of statistical dependency which tell us how much the knowledge of a random variable tells about another one (Hernández-Lemus and Escareño, 2012).

Often GRNs are approximated by the use of the so-called gene co-expression networks (GCNs) which are gene-gene association networks, generally reported as undirected graphs (Baca-López et al., 2009; Hernández-Lemus et al., 2009). In GCNs genes are connected whenever a significant co-expression association between them exists. GCNs are often built from gene expression data by calculating co-expression values in terms of pairwise gene similarity scores (such as MI, Pearson correlation, covariances and other similar scores) and later choosing a significance threshold often based in some form of bootstrapping of the underlying experimental data or by fitting (or mimicking) structural parameters of the actual networks (such as the number of total connections, the ratio of nodes to links, etc.). Other strategies for GCN inference include edge removal based on gene triplets analysis (e.g., ARACNE) (Lachmann et al., 2016; Margolin et al., 2006). GCNs are powerful analytical tools to gather biologically relevant information, useful for instance in the identification of genes not yet associated with explicit biological processes (Alcalá-Corona et al., 2018a, b; de Anda-Jáuregui et al., 2019; Drago-García et al., 2017).

Despite the fact that reverse engineering of biological networks is an enormous theoretical and computational challenge (Banf and Rhee 2017), we are progressed to the point that when appropriate data sources ara available, there are network inference method whose statistical power allows not only for a proper structural reconstruction of the networks but even provide clues about their dynamic behavior (Oates and Mukherjee, 2012). Of particular relevance is the analysis of network dynamics in the context of GRNs (Hecker et al., 2009) since it is in this context that the full potential of GRNs/GCNs to unveil biological clues is revealed.

However, due to a set of limitations mostly arising from the complex, noisy nature of high-throughput gene expression experiments and the so-called dimensionality curse (much larger feature space than the number of samples) validation of GRNs often requires the use of *gold standards* (i.e., sets of interactions validated with a given level of certainty) and the use of statistical thresholds to quantitatively evaluate the adherence of the GRN to such standards, or in some cases perturbation analysis of the biological consequences to asses the network under study. In recent times, a novel approach to validation—a *silver standard*, so to speak—has been developed in the form of what has been called *the wisdom of crowds*, i.e., the notion that inferring a given problem network by using a broad range of different methods *independently* (often in the form of a competition or 'challenge') and latter combining their results may give rise to a much better solution of the inference problem than every single attempt (Marbach et al., 2012).

4.2 Network Databases, Literature Mining, Automated and Manual Curation

Aside from probabilistic and statistical approaches to modeling high-throughput data, biological networks may also be constructed by curation, either directly from experiments measuring the interactions and integrating this knowledge on a network or by resorting to mine the literature or databases. As we previously stated, PPI networks are often build from experimental sources, from these, one that has resulted extremely important is the use of the yeast 2 hybrid (Y2H) method in which protein *baits* are produced in a yeast system for every protein in our desired sampling space. Y2H is an *in vivo* method, that has been considered suitable to determine both transient and stable interactions. It consists in screening the protein of interest against a library of potential interacting protein partners through the activation of a reporter gene—usually the gene Gal4 in the yeast Saccharomyces cerevisiae–. Y2H is affordable, fast and has low requirements, however its use has been object of a recent debate by considering the method not completely reliable in terms of yielding high numbers of false positive identifications. Other methods commonly used for *in vitro* measurements of PPIs are tandem affinity purification and mass spectroscopy (TAP-MS), protein microarrays (Ab-chips), affinity chromatography, XRat christallography and NMR spectroscopy (Tieri et al., 2019).

It is feasible to extract small GRNs by directed transcription factor binding affinity assays, however this results unaffordable to scale up to large size networks due to technical and logistic reasons. In the case of metabolic networks it is possible—yet costly, except for small model systems—to construct them by direct experimental measurements of proteomics/metabolomics/ fluxomics mass spectrometry. In general, however, since a large number of metabolic reactions and pathways are actually well annotated—since they have been experimentally probed for a long time—most metabolic networks are actually build from mining, either biochemical databases or the biomedical literature in an approach known as bibliomics (Grivell, 2002; Rihm et al., 2003). The curation procedure has been traditionally performed by manual or at most semi-automated methods, heavily dependent on the reliability of groups of *curators* and needing large double- and triple-check locks. Recently, however with the advent of sophisticated computational linguistics and natural language processing methods, automated data mining has become a reliable way to construct biological networks (Ilkka, 2010; Wilson et al., 2018).

5 BIOINFORMATICS OF NETWORK ANALYSIS

The quintessential quest for truth in biology is perhaps a desired relationship between *structure* and *function*. This challenge has not changed with the advent of network biology but has indeed been incorporated into the very tenets of biological network analysis. In this regard, once that a given biological network has been constructed one is confronted with the study of its structure—often synonymous with the *topological structure* as we have seen along this chapter—and its function—which depending on the specific type of bionetwork may involve several types of *enrichment* analyses (see related chapter in this book), the network dynamics, or the time dependent mapping leading to biological function–.

5.1 Topological Analysis

As we have seen in the introduction, the determination of graph-theoretical topological parameters allows the characterization of biological networks (Assenov, 2006). As the network become larger, computing the topological parameters may become computationally challenging due to combinatorial constraints. This has led to the development of computationally efficient methods to compute the topological parameters of networks (Assenov et al., 2008).

Sometimes these computational algorithms have been incorporated into general purpose network analysis suites (Doncheva et al., 2012; Winterbach et al., 2013). Such is the case with Cytoscape ((https://cytoscape.org/)) (Shannon et al., 2003), the Network Analysis Profiler, NAP (https://www.networkanalyst.ca.) (Theodosieu et al., 2017) or the multinetwork topological analysis comparison tool CatbNet (https://github.com/LBBSoft/CatbNet) (Pournoor et al., 2019). If the user has more in-depth bioinformatics experience, more sophisticated network topological analysis can be performed with the use of programming tools that will be shortly presented.

5.2 Functional Analysis

Once the structural features of a biological network have been established, the next quest is to determine what are the consequences of these structures for the actual biological functions of the systems under consideration. This is often done by means of what has been called enrichment analyses (García-Campos et al., 2015) which is is commonly directed towards determination of statistical over representation of biological subnetworks and pathways within our networks (Tatarinova and Nikolsky, 2017). Several online and offline tools are available for these kinds of analyses, among these we can mention DAVID (https://david.ncifcrf.gov/) (Jiao et al., 2012) that is quite commonly used though is a bit outdated (last update 2012), as well as WebGESTALT (http://www.webgestalt.org/) (Wang et al., 2017), and OmicsNet (https://www.omicsnet.ca/) (Zhou and Xia, 2018). A number of programming interfaces can also be used to perform enrichment analysis, such as the BioNet R-package (Beisser et al., 2010).

Once the topological and functional network analyses have been performed there is a need to integrate the information derived from both sources. This is often done based on the experience and general knowledge of principal investigators and researchers. Recently, a set of systematic guidelines have been developed to this end (de Anda-Jáuregui, 2019).

5.3 Programming Tools, Interfaces for Visualization and Analysis of Biological Networks

There is life beyond web-based and GUI-based network analysis tools, plenty of it. But it comes with a cost. You need to do some actual programming, but not all. There is a myriad different libraries and packages in the main scientific (and all-purpose) programming languages devoted to network analysis, both structural and functional. All four more widely used bioinformatic-related languages (R, Python, Perl and the recently risen Julia) have libraries devoted to biological network analysis. In R you have the large Bioconductor repository (https://www.bioconductor.org/) which as of June 2020 reported a staggering 7347 entries for network analysis tools (https://www.bioconductor.org/help/search/index.html?q=network/). Important instances among these are the iGraph library (Csardi et al., 2006) (also with a Python version) and the multilayer network analysis suite MuxViz (http://muxviz.net/), (de Domenico et al., 2015).

In Python, you have the network suite of algorithms and libraries bundled as NetworkX (https://networkx.github.io/), (Hagberg et al., 2008) and the analysis and visualization Graphtool library (https://graph-tool.skewed.de/) (Peixoto, 2017). As well as the general purpose bioinformatics hub BioPython (https://biopython. org/".

The BioPerl repository (https://bioperl.org/), has also some packages ready for their use in biological network analysis. Unfortunately, most of them were made considering directed acyclic graphs (DAGs) which are useful in the phylogenetics and bayesian network arenas but quite limited to deal with complex biological networks (i.e., networks with many loops). Finally, in the case of BioJulia https://biojulia.net/, a recently formed repository, to date has no native network analysis tools but in some instances is able to import some of the NetworkX algorithms.

Aside from theses repository resources, we must also mention Gephi, a standalone Java network visualization suite (https://gephi.org/), (Bastian, et al., 2009) that has some analytical built-in capabilities.

6 CONCLUDING REMARKS

As the fields of Network Biology and Network Medicine are becoming well established within the scientific community—with impacts even in the clinical setting by means of network approaches to personalized medicine and translational bioinformatics—it becomes relevant for researchers in biology to become acquainted with the main concepts, theoretical foundations, methods and bioinformatic tools of biological networks. The aim of this chapter is precisely to serve as a gentle introduction to a very complex (yet compelling and powerful) subject, guiding the readers through a journey of discovery of the field. This is a dauntingly challenging endeavor due to the broad range of concepts and applications involved. For this reason, this chapter is far from a completed mission. The extensive literature included—and our deliberate effort to cite it with a biological context in mind—is intended to serve as a guided continuation, a sort of road map for those in search of more in depth understanding of biological networks.

Acknowledgements

Figures 2, 4 and 7 were generated using **BioRender**, https://biorender.com/.

REFERENCES

Abedini, J.A., S. Handa, S. Edwards, B. Chorley and H. El-Masri (2019). Identification of differentially expressed genes and networks related to hepatic lipid dysfunction. Tox. Appl. Pharm. 382: 114757.

Ajelli, M., B. Gonçalves, D. Balcan, V. Colizza, H. Hu, J.J. Ramasco, et al. (2010). Comparing large-scale computational approaches to epidemic modeling: Agent-based versus structured metapopulation models. BMC Infectious Diseases. 10(1): 190.

Alcalá-Corona, S.A., J. Espinal-Enríquez, G. De Anda Jáuregui and E. Hernandez-Lemus (2018a). The hierarchical modular structure of her2+ breast cancer network. Front. Physiol. 9: 1423.

Alcalá-Corona, S.A., G. de Anda-Jáuregui, J. Espinal-Enriquez, H. Tovar and E. Hernández-Lemus (2018b). Network modularity and hierarchical structure in breast cancer molecular subtypes. pp. 352–358. *In*: International Conference on Complex Systems. Springer.

Alshabi, A.M., B. Vastrad, I.A. Shaikh and C. Vastrad (2019). Exploring the molecular mechanism of the drug-treated breast cancer based on gene expression microarray. Biomolecules 9(7): 282.

Assenov, Y. (2006). Topological Analysis of Biological Networks, Ph.D. thesis. Max Planck Institute for Informatics.

Assenov, Y., F. Ramírez, S.-E. Schelhorn, T. Lengauer and M. Albrecht (2008). Computing topological parameters of biological networks. Bioinformatics. 24(2): 282–284.

Baca-López, K., E. Hernández-Lemus, M. Mayorga (2009). Information-theoretical analysis of gene expression data to infer transcriptional interactions. Revista Mexicana de Física. 55(6): 456–466.

Balcan, D., V. Colizza, B. Gonçalves, H. Hu, J.J. Ramasco and A. Vespignani (2009). Multiscale mobility networks and the spatial spreading of infectious diseases. PNAS. 106(51): 21484–21489.

Balcan, D., B. Gonçalves, H. Hu, J.J. Ramasco, V. Colizza and A. Vespignani (2010). Modeling the spatial spread of infectious diseases: The global epidemic and mobility computational model. J. Comput. Sci. 1(3): 132–145.

Banf, M. and S.Y. Rhee (2017). Computational inference of gene regulatory networks: Approaches, limitations and opportunities. Biochimica et Biophysica Acta (BBA)-Gene Regulatory Mechanisms. 1860(1): 41–52.

Barabási, A.-L. (2003). Linked: The New Science of Networks. Perseus Books Group.

Barabasi, A.-L. and Z.N. Oltvai (2004). Network biology: Understanding the cell's functional organization. Nat. Rev. Genet. 5(2): 101–113.

Barabási, A.-L., N. Gulbahce and J. Loscalzo (2011). Network medicine: A network-based approach to human disease. Nat. Rev. Genet. 12(1): 56–68.

Barabási, A.-L. (2016). Network Science. Cambridge University Press.

Barel, G. and R. Herwig. (2018). Network and pathway analysis of toxicogenomics data. Front. Genet. 9: 484.

Barrett, T., D.B. Troup, S.E. Wilhite, P. Ledoux, D. Rudnev, C. Evangelista, et al. (2009). Ncbi geo: Archive for high-throughput functional genomic data, Nucleic Acids Res. 37(Suppl 1): D885–D890.

Barrios-Rodiles, M., K.R. Brown, B. Ozdamar, R. Bose, Z. Liu, R.S. Donovan, et al. (2005). High-throughput mapping of a dynamic signaling network in mammalian cells. Science. 307(5715): 1621–1625.

Bascompte, J. and D.B. Stouffer (2009). The assembly and disassembly of ecological networks. Philosophical Transactions of the Royal Society B: Biological Sciences. 364(1524): 1781–1787.

Basler, G., Z. Nikoloski, A. Larhlimi, A.-L. Barabási and Y.-Y. Liu (2016). Control of fluxes in metabolic networks. Genome Res. 26(7): 956–968.

Bastian, M., S. Heymann and M. Jacomy (2009). Gephi: An open source software for exploring and manipulating networks. In: Third international AAAI conference on weblogs and social media.

Beguerisse-Díaz, M., G. Bosque, D. Oyarzún, J. Picó and M. Barahona (2018). Flux-dependent graphs for metabolic networks, NPJ yst. Biol. Appl. 4(1): 1–14.

Beisser, D., G.W. Klau, T. Dandekar, T. Müller and M.T. Dittrich (2010). Bionet: An R-package for the functional analysis of biological networks. Bioinformatics. 26(8): 1129–1130.

Bollobás, B. and B. Béla (2001). Random Graphs, no. 73. Cambridge University Press.

Breuer, M., T.M. Earnest, C. Merryman, K.S. Wise, L. Sun, M.R. Lynott, et al. (2019). Essential metabolism for a minimal cell. Elife. 8: e36842.

Brown, K.R., D. Otasek, M. Ali, M.J. McGuffin, W. Xie, B. Devani, et al. (2009). Navigator: Network analysis, visualization and graphing toronto. Bioinformatics. 25(24): 3327–3329.

Cagney, G. and A. Emili (2011). Network Biology: Methods and Applications. Springer.

Cheng, F., R.J. Desai, D.E. Handy, R. Wang, S. Schneeweiss, A.-L. Barabási, et al. (2018). Network-based approach to prediction and population-based validation of *in silico* drug repurposing. Nat. Commun. 9(1): 1–12.

Chiang, G.G. and R.T. Abraham (2007). Targeting the mtor signaling network in cancer. Trends Mol. Med. 13(10): 433–442.

Chinazzi, M., J.T. Davis, M. Ajelli, C. Gioannini, M. Litvinova, S. Merler, et al. (2020). The effect of travel restrictions on the spread of the 2019 novel coronavirus (Covid-19) outbreak. Science. 368(6489): 395–400.

Cho, D.-Y., Y.-A. Kim and T.M. Przytycka (2012). Network biology approach to complex diseases. PLoS Comput. Biol. 8(12).

Cohen Jr, M.M. (2003). The hedgehog signaling network. Am. J. Med. Genet. Part A. 123(1): 5–28.

Courtois-Cox, S., S.M.G. Williams, E.E. Reczek, B.W. Johnson, L.T. McGillicuddy, C.M. Johannessen, et al. (2006). A negative feedback signaling network underlies oncogene-induced senescence. Cancer Cell. 10(6): 459–472.

Covert, M.W., N. Xiao, T.J. Chen and J.R. Karr (2008). Integrating metabolic, transcriptional regulatory and signal transduction models in *Escherichia coli*. Bioinformatics. 24(18): 2044–2050.

Csardi, G., T. Nepusz, et al. (2006). The igraph software package for complex network research. Inter. Journal, Complex Systems. 1695(5): 1–9.

de Anda-Jáuregui, G., R.A. Mejía-Pedroza, J. Espinal-Enríquez and E. Hernández-Lemus (2015). Crosstalk events in the estrogen signaling pathway may affect tamoxifen efficacy in breast cancer molecular subtypes. Comput. Biol. Chem. 59: 42–54.

de Anda-Jáuregui, G., S.A. Alcalá-Corona, J. Espinal-Enríquez and E. Hernández-Lemus (2019). Functional and transcriptional connectivity of communities in breast cancer co-expression networks. Appl. Network Sci. 4(1): 22.

de Anda-Jáuregui, G. (2019). Guideline for comparing functional enrichment of biological network modular structures. Appl. Network Sci. 4(1): 13.

de Domenico, M., M.A. Porter and A. Arenas (2015). Muxviz: A tool for multilayer analysis and visualization of networks. J. Complex Networks. 3(2): 159–176.

Dennis, G., B.T. Sherman, D.A. Hosack, J. Yang, W. Gao, H.C. Lane, et al. (2003). David: Database for annotation, visualization, and integrated discovery. Genome Biol. 4(9): R60.

Doncheva, N.T., Y. Assenov, F.S. Domingues and M. Albrecht (2012). Topological analysis and interactive visualization of biological networks and protein structures. Nat. Protoc. 7(4): 670.

Drago-García, D., J. Espinal-Enríquez and E. Hernández-Lemus (2017). Network analysis of emt and met micro-rna regulation in breast cancer. Sci. Rep. 7(1): 1–17.

Duarte, N.C., S.A. Becker, N. Jamshidi, I. Thiele, M.L. Mo, T.D. Vo, et al. (2007). Global reconstruction of the human metabolic network based on genomic and bibliomic data. PNAS. 104(6): 1777–1782.

Dubitzky, W., O. Wolkenhauer, H. Yokota and K.-H. Cho (2013). Encyclopedia of Systems Biology. Springer Publishing Company, Incorporated.

Erdös, P. and A. Rényi (1959). On random graphs. Publ. Math. 6: 290–297.

Erdös, P. and A. Rényi (1961). On the strength of connectedness of a random graph. Acta Mathematica Hungarica. 12(1-2): 261–267.

Fisher, C.P., N.J. Plant, J.B. Moore and A.M. Kierzek (2013). Qsspn: Dynamic simulation of molecular interaction networks describing gene regulation, signalling and whole-cell metabolism in human cells. Bioinformatics. 29(24): 3181–3190.

Franceschini, A., J. Lin, C. von Mering and L.J. Jensen (2016). Svd-phy: Improved prediction of protein functional associations through singular value decomposition of phylogenetic profiles. Bioinformatics. 32(7): 1085–1087.

García-Campos, M.A., J. Espinal-Enríquez and E. Hernández-Lemus (2015) Pathway analysis: State of the art. Front. Physiol. 6.

Ghiassian, S.D., J. Menche and A.-L. Barabási (2015). A disease module detection (diamond) algorithm derived from a systematic analysis of connectivity patterns of disease proteins in the human interactome, PLoS Comput. Biol. 11(4).

Ghiassian, S.D., J. Menche, D.I. Chasman, F. Giulianini, R. Wang, P. Ricchiuto, et al. (2016). Endophenotype network models: Common core of complex diseases. Sci. Rep. 6: 27414.

Gibson, D.G., J.I. Glass, C. Lartigue, V.N. Noskov, R.-Y. Chuang, M.A. Algire, et al. (2010). Creation of a bacterial cell controlled by a chemically synthesized genome. Science. 329(5987): 52–56.

Gilbert, E.N. (1959). Random graphs. The Annals of Mathematical Statistics. 30(4): 1141–1144.

Gomez-Cabrero, D., J. Menche, C. Vargas, I. Cano, D. Maier, A.-L. Barabási, et al. (2016). From comorbidities of chronic obstructive pulmonary disease to identification of shared molecular mechanisms by data integration. BMC Bioinformatics. 17(15): 441.

Grivell, L. (2002). Mining the bibliome: Searching for a needle in a haystack? EMBO Reports. 3(3): 200–203.

Guan, X., Y. Yao, G. Bao, Y. Wang, A. Zhang and X. Zhong (2020). Diagnostic model of combined cerna and DNA methylation related genes in esophageal carcinoma. PeerJ. 8: e8831.

Guney, E., J. Menche, M. Vidal and A.-L. Barábasi (2016). Network-based in silico drug efficacy screening. Nat. Commun. 7: 10331.

Guo, T., D. Hou and D. Yu (2019). Bioinformatics analysis of gene expression profile data to screen key genes involved in intracranial aneurysms. Mol. Med. Rep. 20(5): 4415–4424.

Hagberg, A., P. Swart and D.S Chult (2008). Exploring network structure, dynamics, and function using networkx. Tech. Rep., Los Alamos National Lab. (LANL), Los Alamos, NM (United States).

He, Z., X. Duan and G. Zeng (2019). Identification of potential biomarkers and pivotal biological pathways for prostate cancer using bioinformatics analysis methods. PeerJ. 7: e7872.

Hecker, M., S. Lambeck, S. Toepfer, E. van Someren and R. Guthke (2009). Gene regulatory network inference: Data integration in dynamic modelsa review. Biosystems. 96(1): 86–103.

Hernández-Lemus, E., D. Velázquez-Fernández, J.K. Estrada-Gil, I. Silva-Zolezzi, M.F. Herrera-Hernández, G. Jiménez-Sánchez (2009). Information theoretical methods to deconvolute genetic regulatory networks applied to thyroid neoplasms. Physica A: Statistical Mechanics and its Applications 388(24): 5057–5069.

Hernández-Lemus, E. (2012). Nonequilibrium thermodynamics of cell signaling. J. Thermodyn. 2012: 1–11. Article ID 432143.

Hernández-Lemus, E. and C.R. Escareño (2012). The role of information theory in gene regulatory network inference. pp. 109–144. *In*: P. Deloumeaux and J.D. Gorzalka (eds). Information Theory: New Research. Mathematics Research, Developments Series, Nova Science Publishers, Inc.

Herrgård, M.J., B.-S. Lee, V. Portnoy and B.Ø. Palsson (2006). Integrated analysis of regulatory and metabolic networks reveals novel regulatory mechanisms in saccharomyces cerevisiae. Genome Res. 16(5): 627–635.

Hitomi, J., D.E. Christofferson, A. Ng, J. Yao, A. Degterev, R.J. Xavier, et al. (2008). Identification of a molecular signaling network that regulates a cellular necrotic cell death pathway. Cell. 135(7): 1311–1323.

Ilkka, H. (2010). Biodata Mining and Visualization: Novel Approaches, Vol. 5. World Scientific.

Jean-Quartier, C., F. Jeanquartier and A. Holzinger (2020). Open data for differential network analysis in glioma. Int. J. Mol. Sci. 21(2): 547.

Jeong, H., B. Tombor, R. Albert, Z.N. Oltvai and A.-L. Barabási (2000). The large-scale organization of metabolic networks. Nature. 407(6804): 651.

Jiang, W.-D. and P.-C. Yuan (2019). Molecular network-based identification of competing endogenous RNAs in bladder cancer. PloS one 14(8).

Jiao, X., B.T. Sherman, D.W. Huang, R. Stephens, M.W. Baseler, H.C. Lane, et al. (2012). David-ws: A stateful web service to facilitate gene/protein list analysis. Bioinformatics. 28(13): 1805–1806.

Kanehisa, M., Y. Sato, M. Furumichi, K. Morishima and M. Tanabe (2019). New approach for understanding genome variations in kegg. Nucleic Acids Res. 47(D1): D590–D595.

Katoh, M. and M. Katoh (2007). Wnt signaling pathway and stem cell signaling network. Clin. Cancer Res. 13(14): 4042–4045.

Kitsak, M., A. Sharma, J. Menche, E. Guney, S.D. Ghiassian, J. Loscalzo, et al. (2016). Tissue specificity of human disease module. Sci. Rep. 6(1): 1–12.

Kontogeorgaki, S., R.J. Sánchez-García, R.M. Ewing, K.C. Zygalakis, B.D. MacArthur (2017). Noise-processing by signaling networks. Sci. Rep. 7(1): 1–9.

Kovács, I.A., K. Luck, K. Spirohn, Y. Wang, C. Pollis, S. Schlabach, et al. (2019). Network-based prediction of protein interactions. Nat. Commun. 10(1): 1–8.

Lachmann, A., F.M. Giorgi, G. Lopez and A. Califano (2016). ARACNe-AP: Gene network reverse engineering through adaptive partitioning inference of mutual information. Bioinformatics. 32(14): 2233–2235.

Lee, D.-S., J. Park, K. Kay, N.A. Christakis, Z.N. Oltvai and A.-L. Barabási (2008). The implications of human metabolic network topology for disease comorbidity. PNAS. 105(29): 9880–9885.

Liu, L., S. Wu, X. Zhu, R. Xu, K. Ai, L. Zhang, et al. (2019). Analysis of cerna network identifies prognostic circrna biomarkers in bladder cancer. Neoplasma. 66(5): 736–745.

Loscalzo, J., A.-L. Barabási and E.K. Silverman (2017). Network Medicine. Harvard University Press.

Ma, S., K.J. Minch, T.R. Rustad, S. Hobbs, S.-L. Zhou, D.R. Sherman, et al. (2015). Integrated modeling of gene regulatory and metabolic networks in mycobacterium tuberculosis. PLoS Comput. Biol. 11(11): e1004543.

Marbach, D., J.C. Costello, R. Küffner, N.M. Vega, R.J. Prill, D.M. Camacho, et al. (2012). Wisdom of crowds for robust gene network inference. Nat. Methods. 9(8): 796.

Margolin, A.A., I. Nemenman, K. Basso, C. Wiggins, G. Stolovitzky, R. Favera, et al. (2006). ARACNE: An algorithm for the reconstruction of gene regulatory networks in a mammalian cellular context. BMC Bioinformatics. 7(Suppl 1): S7.

Martin, D.E. and M.N. Hall (2005). The expanding tor signaling network. Curr. Opin. Cell Biol. 17(2): 158–166.

Menche, J., A. Sharma, M. Kitsak, S.D. Ghiassian, M. Vidal, J. Loscalzo, et al. (2015). Uncovering disease-disease relationships through the incomplete interactome. Science. 347(6224): 1257601.

Menche, J., E. Guney, A. Sharma, P.J. Branigan, M.J. Loza, F. Baribaud, et al. (2017). Integrating personalized gene expression profiles into predictive disease-associated gene pools. NPJ Syst. Biol. Appl. 3(1): 1–10.

Meric-Bernstam, F. and A.M. Gonzalez-Angulo. (2009). Targeting the mtor signaling network for cancer therapy. J. Clin. Oncol. 27(13): 2278.

Montoya, J.M., S.L. Pimm and R.V. Solé (2006). Ecological networks and their fragility. Nature. 442(7100): 259–264.

Oates, C.J. and S. Mukherjee (2012). Network inference and biological dynamics. The Annals of Applied Statistics. 6(3): 1209.

Olayioye, M.A., R.M. Neve, H.A. Lane and N.E. Hynes (2000). The erbb signaling network: Receptor heterodimerization in development and cancer. The EMBO J. 19(13): 3159–3167.

Oliver, N., B. Lepri, H. Sterly, R. Lambiotte, S. Delataille, M. de Nadai, et al. (2020). Mobile phone data for informing public health actions across the Covid-19 pandemic life cycle. Sci Adv. 6(23): eabc0764.

Oughtred, R., C. Stark, B.-J. Breitkreutz, J. Rust, L. Boucher, C. Chang, et al. (2019). The biogrid interaction database: 2019 update. Nucleic Acids Res. 47(D1): D529–D541.

Pastor-Satorras, R. and A. Vespignani (2001). Epidemic spreading in scale-free networks. Phys. Rev. Lett. 86(14): 3200.

Peixoto, T.P. (2017) The graph-tool python library, figsharedoi:10.6084/m9. figshare.1164194. URL http://figshare.com/articles/graph_tool/1164194

Pocock, M.J., D.M. Evans and J. Memmott (2012). The robustness and restoration of a network of ecological networks. Science. 335(6071): 973–977.

Pournoor, E., N. Elmi and A. Masoudi-Nejad (2019). Catbnet: A multi network analyzer for comparing and analyzing the topology of biological networks. Current Genomics. 20(1): 69–75.

Pouryahya, M., J.H. Oh, J.C. Mathews, J.O. Deasy and A.R. Tannenbaum (2018). Characterizing cancer drug response and biological correlates: A geometric network approach. Sci. Rep. 8(1): 1–12.

Ravasz, E., A.L. Somera, D.A. Mongru, Z.N. Oltvai and A.-L. Barabási (2002). Hierarchical organization of modularity in metabolic networks. Science. 297(5586): 1551–1555.

Rhodes, D.R., J. Yu, K. Shanker, N. Deshpande, R. Varambally, D. Ghosh, et al. (2004). Oncomine: A cancer microarray database and integrated data-mining platform. Neoplasia. 6(1): 1.

Rihm, B.H., S. Vidal, C. Nemurat, S. Vachenc, S. Mohr, F. Mazur, et al. (2003). From transcriptomics to bibliomics. Med. Sci. Monit. 9(8): MT89–MT95.

Rolland, T., M. Taşan, B. Charloteaux, S.J. Pevzner, Q. Zhong, N. Sahni, et al. (2014). A proteome-scale map of the human interactome network. Cell. 159(5): 1212–1226.

Saito, R., M.E. Smoot, K. Ono, J. Ruscheinski, P.-L. Wang, S. Lotia, et al. (2012). A travel guide to cytoscape plugins. Nat. Methods. 9(11): 1069.

Shannon, P., A. Markiel, O. Ozier, N.S. Baliga, J.T. Wang, D. Ramage, et al. (2003). Cytoscape: A software environment for integrated models of biomolecular interaction networks. Genome Res. 13(11): 2498–2504.

Sharma, A., J. Menche, C.C. Huang, T. Ort, X. Zhou, M. Kitsak, et al. (2015). A disease module in the interactome explains disease heterogeneity, drug response and captures novel pathways and genes in asthma. Hum. Mol. Genet. 24(11): 3005–3020.

Shen, Y., J. Liu, G. Estiu, B. Isin, Y. Ahn, D. Lee, et al. (2010). Blueprint for antimicrobial hit discovery targeting metabolic networks, PNAS. 107(3): 1082–1087.

Sole, R.V. and M. Montoya (2001). Complexity and fragility in ecological networks. Proceedings of the Royal Society of London. Series B: Biological Sciences. 268(1480): 2039–2045.

Sonawane, A.R., S.T. Weiss, K. Glass and A. Sharma (2019). Network medicine in the age of biomedical big data. Front. Genet. 10.

Stitt, M., R. Sulpice and J. Keurentjes (2010). Metabolic networks: How to identify key components in the regulation of metabolism and growth. Plant Physiol. 152(2): 428–444.

Szklarczyk, D., J.H. Morris, H. Cook, M. Kuhn, S. Wyder, M. Simonovic, et al. (2016). The STRING database in 2017: Quality-controlled protein–protein association networks, made broadly accessible. Nucleic Acids Res. 45(D1): D362–D368.

Szklarczyk, D., A.L. Gable, D. Lyon, A. Junge, S. Wyder, J. Huerta-Cepas, et al. (2019). String v11: protein–protein association networks with increased coverage, supporting functional discovery in genome-wide experimental datasets. Nucleic Acids Res. 47(D1): D607–D613.

Tang, Z., C. Li, B. Kang, G. Gao, C. Li and Z. Zhang (2017). Gepia: A web server for cancer and normal gene expression profiling and interactive analyses. Nucleic Acids Res. 45(W1): W98–W102.

Tatarinova, T.V. and Y. Nikolsky (2017). Biological Networks and Pathway Analysis. Springer.

Theodosiou, T., G. Efstathiou, N. Papanikolaou, N.C. Kyrpides, P.G. Bagos, I. Iliopoulos, et al. (2017). Nap: The network analysis profiler, a web tool for easier topological analysis and comparison of medium-scale biological networks. BMC Research Notes. 10(1): 278.

Tieri, P., L. Farina, M. Petti, L. Astolfi, P. Paci and F. Castiglione (2019). Network inference and reconstruction in bioinformatics. pp. 805–813. *In*: S. Ranganathan, M. Gribskov, K, Nakai and C. Schönbach (eds). Encyclopedia of Bioinformatics and Computational Biology, Vol. 2. Academic Press.

Vespignani, A., H. Tian, C. Dye, J.O. Lloyd-Smith, R.M. Eggo, M. Shrestha, et al. (2020). Modelling Covid-19. Nat. Rev. Phys. 1–3.

Vidal, M., M.E. Cusick and A.-L. Barabási (2011). Interactome networks and human disease. Cell. 144(6): 986–998.

Vinayagam, A., T.E. Gibson, H.-J. Lee, B. Yilmazel, C. Roesel, Y. Hu, et al. (2016). Controllability analysis of the directed human protein interaction network identifies disease genes and drug targets. PNAS. 113(18): 4976–4981.

Wagner, A. (2012). Metabolic networks and their evolution. pp. 29–52. *In*: O.S. Soyer (ed.). Evolutionary Systems Biology. Springer.

Walhout, M., M. Vidal and J. Dekker (2012). Handbook of Systems Biology: Concepts and Insights. Academic Press. 2012.

Wang, J., J. Zhong, G. Chen, M. Li, F.-X. Wu and Y. Pan (2014). Clusterviz: A cytoscape app for cluster analysis of biological network. IEEE/ACM Transactions on Computational Biology and Bioinformatics. 12(4): 815–822.

Wang, J., S. Vasaikar, Z. Shi, M. Greer and B. Zhang (2017). Webgestalt 2017: A more comprehensive, powerful, flexible and interactive gene set enrichment analysis toolkit. Nucleic Acids Res. 45(W1): W130–W137.

Wang, L., B. Wang, J. Liu and Z. Quan (2019). Construction and analysis of a spinal cord injury competitive endogenous rna network based on the expression data of long noncoding, micro-and messenger RNAs. Mol. Med. Rep. 19(4): 3021–3034.

Wang, S., H. Wang, W. Liu and B. Wei (2019). Identification of key genes and pathways associated with sex differences in osteoarthritis based on bioinformatics analysis. BioMed. Research International.

Wen, C., G. Xu, S. He, Y. Huang, J. Shi, L. Wu, et al. (2020). Screening circular rnas related to acquired gefitinib resistance in non-small cell lung cancer cell lines. J. Cancer. 11(13): 3816–3826.

Wilson, S., A.D. Wilkins, M.V. Holt, B.K. Choi, D. Konecki, C.-H. Lin, et al. (2018). Automated literature mining and hypothesis generation through a network of medical subject headings. bioRxiv. 403667.

Winterbach, W., P. Van Mieghem, M. Reinders, H. Wang and D. de Ridder (2013). Topology of molecular interaction networks. BMC Systems Biology. 7(1): 90.

Woodward, G., B. Ebenman, M. Emmerson, J.M. Montoya, J.M. Olesen, et al. (2005). Body size in ecological networks. Trends Ecol. Evol. 20(7): 402–409.

Wu, Q., B. Zhang, Y. Sun, R. Xu, X. Hu, S. Ren, et al. (2019). Identification of novel biomarkers and candidate small molecule drugs in non-small-cell lung cancer by integrated microarray analysis. Onco. Targets Ther. 12: 3545.

Wu, R., H. Wang, X. Lv, X. Shen and G. Ye (2020). Rapid action of mechanism investigation of yixin ningshen tablet in treating depression by combinatorial use of systems biology and bioinformatics tools. J. Ethnopharmacol. 112827.

Xia, J., E.E. Gill and R.E. Hancock (2015). Networkanalyst for statistical, visual and network-based meta-analysis of gene expression data. Nat. Protoc. 10(6): 823.

Yilmaz, L.S. and A.J. Walhout (2017). Metabolic network modeling with model organisms. Curr. Opin. Chem. Biol. 36: 32–39.

Zhang, J., M. Litvinova, Y. Liang, Y. Wang, W. Wang, S. Zhao, et al. (2020). Changes in contact patterns shape the dynamics of the Covid-19 outbreak in china. Science.

Zhang, J., M. Litvinova, W. Wang, Y. Wang, X. Deng, X. Chen, et al. (Missing). Evolving epidemiology and transmission dynamics of coronavirus disease 2019 outside hubei province. China: A Descriptive and Modelling Study, The Lancet Infectious Diseases.

Zhou, X., J. Menche, A.-L. Barabási and A. Sharma (2014). Human symptoms–disease network. Nat. Commun. 5(1): 1–10.

Zhou, G. and J. Xia (2018). Omicsnet: A web-based tool for creation and visual analysis of biological networks in 3d space. Nucleic Acids Res. 46(W1): W514–W522.

CHAPTER 14

Bioinformatics of Functional Categories Enrichment

Laura Gómez-Romero[1,*], Hugo Tovar[1]
and Enrique Hernández-Lemus[1,2]

[1]Computational Genomics Division, National Institute of Genomic Medicine, Mexico
[2]Center for Complexity Sciences, Universidad Nacional Autónoma de México, Mexico

1 ANNOTATION SOURCES

The annotation of a gene is composed by all the biological features that belong to that specific gene. For example, a gene can be annotated to belong to a specific pathway, it can be annotated to have a specific functional domain, it can be annotated to be the target of a specific regulator, it can be annotated to be expressed in a specific tissue and so on. No single resource is able to maintain all of the biological aspects since most annotations have very specific curation processes. So, most annotations are kept in separate databases that are hosted and maintained by different research groups. As can be expected, all hypothesis or conclusions derived from functional enrichment methods depend on the annotation used. Table 1 shows a list of databases hosting specific annotations. Some of them, such as GO and KEGG, host a broad category of terms and species and have been implemented by most of the software devoted to perform functional enrichment analysis. Other resources are limited in the species for which they keep functional information.

From all the annotation listed, GO is the most popular one because of the wide spectrum of its annotations and its interoperability. So, we will invest some time to explain what are the GO annotations, how are they created, what kind of features do they have and what kind of changes do they suffer through time.

*Corresponding author: *lgomez@inmegen.gob.mx*

1.1 GO: Gene Ontologies

There are several definitions for *ontology* across the literature: (i) an informal conceptual system, (ii) a specification of a "conceptualization", (iii) a representation of a conceptual system via a logical theory and (iv) a vocabulary used by a logical theory (Guarino and Giaretta, 1995). The basic and common idea between all these definitions is that ontologies provide vocabulary and concepts for a specific domain of knowledge that can be used to establish a ground-truth to facilitate the communication between experts.

Table 1   Features of databases hosting specific annotations

Database	Scope	Annotations	Website
GO (Consortium, 2019)	Ontologies for biological process, molecular functions and cellular components	7,765,270 annotations, 4593 species	http://geneontology.org/ http://amigo.geneontology.org/
KEGG (Kanehisa and Goto, 2000)	Biological pathways	708,399 pathways, 6542 species	https://www.kegg.jp/kegg/
Pfam (El-Gebali et al., 2019)	Protein families and domains	1,203,163 organisms	https://pfam.xfam.org/
TRANSFAC (Wingender et al., 1996)	Regulatory interactions, transcription factors and regulated genes	300 Eukaryotic species	http://gene-regulation.com
GTEx (Carithers et al., 2015)	Tissue-specific gene expression and regulation	54 non-diseased human tissues	https://www.gtexportal.org/
OMIM (Hamosh et al., 2005)	Human genes and genetic disorders	16,275 genes	https://omim.org/
REACTOME (Jassal et al., 2020)	Biological pathways	2362 human pathways	https://reactome.org/
INTERPRO (Mitchell et al., 2019)	Protein families, domains and sequences	1 million organisms	https://www.ebi.ac.uk/interpro/
STRING (Szklarczyk et al., 2019)	Protein-protein interactions	5090 species	https://string-db.org/
Uniprot (Consortium, 2019)	Protein sequence and functional data	1,203,163 annotations	https://www.uniprot.org/

According to the Gene Ontology Consortium (GOC), the GO project has three major goals: (i) to develop a set of controlled, structured vocabularies known as ontologies to describe key domains of molecular biology, including gene product attributes and biological sequences; (ii) to apply GO terms in the annotation of sequences, genes or gene products in biological databases; and to provide a centralized public resource allowing universal access to the ontologies, annotation data sets and software tools developed to be used with GO data (Consortium, 2004).

The GO annotations are divided into three broad categories: (a) *molecular function* which describes the gene activities at the molecular level, (b) *biological process* which describes ordered assembles of molecular functions or biological programs that are carried out by a gene and (c) *cellular component* which describes locations relative to cellular structure and compartments.

The GO is organized as a directed acyclic graph (DAG) (Khatri and Drăghici, 2005). A DAG is formed by a finite number of nodes and edges with no directed cycles, so a path starting from node x can not reach x again for any node in the network. In this representation the nodes are terms in the ontology and the edges are relationships between them. The directed structure of the graph implies that the relationships are always from the type "is part of" or "is a type of" from the leafs to the root of the network. Figure 1 (taken from http://geneontology.org/docs/ontology-documentation/) represents a small fraction of the GO tree under the category GO:0008152 "metabolic process". This GO:0008152 is part of the GO:biological process.

From this tree we can know that hexose biosynthetic process GO:0019319 is a type of hexose metabolic process GO:0019318 that is a type of monosaccharide metabolic process GO:0005996 that is a type of small molecule metabolic process GO:0044281 that is a type of metabolic process GO:008152. Notice that we decided to follow the extreme left path but there are multiple paths from GO:0019319 to GO:008152. A child GO can have multiple parents what indicates that a specific process can be catalogued as a type of several more general processes. Another generality is that terms closer to the root of the three are more general than terms far away from the root. A parent node is always more general than a child node.

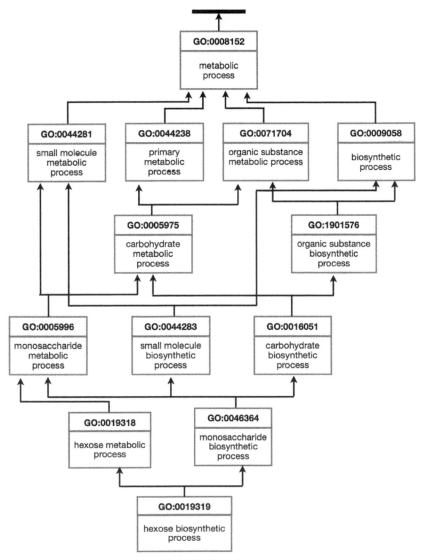

Figure 1 GO DAG structure for the GO:0019319. Each box (node) represents a GO term and the arrows are relationships between GO terms. Each arrow is drawn from a child GO term to its parent(s) GO term(s).

This structure is important because when a gene is associated with a specific term, a relationship between such gene and the term's parent will be automatically inferred. When a new GO is added the consistency between not only its direct parent but all its indirect parents is verified (Rhee et al., 2008). This also results in a very important consequence, a gene can belong to multiple GO categories. A gene annotated with the GO:0019319 will be annotated with each one of the GOs shown at Fig. 1.

Keeping up to date the GO database is one of the tasks carried out by the GO Consortium. Their work has been described in several research articles (Balakrishnan et al., 2013; Blake, 2013; Consortium, 2012; Du Plessis et al., 2011; Rhee et al., 2008). In the curation process, the source of the information is always highly valuable. The GO evidence code will indicate how the annotation to a particular term is supported. A GO annotation will always include an evidence code. As technology advances more experimental codes are added to the catalog to account for new technologies; for example, a 'high throughput' experimental evidence code has been recently added to the catalog per each experimental evidence code, now the catalog includes the evidence code "Inferred from High Throughput Expression Pattern" in addition to the classic "Inferred from Expression Pattern". The following is a list of all broad classifications for the evidence codes:

- **Experimental evidence.**   It indicates that the results from an experiment directly support the annotation.
- **Phylogenetic evidence.**   These annotations are derived from an explicit model of gain and loss of gene function at specific branches in a phylogenetic tree.
- **Computational evidence.**   It indicates that the evidence was obtained from an in-silico experiment such as sequence or structural similarity, sequence orthology, or inference from the genomic context.
- **Author statements.**   These annotations are made on the basis of a statement made by the author of the original research paper.
- **Curatorial statements.**   It indicates that the annotation was made by a curator but it does not fit into one of the other evidence code classifications.
- **Electronic annotations.**   These correspond to automatically generated annotations. These annotations are the only ones that are not manually reviewed and they can not be traced to an experimental source. The evidence code for these annotations is "Inferred from Electronic Annotation" (IEA).

The process of manual curation is of utmost importance. During this process a curator reads the full texts of original literature and captures detailed data on the database such as sequence and function. This detailed information can be used by automated pipelines to infer function based on sequence similar or orthology. These automated functional inferences provide functional characterization for poorly studied species or even for poorly studied genes of highly studied species (Huntley et al., 2014). However, it is important to be aware that most GO annotations belong to the category of automatically generated annotations and that this phenomenon does not affect all species equally. In a 2008 review there reported more than 15 millions annotation with the IEA evidence code compared to roughly 700,000 from any other evidence code. They also compared how this phenomenon is reflected across several species; in the case of *Sacharomyces pombe* 100% of its genes have been annotated and 90.9% of its genes have an experimental annotation; in the other extreme only 39.2% of the cow genes have been annotated and only 0.4% of its genes are associated with an experimental annotation (Rhee et al., 2008). Although we expect the specific numbers to have changed over time, we expect the same tendency to remain.

The GO annotations are updated to remain in line with current knowledge as new discoveries are made and more functional relationships are assigned. So, GOs are always evolving as our knowledge on biological function expands. Alteration in GO annotations could involve small changes such as update a definition or add a child term or it may involve a comprehensive reorganization of a specific part of the ontology if there is a global change in some area of the underlying biology. Also, the relationships between the terms can be updated to reflect novel knowledge. Finally, some terms can become obsolete and must be removed from the ontology. Several mechanisms to verify the correctness of the ontology have been developed. For example, most terms are taxon neutral but some terms have taxon restrictions as they can be annotated only to specific taxa; also, there is an annotation blacklist specifying protein: GO term combinations that should not exist. These restrictions are verified when new terms or relationships are incorporated into the ontology (Huntley et al., 2014).

The AmiGO browser is a resource created by the GO software group. In this browser any user can explore the annotations, look for all genes annotated with a specific term, look for all the annotations of a specific gene or use the Term Enrichment Service to do a functional enrichment analysis. The GO project is a community project as GO users can report problems in the annotation or they can request specific novel features to be implemented in the AmiGO browser.

2 ENRICHMENT ANALYSIS STRATEGIES AND STATISTICS

The final result from a high throughput expression experiment usually is a list of genes and expression values. For each gene a differential expression value can be obtained that summarizes how much its expression changes across paired conditions. The differential expression is commonly used to order the genes by relevance but can be obtained only if the experiment included samples from at least two biological conditions.

A functional enrichment analysis is usually applied to extract relevant biological information either from the complete list of genes and expression values or from the filtered list of relevant genes. The enrichment analysis strategies have been classified into four categories according to several authors. A summary of the classification proposed by two authors is presented in Table 2 (Curtis et al., 2005; Huang et al., 2009a).

Table 2 General description for each of the functional enrichment strategies proposed by different authors

Huang et al., 2009a	Curtis et al., 2005	Description	Limitations
Singular Enrichment Analysis (SEA)	Enrichment	It takes the list of relevant genes and test for the enrichment of each annotation term. All enriched annotation terms are reported	It does not use the complete information of the experiment. Relationships between annotation terms are not considered.
Modular Enrichment Analysis (MEA)		It uses the same enrichment strategy than in SEA but incorporates additional algorithms to consider term-to-term relationships	It does not use the complete information of the experiment.
Gene Set Enrichment Analysis (GSEA)	Gene Set Enrichment Analysis (GSEA)	The list of all genes from an experiment is sorted according to a quantitative metric. GSEA tests if the members of a gene set tend to occur toward the top (or bottom) of the list of genes	It needs a quantitative measure to summarize the biological importance of each gene.
	Scoring Enrichment	A list of relevant genes is compared with a list of genes from each annotation term. The enrichment is determined by a score, the score is proportional to the number of shared terms (hits).	The results depend on the hit-counting method

2.1   Singular Enrichment Analysis

The fundamental idea of this type of analysis is to find the statistically enriched pathways from a list of either relevant or interesting genes. For each pathway, a comparison between the number of expected genes in the list of relevant genes drawn by chance and the number of observed genes is used to grant the statistical significance of the enrichment (Khatri and Drăghici, 2005). An example illustrating the process is show in Fig. 2. The expected number of genes will depend on the background model. Besides, different statistical models can be used to calculate the significance of the enrichment. These two aspects will be discussed in detail in the following sections.

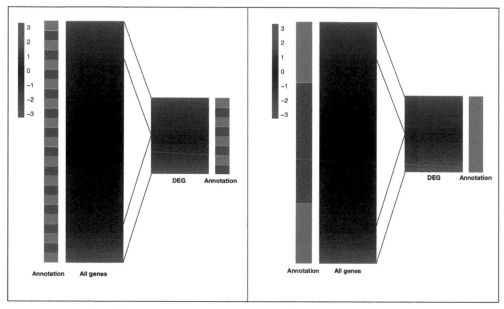

Figure 2   Singular Enrichment Analysis. In both panels, the color scale (red to green) represents the differential expression values; bright red indicates sub expression while bright green indicates over expression. The colors at the annotation bar represent the annotation label for a specific annotation category; e.g., blue = apoptosis genes, orange = no apoptosis genes. The two bars at the left of each panel show the annotation label and differential expression value for each gene measured in the experiment. The two bars at the right of each panel show the differential expression value and annotation label only for the differentially expressed genes (DEGs). The left panel corresponds to an experiment in which there is no enrichment for apoptosis genes over the DEGs. The right panel corresponds to an experiment in which there is a clear enrichment for apoptosis genes over the DEGs.

2.1.1   Selection of background model

The background model should reflect which genes could have been chosen to be in the list of relevant genes, e.g., differentially expressed genes. Imagine you are studying an organism that has 1000 genes annotated as apoptosis genes along with a plethora of genes related with other biological processes. You perform a targeted study in which you measure the expression of only 500 of those 1000 genes along with many other genes. At the end of the experiment, it turns out that those 500 apoptosis genes are differentially expressed. The answer to the question: how many of the total apoptosis genes are differentially expressed in your experiment? depends on the definition of the background model. If you consider 1000 as the total number of apoptosis genes, the answer would be 50%; however, this would be a misleading answer because not all the genes were interrogated in the experiment and, as a consequence, not all the gens could have been chosen as differentially expressed. An answer closer to the truth would be 500 differentially expressed genes out of 500 analyzed genes. Even now, it would be a closer answer, not an exact answer, because the knowledge about biological function is not complete and there could be some annotation bias in the analysis.

As illustrated by the previous example, the background model is a critical factor that could directly bias the conclusions drawn from any functional enrichment analysis. A very good rule of thumb is to set up the background model to the pool of genes that could be selected for the set of relevant genes, i.e., all genes in a genome in the case of a high throughput expression experiment, all genes included in a commercial microarray or the subset of genes chosen by a specific user in a targeted experiment. Although this is a very good approximation, it is not perfect as some technical bias could occlude the detection of specific sequences or genes. The selection of the adequate background model is important as larger backgrounds tend to give more significant *p*-values compared with smaller backgrounds. However, it has been shown that if the same dataset is analyzed with different backgrounds models the ranking of the enriched categories remains practically constant. So, the functional conclusions will remain stable even if different backgrounds were chosen although in some cases the enriched annotation terms would not reach statistical significance (Huang et al., 2009a).

2.1.2 Statistical models

In this section we will explain some statistical models commonly used for SEA, including the binomial test, fisher's exact test and chi-squared test.. A binomial distribution counts the number of successes, *k*, in *n* independent Bernoulli trials with a fixed probability of success *p*. A Bernoulli trial is an event in which only two outcomes are possible, a success with probability *p* and a failure with probability $1 - p$. So, if we take *n* as the size of the relevant gene list, and we define *p* as the probability of a gene to belong to the *Y* annotation term then we could calculate the probability of having *k* or more genes annotated as *Y* only by chance in our gene list. The probability function of the binomial distribution is defined by:

$$P(X = k) = \binom{n}{k} p^k (1 - p)^{n-k}, 0 \le p \le 1$$

where $k = 0, 1, 2, ..., n$, $\binom{n}{k} = \dfrac{n!}{k!(n-k)!}$ is the set of all *k*-combinations of a set with *n* elements, *p* is the success probability, *k* is the number of successes and *n* is the number of Bernoulli trials.

A practical example: let's assume that the relevant genes list contains differentially expressed genes and we are interested in calculating if there is an enrichment of a specific annotation term, e.g., cell cycle. First, we should define what is the probability of a gene being annotated as a cell cycle gene; this probability is going to depend on how many genes are annotated as cell cycle genes and how many total genes there are. The total number of genes is going to depend on the background model. After that, we only need to know how many genes of our list are annotated as cell cycle genes. Once we have these two values, we can use the binomial distribution to calculate the probability of obtaining that specific proportion (or a more extreme one) of genes annotated as cell cycle genes among the differentially expressed genes just by chance. This probability is interpreted as the statistical significance (*p*-value) of the enrichment. A very low probability tell us that obtaining such configuration by chance would be very rare. Terms with probability below the statistical significance threshold (usually 0.05 or 0.01) are deemed as enriched. Hopefully, these terms provide biological insights into the phenomena under study.

The binomial approximation assumes that the probability *p* stays fixed. This is true when the number of elements in the background model is large (large reference, such as genome-wide expression experiments) because picking a specific gene does not change dramatically the proportions of the remaining genes in each category. However, for small references (such as targeted microarrays) the proportion of remaining genes in each functional class could change dramatically between the first gene being chosen and the last one. In these cases, the hypergeometric distribution or the chi-squared distribution are better suited statistical models (Qureshi and Sacan, 2013; Rivals et al., 2007).

Table 3   General description of a 2×2 contingency table considered by the hypergeometric distribution

	Number of objects drawn	Number of objects not drawn	Total
with feature	k	$K - k$	K
with no feature	$n - k$	$N + k - n - K$	$N - K$
total	n	$N - n$	N

The hypergeometric distribution describes the probability of drawing k successes, defined as drawing an object with a special feature, in n draws from a finite population of size N that contains exactly K objects with that feature. So, it is clear how the hypergeometric distribution describes exactly the phenomena we are studying, i.e., the exact probability of having k genes annotated as Y in a list of size n if the special feature is seen as the specific annotation term (Y), the n draws are considered as the n genes selected in the relevant list and the N and K parameters are defined from the background model. All this information can be represented in a 2×2 contingency table as shown in Table 3. The most important difference between the binomial distribution and the hypergeometric distribution is that the draws are considered with replacement and without replacement, respectively. So, the hypergeometric distribution approximates to the binomial distribution at a high number of samples (Curtis et al., 2005).

The probability mass function of the hypergeometric distribution is defined by:

$$P(X = k) = \frac{\binom{K}{k}\binom{N - K}{n - k}}{\binom{N}{n}}$$

This probability is an exact metric that describes the probability of having this exact arrangement of the data: i.e., the exact number of annotated genes in a list of the exact size as our relevant list. There are $\binom{N}{n}$ possible samples. Of these $\binom{K}{k}$ is the number of ways of choosing k elements in a sample of size K and $\binom{N-K}{n-k}$ is the number of choosing $n - k$ elements in a sample of size $N - K$. And because these two samplings are independent there are $\binom{K}{k}\binom{N-K}{n-k}$ total combinations.

The Fisher's exact test is based on the hypergeometric distribution. And it is used to calculate the statistical significance of the association between two variables. As part of the Fisher's exact test, the above calculation is done for all combinations more extreme than the one observed in the data (Hoffman, 2015). Once again, a low probability implies that it would be very rare to have the observed rearrangement only by chance. So, low probability terms are flagged as enriched.

Finally, the chi-squared test also relies on a 2×2 contingency table to calculate the difference between the observed and expected values for each annotation term (Khatri et al., 2004). The observed values for each pathway are stored in a such table. Then, the expected values based on the observed marginal probabilities are calculated. After this, the test statistic is computed as defined by the following formula:

$$\chi^2 = \sum_{i=1}^{r} \sum_{j=1}^{c} \frac{(O_{i,j} - E_{i,j})^2}{E_{i,j}}$$

where r and c equals the number of rows and columns in the contingency table, respectively, and $O_{i,j}$ and $E_{i,j}$ is the observed value and expected value at cell i, j, respectively. The χ^2

statistic is then located in the chi-squared distribution table with one degree of freedom and it is translated into a significance value or p-value. The degrees of freedom are calculated by the formula $(r - 1) * (c - 1)$. In a 2×2 contingency table, this always equals 1. The resulting *p*-value describes the probability of observe deviations as large as the ones being observed in the current experiment by chance. A cartoon example of the whole procedure is shown in Fig. 3.

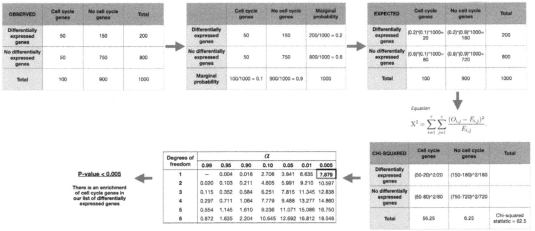

Figure 3 Chi-squared statistical test. This is a step-by-step cartoon example about how the chi-squared test is performed. Let's assume we have an experiment in which 200 genes were differentially expressed, 50 of those genes are cell cycle genes. In our background model there are 1000 total genes, 100 of those genes are cell cycle genes. Using all this information we can fill the 'observed' table. Now, we can calculate the marginal probabilities that tell us that 20% of the total genes were differentially expressed and that 10% of the total genes are cell cycle genes. Using these marginal probabilities we can compute the number of 'expected' hits for each cell in our 2×2 'expected' contingency table. Now, we are ready to compute the chi-squared statistic. We can now look for the chi-squared value in a chi-squared distribution table with one degree of freedom. We see that our chi-squared value is much higher than 7.8, what corresponds to $\alpha < 0.005$. α is the significance value and can be interpreted as the probability of having deviations as large as the ones observed in the data by chance.

The chi-squared statistic is simple to calculate and the interpretation is very straightforward. However, it is an approximate test and it is restricted to situations in which all four values in the 2×2 contingency table are higher than five (e.g., differentially expressed genes that are cell-cycle genes). The Fisher's exact test is an alternative when there is at least one very small observed value (Beißbarth and Speed, 2004).

Some enrichment tools have incorporated specific analysis to highlight the statistical significance of enriched functional categories. AgriGO computes *p*-values for 99 lists of randomly selected genes of the same size as the list of relevant genes. In its website the *p*-value's distribution for each enriched term is shown, in this plot the *p*-values for the observed list and the 99 random lists are displayed allowing a visual inspection of the significance of the enrichment and decreasing the false positive rate (Tian et al., 2017).

Other tools have incorporated *ad hoc* statistics. Enrichr, an interactive and collaborative enrichment tool, computes the statistical significance of the enrichment by the Fisher's exact test and by an internally developed test statistic. This novel statistic measures the deviation of the Fisher's exact test from the expected rank. To calculate this deviation, a large number of random lists are analyzed to compute a mean rank, variance and standard deviation for each term in each gene-set library. Then a z-score for the deviation from this expected rank is calculated for each functional category. These z-scores are defined as the new scores to define the statistical significance of each term. The authors claim that this "corrected" score outperforms the classical Fisher's exact test. As part of Enrichr, the authors created 35 gene-set libraries; some of them are borrowed from resources such as ChEA, TRANSFAC, ENCODE, KEGG, OMIM, GeneSigDB, Mouse and Human Gene Atlases, Cancer Cell Line Encyclopedia and some of them are newly created and only available in Enrichr (Chen et al., 2013).

A clear limitation of Singular Enrichment Analysis is that it only takes into account the preselected list of relevant genes and it does not consider the expression values for all the other genes tested during the experiment. Besides, the functional relationships between related terms can be difficult to highlight since the results usually are presented as a linear tabular format. Also, this kind of analysis assumes that a good gene list will present the following attributes (Huang et al., 2009b):

- Many important biologically relevant genes (for the specific phenomenon under study) were tested.
- Reasonable number of tested genes are not on the list of relevant genes (expression is not extremely low or high for most genes).
- A significant portion of relevant genes (differentially expressed) are involved in certain interesting biological process. This point is very important as it is known that in some cases the over-expression or sub-expression of very few genes could have a profound biological impact.
- A relevant list should have consistently more enriched biology than a random list of the same size.
- A relevant list should be reproducible between different experiments studying the same biological phenomena.

As explained throughout the section, in SEA analysis the enrichment for each functional category is independently tested. So, an important downstream step in the analysis is to correct by multiple-testing, why is it necessary and how it is done will be explained in the section "Statistical methods to adjust the p-values by multiple testing".

2.2   Modular Enrichment Analysis (MEA)

As explained earlier, the classic SEA methods assume independence between each annotation term and they test all of them for enrichment. However, annotation terms are not completely independent. MEA inherits the basic enrichment statistics used in SEA but considers relationships between terms. An implementation of this kind of analysis is seen in DAVID (Huang et al., 2009b). DAVID groups functionally related annotations in classes. This relatedness is obtained trough the mining of complex biological co-occurrences found in heterogenous annotation terms. Another tool, EnrichNet, computes a network similarity score (Xd-score). The Xd scores measure network interconnectivity between the list of relevant genes and the pathways mapped to the corresponding molecular interaction network (Glaab et al., 2012).

2.3   Gene Set Enrichment Analysis (GSEA)

Also, as explained in Section 2.1, SEA focuses on the analysis of a preselected gene list, which could result in several limitations: (i) after correcting for multiple testing no pathway may meet the threshold to reach statistical significance, (ii) in the other hand, one could end up with a long list of statistically enriched pathways with no outstanding biological unifying theme, (iii) some important biological behaviors can be missed, e.g., an uniformly but modest increase in expression in all the genes of a specific pathway and (iv) one could face lack of reproducibility between the relevant list genes obtained by studying the same biological phenomenon.

GSEA overcome these limitations. This method focuses on gene sets (S) defined as groups of genes that share biological properties, such as function, chromosomal location or regulation.

It uses the whole set of genes measured by any given experiment (L). According to GSEA's creators "The goal of GSEA is to determine whether members of a gene set S tend to occur toward the top (or bottom) of the list L, in which case the gene set is correlated with the phenotypic class distinction" (Subramanian et al., 2005). An example illustrating this type of analysis is shown in Fig. 4.

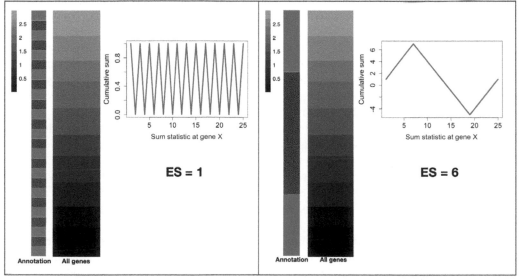

Figure 4 Gene Set Enrichment Analysis. In both panels, the color scale (black to bright purple) represents the absolute values for differential expression (any other quantitative metric could be used); black indicates no change in expression and bright purple indicates a large change in expression in either direction. The colors at the annotation bar represent the annotation label for a specific gene set; blue = that gene belongs to the gene set, orange = that gene does not belong to the gene set. The two bars at the left of each panel show the annotation label and absolute differential expression value for each gene measured in the experiment. The plot at the right of each panel show the sum statistic across all genes in the experiment. The ES (the maximum value of the cumulative sum statistic) is shown in each case. The left panel corresponds to an experiment in which there is no functional relationship between that gene set and the experiment. The right panel corresponds to an experiment in which there is functional relationship between that gene set and the experiment.

Similar to SEA, GSEA is divided into three processes: the calculation of an enrichment score (ES), the estimation of the significance level of the ES and the adjustment for multiple hypothesis testing.

An important preprocessing step consists in ranking the whole list of genes based on a quantitative criterion. Ideally, this criterion should be related with the biological importance of each gene for the biological phenomenon under study. Expression or differential expression values are usually treated as such quantitive measure however concerns have been raised about the correctness of this assumption. Once the list of genes has been ranked one can proceed to calculate the ES. The ES is calculated with the following algorithm per each gene set S:

1. Initialize the sum statistic to zero
2. Start by the top of the ranked list L
3. If the gene at that position of the list belongs to the gene set increase in x your sum statistic. If the gene at that position of the list does not belong to the gene seat decrease in y your sum statistic.
4. Move one position downwards in the ranked list L
5. Repeat 3 and 4 until you reach the end of the ranked list L
6. Repeat 3

The ES is the maximum deviation from zero encountered in the analysis. The *leading-edge* subset are those genes in the gene set S that appear in the gene list L at, or before, the ES is reached. The *leading-edge subset* has been interpreted as the core of genes from the gene set S that produces the enrichment signal.

A permutation procedure is used to estimate the significance level of the ES. The phenotype labels are permuted and the ES for each gene set is recomputed from the shuffled data. The ES obtained from the permuted data generates a null distribution for the ES. The *p*-value is then calculated by comparing the experimental ES to this null distribution. The phenotype-based permutation permits the conservation of the complex correlation structure of the expression data. However, if there are very few samples, the permutation of phenotype labels is not enough to generate a robust null distribution. In such cases, the genes can be permuted, e.g., the genes are randomly assigned to all gene sets maintaining only the gene sets' size. This procedure should never be the first choice since the structure of the expression data is lost.

At the end, the ES is normalized to account for the size of each gene set. Moreover, adjustment for multiple testing is further applied since multiple gene sets are being independently tested.

The creators of GSEA defined their own statistic to correct by multiple testing. They defined a FDR statistic as the ratio of two distributions: (1) the actual ES versus the ESs for all gene sets against all permutations of the dataset and (2) the actual ES versus the ESs of all gene sets against the actual dataset.

An indispensable piece of information required by GSEA are the gene sets of functionally related genes. Along with the method, the creators of GSEA made freely available more than 1000 gene sets (Subramanian et al., 2005; Subramanian et al., 2007; Mootha et al., 2003; Liberzon et al., 2011). This datasets along with the desktop tool can be downloaded from the BROAD Institute website. The available datasets are hosted in MSigDB. At this website the user can browse any gene set, examine the annotations associated with any gene set, compute the overlaps between gene sets, look at expression profiles of a gene set or download all existing gene sets. The current available gene sets are:

- Hallmark gene sets. This represents well-defined biological states or process. The genes of each of these gene sets form coherently expressed signatures.
- Positional gene sets. For each human chromosome and cytogenetic band.
- Curated gene sets. These have been derived from pathway databases, publications in PubMed and knowledge of domain experts.
- Regulatory target gene sets. These are based on target predictions for microRNAs and predicted transcription factor binding sites.
- Computational gene sets. These have been derived from mining large collections of cancer-oriented microarray data.
- GO gene sets. Genes annotated in the same GO term.
- Oncogenic gene sets. From microarray gene expression data from cancer gene perturbations.
- Immunologic gene sets. From microarray gene expression data from immunologic studies.

As can be seen, incredible curation efforts have been directed towards the creation of a comprehensive catalog of gene sets covering a broad spectrum of biological aspects beyond function. Nevertheless, the GSEA method can be applied to any custom gene set created to cover any special need.

Although GSEA is a powerful method it requires a quantitative value to summarize the biological importance for each gene on the gene list. This summary value could be challenging to define if the study involves multiple variants simultaneously, e.g., disease/normal, different periods in time, different tissues, age, sex, different treatments. In such cases, additional statistical methods should be implemented to deal with the variance and batch effects.

2.4 Scoring Enrichment

This enrichment strategy has not been widely applied. The score of the enrichment is calculated by counting the number of genes that are shared between a relevant list of genes and a specific pathway. The number of shared genes is proportional to the score and a higher score means higher enrichment. To calculate the statistical significance of the enrichment, random lists are created and the scores are calculated to create a null distribution. To our knowledge, only two works have applied this strategy. Doniger, et. al. applied the described principle to calculate a z-score associated with their hit count (Doniger et al., 2003). Choi, et. al. described a statistical metric that takes into account the hierarchical structure of GO terms; they computed an odds ratio between the odds of dysregulation of the GO term to the odds of dysregulation of the broad category to which the GO term belongs (Choi et al., 2004).

3 STATISTICAL METHODS TO ADJUST THE P-VALUES BY MULTIPLE TESTING

During functional profiling analysis a researcher could focus on two general strategies. A hypothesis-generating strategy; i.e., the researcher has no previous hypothesis about which pathway or gene set is associated with the biological condition being studied. A hypothesis-driven analysis; i.e., the researcher is interested in wether there exist an association with a specific process. In the hypothesis-driven scenario no multiple testing correction is needed because only one test is being performed.

However all the analysis described in this chapter are hypothesis-generating strategies. Statistical analysis are done to pinpoint a significant enrichment between a relevant gene list and each possible functional category or to find statistical associations between a complete gene list and each possible gene set. In both cases, a statistical value is calculated to reflect the significance of the finding. This statistic is usually associated with the probability of finding a configuration at least as extreme as the one seen in the data by chance. Usually a nominal significance value of 0.05 is chosen. This significance value means that 5% of the times the researcher will get a configuration as rare as the observed just by chance; indicating that 5% of the times the researcher will categorize either a pathway or a gene set as significant when it is not. So, by using a nominal significance value of 0.05 the researcher will be accepting a 5% rate of false positive assignments. A lower nominal significance value can be used if the precision of the assignment needs to be increased, e.g., a nominal significance value of 0.01 will allow a 1% rate of false positive assignment.

However, if any experiment is repeated a big enough number of times, rare configurations will do happen. For example, let's assume that 100 statistical tests are performed and that for each test a p-value of 0.01 is calculated. For each independent test this implies that there is a probability of 0.01 of having a configuration as rare as the one observed, i.e., it is probable that 1 out of 100 experiments will have a configuration as rare as the one observed. So, in each independent test our conclusion would be that the enrichment is statistically significant and the observed configuration is not produced only by chance. However, if we take into account that we performed 100 statistical tests, the p-value of 0.01 tell us that it is very probable to have at least one test in which the observed configuration was indeed produced by chance. Because of this, we would have included at least one false positive in the 100 hundred tests that were defined as statistical significant based on their non-adjusted p-value. In conclusion, the plain statistical significance values are misleading because, if no other piece of information is taken into account, they may indicate statistical significance of an enrichment even though any particular enrichment value can appear just by chance if an experiment is repeated enough times.

There are several strategies to reduce the impact of multiple testing. One strategy is to remove terms with no genes present in the list being analyzed. Another strategy is to remove rare terms that may not be able to reach statistical significance. A last strategy is to initially examine only very broad annotations; this could be achieved by using the GO Slim terms, which are a set of high-level annotation released by the GO consortium.

There are multiple ways of adjusting the p-values by multiple testing. The most widely used methods are described in the following subsections. All of these methods are designed to control the type I error, which happens when the null-hypothesis is incorrectly rejected. In our specific topic, this implies that the flag enrichment has been turned on even when the observed configuration was produced only by chance. At the end of this section, a discussion about the different methods is provided.

3.1 Bonferroni Correction

This method was proposed by Holm in 1979. The Bonferroni correction method is widely used because of their simplicity (Holm, 1979). It dictates that to account for the multiple-testing effect the unadjusted p-value of each test must be divided between the number of total tests. So, the adjusted p-value will be given by:

$$p_k^{Bonferroni} = p_k N$$

where p_k is the unadjusted p-value of test k, N is the number of total tests and $p_k^{Bonferroni}$ is the adjusted p-value by the Bonferroni correction method (Vickerstaff et al., 2019).

3.2 Holm Method

This method is considered as a step-down method. The unadjusted p-values are ordered from smallest $p(1)$ to largest $p(M)$ and each unadjusted p-value is adjusted by:

$$p_k^{Holm} = (M - k + 1) p_k$$

where $k = 1, \ldots, M$ is the rank of the corresponding p-value, p_k is the unadjusted p-value of test k, and p_k^{Holm} is the adjusted p-value by the Holm correction method.

To determine the statistically significant terms, each adjusted p-value is compared with the nominal significance value starting with the smallest one (the most significant value). The procedure is repeated until a p-value greater than the nominal significance value is reached in the jth test. This will result in tests from 1 to j deemed as significant and tests from $j + 1$ to M deemed as not significant (Holm, 1979).

3.3 Hochberg Method

This method is similar to the Holm method, but it works in the opposite direction. So, it is considered as a step-up method. The unadjusted p-values are ranked from largest $p(1)$ to smallest $p(M)$ and each p-value is adjusted by:

$$p_k^{Hochberg} = (M - k + 1) p_k$$

where $k = 1, \ldots, M$ is the rank of the corresponding p-value, p_k is the unadjusted p-value of test k, and $p_k^{Hochberg}$ is the adjusted p-value by the Hochberg correction method.

To determine the statistically significant terms, each adjusted p-value is compared with the nominal significance value starting with the largest one (the least significant value). The procedure is repeated until a p-value lower than the nominal significance value is reached in the jth test. This will result in tests from 1 to j deemed as not significant and tests from $j + 1$ to M deemed as significant (Hochberg, 1988).

3.4 Hommel Method

The unadjusted p-values are ranked from largest $p(M)$ to smallest $p(1)$. M is the largest rank that is equal to the number of tests. Then l is calculated. l is defined as the largest integer for which:

$$p(M - l + j) > \frac{j_\alpha}{l}$$

for all $j = 1, \ldots, l$. j indicates the jth test and j_α corresponds to the p-value of the jth test. If no j exists then all tests are considered as statistically significant; otherwise all outcomes with

$$p_i \leq \frac{\alpha}{j}$$

Can be considered statistically significant, where α is the nominal significance value $j = 1, \ldots, M$; $i = 1, \ldots, M$ (Hommel, 1988).

3.5 Benjamini & Hochberg Method (BH)

This method was developd to control the percentage of false discoveries (FDR) in the data.

Similar to the Holm method, the unadjusted p-values are ranked from smallest $p(1)$ to largest $p(M)$. So, the smallest value has rank 1, the second smallest rank 2 and so on, until that the largest p-value has rank M. The adjusted p-values will be defined by:

$$p_k^{BH} = \frac{k}{M} Q$$

where $k = 1, \ldots, M$ is the rank of the corresponding p-value, M is largest rank that is equal to the number of tests and Q is the false discovery rate. Q is chosen by the user, and it is usually set to 0.05. The tests for which the adjusted p-values are still smaller than the nominal significance value are considered as statistically significant.

There is another formulation to explain how the Benjamini & Hochberg method works. This formulation will be useful to understand the Benjamini & Yekutieli method.

Set a FDR threshold, Q. For a given Q, find the largest k such that:

$$p_k \leq = \frac{k}{M} Q$$

This will result in tests from 1 to k considered as significant and tests from $k + 1$ to M considered as not significant.

3.6 Benjamini & Yekutieli Method (BY)

The Benjamini & Yekutieli method takes into account that the tests are not always completely independent (Yekutieli and Benjamini, 1999). It is a derivation from the Benjamini & Hochberg method. It is based on finding the largest k such that:

$$p_k \leq = \frac{k}{M * c(M)} Q$$

where M are the number of tests, $c(M)$ will account for test dependence. $c(M) = 1$ if the tests are independent or positively correlated, notice that in this case the formulation is reduced to the BH test.

Under arbitrary dependence:

$$c(M) = \sum_{i=1}^{M} \frac{1}{i}$$

where $i = 1, \ldots, k$

3.7 Discussion about the different Correction Methods

The Bonferroni method has been widely applied. However when high throughput experiments are performed in which almost the whole genome is interrogated this method becomes very restrictive as a very large number of annotations or gene sets are tested, for example GO has more than 7 million annotations terms. Besides, Bonferroni correction assumes independence between the methods. This assumption is clearly violated by GO categories because one gene can belong to more than one GO category.

The number of tests can be reduced by only testing the functional categories with at least one gene in the selected gene list. If the number of tests is reduced Bonferroni correction is a good option. However, if a big number of unrelated categories are tested, Holm's correction method is a good choice (Khatri and Drăghici, 2005).

If there are several not independent functional categories, the FDR-based methods are the best choice. Also, the FDR methods are recommended if there is a large number of tests since they are less conservative although there is an associated loss of power (Rhee et al., 2008).

4 SUMMARY OF STRATEGIES IMPLEMENTED BY DIFFERENT TOOLS

There exist a large number of tools devoted to do functional enrichment. A review of the open-source tools that are currently maintained is presented in Tables 4 and 5. As part of this research, we realized that a lot of tools are not currently maintained or are very limited in functionality (these tools are not included in Table 4).

Table 4 General characteristics of functional enrichment tools

Tool	Class	Statistical Model	Multiple Test Correction	Background Model/Gene Sets
FunSpec	SEA	Hypergeometric	Bonferroni	Yeast
FuncAssociate	SEA	Fisher's exact test	Permutations	Ensembl and refseq genes, uniprot, affimetrix microarrays
GeneMerge	SEA	Hypergeometric	FDR	Custom
CLENCH	SEA	Hypergeometric, chi-square, binomial	FDR	*Arabidopsis thaliana* genes
GO:TermFinder	SEA	Hypergeometric	Bonferroni, FDR	Whole genome, custom list. GO supported species
GOStat	SEA	Hypergeometric	No correction is performed	Whole genome, custom list. GO supported species
BiNGO	SEA	Hypergeometric, binomial	Bonferroni, BH	GO supported species
Funrich	SEA	Hypergeometric test	Bonferroni, BH	UniProt supported species, custom list

Table 4. Contd. ...

Table 4 General characteristics of functional enrichment tools (Contd. ...)

Tool	Class	Statistical Model	Multiple Test Correction	Background Model/Gene Sets
WebGestalt	SEA, GSEA and MEA	SEA: Hypergeometric; GSEA: Permutation	SEA: BH, BY, bonferroni, Holm and Hommel; GSEA: top-enriched gene sets	affymetrics, illumina and Agilent microarrays, whole genomes for GO supported species
WEGO	SEA	Chi-squared	No correction is performed	Genome for 9 species
Enrichr	SEA	Fisher's exact test	BH	Permutation from random gene lists
agriGO	SEA, GSEA	SEA: Hypergeometric, chi-square and Fisher's exact test. GSEA: Permutation	BH, BY, bonferroni, Holm, Hommel and Hochberg	SEA: Genome for 45 species (agricultural value); GSEA: GO annotations
g:Profiler	SEA, GSEA	Hypergeometric	Bonferroni; BH	SEA: Ensembl supported species: whole genome, only annotated genes or custom; GSEA: Gene sets from GO, KEGG, Reactome, miRTar- Base, TRANSFAC, Human Protein Atlas, CORUM, Human Phenotype Ontology
GOEAST	SEA	Hypergeometric, Fisher's exact test, chi-squared	BH, BY, bonferroni, Hommel and Hochberg	Genome for more than 70 species
DAVID	SEA MEA	Modified Fisher's Exact	BH	Only human. Whole genome or custom list
T-profiler	GSEA	T-test	No correction is performed	Two organisms, three gene sets for each organism
GeneTrail	GSEA	Hypergeometric, Kolmogorov-Smirnov	BH, BY, bonferroni, Holm, Hommel and Hochberg	Gene sets from GO KEGG, Reactome, SMPDB, miRDB, miR-TarBase, GWAS, PHEWAS
topGO	MEA	Fisher's exact test, Kolmogorov-Smirnov, t-test	BH, BY, bonferroni, Holm, Hommel and Hochberg	GO supported species, microarrays annotated at Bioconductor
GeneCodis	MEA	Hypergeometric, chi-squared	BH	15 organisms
Enrichnet	MEA	Fisher's exact test, Pearson correlation	Not specified	Only human. Pathways obtained from KEGG, BioCarta, Reactome, WikiPathways, GO, NCI Pathway DB
GSEA	GSEA	Permutation	Modified FDR	More than 1000 human gene sets
Gorilla	SEA and GSEA	SEA: Hypergeometric; GSEA: mHG statistic	No correction is performed	SEA: custom. GSEA: GO annotation for 9 organisms

Table 5 Website for each functional enrichment tools

Tool	Webpage
FunSpec	http://funspec.med.utoronto.ca/
FuncAssociate	http://llama.mshri.on.ca/funcassociate/
GeneMerge	http://www.genemerge.net/ (standalone)
GO::TermFinder	https://metacpan.org/pod/GO::TermFinder (CPAN package)
GOStat	Bioconductor package
BiNGO	https://www.psb.ugent.be/cbd/papers/BiNGO/Home.html (Cytoscape plugin)
Funrich	http://www.funrich.org/ (standalone)
WebGestalt	http://www.webgestalt.org/
WEGO	http://wego.genomics.org.cn/
Enrichr	http://amp.pharm.mssm.edu/Enrichr/
agriGO	http://bioinfo.cau.edu.cn/agriGO/index.php
g:Profiler	https://biit.cs.ut.ee/gprofiler/gost
GOEAST	http://omicslab.genetics.ac.cn/GOEAST/
DAVID	https://david.ncifcrf.gov/home.jsp
T-profiler	http://www.t-profiler.org/
GeneTrail	http://genetrail.bioinf.uni-sb.de/
topGO	Bioconductor package
GeneCodis	https://genecodis.genyo.es/
Enrichnet	http://www.enrichnet.org/
GSEA	https://www.gsea-msigdb.org/gsea/index.jsp (standalone)
Gorilla	http://cbl-gorilla.cs.technion.ac.il/help.html

5   GENERAL LIMITATIONS

5.1   Comparison between Tools

As observed in Table 4, there is a huge variety of available tools. Although several reviews exist to explain the underlying statistical methods, there is no comprehensive comparison of the enrichment results obtained by the different methodologies. In 2005, Curtis et. al. compared the similarity of the results obtained by using SEA based on z-scores, SEA based on the binomial distribution and GSEA using pathways from GenMAPP (this tool is no supported anymore) and KEGG. Their general conclusion indicated a similar number of significant enriched pathways with very close p-value distributions between the two SEA strategies. On the other hand, they reported some overlap between GSEA and SEA results although there was an increase on down-regulated pathways in GSEA results. Although informative, these results could be out of date since they were obtained from expression values derived from microarray technology; a technology that is being replaced rapidly by high throughput RNA sequencing (Curtis et al., 2005).

More recently, the authors of GOSSIP (a functional enrichment tool that is no supported anymore) reported a comprehensive performance test across several correction techniques. They compared the discovery sensitivity and specificity. They concluded that overly conservative approaches may not importantly improve specificity but they could have a negative impact on sensitivity (Blüthgen et al., 2005).

5.2   ID Mapping

A serious caveat in functional enrichment analysis is the lack of a unified homogeneous resource to ligate all different types of identifiers. Each annotation database is organized in a unique way and each database curation team take care of their internal concordance and quality. As a consequence, some times no direct connection can be established between the genes or proteins identifiers from different databases. Each human gene could have an Entrez Gene ID and Refseq ID (NCBI), HGNC symbol (HUGO Gene Nomenclature Committee), ENSEMBL ID (ENSEMBL). Also a gene could be translated into multiple proteins, and each protein could have a UniProt ID and a PIR-ID. The connections between all these identifiers is not always straightforward.

A variety of tools have been created to address such issue: Onto-Translate, MatchMiner, IDConverter an DAVID ID Converter are just a few examples (Huang et al., 2009a). Nevertheless, improvements in the field are still required.

5.3 Annotation Bias

An enrichment can only be detected if there is a functional annotation available. So, an invisible and unavoidable bias will exist as long as the knowledge about biological function is incomplete. Besides, the discoveries made with enrichment strategies will be biased towards the functions or even towards the pathways that are most studied. For example, most annotated genes are protein-coding genes so the functional enrichments regarding other genetic elements such as smallRNAs or long non coding RNAs will be limited. Also, some genes are present in a lot of functional categories. Indeed, the gene frequency across different functional categories follows a power law; most genes are annotated as part of few functional classes but there are few genes that are annotated as part of a lot of functional classes. This will result in some genes appearing more often on the statistically enriched terms.

A clear blind spot for functional enrichment strategies are unknown functions of known genes, as only the known functions will be related with such genes. On the other hand, there are genes that are involved in more than one biological process and their dysregulation affect those biological process differentially, however they are weighted the same across all pathways by the functional enrichment metrics. Another limitation arises from imprecise or incorrect annotation derived either from manual curation or from automated processes.

Although most enrichment tools are based on GO annotation, there are some efforts to create novel annotations. The authors of the tool Enrichr have created more than 30,000 gene libraries divided into six categories: transcription, pathways, ontologies, diseases/drugs, cell types and miscellaneous. These libraries contain functional related genes and are used by Enrichr to perform SEA (Chen et al., 2013).

Besides, in some cases, specific annotation sources can be used for very particular purposes. For example, the phenotypes observed in loss-of-function mutant mice can be broadly compared with human phenotypes. As part of the Knockout Mouse Phenotyping Program (KOMP2) an important number of mouse genes have been and will be mutated and their phenotypic effects translated into a structured ontology (the Mammalian Phenotype Ontology). This resource could be specifically applied to the functional enrichment analysis in the case of structural variants that could have a loss of function effect in human genes (Webber, 2011).

5.4 Statistical Bias

It is known that the size of the relevant gene list, the size of each gene set or the number of genes annotated in each functional annotation term will impact the calculated p-value in a functional enrichment test. A larger gene list will result in more significant p-values to slightly enriched terms as well as terms with a smaller number of genes (more specific terms). On the other hand, the statistical power will be reduced to detect largely enriched terms and more general terms (with a large number of genes). So, at the end of the day, the annotation terms deemed as significant may be dependent on the size of the relevant gene list. In the case of the Fisher's exact test, the ranking of the significance values is affected not only by the size of the relevant gene list but by the size of each annotation term. Annotation terms with few genes are ranked higher if the relevant gene list have few genes and there is at least one shared term (Chen et al., 2013).

Most of the statistical metrics described in this chapter assume independence between the genes and independence between annotation terms. Also, they assume that the annotation is complete and that the total number of genes in each functional category is known. However, it is clear that none of these assumptions hold in a real biological situation. The change in expression in one gene is almost never independent from the change in expression in other genes. Annotation categories are not independent, indeed, they are largely redundant, and even some very specific annotation terms are a complete subset of broader terms. Besides, biological processes are not independent between each other as they share transporters, regulators or enzymes. Indeed, some genes can have multiple functions and they can be involved in more than one biological process. No statistical method is able to contend with all these complex factors. Therefore, there is no absolute interpretation for p-values and they are usually seen as a scoring system that is used to highlight possible relevant annotation terms.

Another important limitation on the statistical analysis is that a lot of tools only look for enrichment of functional terms but they ignore the statistical depletion of functional categories which could also be relevant in the biological description of the phenomena under study.

6 CONCLUDING REMARKS

Functional enrichment analysis is used as a discovery strategy to highlight relevant biological features such as biological processes, celular locations, regulation, structural properties or molecular functions associated with a specific biological trait. In this chapter, a detailed description of the most common annotations, the mathematical methods and statistical models underlying such analysis were provided. We think that this knowledge would be useful to any researcher facing the problem of choosing the best strategy to do a functional enrichment analysis on his/her own data. It is important to say, that enriched annotation terms or gene sets with statistically significant enrichment scores, will act as indicators, the interpretation of how is this connected to the relevant biological trait will still be the responsibility of the researcher conducting the analysis.

REFERENCES

Balakrishnan, R., M.A. Harris, R. Huntley, K. Van Auken and J.M. Cherry (2013). A guide to best practices for Gene Ontology (GO) manual annotation. Database. bat054. doi: 10.1093/database/bat054.

Beißbarth, T. and T.P. Speed (2004). Gostat: Find statistically overrepresented gene ontologies within a group of genes. Bioinformatics. 20(9): 1464–1465.

Blake, J.A. (2013). Ten quick tips for using the gene ontology. PLoS Comput. Biol. 9(11): e1003343.

Blüthgen, N., K. Brand, B. Cajavec, M. Swat, H. Herzel, D. Beule, et al., (2005). Biological profiling of gene groups utilizing gene ontology. Genome Informatics. 16(1): 106–115.

Carithers, L.J., K. Ardlie, M. Barcus, P.A. Branton, A. Britton, S.A. Buia, et al., (2015). A novel approach to high-quality postmortem tissue procurement: the gtex project. Biopreservation and Biobanking. 13(5): 311–319.

Chen, E.Y., C.M. Tan, Y. Kou, Q. Duan, Z. Wang, G.V. Meirelles, et al., (2013) Enrichr: Interactive and collaborative HTML5 gene list enrichment analysis tool. BMC Bioinformatics. 14 (1): 128.

Choi, J.K., J.Y. Choi, D.G. Kim, D.W. Choi, B.Y. Kim, K.H. Lee, et al., (2004). Integrative analysis of multiple gene expression profiles applied to liver cancer study. FEBS Lett. 565(1-3): 93–100.

Consortium, G.O. (2004). The gene ontology (go) database and informatics resource. Nucleic Acids Research. 32(suppl 1): D258–D261.

Consortium, G.O. (2012). Gene ontology annotations and resources. Nucleic Acids Research. 41(D1): D530–D535.

Consortium, G.O. (2019). The gene ontology resource: 20 years and still going strong. Nucleic Acids Research. 47(D1): D330–D338.

Consortium, U. (2019). Uniprot: A worldwide hub of protein knowledge. Nucleic Acids Research. 47(D1): D506–D515.

Curtis, R.K., M. Orešič and A. Vidal-Puig (2005). Pathways to the analysis of microarray data. TRENDS in Biotechnology. 23(8): 429–435.

Doniger, S.W., N. Salomonis, K.D. Dahlquist, K. Vranizan, S.C. Lawlor, B.R. Conklin (2003). Mappfinder: Using gene ontology and genmapp to create a global gene-expression profile from microarray data. Genome Biology. 4(1): R7.

Du Plessis, L., N. Škunca and C. Dessimoz (2011). The what, where, how and why of gene ontology—A primer for bioinformaticians. Briefings in Bioinformatics. 12(6): 723–735.

El-Gebali, S., J. Mistry, A. Bateman, S.R. Eddy, A. Luciani, S.C. Potter, et al., (2019). The pfam protein families database in 2019. Nucleic Acids Research. 47(D1): D427–D432.

Glaab, E., A. Baudot, N. Krasnogor, R. Schneider and A. Valencia (2012). Enrichnet: Network-based gene set enrichment analysis. Bioinformatics. 28(18): i451–i457.

Guarino, N. and P. Giaretta (1995). Ontologies and knowledge bases. Towards Very Large Knowledge Bases. 1–2.

Hamosh, A., A.F. Scott, J.S. Amberger, C.A. Bocchini and V.A. McKusick (2005). Online mendelian inheritance in man (omim), a knowledgebase of human genes and genetic disorders. Nucleic Acids Research. 33(suppl 1): D514–D517.

Hochberg, Y. (1988). A sharper bonferroni procedure for multiple tests of significance. Biometrika. 75(4): 800–802.

Hoffman, J.I. (2015). Biostatistics for Medical and Biomedical Practitioners. Academic Press.

Holm, S. (1979). A simple sequentially rejective multiple test procedure. Scandinavian Journal of Statistics. 65–70.

Hommel, G. (1988). A stagewise rejective multiple test procedure based on a modified bonferroni test. Biometrika. 75(2): 383–386.

Huang, D.W., B.T. Sherman and R.A. Lempicki (2009a). Bioinformatics enrichment tools: Paths toward the comprehensive functional analysis of large gene lists. Nucleic Acids Research. 37(1): 1–13.

Huang, D.W., B.T. Sherman, R.A. Lempicki (2009b). Systematic and integrative analysis of large gene lists using DAVID bioinformatics resources. Nat. Protoc. 4(1): 44–57.

Huntley, R.P., T. Sawford, M.J. Martin and C. O'Donovan (2014). Understanding how and why the gene ontology and its annotations evolve: The go within uniprot GigaScience. 3(1): 2047–217X.

Jassal, B., L. Matthews, G. Viteri, C. Gong, P. Lorente, A. Fabregat, et al., (2020). The reactome pathway knowledgebase. Nucleic Acids Research. 48(D1): D498–D503.

Kanehisa, M. and S. Goto (2000). Kegg: Kyoto encyclopedia of genes and genomes. Nucleic Acids Research. 28(1): 27–30.

Khatri, P., P. Bhavsar, G. Bawa and S. Draghici (2004). Onto-tools: An ensemble of web-accessible, ontology-based tools for the functional design and interpretation of high-throughput gene expression experiments. Nucleic Acids Research. 32(suppl 2): W449–W456.

Khatri, P. and S. Drăghici (2005). Ontological analysis of gene expression data: Current tools, limitations, and open problems. Bioinformatics. 21(18): 3587–3595.

Liberzon, A., A. Subramanian, R. Pinchback, H. Thorvaldsdóttir, P. Tamayo and J.P. Mesirov (2011). Molecular signatures database (MSIGDB) 3.0. Bioinformatics. 27(12): 1739–1740.

Mitchell, A.L., T.K. Attwood, P.C. Babbitt, M. Blum, P. Bork, A. Bridge, et al., (2019). Interpro in 2019: Improving coverage, classification and access to protein sequence annotations. Nucleic Acids Research. 47(D1): D351–D360.

Mootha, V.K., C.M. Lindgren, K.-F. Eriksson, A. Subramanian, S. Sihag, J. Lehar, et al., (2003). Pgc1-responsive genes involved in oxidative phosphorylation are coordinately downregulated in human diabetes. Nature Genetics. 34(3): 267–273.

Qureshi, R. and A. Sacan (2013). Weighted set enrichment of gene expression data. BMC Systems Biology. 7(S4): S10.

Rhee, S.Y., V. Wood, K. Dolinski and S. Draghici (2008). Use and misuse of the gene ontology annotations. Nature Reviews Genetics. 9(7): 509–515.

Rivals, I., L. Personnaz, L. Taing and M.-C. Potier (2007). Enrichment or depletion of a go category within a class of genes: Which test? Bioinformatics. 23(4): 401–407.

Subramanian, A., P. Tamayo, V.K. Mootha, S. Mukherjee, B.L. Ebert, M.A. Gillette, et al., (2005). Gene set enrichment analysis: A knowledge-based approach for interpreting genome-wide expression profiles. Proceedings of the National Academy of Sciences. 102(43): 15545–15550.

Subramanian, A., H. Kuehn, J. Gould, P. Tamayo and J.P. Mesirov (2007). GSEA-P: A desktop application for gene set enrichment analysis. Bioinformatics. 23(23): 3251–3253.

Szklarczyk, D., A.L. Gable, D. Lyon, A. Junge, S. Wyder, J. Huerta-Cepas, et al. (2019). String v11: Protein–protein association networks with increased coverage, supporting functional discovery in genome-wide experimental datasets. Nucleic Acids Research. 47(D1): D607–D613.

Tian, T., Y. Liu, H. Yan, Q. You, X. Yi, Z. Du, et al., (2017). Agrigo v2. 0: A go analysis toolkit for the agricultural community, 2017 update. Nucleic Acids Research. 45(W1): W122–W129.

Vickerstaff, V., R.Z. Omar and G. Ambler (2019). Methods to adjust for multiple comparisons in the analysis and sample size calculation of randomised controlled trials with multiple primary outcomes. BMC Medical Research Methodology. 19(1): 129.

Webber, C. (2011). Functional enrichment analysis with structural variants: Pitfalls and strategies. Cytogenetic and Genome Research. 135(3-4): 277–285.

Wingender, E., P. Dietze, H. Karas and R. Knüppel (1996). Transfac: A database on transcription factors and their dna binding sites. Nucleic Acids Research. 24(1): 238–241.

Yekutieli, D. and Y. Benjamini (1999). Resampling-based false discovery rate controlling multiple test procedures for correlated test statistics. Journal of Statistical Planning and Inference. 82(1-2): 171–196.

CHAPTER 15

Bioinformatics of Meta-analyses of Genomic Data

Aditya Saxena

Department of Computer Engineering & Applications,
Institute of Engineering & Technology,
GLA University, Mathura 281 406 U.P. India

1 INTRODUCTION

With the advent of DNA microarray, and sequencing technologies, it is now possible to profile genome-scale transcript abundance across conditions of biological interest. These transcriptomic read-outs (both coding, as well as non-coding) have potential to explicate the underlying physiological and pathophysiological processes at the cellular level and to abridge the genome-to-phenome relationships. However, variability in gene expressions across samples belonging to the same class, combined with the technical limitation of these technologies, makes it a daunting task to relate molecular processes with end-phenotypes.

Statistical meta-analysis is a process of integrating multiple related studies with an objective to generalize the results of single study experiments with more statistical power (Ramasamy et al., 2008). These analysis help to identify robust molecular signature and hence provide new biological insight. Various R/Bioconductor-based packages as well as web-based tools are now available to carry out meta-analysis of GWAS, and transcriptomic data. In this chapter, an attempt has been made to present some basic concepts of statistical meta-analysis with reference to gene expression studies, and the software options available for these tasks.

2 PROBLEMS IN SINGLE STUDY GENOMIC EXPERIMENTS

Gene expression technologies suffer with a major design issue—expression of hundreds of thousands of genes have to measure in a small number of samples. In addition, biological and

*Corresponding author: aditya.saxena@gla.ac.in

technical variability coupled with high experimental cost of these studies necessitate the need to develop methods of statistical meta-analysis in bioinformatics. Through meta-analysis, we can increase the statistical power to obtain a more precise estimate of gene expression differentials, and assess the heterogeneity of the overall estimates.

The main induction towards the development of these methods in functional genomics lies in the availability of large public repositories of gene expression data such as Gene Expression Omnibus (GEO) (Clough and Barrett, 2016), and Array Express (Parkinson et al., 2007) etc. Indeed to carry out integrative meta-analysis directly from GEO database, a web-based tool, ImaGEO (Toro-Domínguez et al., 2018) has been developed which require only GEO series number. Meta-analysis of this vast amount of data enables us to extract new and valuable biomedical insights beyond we could get from the original publication using single-study centric approach.

3   STEPS IN A META-ANALYSIS

The procedure of meta-analysis is based on the end objectives of study, however, a typical meta-analysis may broadly constitute following steps:

3.1   Identification of Studies for Meta-analysis

A common method to identify relevant studies for meta-analysis is 'keyword search' in PubMed/ Google, NCBI-GEO or ENA-Array Express databases. These databases also provide options for advance search to specify disease/MeSH (Medical Subject Headings), species, and platform type etc. recently a repository and search engine for bioinformatics datasets—Datasets2Tools (Torre et al., 2018) has been launched to indexes gene expression studies available at GEO and therefore is a very useful resource to select relevant studies. The next step should be to carefully read the associative publications to identify study objectives, inclusion and exclusion criteria, and salient findings. A final decision should then be taken whether the given study may contribute to our objective of meta-analysis or may have counter-intuitive results.

In some cases, study dataset may comprise more than one case groups. In these situations, it is advisable to pair it into sub-sets comprising one control group and one case group, i.e., if a study includes samples from normal glucose tolerant (NGT), insulin resistant (IR), and type 2 diabetics (T2D); pair NGT with IR, and T2D separately and construct two sub-sets.

3.2   Obtaining Gene Expression Matrices

Obtain the feature-level extraction files such as CEL, GRP, etc. from the database and transform them into gene expression data-matrices comprising samples in columns and gene-level normalized expression values into rows. The best way to obtain these matrices is to use R-based bioconductor packages such as *affy, limma, beadarray, lumi,* and then normalize those using *rma, gcrma, mas5, limma,* and *beadarray* packages depending upon the microarray platform. Furthermore, GEO also provides series matrix files in 'coma-separated values' format for direct use.

In case of RNA-seq data, obtaining gene-level count matrix from raw FASTQ file requires command line-based bioinformatics pipelines with high-end computational resources or web-based galaxy framework (Afgan et al., 2018). Recently a Google chrome extension—ARCHS4 (Lachmann et al., 2018) has been launched to provide direct access to gene counts from HiSeq 2000, HiSeq 2500 and NextSeq 500 platforms for human and mouse experiments deposited to GEO and SRA. This development really streamlined the process to use RNA-seq data for meta-analysis. Next, each dataset's probe ids/identifiers must be collapsed into common identifiers such as official gene symbols/Entrez id and each sample must be annotated with a class label.

3.3 Preprocessing of Datasets

The next step is to check and correct for any batch effects (Johnson and Li 2007) among datasets, especially in large studies. Unsupervised visualization such as Principal Component Analysis (PCA) or density plot may help to identify any grouping caused by experimental factors. If it is significant, we can use an R Package SVA (Leek et al., 2012) for removing batch effects and other unwanted variation in high-throughput experiments which provide a function *combat*. It uses parametric or non-parametric empirical bayes frameworks for adjusting data for batch effects; users are returned a corrected expression matrix and now the input data for meta-analysis may be assumed to be cleaned.

3.4 Choosing a Meta-analysis Technique

There are different gene-level meta-analysis approaches depending upon microarray experiment design and the objective of meta-analysis. The best tool is NetworkAnalyst (Xia et al., 2015) that allow meta-analysis over multiple gene expression datasets using their summary-level data (i.e., P-values, fold changes (FCs) or effect sizes, vote counting, and direct merging); it first extracts these values and then identify genes based on their statistical integration. Effect size and P-values-based integration is recommended for general meta-analysis and vote counting, and direct merging is generally used for exploratory purposes. Another R-based program *GeneMeta* (Lusa et al., 2020) implements t-test based procedures for meta-analysis. It estimates the within study variability (σ) and between study variability (τ), and if $\tau = 0$, it uses a fixed effect model (FEM) or otherwise, random effects model (REM). Another R-package metaMA proposes a method to calculate moderated effect sizes or p-values from standard and moderated t-tests. *metaMA* can enhance sensitivity by using shrinkage approaches when the number of samples is small in each individual study.

3.5 Bioinformatics Approaches for Functional Interpretations

The results of meta-analysis generated two types of outputs: a combined normalized gene expression matrix adjusted for batch effects, and a meta-gene signature comprising genes with statistically significant expression differences between classes. The expression matrix might be used for supervised/unsupervised clustering, creation of co-expression networks and/or to find modules of co-expressed genes using weighted gene correlation network analysis (WGCNA) (Langfelder and Horvath, 2008). Meta-signature of genes can be used for gene ontology- or pathway-based enrichment analysis or can be mapped on a global protein-protein interaction network to create condition-specific sub-networks for network-based enrichment analysis such as identification of disease-modules (Barabási et al., 2010), genes with best degree- or bottleneck-centrality, etc.

Additionally, network pharmacology approaches (Hao et al., 2018) can be used to pin-point most important metabolic or cell signaling pathway enriched by meta-genes, its interaction with other pathways and selection of suitable drug targets for further follow-up.

In short, meta-analysis is a very powerful technique to derive new hypothesis and knowledge from high-throughput biological data. However, the validity of meta-genes should be checked using low-throughput experiments such as real time PCR, western blot, immunohistochemistry, etc.

REFERENCES

Afgan, E., D. Baker, B. Batut, M. Van Den Beek, D. Bouvier, M. Čech, et al. (2018). The Galaxy platform for accessible, reproducible and collaborative biomedical analyses: 2018 update. Nucleic Acids Research. 46(W1).

Barabási, A.L., N. Gulbahce and J. Loscalzo (2010). Network medicine: A network-based approach to human disease. Nature Reviews Genetics. 12(1): 56–68.

Clough, E. and T. Barrett (2016). The gene expression omnibus database. Methods in Molecular Biology Statistical Genomics. 93–110.

Hao, T., Q. Wang, L. Zhao, D. Wu, E. Wang and J. Sun (2018). Analyzing of molecular networks for human diseases and drug discovery. Curr. Top. Med. Chem. 18(12): 1007–1014.

Johnson, W.E. and C. Li (2007). Adjusting Batch Effects in Microarray Experiments with Small Sample Size Using Empirical Bayes Methods. Batch Effects and Noise in Microarray Experiments: 113–129.

Lachmann, A., D. Torre, A.B. Keenan, K.M. Jagodnik, H.J. Lee, L. Wang, et al. (2018). Massive mining of publicly available RNA-seq data from human and mouse. Nat. Commun. 9(1).

Langfelder, P. and S. Horvath (2008). WGCNA: An R package for weighted correlation network analysis. BMC Bioinformatics. 9: 559.

Leek, J.T., W.E. Johnson, H.S. Parker, A.E. Jaffe, and J.D. Storey (2012). The sva package for removing batch effects and other unwanted variation in high-throughput experiments. Bioinformatics. 28(6): 882–883.

Lusa, L., R. Gentleman and M. Ruschhaupt (2020). GeneMeta: Meta-analysis for high-throughput experiments. R package version 1.60.0.

Parkinson, H., M. Kapushesky, M. Shojatalab, N. Abeygunawardena, R. Coulson, A. Farne, et al. (2007). ArrayExpress—A public database of microarray experiments and gene expression profiles. Nucleic Acids Res. 35 (Database).

Ramasamy, A., A. Mondry, C.C. Holmes and D.G. Altman (2008). Key issues in conducting a meta-analysis of gene expression microarray datasets. PLoS Medicine. 5(9).

Toro-Domínguez, D., J. Martorell-Marugán, R. López-Domínguez, A. García-Moreno, V. González-Rumayor, M.E. Alarcón-Riquelme, et al. (2018). ImaGEO: Integrative gene expression meta-analysis from GEO database. Bioinformatics. 35(5): 880–882.

Torre, D., P. Krawczuk, K.M. Jagodnik, A. Lachmann, Z. Wang, L. Wang, et al. (2018). Datasets2Tools, repository and search engine for bioinformatics datasets, tools and canned analyses. Sci. Data. 5(1).

Xia, J., E.E. Gill and R.E.W. Hancock (2015). NetworkAnalyst for statistical, visual and network-based meta-analysis of gene expression data. Nat. Protoc. 10(6): 823–844.

CHAPTER 16

Clinical Data Integration with Cancer Genomics: Insights Into Computational and Quantitative Methods

Tábata Barbosa, Felipe Rojas-Rodríguez, Janneth Gonzalez and Andres Felipe Aristizabal-Pachón*

Laboratorio de Bioquímica Experimental y Computacional,
Departamento de Nutrición y Bioquímica, Facultad de Ciencias,
Pontificia Universidad Javeriana, Bogotá D.C, Colombia

1   INTRODUCTION

Increasing application of next generation sequencing (NGS) methods have become a recurrent clinical procedure for cancer patients, making possible to increase patient-specific data. Due to an increase in cancer data a considerable fraction is publicly available in databases such as Genomic Data Commons (GDC, 2016) and International Cancer Genome Consortium (ICGC, 2011). These large genomic repositories have been essential for the storage and distribution of genomic, functional and clinical data. Nevertheless, it is worth a notice that the availability of clinical data is subject to several practical accessibility restrictions derived from privacy of patients. One approach to overcome clinical distribution was implemented by the MIMIC-III clinical database for intensive care units (Johnson et al., 2016) highlighting the role of full anonymity and patient consent for data accessibility. When possible, using such publicly available data has proved to be essential for the identification of new mutations associated with cancer variants, molecular markers through genomic-clinical association and functional variants associated with differential response to chemotherapy (Chen et al., 2019). Parallel to

*Corresponding author: andres_aristizabal@javeriana.edu.co

the development of NGS, molecular insights into cancer biology and therapy have emerged taking advantage of the molecular landscape of cancer (Angus et al., 2019). Identification of molecular variants and risk prediction by molecular signatures is essential to underlie potential early diagnosis of cancer (Michailidou et al., 2017). Precision oncology represents a cornerstone towards cancer prevention, increment in the positive response rate, reduced therapy-related side effects and life quality improvement (Patel, 2018).

In this matter it is important to highlight the essential role of experimental research towards cancer biology and therapy. Nevertheless, computational approaches tend to overcome specific restrictions such as population dynamics, mutation correlation and data analysis in a big scale. In order to take advantage of the data available to improve precision medicine in cancer, it is necessary to apply computational and quantitative methods (Sepulveda, 2020). Such necessity have led to unprecedented advancement in computational and theoretical biology, integrating methods from engineering, economy, statistics and mathematics to develop new approaches for molecular data analysis. One of the big challenges facing cancer prediction and prevention is the application of machine learning and statistics to heterogeneous data such as in the case of molecular omics data and phenotypical data. Moreover, implementation of novel mathematical and statistical models in biology and medicine depends upon data quality and density. Sample quality is a bottleneck for genomic data analysis considering that from sample purity and sample conservation methods to clinical data acquisition, non-standard reservoirs and collection frameworks affects the decision making related to the patient's standard care and the research associated with the data. In terms of data density, the issues arise at the analysis level where some of the most robust models available tend to rely upon enormous data samples that are challenging in the context of cancer. Even though research initiatives such as the Pan-Cancer Analysis of Whole Genomes (PCAWG), the International Cancer Genome Consortium (ICGC), the Cancer Genome Atlas (TCGA), Breast Cancer Association Consortium (BCAC), the Ovarian Cancer Association Consortium (OCAC), the Prostate Cancer Association Group to Investigate Cancer Associated Alterations in the Genome (PRACTICAL) and the Consortium of Investigators of Modifiers of BRCA1/2 (CIMBA), among others.

With all these initiatives in mind, bioinformatic approaches became critical for both the analysis of vast and complex molecular data as well as the connection between mathematics and statistics with biological problems. Also, advances in bioinformatics depend upon the application of both private and open source code, highlighting the increase of specialized methods and algorithms implemented in R and Python due to an active collaborative community. Such active community led to an important number of advances in cancer genomic integration with clinical data (Sepulveda, 2020). Even though a considerable number of methods have been developed in cancer and its application for personalized medicine, it is necessary to improve the analysis and identification of typical genomic features such as single nucleotide variants (SNV), insertions and deletions (indels) or copy number variants (CNV), identification of molecular markers and patient classification (Chen et al., 2019).

Additional to the augmented capacity of genomic data analysis, inheritable variability of clinical data challenges the current and typical analytical methods such as regression models and descriptive statistics. Pathology and radiology reports, heterogeneity of physician's notes and clinical tests present a challenge for curation and quantification. Data curators rise as a fundamental role in the big data of cancer research considering that normalization and homogeneity of clinical and molecular data. It is important to highlight that cancer patient clinical data heterogenicity is related to ethnicity, development stage of the tumor, tumor type, molecular subpopulation and type/stage of treatment. Computational pipelines considering clinical test heterogeneity integrated with genomic features offer a powerful tool to study cancer progression. Additionally, another challenge associated with data collection is the intra-tumor heterogenicity of neoplastic diseases such as cancer (Sun and Yu, 2015). From the tumor microenvironment to the lineages of mutagenesis within a tumor, both clinical (samples, markers and radio imaging) and molecular (tissue, stage of development and signatures) features can vary. For that reason, we focus this chapter to the advances across clinico-genomics, patient classification and prevention based on breast cancer clinical data. By reviewing the current methods used in clinical data integration with cancer genomics, we aim to present a conceptual framework to improve the integration of non-homogeneous data in cancer research as well as predict the potential diagnosis based on molecular marks. Clinical integration with genomic data is essential to improve preventive therapies, diagnosis and personalized treatment in cancer.

2 CANCER CLINICOGENOMICS

Examples of initiatives for cancer genomics association with genomics data is the xT 500 cohort analysis from patient data deposited in the Tempus platform. Through analytical tools, molecular, clinicaltreatment and outcomes data are being integrated for individual patients. Also, these data analyses provide researchers and physicians insights into profiles of patients with a similar clinical and molecular context (Beaubier et al., 2019). Databases play a crucial role in the use of cancer genome data for research in the understanding of the molecular mechanisms underlying cancer stages. These platforms have turned indispensable due to their associated tools for data query, visualization and analysis while providing public access to this massive genomic information. Some recurrent databases for cancer investigation employing genomics data include the following:

The Catalogue of Somatic Mutations in Cancer (COSMIC) is a public database that comprises manually curated data of mutation profiles across the range of human cancers. COSMIC v90 (2019) includes data from 39.2 million coding mutations across 1.4 million samples. This data, which is updated every three months, incorporates the genetics of drug resistance as well as clinical details from patients (Forbes et al., 2017). COSMIC website has tools for data query such as a genome browser, gene pages, cancer browser, fusion genes, drug resistance data, mutational signatures, copy number analysis (CONAN) and Hallmarks of cancer. Some ongoing projects from COSMIC are the Cancer Gene Census, where driver genes are described for each cancer type, the Cell Lines Project, released to develop a genetic and genomic characterization of cancer cell lines for an improvement in their utility, and COSMIC-3D which displays three-dimensional protein structures and relates this conformation with functional consequences (Tate et al., 2019). File downloading requires the researcher to login without a fee. The downloads of somatic mutations files can be filtered by gene, sample or cancer type (Tate et al., 2019). For further information about COSMIC you can visit the frequently asked questions page of the database (https://cancer.sanger.ac.uk/cosmic/help/faq).

The gene expression profiling interactive analysis (GEPIA) web server holds data from 9736 tumors and 8587 normal samples from the Cancer Genome Atlas (TCGA) project and the Genotype-Tissue Expression (GTEx) project. GEPIA integrates data available at the GDC (where data from the TCGA samples resides) and the Genotype-Tissue Expression (GTEx) project, which derives in applications for differential expression analysis (Saha et al., 2019). GEPIA has enabled a tool for researchers that has resulted in identification of biomarkers, classification of cancer subtypes and improvement of oncotherapy (http://gepia2.cancer-pku.cn; Tang et al., 2019).

The cBioPortal for Cancer Genomics is an open-access platform for visualizing and analyzing multidimensional cancer genomics data (Cerami et al., 2012). The interface allows users to explore genetic alterations such as somatic mutations, DNA copy-number alterations (CNAs), DNA methylation, protein abundance, phosphoprotein abundance, mRNA and miRNA expression across samples (Gao et al., 2013). Datasets exploration can be performed, as well as querying of single cancer studies, individual patients or samples in depth. Group comparison of clinical and genomic data from these patients or samples is possible when the user defines groups based on clinical or genomic elements (Cerami et al., 2012). Onco Query Language (OQL) is highly recommended for an advanced cancer genomic data visualization. Through the implementation of keywords and commands, specific genetic alterations can be included in a query (Gao et al., 2013). For further information related to this language like syntax, modifiers, and usage, you can visit the Introduction to OQL page from cBioPortal (https://www.cbioportal.org/oql).

Gene Expression Omnibus (GEO) distributes high-throughput functional genomic data from more than 3 million samples (Clough and Barret, 2016). Exploration can be made from the Repository Browser, from the curated Dataset Browser, from Tools or by searching a Keyword or a specific GEO accession number at the home page (https://www.ncbi.nlm.nih.gov/geo/). Quickly query construction of GEO datasets, a study-level database or GEO profiles, a gene-level database can be performed with free text or by typing terms, fields and Boolean operators in the search box.

Some methods that have been suggested to exploit the results that have been achieved, machine learning algorithms are suited to handle genomics robust data. Nonetheless, the effectiveness of these algorithms rely on how the input is computed given its full data-driven processing. Deep learning as a subdiscipline of machine learning has grown crucial for NGS cancer data analysis because of its end-to-end models. Deep learning approaches are key to extensive genomic profiling for molecular phenotypes prediction from sequences and in biomarkers discovery. Deep neural networks improve prediction accuracy through detecting relevant features in high dimensional data (Eraslan et al., 2019).

3   GENOMIC ASSOCIATION AND PREDICTION BASED ON ROUTINE CLINICAL DATA

Clinical characterization for breast cancer patients frequently involves tumor morphological assessment, testing for oestrogen and progesterone receptors (ER and PR respectively) as well as testing for human epidermal growth factor receptor 2 (HER2) (Pereira et al., 2016). G-band karyotyping, fluorescence *in situ* hybridization (FISH), PCR, RNA sequencing (RNA-seq) and whole-genome sequencing (WGS) are methods frequently performed in the clinic for cancer genome characterization, especially for structural variants (SVs) identification (Dixon et al., 2018). Nonetheless, this characterization is often a challenge because of cancer intra-tumor genomics heterogeneity and instability, which has implications for precision oncology and cancer research (Ben-David et al., 2019). The cohort study METABRIC (Molecular Taxonomy of Breast Cancer International Consortium) integrates analysis of somatic copy number aberrations (CNAs) and gene expression profiles in 2000 breast cancer tumors. METABRIC achieved reclassification of breast cancer into ten integrative clusters (IntClust) for breast cancer subtypes and their molecular drivers (Mukherjee et al., 2018).

4   CANCER GENOMICS AND PHARMACODYNAMICS

Several cases of cancer genomics identification have revealed the presence of in-frame fusion genes such as RET and NTRK3 in several cancer types as therapeutically targetable for drug treatment (Amatu et al., 2016; Mologni, 2011). Current cancer treatments have been facing drug resistance though mechanisms such as drug inactivation, alteration of drug targets, drug efflux, DNA damage repair, cell death inhibition, epithelial-mesenchymal transition and metastasis among other molecular mechanisms driven by epigenetics (Housman et al., 2014).

Drug resistance prediction computational methods are ongoing. These methods are developed according to the target in which relies the effort for identifying drug resistance; for example, for protein targets, analysis of three-dimensional (3D) structures are frequently employed (Liu et al., 2020). The discovery and production of a new generation of cancer drugs is inherent in a context where drug resistance is taking advantage.

Human cancer cell lines are a pillar for drug discovery. The Cancer Cell Line Encyclopedia project (CCLE) conducts a genetic and pharmacological characterization for over 1400 cell lines with public access. Recently CCLE genomic data has been used to perform a systematic metabolic analysis to understand cancer diversity (Li et al., 2019). Prediction of drug resistance is an ongoing effort that has been approached from computational methods (Liu et al., 2020). An example of this approach was developed using PRISM (profiling relative inhibition simultaneously in mixtures), a molecular barcoding method to test 4518 drugs against 578 human cancer cell lines through unsupervised clustering of compound viability profiles using the uniform manifold approximation and projection (UMAP) method (Corsello et al., 2020). The findings and datasets of the study are publicly available at Depmap (https://depmap.org/repurposing/).

Another public knowledgebase that joined the pursuit of cancer drug prediction is canSAR (http://cansar.icr.ac.uk/). This portal integrates biological, chemical, pharmacological and clinical data in order to identify cancer biomarkers, set up validation of targets and enable drug discovery predictions through machine learning (Tym et al., 2016). 3D structure-based, ligand-based and network-based orthogonal druggability calculations are updated each week. Also, a 'disease synopsis' is provided by canSAR, where each cancer type or subtype is attached with data of the number of drugs and clinical trials developed in patient cohorts and cell line models (Coker et al., 2019). This combination of druggability assessments and summarization enables users to do prior consideration of a target's viability for cancer pharmacological prospection.

Therapeutically applicable research to generate effective treatment (TARGET) uses large-scale genomic data and clinical data to find molecular variations that are related to childhood cancer developing for drug advancement. TARGET allows exploration of mutations, genes and pathways across histotypes and relates the somatic variants analyzed in pediatric pan-cancer studies performed in developing mesodermic tissues (Ma et al., 2018).

TARGET has open data such as clinical information, tissue pathology data, copy number alterations, sequence data of single amplicons and mutations, and controlled access data such as specific genotype or phenotype data for each case, information linking all sequence traces to a patient and raw sequences files from a patient, which requires Data Use Certification. The Office of Cancer Genomics from the National Institutes of Health (NIH) offers guidelines for searching and downloading the TARGET large-scale genomic data (OCG, 2017). This portal can be accessed from https://ocg.cancer.gov/programs/target/using-target-data.

NGS technologies are used to inform physicians for the decision making process in cancer therapy, to help determination of targets for immunotherapy with engineered T cells, to crack tumour-immune cell interactions and for neoantigens discovery for therapeutic cancer vaccination (Finotello et al., 2019). Detection of SVs patterns in cancer data integrates optical mapping, high-throughput chromosome conformation capture (Hi-C) and whole genome sequencing. Recurrent inversions, deletions, duplications, and translocations end up in oncogenes proliferation, thus supplying targets for drug therapy (Dixon et al., 2018). Oncomine database contains 715 datasets and 86,733 samples which integrates high-throughput cancer profiling data from multiple cancer types and experiments. This platform offers curated data that can be used to identify novel targets for drug development (Saha et al., 2019). Project DRIVE provides gene dependence profiles from 400 cell lines and can be used in combination with large complex data to discover novel pathway components. DRIVE functional genomics complement the molecular characterization by TCGA and ICGC which together assist in the detection of new drugs for cancer treatment (McDonald et al., 2017).

5 CONCLUSIONS

In this chapterwe presented some NGS-based free bioinformatic resourcethat may be used by the scientific communityin their research projects aimed to find the genetic basis of cancer. These resources may be able to improve development of more efficient and accurate susceptibility, diagnostic and prognostic biomarkers, as well as develop safe and more effective treatments.

This chapter set out some databases with cancer genomic data such as the Catalogue of Somatic Mutations in Cancer (COSMIC), Gene Expression Profiling Interactive Analysis (GEPIA), Gene Expression Omnibus (GEO) and cBioPortal. Each of these databases offer a set of special tools, allowing users to perform different kinds of data analysis and visualization. Furthermore, it showed approaches used in cancer genetics studies, which allow to identify association between genomic data and patient clinical information.

In rare type of cancers, there is difference in the survival rate compared to the common type of cancers. These types of cancer often fail having an appropriate size cohort of patients and a sufficiently large set of data for a genomic study. Refinement of bioinformatics tools allows to increase the power to detect genomic factors associated with rare cancers (Abbas-Aghababazadeh et al., 2019).

REFERENCES

Abbas-Aghababazadeh, F., Q. Mo, and B.L. Fridley. (2019). Statistical genomics in rare cancer. Semin. Cancer Biol. 61: 1–10. https://doi.org/10.1016/j.semcancer.2019.08.021

Amatu, A., A. Sartore-Bianchi and S. Siena (2016). NTRK gene fusions as novel targets of cancer therapy across multiple tumour types. ESMO Open. 1(2): e000023. doi: 10.1136/esmoopen-2015–000023.

Angus, L., M. Smid, S.M. Wilting, et al. (2019). The genomic landscape of metastatic breast cancer highlights changes in mutation and signature frequencies. Nat. Genet. 51: 1450–1458.

Ben-David, U., R. Beroukhim and T.R. Golub (2019). Genomic evolution of cancer models: Perils and opportunities. Nat. Rev. Cancer. 19(2): 97–109.

Beaubier, N., M. Bontrager, R. Huether, C. Igartua, D. Lau, R. Tell, et al. (2019). Integrated genomic profiling expands clinical options for patients with cancer. Nat. Biotechnol. 37(11): 1351–1360.

Cerami, E., J. Gao, U. Dogrusoz, B.E. Gross, S.O. Sumer, B.A. Aksoy, et al. (2012). The cBio cancer genomics portal: An open platform for exploring multidimensional cancer genomics data. Cancer Discovery. 2(5): 401–404.

Chen, H.Z., R. Bonneville and S. Roychowdhury (2019). Implementing precision cancer medicine in the genomic era. Semin. Cancer Biol. 55: 16–27.

Clough, E. and T. Barrett. (2016). The gene expression omnibus database. Methods Mol. Biol. 1418: 93–110.

Coker, E., C. Mitsopoulos, J. Tym, A. Komianou, C. Kannas, P. Di Micco, et al. (2019). canSAR: Update to the cancer translational research and drug discovery knowledgebase. Nucleic Acids Res. 8: 47(D): D917–D922.

Corsello, S.M., R.T. Nagari, R.D. Spangler, J. Rossen, M. Kocak, J.G. Bryan, et al. (2020). Discovering the anticancer potential of non-oncology drugs by systematic viability profiling. Nat Cancer. 1(2): 235–248. doi:10.1038/s43018–019–0018–6.

Dixon, J.R., J. Xu, V. Dileep, Y. Zhan, F. Song, V.T. Le, et al. (2018). Integrative detection and analysis of structural variation in cancer genomes. Nat. Genet. 50(10): 1388–1398. https://doi.org/10.1038/s41588-018-0195-8

Eraslan, G., Z. Avsec, J. Gagneur and F.J. Theis (2019). Deep learning: New computational modelling techniques for genomics. Nat. Rev. Genet. 20(7): 389–403.

Finotello, F., D. Rieder, H. Hackl and Z. Trajanoski (2019). Next-generation computational tools for interrogating cancer immunity. Nat. Rev. Genet. 20(12): 724–746.

Forbes, S.A., D. Beare, H. Boutselakis, S. Bamford, N. Bindal, J. Tate, et al. (2017). COSMIC: Somatic cancer genetics at high-resolution. Nucleic Acids Res. 45(D1): D777–D783.

Gao, J., B.A. Aksoy, U. Dogrusoz, G. Dresdner, S.O. Sumer, Y. Sun, et al. (2013). Integrative analysis of complex cancer genomics and clinical profiles using the cBioPortal. Sci Signal. 6(269): pl1.

Housman, G., S. Byler, S. Heerboth, K. Lapinska, M. Longacre, N. Snyder, et al. (2013). Drug resistance in cancer: An overview. Cancers. 6: 1769–1792.

Johnson, A., T. Pollard, L. Shen, et al. (2016). MIMIC-III, a freely accessible critical care database. Sci. Data. 3: 160035.

Li, H., S. Ning, M. Ghandi, G.V. Kryukov, S. Gopal, A. Deik, et al. (2019). The landscape of cancer cell line metabolism. Nat. Med. 25(5): 850–860.

Liu, J., J. Pei and L. Lai (2020). A combined computational and experimental strategy identifies mutations conferring resistance to drugs targeting the BCR-ABL fusion protein. Commun. Biol. 3: 18. doi:10.1038/s42003-019-0743-5.

Ma, X., Y. Liu, L.B. Alexandrov, M.N. Edmonson, C. Gawad and J. Zhang (2018). Pan-cancer genome and transcriptome analyses of 1,699 paediatric leukaemias and solid tumours. Nature. 555(7696): 371–376. doi:10.1038/nature25795.

McDonald, E.R., A. de Weck, M.R. Schlabach, E. Billy, K.J. Mavrakis, G.R. Hoffman, et al. (2017). Project DRIVE: A compendium of cancer dependencies and synthetic lethal relationships uncovered by large-scale, deep RNAi screening. Cell. 170(3): 577–592. e10. https://doi.org/10.1016/j.cell.2017.07.005

Michailidou, K., S. Lindström, J. Dennis, J. Beesley, S. Hui, S. Kar, et al. (2017). Association analysis identifies 65 new breast cancer risk loci. Nature. 551(7678): 92–94.

Mologni, L. (2011). Development of RET kinase inhibitors for targeted cancer therapy. Curr. Med. Chem. 18(2): 162–175. doi:10.2174/092986711794088308.

Mukherjee, A., R. Russell, S.-F. Chin, B. Liu, O.M. Rueda, H.R. Ali, et al. (2018). Associations between genomic stratification of breast cancer and centrally reviewed tumour pathology in the METABRIC cohort. NPJ Breast Cancer. 4: 5. doi:10.1038/s41523–018–0056-8.

Patel, J. (2018). Lessons in practicing cancer genomics and precision medicine. Expert Review of Precision Medicine and Drug Development. 3(5): 287–298. doi:10.1080/23808993.2018.1526081.

Pereira, B., S.-F. Chin, O.M. Rueda, H.-K.M. Vollan, E. Provenzano, H.A. Bardwell, et al. (2016). The somatic mutation profiles of 2,433 breast cancers refine their genomic and transcriptomic landscapes. Nat. Commun. 7(1): 11479. https://doi.org/10.1038/ncomms11479

Saha, S.K., S.M.R. Islam, K.S. Kwak, M.S. Rahman and S.G. Cho (2019). PROM1 and PROM2 expression differentially modulates clinical prognosis of cancer: A multiomics analysis. Cancer Gene Ther. 27(3-4): 147–167.

Sepulveda, J.L. (2020). Using R and bioconductor in clinical genomics and transcriptomics. J. Mol. Diagn. 22(1): 3–20.

Sun, X.X. and Q. Yu (2015). Intra-tumor heterogeneity of cancer cells and its implications for cancer treatment. Acta Pharmacologica Sinica. 36(10): 1219–1227.

Tang, Z., B. Kang, C. Li, T. Chen and Z. Zhang .(2019). GEPIA2: An enhanced web server for large-scale expression profiling and interactive analysis. Nucleic Acids Res. 47(W1): W556–W560.

Tate, J.G., S. Bamford, H.C. Jubb, Z. Sondka, D.M. Beare, N. Bindal, et al. (2019). COSMIC: The catalogue of somatic mutations in cancer. Nucleic Acids Res. 47(D1): D941–D947.

Tym, J., C. Mitsopoulos, E. Coker, P. Razaz, A. Schierz, A. Antolin, et al. (2016). canSAR: An updated cancer research and drug discovery knowledgebase. Nucleic Acids Res. 44(D1): 4: D938–D943.

CHAPTER 17

Bioinformatics of Correction of Multiple Testing: An Introduction for Life Scientists

(in Bioinformatics and Human Genomics Research)

Antonio Carvajal-Rodríguez

Departamento de Bioquímica, Genética e Inmunología y Centro de Investigación Mariña (CIM-UVIGO), Universidade de Vigo, Vigo, Spain

1 INTRODUCTION

Over the past years, biologists are generating data on a massive scale due to technologies such as microarray and high-throughput sequencing. In this biological big data era in which large numbers of hypotheses are simultaneously tested, even on the scale of hundreds of thousands or millions, the multiple testing correction has become of great importance.

Multiple hypothesis testing becomes standard in many scientific areas such as pharmacogenetics, genomics and proteomics. For example, understanding the genetic basis for a certain disease implies testing the expression of thousands of genes between different groups of patients. Thus, the interest for multiple testing procedures (MTPs) and the trade-off between false positive error and statistical power becomes key in current research.

There is a large number of approaches for multiple testing correction. In this review we just outline the basic concepts and strategies. More detailed and complete descriptions are reviewed elsewhere (Goeman and Solari, 2014; Kang, 2020a; Korthauer et al., 2019; MacDonald et al., 2019; Rudra et al., 2019; Tamhane and Gou, 2018). The present chapter is organized in six sections including this Introduction. Section 2 gives an informal overview about the principal multiple testing strategies and their utility under different research scenarios. Section 3 provides

---

*Corresponding author: *acraaj@uvigo.es*

commented definitions of important concepts. Section 4, provides a more formal and extended technical description, with formulae and algorithms for the different methods described in Section 2. Section 5 briefly, sketches some recent approaches for multiple testing correction. Finally, Section 6 concludes the previous sections.

2 MULTIPLE TESTING CORRECTION OVERVIEW

The scientific method works with proposed explanations for a phenomenon under study. These explanations are called scientific hypotheses provided they can be tested in some way. A test is a rule for deciding whether to accept or reject a hypothesis. The hypothesis under test is called the main or null hypothesis.

Consider an experiment that compares the expression levels of a certain gene in two groups, cases and controls, with sample size $n = 20$ each. According to the null hypothesis, the gene expression is equal between cases and controls. Meanwhile the rejection of the null hypothesis implies that there are differences in the gene expression between cases and controls. Let us consider a test for the hypothesis of equal gene expression, if we perform the test at level α, the risk of rejecting the null hypothesis of equal gene expression when it is true, has a probability of α which is called the type I error probability (Larson, 1982).

Hypotheses testing (Neyman-Pearson sense) consists in applying a rule to a function of the observed data for deciding whether to accept or reject an hypothesis. In applying that rule, the researcher decides in advance the maximum type I error rate (α) that she/he considers acceptable.

In summary, when we perform a single test, two types of errors can occur. The type I error, or false positive, is committed when rejecting a true null hypothesis; the type II error, or false negative, is committed when accepting a false null hypothesis (Table 1). Thus, type I error is controlled by the user of the test by means of the value α decided before performing the test. For example, defining $\alpha = 0.05$ means that type I error of the test is being controlled to have probability equal or less than 0.05.

Table 1 Possible outcomes when testing a null hypothesis H_0

	H_0 *True*	H_0 *False*
Reject H_0	Type I error	No error
Accept H_0	No error	Type II error

Nowadays, high-throughput experiments involve not one single but thousands of statistical tests. The problem of multiple testing correction consists in that if we compare the expression of thousands of genes and, as in single testing, we fix the type I error to 0.05 for each test, we can be sure that we will have a bunch of false positives (aka false discoveries). Consequently, we need to control type I error for the whole set of tests in some way similarly as the acceptance level α controls type I error for the single test. Of course, in addition to microarray expression studies there are many other scenarios where the same or a similar problem arises, as the genome wide association studies, and in general the comparison issues that raises from the analysis of omics data related to research on therapies, vaccines, diagnostics, etc. Under all these settings we require multiple testing correction to deal with type I error because this kind of error has the risk of disseminating misleading scientific results.

When performing multiple tests there are more than one definition for the type I error rate in the family of tests. We may consider two different definitions. First option considers the distribution of the number (not a proportion) of individual type I errors; an example of this is the family-wise error rate (FWER). The second option considers the distribution of the false discovery proportion (FDP); an example of this is the average of the FDP also called the false discovery rate (FDR).

The family-wise error rate, FWER, is the probability of at least one type I error in the family of tests, that is (see Table 2) FWER $= \Pr(V \geq 1)$, where V is the number of false positives. The FDP is the proportion of type I errors among the rejected hypotheses, i.e., FDP $= V/R$, with the convention of taking FDP $= 0$ when $R = 0$ (Dudoit and Laan, 2008). The FDR is the expectation of the FDP but the convention of FDP $= 0$, when $R = 0$ requires FDR defined as FDR $= E[V/R \mid R > 0] \times \Pr(R > 0)$.

Table 2 Numbers of Type I and II errors when performing M tests of hypotheses

	H_0 *True*	H_0 *False*	*Total*
Reject H_0	V	U	$R = V + U$
Accept H_0	$M_0 - V$	$M_1 - U$	$M - R$
Total	M_0	M_1	$M = M_0 + M_1$

In Table 2 we may appreciate that if from a total of M hypotheses there are M_0 for which the null is true and M_1 for which is false, then after R rejections we may commit V wrong rejections (type I errors) plus U correct rejections. Similarly, for $M - R$ null acceptances, there are $M_1 - U$ acceptances when the null is false (type II errors) and $M_0 - V$ correct null acceptances.

In this work we focus on three main strategies for managing the type I error under the multiple test setting, namely, those controlling the family-wise error rate (FWER), those controlling the false discovery rate (FDR), and those that estimate the false discovery proportion (FDP). In the following sections an overview is given of different methods based on each strategy, their underlying assumptions jointly with their strengths and weaknesses.

2.1   Methods of Controlling the Family-Wise Error Rate (FWER)

The methods explained below work on a set of M p-values obtained from a family of M tests. A common assumption, except for the permutation based methods, is that the p-values are continuous and uniformly distributed in the $(0, 1)$ interval or they are stochastically larger than uniform in the discrete case (Lehmann and Romano, 2005).

2.1.1   FWER and genomics research

Let us continue with our previous example. Consider that we are comparing the expression levels of 1,000 independent genes for two samples, one with 20 cases and other with 20 controls. For each gene we perform the test under a given critical value (see Section 3.1) that has its proper type I error level, say $\alpha' = 0.05$. In this case, the probability of no type I error for each test is $1 - 0.05 = 0.95$, then for the whole family of 1,000 tests, the probability of committing no error is $(1 - \alpha')^{1,000} = 0.95^{1,000} = 5.3 \times 10^{-23}$ and the probability of at least 1 type I error in the family of tests is FWER $= 1 - (1 - \alpha')^{1,000} = 1 - 5.3 \times 10^{-23} \approx 1$.

Therefore, if we perform M tests and want to maintain the type I error below a given rate we need to apply a multiple testing method to guarantee that. Among the many methods available for controlling the type I error rate some of them control directly the FWER (Table 3).

Table 3 FWER control methods with different dependence assumptions and usability in terms of the exploratory or confirmatory nature of the experiments

Method	*Control*	*Dependence assumptions*	*Usability level*	*Software*
Bonferroni	Strong	None	Confirmatory	p.adjust, Myriads v1.2
Holm	Strong	None	Confirmatory	multcomp, Myriads
Hommel	Strong	Positive dependence	Confirmatory	hommel, Myriads v1.2
maxT	Strong	None	Confirmatory	multtest, Myriads v1.2
SGoF	Weak	Independence	Exploratory	sgof, Myriads

2.1.2 Bonferroni

The method of Bonferroni is a single-step procedure that controls FWER at level α by rejecting the set of hypotheses that have p-values not larger than α divided by the total number of tests, i.e., the method rejects hypotheses having p-value $\leq \alpha/M$. This method has strong FWER control which means that it controls the FWER for any combination of true and false null hypotheses. Also, Bonferroni provides FWER control under any dependence structure of the p-values. The method is conservative, i.e., the probability of type I error is usually below the nominal α level.

Bonferroni is used in GWAS analysis because it is assumed that analyzing the whole genome is like performing only 10^6 tests (instead of the very much higher number of SNPs) and under such assumption, the FWER can be controlled by a Bonferroni adjustment with a genome-wide error level $\alpha = 5 \times 10^{-8}$. This assumption is based on the strong local correlations in the genome but the number of tests shouldn't be taken as universal since it depends on the correlation structure of the p-values and the kind of variant analysis we perform onto the genome (Hoggart et al., 2008; Lin, 2019; Sham and Purcell, 2014).

Bonferroni correction can be performed, using the R software, by the p.adjust function of the package stats (R Development Core Team, 2019) or by the package multcomp (Hothorn et al., 2008) and outside the R environment, by the software Myriads in its version v1.2 (Carvajal -Rodríguez, 2018).

2.1.3 Holm (Sequential Bonferroni)

This method is a sequential version of the Bonferroni. It is a step-down procedure, i.e., iterates beginning from the highest test value (smallest p-value). Like Bonferroni, Holm's method has strong FWER control at level α under any dependence structure of the p-values. It is more powerful than Bonferroni and should be in general recommended instead of it.

Regarding the application of the method in genomics, as a FWER control method is specially relevant for confirmatory (non-exploratory) experiments (Fig. 1). However, Holm's is very conservative and when the dependence structure is adequate (see below), more powerful variants should be used (Goeman and Solari, 2014).

Holm's sequential Bonferroni correction can be performed using the R software by the p.adjust function of the package stats (R Development Core Team, 2019) or by the package multcomp (Hothorn et al., 2008) and outside the R environment, by any of the versions of the software Myriads (Carvajal-Rodríguez, 2018).

2.1.4 Hommel

The Hommel method is a step-up procedure, i.e., iterates beginning from the lowest test value (largest p-value). Hommel's method has strong FWER control at level α, it operates under the assumption of independence of p-values or even positive dependence (through stochastic ordering, see Section 4).

Regarding the application of the method in genomics, it has the advantage of being more powerful than the Bonferroni and Holm methods but with the requirement of independence or at least positive dependence in the p-values.

Hommel's correction can be performed using the R software, by the p.adjust function of the package stats (R Development Core Team, 2019) or by the package Hommel (Goeman et al., 2019a) and outside the R environment, by the software Myriads v1.2 (Carvajal-Rodríguez, 2018).

2.1.5 MaxT

MaxT (Westfall and Young, 1993) is a permutation-based method that provides strong FWER control. MaxT does not impose any assumption on the dependence of the data and even the assumption of uniformly distributed *p*-values is not required. Besides, MaxT is more powerful than the Holm and Hommel FWER-control methods. A limitation of the method is that it requires an invariance condition (interchangeability) that means that the distribution of the permuted data set should be identical to the original one. Thus, we cannot always define adequate (holding the invariance condition) permutations for all hypotheses and models. In general, only relatively simple experimental designs allow permutation tests to be used (Goeman and Solari, 2014). Another limitation is the computational cost when the number of tests is large. Thus, a key issue for the computational feasibility of MaxT is the number of permutations required to obtain acceptable accuracy (see Section 4 for details).

MaxT guarantees FWER control while providing more power than other FWER methods, so it is a recommended method for confirmatory (non-exploratory) genomics data analysis when appropriate permutations are available (Fig. 1).

MaxT correction can be performed, using the R software, by the mt.maxT function of the package multtest (Pollard et al., 2005) and outside the R environment, by the software Myriads v1.2 (Carvajal-Rodríguez, 2018).

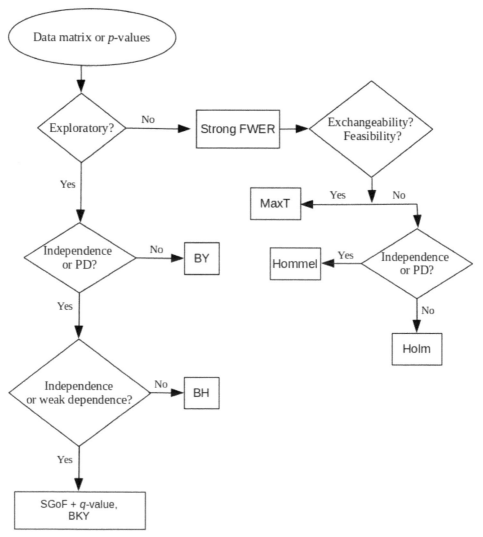

Figure 1 Decision flowchart for multiple testing procedures. PD: positive dependence. (Figure Courtesy, Myriads Manual, Carvajal-Rodríguez, 2018)

2.1.6 SGoF

The Sequential Goodness of Fit (SGoF) method is a step-down FWER-controlling procedure in the weak sense, which means that it has a strict control only under the complete null hypothesis, i.e., when all null hypotheses are true. Unlike methods with strong FWER control, SGoF increases its power with the number of tests and it can detect weak effects (Carvajal-Rodríguez et al., 2009; Carvajal-Rodríguez and de Uña-Álvarez, 2011; de Uña-Álvarez, 2011). However, the method requires the assumption of independence of *p*-values and can be too liberal when large blocks of correlated values are present (Carvajal-Rodríguez, 2018).

SGoF's weak FWER control may be useful if large power is preferred over type I error strong control. This scenario may occur when screening a large number of factors for detecting some important association that can be validated later; or simply when the researcher is primarily interested in an exploratory phase. Of course, when the requirements are confirmatory, only methods that keep strong control should be used (Fig. 1).

SGoF correction can be performed, using the R software, by the SGoF package (Castro-Conde and de Uña-Álvarez, 2014) and outside the R environment, by any of the versions of the software Myriads (Carvajal-Rodríguez, 2018).

2.2 Methods that Control False Discovery Rate (FDR)

In general, FDR control is less conservative and more powerful than FWER, specially when there are many false hypotheses, which makes FDR control a suitable tool for exploratory genomics studies where researchers are interested in selecting sets of promising hypotheses. From herein the FDR control methods are assumed to have strong control unless indicated otherwise. However, it is worth noting a key difference between FWER and FDR controlling procedures that is often omitted. If FWER is controlled at level α for a set of hypotheses then it is also controlled at the same level for any subset, including single hypotheses. This subset property is not true for FDR, which means that for a set with FDR controlled at level α it does not imply that a given subset is controlled at the same level (Finner and Roters, 2001). This is important because it means that the FWER for a set is also the FWER for each hypothesis in the set which is not true in the case of FDR. Thus, the FDR-adjusted *p*-value is a property of the rejected set not of any individual hypothesis (Goeman and Solari, 2014). Therefore, if statements on individual hypothesis are required as in confirmatory (non-exploratory) experiments, the FWER controlling methods should be preferable (Fig. 1).

Table 4 FDR control methods with different dependence assumptions and usability in terms of the exploratory or non-exploratory nature of the experiments

Method	Dependence assumptions	Usability level	Software
BH	Positive dependence	exploratory	p.adjust, Myriads
BY	None	exploratory	p.adjust, Myriads v1.2
BKY	Positive dependence	exploratory	cp4p, Myriads v1.2

2.2.1 Benjamini & Hochberg (BH)

The Benjamini & Hochberg (BH) method (Benjamini and Hochberg, 1995) is a step-up FDR controlling procedure under the assumption of independence of *p*-values or even positive dependence. BH is more powerful than Hommel.

BH correction can be performed, using the R software, by the p.adjust function of the package stats (R Development Core Team, 2019) and outside the R environment, by any of the versions of the software Myriads (Carvajal-Rodríguez, 2018).

2.2.2 Benjamini & Yekutieli (BY)

The Benjamini & Yekutieli (BY) method (Benjamini and Yekutieli, 2001) is a step-up FDR controlling procedure that is valid under any dependence structure. It is more conservative and has less power than the BH procedure, so BY should only be preferred when the dependence structure cannot be guaranteed (Fig. 1).

BY correction can be performed, using the R software, by the p.adjust function of the package stats, (R Development Core Team, 2019) and outside the R environment, by the software Myriads v1.2 (Carvajal-Rodríguez, 2018).

2.2.3 BKY adaptive two-stage method

The BH method controls FDR at level $\pi_0\alpha$, where $\pi_0 = M_0/M$ is the proportion of true nulls. The adaptive BH-like procedures intend to gain power over BH by estimating π_0 in a first step, and controlling FDR over $\pi_0 M$, instead of over M, in the second step. Benjamini, Krieger and Yekutieli (Benjamini et al., 2006) developed one of such procedures (BKY, see Section 4 for details). The BKY method is an adaptive BH-like procedure that controls FDR under independence or positive dependence and even remains conservative with relative good power when the degree of dependence is unknown (Blanchard and Roquain, 2009; Kim and van de Wiel, 2008).

The BKY correction can be performed, using the R software, by the adjust.p function (with pi0.method = "bky" argument) of the package cp4p (Gianetto et al., 2019) and outside the R environment, by the software Myriads v1.2 (Carvajal-Rodríguez, 2018).

2.3 Methods that Estimate the False Discovery Proportion (FDP)

FDR is the expectation of the false discovery proportion (FDP) unconditional on the occurrence of rejections. Under an FDR controlling procedure at level α, if for a subset of hypotheses the expected FDP is less or equal to α, we reject such hypotheses. For the FDP estimation, the procedure is reversed, it starts with the set of hypotheses candidate for rejection and finds an estimate Q for the FDP of that set. It can be argued that knowledge about the FDP is more relevant because it is directly related to the current experiment. That is, if we use any of the procedures of the previous section for controlling FDR at level α, we may obtain a set of rejected hypotheses. In this rejected set, the FDP is in average bounded by α, and the word "average" is key here, meaning that the FDR procedure is only indirectly (in average) describing the error rate of the rejected data. However, if we obtain an estimate of the FDP for a given set of hypotheses, it is a direct description of the error rate committed for such rejections (see FDP vs FDR in Section 4).

2.3.1 Storey's bayesian pFDR-estimation (*q*-values)

From the point of view of a researcher it seems desirable that when all nulls are true ($\pi_0 = 1$), the false discovery rate should be 1 because in this scenario any rejection is obviously a false one. However, the FDR when $\pi_0 = 1$ can be less than one. Even more, the researcher may not be interested in cases where there is no significant test. To solve this requirement the pFDR is defined as the expected FDP when at least one discovery has occurred (Storey, 2003). Defined in this way, and because we cannot control when the discoveries happened or not, the pFDR cannot be controlled a priori, contrary to the FDR in the BH and other FDR controlling procedures. Therefore, the computation of pFDR can be viewed as an FDP estimation (Fan et al., 2012).

The pFDR assumes independency, although seems to work well under weak dependence may have great variance under realistic dependence values (Goeman and Solari, 2014).

For estimating π_0, Storey's method uses a threshold parameter λ so the pFDR estimate has sometimes being called Storey-λ (Blanchard and Roquain, 2009).

Because the pFDR is not controlled a priori, adjusted *p*-values cannot be formally defined but the so-called *q*-values, that give an error measure for each statistic with respect to pFDR (see Section 4). Like the FDR controlling procedures, the Storey-λ FDP estimation lacks the subset property, i.e., the *q*-value is a property of the hypothesis in a given rejection set not of the individual hypotheses.

The Storey-λ *q*-values can be computed, using the R software, by the package *q*-value (Storey et al., 2020) and outside the R environment, by any of the versions of the software Myriads (Carvajal-Rodríguez, 2018).

2.3.2   Significance analysis of microarrays (SAM)

SAM (Tusher et al., 2001) is a method that estimates FDP by a permutation-based variant of the Storey-λ method with $\lambda = 0.5$ (Storey and Tibshirani, 2003a). Because it is permutation-based it adapts to the dependence structure. However, it is a known concern that the estimate of π_0 is less accurate under dependence (Schwartzman and Lin, 2011). See Section 4 for more details. SAM estimates can be computed, using the R software, by the package samr (Tibshirani et al., 2018).

2.3.3   Efrom's bayesian local FDR-estimation

The concept of local-FDR (Efron et al., 2001) solves the problem of lacking the subset property by providing estimates of FDP for individual hypotheses. The approach of Efrom has the additional requirement of assuming that the set of tests follows a mixture distribution of test statistics for the true and false hypotheses with prior probabilities π_0 and $1 - \pi_0$ respectively. Similar to Storey-λ, the local-FDR method suffers high variance in π_0 and in the FDP estimates distribution when the statistics are correlated, in such cases the empirical null distribution estimation should be preferred (Efron, 2007). Local-FDR estimates can be computed, using the R software, by the packages locfdr (Efron et al., 2015) and samr (Tibshirani et al., 2018).

Besides the above point estimates of FDP, there has been recent work on providing confidence intervals for the FDP (Goeman and Solari, 2011; Hemerik et al., 2019; Hemerik and Goeman, 2018). See Sections 4 and 5 for more details.

3   DEFINITIONS

We reproduce some relevant definitions with commentaries as they appear in the Myriads manual (Carvajal-Rodríguez, 2018).

3.1   Test of Hypotheses

A rule for deciding whether to accept or reject a hypothesis. The hypothesis under test is called the main or null hypothesis (Perezgonzalez, 2014; Sokal and Rohlf, 1981). The boundary for deciding between hypotheses is called the critical value of the test. The type I error expected using this critical value is called nominal type I error rate, or simply α level (see below).

3.2   Type I Error

The rejection of a true null hypothesis.

3.3   Nominal Type I Error Rate α

The user-supplied upper-bound for the type I error rate (Greenland, 2019).

3.4 Type II Error

The acceptance of a false null hypothesis.

3.5 Power of a Test

For detecting a true alternative hypothesis is the probability that the test will reject the null hypothesis. In the context of binary classification, e.g., medical testing, it is also called sensitivity or true positive rate. The power is one minus the probability of a type II error.

3.6 Observed *p*-value

Is the probability, under the null hypothesis H_0, that a test statistic would be equal to or more extreme than the observed value. This is equivalent to say that the observed *p*-value is the smallest nominal type I error level of the single hypothesis testing procedure that would allow rejection of H_0 given the test statistic value (Dudoit and Laan, 2008). A more formal and rigorous definition follows. Given a statistical model A and a tested hypothesis H_0, the observed *p-value* is the probability that the test statistic be equal or larger than its observed value in the current sample realization if every model assumption were correct, including H_0 (Greenland et al., 2016).

3.7 Complete Null Hypothesis

When all null hypotheses are true.

3.8 Control in the Weak Sense

Control in the weak sense occurs when the type I error rate is controlled at the specified level only under the complete null hypothesis.

3.9 Control in the Strong Sense

Control in the strong sense occurs when the type I error rate is controlled at the specified level for any combination of true and false null hypotheses.

3.10 Per-Family Error Rate (PFER)

The expected number of type I errors in the family of tests, i.e., PFER $= E(V)$.

3.11 Per-Comparison Error Rate (PCER)

The expected value of the number of type I errors divided by the number of tests, i.e., PCER $= E(V)/M$. If we are performing each test at level α, the PCER is equal or less than α. This is the expected type I error rate, also called EER in (Finner and Roters, 2001). In a multiple testing context, controlling the PCER is like not considering the multiple test setting at all, and consequently is more liberal (anti-conservative) than controlling FWER or FDR (see definitions below).

3.12   Family-Wise Error Rate (FWER)

Is the probability of at least one type I error in the set of tests, i.e., FWER $= \Pr(V \geq 1)$. Controlling the FWER is a conservative strategy which means that the probability of rejecting the null hypotheses is below the nominal α level. There is a generalization of the FWER concept called k-FWER which is the probability of at least k false rejections. Obviously, FWER corresponds to k-FWER with $k = 1$ (Lehmann and Romano, 2005).

3.13   False Discovery Proportion (FDP)

FDP is the (unobserved) proportion of false rejections V among total rejections R, FDP $= V/R$, with the convention of FDP $= 0$ when $R = 0$.

3.14   False Discovery Rate (FDR)

FDR is the FDP averaged over all possible experimental replicates. More technically, it is the expected FDP unconditional on the occurrence of rejections. Because FDP equals 0 when $R = 0$, FDR can be expressed as

$$\text{FDR} = E\left[\frac{V}{R}\middle|R > 0\right] \cdot \Pr(R > 0) \tag{1}$$

as defined in (Benjamini and Hochberg, 1995) but see also (Storey, 2003). We will make explicit some differences between FDR control versus FDP estimation in Section 4.5.

3.15   Positive False Discovery Rate (pFDR)

The expected proportion of false rejections V among the rejections R conditioned on and least one rejection

$$\text{pFDR} = E\left[\frac{V}{R}\middle|R > 0\right] \tag{2}$$

Note that, because we ignore if any rejections will occur, pFDR cannot be controlled at any given threshold (Storey, 2002; 2003). The pFDR and FDR coincide when the number of tests is large enough to guarantee at least one rejection, i.e., $\Pr(R > 0) = 1$. However, under finite sample size $R = 0$ may occur, so in the estimation of pFDR when $R = 0$, the convention of substituting R by 1 is applied (Storey, 2002). Under the complete null, the value of pFDR is 1, provided that some rejection occur. The computation of pFDR can be considered as a point estimate of the FDP (Fan et al., 2012; Goeman and Solari, 2014).

3.16   Subset Property

A FWER-controlling multiple testing procedure (MTP) is said that has the subset property if, when rejecting a set of hypotheses, the FWER control is also guaranteed for any subset including the single hypotheses. An FDR controlling procedure has not necessarily the subset property but if it has, such procedure also controls the FWER at level α. That is, any MTP with the subset property is a FWER controlling procedure (Finner and Roters, 2001; Goeman and Solari, 2014).

4 TECHNICAL DETAILS AND ALGORITHMS

4.1 Assumptions of Multiple Testing Correction Methods

4.1.1 Uniformity

Let us note the M_0 p-values corresponding to true nulls as $q_1, ..., q_{m0}$, then these p-values should be uniformly distributed between 0 and 1, or stochastically greater than uniform if data are discrete, anyway they should satisfy

$$\Pr(q_i \leq t) \leq t \tag{3}$$

Most MTPs require the p-values satisfy (3). However, the uniformity may be only approximate specially for small sample sizes.

4.1.2 Dependence structure

Some MTPs as Bonferroni, Holm, BY, or permutation-based methods do not require any dependence assumption and work under independence or any form of general dependence of the p-values. These methods are in general less powerful. Methods as Hommel and BH, work under independence or some kind of positive dependence called positive dependence through stochastic ordering (PDS, aka positive regression dependence) on the subset of p-values of true null hypotheses (Benjamini and Yekutieli, 2001; Goeman and Solari, 2014; Sarkar, 2008). Methods as Storey-λ require weak positive dependence implying only local correlations (Schwartzman and Lin, 2011). Even methods working with some kind of positive dependence may fail when there are strong correlations in the p-values (Blanchard and Roquain, 2009).

4.2 Adjusted p-values and q-values

Adjusted p-values can be considered as the multiple testing analogous of the single hypothesis test observed p-values. The adjusted p-value $\tilde{p}_m$ of a hypothesis H_m is the smallest α (nominal type I error level measured as FWER or FDR) of the multiple hypotheses testing procedure at which one would reject the hypothesis, given the test statistic value (Dudoit and Laan, 2008; Tamhane and Gou, 2018). However, because of the subset property, the interpretation of the adjusted p-value is different for FWER and FDR controlling methods. In the FWER controlling methods, the adjusted p-value is a property of each single hypothesis, but in the FDR controlling methods the adjusted p-value is a property of the set of rejected hypotheses, not of each hypothesis. The concept of local FDR (Efron et al., 2001) solves this by providing estimates of FDP for individual hypotheses.

The q-value is the minimum pFDR that can occur when rejecting the statistic (Storey, 2002). Often, it is said that q-values are adjusted pFDR p-values, which is technically incorrect because pFDR cannot be controlled by a test procedure (Storey, 2003). Like the adjusted FDR p-values, the q-values are a property of the set of rejected hypotheses, not of each hypothesis.

4.3 FWER Methods

4.3.1 Bonferroni

Bonferroni's method consists of rejecting hypotheses only if they have raw p-value smaller than α/M. This method provides FWER control for the set of M hypotheses at α level under any dependence structure of the p-values. It conservatively controls FWER for any combination of true and false hypotheses, i.e., it controls the FWER at level $\pi_0\alpha$, where π_0 is the unknown proportion of true null hypotheses in the set of tests. Therefore, if there are many false null hypotheses (π_0 is low) the method is very conservative. In general, Bonferroni will be very conservative if the *p*-values are positively correlated and less conservative if the *p*-values are independent or negatively correlated (Goeman and Solari, 2014). The adjusted *p*-value for a test *i* under Bonferroni is min (Mp_i, 1), where p_i is the raw *p*-value.

Algorithm with adjusted p-values

Compute the adjusted *p*-values $\tilde{p}_i = \min\{M \times p_i, 1\}$.

Reject hypotheses with adjusted *p*-value $\tilde{p}_i \leq \alpha$.

4.3.2 Holm

Holm's method works in step-down way by iterating the Bonferroni method as follows. Consider the sorted *p*-values $p_1 \leq p_2 \ldots \leq p_M$ and their corresponding sorted hypotheses. The hypothesis $i(i = 1, \ldots, M)$ will be rejected if its raw *p*-value is smaller than $\alpha/(M - i + 1)$, else the procedure ends.

Like Bonferroni, Holm's procedure has FWER control with the only assumption of uniformity of *p*-values [Eqn (3)]. Holm's method is less conservative and more powerful than Bonferroni and should be used instead (Goeman and Solari, 2014).

Algorithm with adjusted p-values

0. Set $i = 1$.
1. Sort the *p*-values $p_1 \leq p_2 \ldots \leq p_M$.
2. Compute the adjusted *p*-value $\tilde{p}_i = \min\{(M - i + 1) \times p_i, 1\}$.
3. Enforce monotonicity $\tilde{p}_i = \max\{\tilde{p}_h\}$, $h = 1, \ldots, i$.
4. If $i < M$ increase i and repeat from step 2.
5. End.

Reject hypotheses H_i with adjusted *p*-value $\tilde{p}_i \leq \alpha$.

4.3.3 Hommel

Hommel's method is a step-up procedure that has strong FWER control under the assumption of independence of *p*-values or even positive dependence (Goeman and Solari, 2014; Tamhane and Gou, 2018). The classical algorithm for computing Hommel adjusted *p*-values is the Wright algorithm (Wright, 1992) which is time consuming. However, a recent work by (Meijer et al., 2019) provides a linear time algorithm for computing the adjusted *p*-values. Here we present the Hommel step-up adjusted *p*-values as computed from (Wright, 1992).

Algorithm with adjusted p-values

0. Sort the *p*-values $p_1 \leq p_2 \ldots \leq p_M$
1. Initially set $\tilde{p}_i = p_i$ for all *i*.
2. For each $m = M, M - 1, \ldots, 2$ (in that order), do:
   2a. For each $i > (M - m)$ do:
   $$\text{Compute } c_i = (mp_i)/(m + i - M)$$
   2b. $c_{min} = \min\{c_i\}$, $i = M - m + 1, \ldots, M$. // for this subset
   2c. For each $i > (M - m)$ do:
   $$\text{If } \tilde{p}_i < c_{min} \text{ then } \tilde{p}_i = c_{min}$$
   2d. For $i \leq (M - m)$ do:
   (i) $c_i = \min(c_{min}, mp_i)$
   (ii) if $\tilde{p}_i < c_i$ then $\tilde{p}_i = c_i$.
3. End

Reject hypotheses H_i with adjusted *p*-value $\tilde{p}_i \leq \alpha$.

4.3.4 SGoF for weak FWER control

The SGoF procedure is a step-down FWER-control method in the weak sense, i.e., under the complete null hypothesis. It was originally developed in (Carvajal-Rodríguez et al., 2009) and different variants have been developed since then (Carvajal-Rodríguez and de Uña-Álvarez, 2011; Castro-Conde et al., 2017; Castro-Conde and de Uña-Álvarez, 2015a; de Uña-Álvarez, 2012). The adjusted p-values can be computed following the algorithm in (Castro-Conde and de Uña-Álvarez, 2015b). There is also an efficient algorithm that provides an upper-bound for the adjusted p-values which can be useful when the number of tests is very high (Carvajal-Rodríguez, 2018). The statistical properties of the SGoF procedure were described in (de Uña-Álvarez, 2011, 2012).

4.3.5 A note on permutation based multiple testing

Instead of making assumptions about the dependence we can adapt the procedure to the observed dependence structure by using a permutation test. However, it is required that the null invariance condition or exchangeability (Westfall and Troendle, 2008) is satisfied, i.e., shuffling the observations should keep the data just as likely as the original set under the null hypothesis. Also, the power of permutation testing comes with a computational cost for moderate sample sizes when all permutations are performed. Thus, an alternative are Monte Carlo permutation tests that sample a sufficient number of permutations instead of doing all. The number of permutations varies, depending on the kind of test, the response variable, and the sample size n. For example, for the case-control scenario we have $B = n!/(n_1!n_2!)$ permutations of the n_1 case and n_2 control labels. For more details on re-sampling algorithms, the following references may be consulted (Dudoit et al., 2003; Ge et al., 2003; Romano and Wolf, 2005).

4.3.6 MaxT

As we have seen in Section 2, MaxT (Westfall and Young, 1993) is a powerful permutation-based method that provides strong FWER control. It does not impose any assumption on the dependence of the data and even the assumption of uniformly distributed p-values is not required.

A permutation algorithm for step-down maxT adjusted p-values can be found in (Dudoit et al., 2003, Box 2 in Section 2.6) and a recent efficient algorithm for resampling-based step-down adjusted p-values can be found in Algorithm 4.1 in (Romano and Wolf, 2016).

So far, we have reviewed various methods that provide FWER control, there are also generalized step-down methods for controlling k-FWER, the reader is referred to (Romano and Wolf, 2007) for a review of these methods.

4.4 FDR Methods

4.4.1 Benjamini-Hochberg (B-H) FDR-control method

The (unconditional) FDR (Benjamini and Hochberg, 1995) is the expected false discovery proportion (FDP, see Definitions 3.13 and 3.14). It is unconditional because it is not conditioned on the existence of rejections (Zaykin et al., 2000). The Benjamini-Hochberg (BH) is a step-up procedure that controls FDR at a desired level α.

Algorithm with adjusted p-values
    0.   Set $i = M$.
    1.   Sort the p-values $p_1 \leq p_2 \ldots \leq p_M$.
    2.   Compute the adjusted p-value $\tilde{p}_i = \min\{(M/i) \times p_i, 1\}$
    3.   Enforce monotonicity $\tilde{p}_i = \min\{\tilde{p}_h\}$, $h = i, \ldots, M$.
    4.   If $i > 1$ decrease i and repeat from step 2.
    5.   End.
Reject hypotheses H_i with adjusted p-value $\tilde{p}_i \leq \alpha$.

Interestingly, the FDR can be written in terms of specificity and sensitivity (power) (Storey and Tibshirani, 2003b), so

$$\text{FDR} = E\left[\frac{M_0 \cdot (1 - specificity)}{M_0 \cdot (1 - specificity) + M_1 \cdot sensitivity}\right] \tag{4}$$

where M_0 is the number of true null hypotheses and $M_1 = M - M_0$ the number of true alternative hypotheses.

Recalling that the false positive rate $\alpha = 1 -$ specificity, and that sensitivity is 1 minus the probability of type 2 error (β) then we have

$$\text{FDR} = E\left[\frac{M_0\alpha}{M_0\alpha + M_1(1-\beta)}\right]$$

If we divide M_0 and M_1 by M the quotient does not change and so

$$\text{FDR} = E\left[\frac{\pi_0\alpha}{\pi_0\alpha + \pi_1(1-\beta)}\right] \tag{5}$$

where $\pi_0 = M_0/M$ and $\pi_1 = M_1/M = 1 - \pi_0$.

For any given error level α and statistical power $1 - \beta$, FDP increases with π_0 and decreases with π_1. When $\pi_0 = 1$, FDP = 1 so, we can ask, how can FDR, which is the FDP expectation, be controlled at any level when $\pi_0 = 1$? The answer to this important question is given in subsection 4.5.

4.4.2   Benjamini and Yekutieli (BY)

The Benjamini and Yekutieli (BY) method (Benjamini and Yekutieli, 2001) is a step-up FDR controlling procedure that, unlike BH, is valid under any dependence structure. The price for this is that BY has less power than BH, so BY should only be preferred when either independence or positive dependence structure cannot be guaranteed (Fig. 1).

The adjusted p-values for BY can be computed with the same algorithm as for BH just changing step 2 to be

$$\tilde{p}_i = \min\left\{\left(\frac{kM}{i}\right) \times p_i, 1\right\} \text{ with } k = \sum_{j=1}^{M}\frac{1}{j} \qquad .$$

4.4.3   BKY adaptive two-stage method

As seen in Section 2, the BKY method is an adaptive two-stage BH-like procedure that controls FDR under independence or positive dependence with relative good power and conservativeness even when the degree of dependence is unknown (Benjamini et al., 2006; Blanchard and Roquain, 2009; Kim and van de Wiel, 2008).

The adjusted p-values for BKY can be computed with the same algorithm as for BH in two different steps. First, the algorithm of BH is utilized at level $\alpha' = \alpha/(1 + \alpha)$. Let r_1 be the number of rejected hypotheses by BH$_{\alpha'}$ then estimate π_0 as $p_0 = (M - r_1)/M$. If $p_0 = 1$ do not reject any hypothesis and finish; if $p_0 = 0$ rejects all hypotheses and finish; otherwise, perform a second BH at level $\alpha^* = \alpha'/p_0$. In doing so we can compute the adjusted p-values following the BH algorithm just changing the step 2 to be

$$\tilde{p}_i = \min\left\{\left(\frac{(1+\alpha)\,p_0 M}{i}\right) \times p_i, 1\right\}$$

Reject hypotheses H_i with adjusted p-value $\tilde{p}_i \leq \alpha$.

In addition to the BKY method and those reviewed in (Benjamini et al., 2006) there are various other kinds of adaptive procedures, the interested reader may consult (Blanchard and Roquain, 2009; Kang, 2020a).

4.4.4 Weighted FWER and FDR methods

Sometimes there is available meaningful prior information related to the hypotheses being tested so that not all null hypotheses have the same importance. Consequently, weighted multiple hypothesis testing procedures have being developed for FWER as well for FDR control (Genovese et al., 2006; Kang et al., 2009). When the weights are informative these methods are usually more powerful than their unweighted counterparts.

There are in general two strategies for estimating the weights: external weights, where prior information (based on scientific knowledge or prior data) exists for specific hypotheses; and estimated weights, where some informative covariates are used to construct weights (Ignatiadis et al., 2016; Ignatiadis and Huber, 2017; Korthauer et al., 2019; Roeder and Wasserman, 2009).

Usually, the weights must satisfy

$$\frac{1}{M} \sum_{j=1}^{M} w_j = 1 \quad \text{with } w_j \ge 0$$

and the weighted p-values are defined as $\frac{p_i}{w_i}$. Adjusted weighted p-values can be computed for different FWER and FDR procedures, see for example (Genovese et al., 2006; Kang et al., 2009).

4.5 FDP vs FDR

Consider the complete null hypothesis where all nulls are true ($\pi_0 = 1$) or equivalently, all rejections are false, $V = R$ and so FDP $= V/R = 1$. In the previous subsection when talking about BH we have asked, how can FDR, which is the FDP expectation, be controlled at any level when $\pi_0 = 1$? To put it clear, if FDP is 1, how can we assure FDR ≤ 0.05?

First, it is important to recall that FDR is unconditional on the number of rejections (Zaykin et al., 2000). In other words, FDR can be defined as an expectation independently of the observed tests, with or without rejections. It maintains the control because it is an average, so, if we are controlling the FDR at level α we expect that, on an average, the proportion of false discoveries is upper-bounded by α. This average, allow me to insist, is what we call FDR, and is the average what is maintained below α. In the case of the BH procedure, the FDR upper bound is $\pi_0 \alpha$ (Benjamini et al., 2006).

Let's see an example, consider performing an *in silico* experiment or simulation, for which all null hypotheses are true, i.e., the complete null hypothesis ($\pi_0 = 1$). This experiment consists in $M = 100$ independent tests each performed at $\alpha = 0.05$. If we do not apply an MTP, we expect 5 false rejections in 100 tests (PFER = 5). Under the complete null the FDR = FWER $= 1 - (1 - 0.05)^{100} = 0.99$. Furthermore, we repeated the same kind of experiment 1000 times. On each occasion the FWER and FDR is 0.99.

Because of such a high error we decide to control the FDR at 0.05 level applying the BH procedure. However, under the complete null we should be aware that in any experiment in which we have some rejection ($R > 0$) the observed proportion of false discoveries is FDP $= 1$. On the contrary, in the experiments without rejections ($R = 0$), the FDR takes value 0 by definition and so does the FDP. Thus, applying $BH_{0.05}$ we expect that in 95% of our experiments there are no rejection so FDP $= 0$ while 5% have at least one rejection so FDP $= 1$. Then we can compute the expected FDP which is FDR $= E(\text{FDP}) = 0.95 \times 0 + 0.05 \times 1 = 0.05$. This is how the FDR can be controlled at level α when all nulls are true or, in general, at level $\alpha \pi_0$, whatever the combination of nulls and false hypotheses. Under the complete null, at each experiment the observed FDP is 0 or 1, although the FDR is being controlled as an expectation of 0.05.

Let us consider now what happens with pFDR, which is a conditional FDR. The pFDR estimates the FDP for a given rejected set, which means that in our *in silico* lab we will obtain an FDP value for each performed experiment having rejections (Carvajal-Rodríguez and de Uña-Alvarez, 2011; Schwartzman, 2012; Storey, 2003; Zaykin et al., 2000). Under the complete null, the probability α of false rejection, matches the probability of rejection, $\Pr(R > 0) = \alpha$, and recalling the definition of FDR in terms of pFDR, i.e., FDR = pFDR $\times$ $\Pr(R > 0)$ and solving for pFDR, we get pFDR = FDR/$\Pr(R > 0)$ = α/α = 1. It is clear that, given at least one rejection in our experiment, although the BH controls the FDR at level α, we are still committing a pFDR = 1, independently of α and the statistical power.

Whether FDR or pFDR are the quantities of interest has been disputed, e.g., Storey argues that the interest relies in situations where there is at least one rejection. On the other side, (Dudoit et al., 2008) argues that pFDR being equal to one under the complete null hypothesis impedes its control under this testing scenario. Besides, the FDR reduces to the FWER = $\Pr(V > 0)$ under the complete null.

4.6 FDP Estimation Methods

4.6.1 Storey's Bayesian pFDR-estimation (*q*-values)

The pFDR was defined as the expected FDP when at least one discovery has occurred (Storey, 2003; Storey and Tibshirani, 2001). The pFDR can be estimated as pFDR(α) = $p_0 tM/R(t)$, where p_0 is an estimate of π_0 and $R(t)$ is the total number of rejections under probability threshold t. Thus, we only need to estimate π_0. It is worth noting that under certain general conditions, the pFDR can be expressed as a Bayesian posterior probability, where π_0 is the prior for the posterior probability of rejecting a true null (Storey, 2003). We have mentioned in Section 2 that Storey uses a threshold parameter λ for estimating π_0. The value of the parameter λ can be fixed or automatically computed by bootstrap or fitting a cubic spline (Storey and Tibshirani, 2003b; Storey, 2002). Besides λ-estimation, several other methods has been proposed for estimating π_0, some of them have been reviewed in (Carvajal-Rodríguez, 2018; Carvajal-Rodríguez and de Uña-Álvarez, 2011; Friguet and Causeur, 2011; Kang, 2020b). The λ-estimation and related methods assume independence or weak dependence implying local correlations. Under more realistic dependence, the FDP estimation can have very large variance, skewness and bias (Owen, 2005).

Analogous to the FDR adjusted *p*-values, the *q*-value is the minimum pFDR that can occur when the given statistic is rejected for the set of rejection regions (Storey, 2002). As already commented, the *q*-value, although interesting, is a property of the hypothesis within the specific rejected set not of the individual hypothesis itself.

4.6.2 SAM

The significance analysis of microarrays (SAM) method (Tusher et al., 2001) does not control neither estimate FDR but the expected number of false positives PFER = $E(V)$ (Dudoit et al., 2003). This value $E(V)$ divided by the number of rejections R is an estimate of the FDP although its reliability is not clear under general dependence conditions (Blanchard and Roquain, 2009; Goeman and Solari, 2014; Kim and van de Wiel, 2008). The SAM algorithm is given in (Dudoit et al., 2003). The procedure has been recently extended by the addition of upper bounds to the FDP estimation (Hemerik and Goeman, 2018). There is also an extended SAM software R package called confSAM.

4.6.3   Efrom's Bayesian local FDR-estimation (empirical null estimation)

The Benjamini and Hochberg's (1995) false discovery rate (FDR) is based on tail area properties (tail area FDR) while local false discovery rates are FDR based on densities. Given the test statistic t, the model of a mixture density is defined for the unaffected (null) and for the affected treatment of interest

$$f(z) = \pi_0 f_0(t) + \pi_1 f_1(t).$$

The model requires an estimate of the "null density" $f_0(t)$ which is done by empirical null estimation, for example, microarray data structures allow to estimate the density by permutation. The main advantage of the empirical null estimation is the robustness to dependence. The value of the proportion of true nulls π_0 of false hypotheses are estimated from data. However, like previous estimates both the density and π_0 may be highly variable when the p-values are correlated (Efron, 2005).

4.7   Relaxing the Continuity Assumption: Discrete p-values

Classic MTPs, including BH, were developed under the assumption that the p-values are uniformly and continuously distributed when the null is true. However, examples of discrete test statistics are common in genomics and related biomedical sciences (He and Heyse, 2019; Liang, 2016). Methods developed under the assumption of continuity could be too conservative when the p-values are discrete, and may not be as powerful as one would hope for. Several authors have demonstrated the advantages of using discrete information properties when the data is highly discrete, see for example (Westfall and Troendle, 2008; Westfall and Wolfinger, 1997). Discrete version of different MTPs has been developed both for FWER (Castro-Conde et al., 2017; He and Heyse, 2019; Zhu and Guo, 2020) and for FDR control and estimation (Chen, 2020; Chen and Sarkar, 2020; Döhler, 2018; Liang, 2016).

5   RECENT DEVELOPMENTS

In recent years, several multiple testing improvements indicate the strength of the field within the big biological data context. Regarding computational efficiency, new algorithms were recently proposed, e.g., for the Hommel's procedure in linear time (Meijer et al., 2019) or for resampling-based step-down adjusted p-values (Romano and Wolf, 2016), or the generalized FWER error control (k-FWER) and false positives and negatives control (Song and Fellouris, 2019). Regarding FDR, some new weighted covariate methods as IHW (Ignatiadis et al., 2016) that reduces to the BH procedure when the covariate is completely uninformative; similarly, BL (Boca and Leek, 2018) reduces to the Store's q-value; also, the functional FDR incorporates informative variables when available, for computing FDR and q-values (Chen et al., 2019). Some of these new FDR methods has been recently benchmarked in (Korthauer et al., 2019).

The estimation of FDP under strong dependence has been recently studied (Fan et al., 2019, 2012; Fan and Han, 2017). Another avenue of research come from the adaptive control of FWER and FDR by assuming dependency structure by blocks (Guo and Sarkar, 2019), or by estimation of confidence bounds for the false discovery proportion (Goeman et al., 2019b; Goeman and Solari, 2011; Hemerik and Goeman, 2018). Also, when there are logical relations among the hypotheses, the control can be exerted by hierarchically ordering the hypotheses and by graphical approaches (Tamhane and Gou, 2018). The different types of prior information, e.g., weights, dependence structure, proportion of nulls, hypotheses subgroups, can be combined for FDR control of grouped hypotheses (Ramdas et al., 2019).

Within the field of integrative genomics, the simultaneous analysis of multiple data sets boosted the extension of MTPs for multivariate p-values (Chi, 2008; Phillips and Ghosh, 2014; Richardson et al., 2016; Rudra et al., 2019; Xia et al., 2019). Last but not least, multiple hypotheses testing can also be done using the Bayesian counterpart of p-values, the Bayes factors so called e-values, and different procedures have been recently proposed under this setting (Vovk and Wang, 2019a,b).

6 CONCLUSIONS

We have reviewed classical and some of the most important methods for controlling type I error in multiple hypotheses testing. Though there is plenty of different methods, the main avenue for controlling type I error goes through FWER or FDR control and/or false discovery proportion (FDP) estimation. Meanwhile, we provided a map for deciding the best strategy depending on the research interest, either exploratory or confirmatory, the assumptions that can be made, the availability of prior information and the kind of statistical test. We either explicitly gave or referenced, some well-known algorithms for computing the adjusted p-values.

In addition, we made explicit some key differences between methods often omitted in the literature. First, FDR control may be less conservative than FWER which makes FDR control a suitable tool for exploratory genomics studies where we are interested in selecting sets of promising hypotheses; even more, if independence or weak dependence is guaranteed, the SGoF method can be a valuable and powerful exploratory alternative. On the contrary, FWER strong control is specially relevant for confirmatory (non-exploratory) experiments. Obviously, when possible, the most powerful and flexible FWER controlling variant, MaxT, should be used; alternatively, if permutation techniques are not allowable but the dependence structure is adequate, the Hommel's procedure is a good option also.

Second, the subset property states that, if FWER is controlled at level α for a set of hypotheses then it is also controlled at the same level for any subset. This means that we can associate the FWER control to a single hypothesis so that by rejecting hypothesis i, the type I error is bounded by α. The same subset property is not true for FDR, so that for a set with FDR controlled at level α, it does not mean that a given subset, e.g., a single hypothesis, is controlled at the same level. While the local FDR point estimate variants have the subset property, they are less powerful and more challenging to estimate accurately.

Third, recall that FDR is the FDP expectation and only controls the false positive rate in average which implies that the actual proportion of false discoveries in the rejected set can be substantially larger than the desired level, especially if the proportion of true nulls is large, e.g., under the complete null, the percentage of false discoveries may be 100% under an FDR control of 5%. The pFDR and q-value improves power over FDR procedures (as BH and BY) because, like adaptive methods, estimate the proportion of true nulls π_0 to control false positives from this proportion. Because pFDR is conditioned on occurrence of rejections it is more suited to error estimation than to error control; there are several techniques for FDP estimation providing an alternative strategy for managing type I error.

Finally, multiple testing is a very active research field, it seems that multiple testing procedures and p-value (and e-value) adjustment are here to stay. They are already important contributors for enhancing the reproducibility and reliability of scientific research.

Acknowledgements

I wish to thank Sonia Prado and Pili Alvariño for their comments on the manuscript. This research was supported by the Ministerio de Economía y Competitividad (CGL2016-75482-P) and Xunta de Galicia (Grupo de Referencia Competitiva, ED431C 2020/05, Centro Singular de Investigación de Galicia accreditation 2019-2022), and by the European Union (European Regional Development Fund - ERDF, "Unha maneira de facer Europa")

REFERENCES

Benjamini, Y. and Y. Hochberg (1995). Controlling the False Discovery Rate: A Practical and Powerful Approach to Multiple Testing. Journal of the Royal Statistical Society. Series B (Methodological). 57: 289–300.

Benjamini, Y. and D. Yekutieli (2001). The control of the false discovery rate in multiple testing under dependency. The Annals of Statistics. 29: 1165–1188.

Benjamini, Y., A. Krieger and D. Yekutieli (2006). Adaptive linear step-up procedures that control the false discovery rate. Biometrika. 93: 491–507.

Blanchard, G. and E. Roquain (2009). Adaptive False Discovery Rate Control under Independence and Dependence. Journal of Machine Learning Research. 10: 2837–2871.

Boca, S.M. and J.T. Leek (2018). A direct approach to estimating false discovery rates conditional on covariates. PeerJ. 6: e6035. https://doi.org/10.7717/peerj.6035.

Carvajal-Rodríguez, A., J. de Uña-Álvarez and E. Rolan-Alvarez (2009). A new multitest correction (SGoF) that increases its statistical power when increasing the number of tests. BMC Bioinformatics. 10: 209.

Carvajal-Rodríguez, A. and J. de Uña-Álvarez (2011). Assessing significance in high-throughput experiments by sequential goodness of fit and q-value estimation. PLoS One. 6: e24700.

Carvajal-Rodríguez, A., (2018). Myriads: p-value-based multiple testing correction. Bioinformatics. 34: 1043–1045.

Castro-Conde, I. and J. de Uña-Álvarez (2014). sgof: An R Package for Multiple Testing Problems. The R Journal. 6: 96–113.

Castro-Conde, I. and J. de Uña-Álvarez (2015a). Power, FDR and conservativeness of BB-SGoF method. Computational Statistics. 30: 1143–1161.

Castro-Conde, I. and J. de Uña-Álvarez (2015b). Adjusted p-values for SGoF multiple test procedure. Biometrical Journal. 57: 108–122.

Castro-Conde, I., S. Döhler and J. de Uña-Álvarez (2017). An extended sequential goodness-of-fit multiple testing method for discrete data. Stat Methods Med Res. 26: 2356–2375.

Chen, X., D.G. Robinson and J.D. Storey (2019). The functional false discovery rate with applications to genomics. Biostatistics.

Chen, X. (2020). False discovery rate control for multiple testing based on discrete p-values. Biom. J. 62(4): 1060–1079.

Chen, X. and S.K. Sarkar (2020). On Benjamini–Hochberg procedure applied to mid p-values. Journal of Statistical Planning and Inference. 205: 34–45.

Chi, Z., (2008). False discovery rate control with multivariate p-values. Electron. J. Statist. 2: 368–411.

de Uña-Álvarez, J. (2011). On the Statistical Properties of SGoF Multitesting Method. Stat. Appl. Genet. Mol. Biol. 10(1): 18.

de Uña-Álvarez, J. (2012). The Beta-Binomial SGoF method for multiple dependent tests. Stat. Appl. Genet. Mol. Biol. 11: 1–32.

Döhler, S., (2018). A discrete modification of the Benjamini–Yekutieli procedure. Econometrics and Statistics. 5: 137–147.

Dudoit, S., J.P. Shaffer and J.C. Boldrick (2003). Multiple Hypothesis Testing in Microarray Experiments. Statist. Sci. 18: 71–103.

Dudoit, S., H.N. Gilbert and M.J. van der Laan (2008). Resampling-based empirical bayes multiple testing procedures for controlling generalized tail probability and expected value error rates: Focus on the false discovery rate and simulation study. Biom. J. 50: 716–744.

Dudoit, S. and M.J. van der Laan, (2008). Multiple Testing Procedures with Applications to Genomics. Springer Series in Statistics. Springer, New York.

Efron, B., R. Tibshirani, J.D. Storey and V. Tusher (2001). Empirical Bayes Analysis of a Microarray Experiment. Journal of the American Statistical Association. 96: 1151–1160.

Efron, B. (2005). Local false discovery rates.

Efron, B. (2007). Correlation and Large-Scale Simultaneous Significance Testing. Journal of the American Statistical Association. 102: 93–103.

Efron, B., B. Turnbull, B. Narasimhan and K. Strimmer (2015). locfdr: Computes Local False Discovery Rates.

Fan, J., X. Han, and W. Gu (2012). Estimating False Discovery Proportion Under Arbitrary Covariance Dependence. J. Am. Stat. Assoc. 107: 1019–1035.

Fan, J. and X. Han (2017). Estimation of the false discovery proportion with unknown dependence. Journal of the Royal Statistical Society: Series B (Statistical Methodology). 79: 1143–1164.

Fan, J., Y. Ke, Q. Sun, and W.X. Zhou (2019). FarmTest: Factor-Adjusted Robust Multiple Testing with Approximate False Discovery Control. J. Am. Stat. Assoc. 114(528): 1880–1893.

Finner, H. and M. Roters (2001). On the False Discovery Rate and Expected Type I Errors. Biometrical Journal. 43: 985–1005.

Friguet, C. and D. Causeur (2011). Estimation of the proportion of true null hypotheses in highdimensional data under dependence. Computational Statistics & Data Analysis. 55: 2665– 2676.

Ge, Y., S. Dudoit and T.P. Speed (2003). Resampling-based multiple testing for microarray data hypothesis. Test. 12: 1–44.

Genovese, C.R., K. Roeder and L. Wasserman (2006). False Discovery Control with p-Value Weighting. Biometrika. 93: 509–524.

Gianetto, Q.G., F. Combes, C. Ramus, C. Bruley, Y. Couté and T. Burger (2019). cp4p: Calibration Plot for Proteomics.

Goeman, J.J. and A. Solari (2011). Multiple Testing for Exploratory Research. Statist. Sci. 26: 584–597.

Goeman, J.J. and A. Solari (2014). Multiple hypothesis testing in genomics. Statistics in Medicine. 33: 1946–1978.

Goeman, J., Meijer, Rosa, Krebs and Thijmen (2019a). hommel: Methods for Closed Testing with Simes Inequality, in Particular Hommel's Method. R package version, 1.

Goeman, J., R. Meijer, T. Krebs and A. Solari (2019b). Simultaneous control of all false discovery proportions in large-scale multiple hypothesis testing. Biometrika. 106: 841–856.

Greenland, S., S.J. Senn, K.J. Rothman, J.B. Carlin, C. Poole, S.N. Goodman, et al., (2016). Statistical tests, P-values, confidence intervals, and power: A guide to misinterpretations. European Journal of Epidemiology. 31: 337–350.

Greenland, S., (2019). Valid P-Values Behave Exactly as They Should: Some Misleading Criticisms of P-Values and Their Resolution With S-Values. The American Statistician. 73: 106–114.

Guo, W. and S. Sarkar (2019). Adaptive controls of FWER and FDR under block dependence. Journal of Statistical Planning and Inference.

He, L. and J.F. Heyse (2019). Improved power of familywise error rate procedures for discrete data under dependency. Biometrical Journal. 61: 101–114.

Hemerik, J. and J.J. Goeman (2018). False discovery proportion estimation by permutations: confidence for significance analysis of microarrays. Journal of the Royal Statistical Society: Series B (Statistical Methodology). 80: 137–155.

Hemerik, J., A. Solari and J.J. Goeman (2019). Permutation-based simultaneous confidence bounds for the false discovery proportion. Biometrika. 106: 635–649.

Hoggart, C.J., T.G. Clark, M.D. Iorio, J.C. Whittaker and D.J. Balding (2008). Genome-wide significance for dense SNP and resequencing data. Genetic Epidemiology. 32: 179–185.

Hothorn, T., F. Bretz and P. Westfall (2008). Simultaneous inference in general parametric models. Biometrical Journal. 50: 346–363.

Ignatiadis, N., B. Klaus, J. Zaugg and W. Huber (2016). Data-driven hypothesis weighting increases detection power in genome-scale multiple testing. Nat Methods. 13: 577–580.

Ignatiadis, N. and W. Huber (2017). Covariate powered cross-weighted multiple testing with false discovery rate control [WWW Document]. URL /paper/Covariate-powered-cross-weightedmultiple-testing-Ignatiadis-Huber/0021dcbefe3bdc7a00ea347894d26cb54ca187d8 (accessed 2.15.20).

Kang, G., K. Ye, N. Liu, D.B. Allison and G. Gao (2009). Weighted Multiple Hypothesis Testing Procedures. Stat Appl Genet Mol Biol. 8.

Kang, J., (2020a). Two-stage false discovery rate in microarray studies. Communications in Statistics-Theory and Methods. 49: 894–908.

Kang, J., (2020b). Comparison of methods for the proportion of true null hypotheses in microarray studie. Communications for Statistical Applications and Methods. 27: 141–148.

Kim, K.I. and M. van de Wiel (2008). Effects of dependence in high-dimensional multiple testing problems. BMC Bioinformatics. 9: 114.

Korthauer, K., P.K. Kimes, C. Duvallet, A. Reyes, A. Subramanian, M. Teng, et al. (2019). A practical guide to methods controlling false discoveries in computational biology. Genome Biology. 20: 118.

Larson, H.J., (1982). Introduction to Probability Theory and Statistical Inference, Wiley series in probability and mathematical statistics: Probability and mathematical statistics. Wiley.

Lehmann, E.L. and J.P. Romano (2005). Generalizations of the familywise error rate. Ann. Statist. 33: 1138–1154.

Liang, K. (2016). False discovery rate estimation for large-scale homogeneous discrete p-values. Biometrics. 72: 639–648.

Lin, D.Y., (2019). A simple and accurate method to determine genomewide significance for association tests in sequencing studies. Genetic Epidemiology. 43: 365–372.

MacDonald, P.W., K. Liang and A. Janssen (2019). Dynamic adaptive procedures that control the false discovery rate. Electronic Journal of Statistics. 13: 3009–3024.

Meijer, R.J., T.J.P. Krebs and J.J. Goeman (2019). Hommel's procedure in linear time. Biometrical Journal. 61: 73–82.

Owen, A.B., (2005). Variance of the Number of False Discoveries. Journal of the Royal Statistical Society. Series B (Statistical Methodology). 67: 411.

Perezgonzalez, J.D., (2014). A reconceptualization of significance testing. Theory & Psychology. 24: 852–859.

Phillips, D. and D. Ghosh (2014). Testing the disjunction hypothesis using Voronoi diagrams with applications to genetics. The Annals of Applied Statistics. 8: 801–823.

Pollard, K., S. Dudoit and M.J. van der Laan (2005). Multiple Testing Procedures: R multtest Package and Applications to Genomics, Bioinformatics and Computational Biology Solutions Using R and Bioconductor. Springer.

R Development Core Team, (2019). R: A language and environment for statistical computing. Vienna, Austria.

Ramdas, A.K., R.F. Barber, M.J. Wainwright and M.I. Jordan (2019). A unified treatment of multiple testing with prior knowledge using the p-filter. The Annals of Statistics. 47: 2790–2821.

Richardson, S., G.C. Tseng and W. Sun (2016). Statistical Methods in Integrative Genomics. Annual Review of Statistics and Its Application. 3: 181–209.

Roeder, K. and L. Wasserman (2009). Genome-Wide Significance Levels and Weighted Hypothesis Testing. Stat Sci. 24: 398–413.

Romano, J.P. and M. Wolf (2005). Exact and Approximate Stepdown Methods for Multiple Hypothesis Testing. Journal of the American Statistical Association. 100: 94–108.

Romano, J.P. and M. Wolf (2007). Control of generalized error rates in multiple testing. Ann. Statist. 35: 1378–1408.

Romano, J.P. and M. Wolf (2016). Efficient computation of adjusted p-values for resampling-based stepdown multiple testing. Statistics & Probability Letters. 113: 38–40.

Rudra, P., E. Cruz-Cortés, X. Zhang and D. Ghosh (2019). Multiple testing approaches for hypotheses in integrative genomics. WIREs Computational Statistics n/a, e1493.

Sarkar, S.K., (2008). On Methods Controlling the False Discovery Rate. Sankhyā: The Indian Journal of Statistics, Series A (2008-). 70: 135–168.

Schwartzman, A. and X. Lin (2011). The effect of correlation in false discovery rate estimation. Biometrika. 98: 199–214.

Schwartzman, A., (2012). Comment: FDP vs FDR and the Effect of Conditioning. Journal of the American Statistical Association. 107: 1039–1041.

Sham, P.C. and S.M. Purcell (2014). Statistical power and significance testing in large-scale genetic studies. Nat Rev Genet. 15: 335–346.

Sokal, R.R. and F.J. Rohlf (1981). Biometry, Second. ed. W. H. Freeman and Co., New York.

Song, Y. and G. Fellouris (2019). Sequential multiple testing with generalized error control: An asymptotic optimality theory. Ann. Statist. 47: 1776–1803.

Storey, J.D. and R. Tibshirani (2001). Estimating false discovery rates under dependence, with applications to DNA microarrays. Technical Report 2001–2028, Department of Statistics, Stanford University.

Storey, J.D., (2002). A Direct Approach to False Discovery Rates. Journal of the Royal Statistical Society. Series B (Statistical Methodology). 64: 479.

Storey, J., (2003). The positive false discovery rate: A Bayesian interpretation and the q-value. The Annals of Statistics. 31: 2013–2035.

Storey, J. and R. Tibshirani (2003a). SAM Thresholding and False Discovery Rates for Detecting Differential Gene Expression in DNA Microarrays, in: Parmigiani, G., Garrett, E.S., Irizarry, R.A., Zeger, S.L. (Eds.), The Analysis of Gene Expression Data: Methods and Software, Statistics for Biology and Health. Springer, New York, NY, pp. 272–290.

Storey, J. and R. Tibshirani (2003b). Statistical significance for genomewide studies. Proc Natl Acad Sci U.S.A. 100: 9440–5.

Storey, J.D., A.J. Bass, A. Dabney, D. Robinson and G. Warnes (2020). qvalue: Q-value estimation for false discovery rate control. Bioconductor version: Release (3.10).

Tamhane, A.C. and J. Gou (2018). Advances in p-Value Based Multiple Test Procedures. Journal of Biopharmaceutical Statistics. 28: 10–27.

Tibshirani, R., M.J. Seo, G. Chu, B. Narasimhan and J. Li (2018). Package 'samr': Significance Analysis of Microarrays for differential expression analysis, RNAseq data and related problems. Version 3.0.

Tusher, V.G., R. Tibshirani and G. Chu (2001). Significance analysis of microarrays applied to the ionizing radiation response. Proceedings of the National Academy of Sciences. 98: 5116–5121.

Vovk, V. and R. Wang (2019a). Combining e-values and p-values (SSRN Scholarly Paper No. ID 3504009). Social Science Research Network, Rochester, NY.

Vovk, V. and R. Wang (2019b). True and false discoveries with e-values. arXiv preprint arXiv:1912.13292.

Westfall, P.H. and S.S. Young (1993). Resampling-Based Multiple Testing: Examples and Methods for p-Value Adjustment. Wiley, New York.

Westfall, P.H. and R.D. Wolfinger (1997). Multiple Tests with Discrete Distributions. The American Statistician. 51: 3–8.

Westfall, P.H. and J.F. Troendle (2008). Multiple Testing with Minimal Assumptions. Biometrical Journal. 50: 745–755.

Wright, S.P., (1992). Adjusted P-Values for Simultaneous Inference. Biometrics. 48: 1005–1013.

Xia, Y., L. Li, S.N. Lockhart and W.J. Jagust (2019). Simultaneous Covariance Inference for Multimodal Integrative Analysis. Journal of the American Statistical Association. 0: 1–13.

Zaykin, D.V., S.S. Young and P.H. Westfall (2000). Using the false discovery rate approach in the genetic dissection of complex traits: a response to Weller et al. Genetics. 154: 1917–8.

Zhu, Y. and W. Guo (2020). Family-wise error rate controlling procedures for discrete data. Stat. Biopharm. Res. 12: 117–128.

Index

Milton Keynes UK
Ingram Content Group UK Ltd.
UKHW05202614102\4
449569UK00016B/718